Complex Total Laparoscopic Hysterectomy (TLH) with Newer Approaches in Bladder Dissection

Springer Nature More Media App

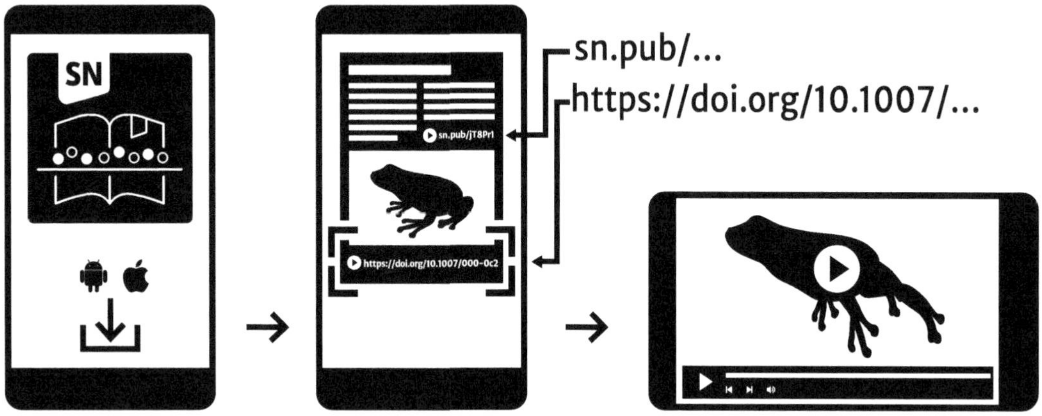

1. Download → 2. Scan Link → 3. Enjoy Video

Support: customerservice@springernature.com

Nutan Jain
Editor

Complex Total Laparoscopic Hysterectomy (TLH) with Newer Approaches in Bladder Dissection

Springer

Editor
Nutan Jain
Department of Gynaecology, IVF and Laparoscopic Surgery
Vardhman Hospital
Muzaffarnagar, Uttar Pradesh, India

This work contains media enhancements, which are displayed with a "play" icon. Material in the print book can be viewed on a mobile device by downloading the Springer Nature "More Media" app available in the major app stores. The media enhancements in the online version of the work can be accessed directly by authorized users.

ISBN 978-981-97-3225-8 ISBN 978-981-97-3226-5 (eBook)
https://doi.org/10.1007/978-981-97-3226-5

This Springer imprint is published by the registered company Springer Nature Singapore Pte Ltd.
The registered company address is: 152 Beach Road, #21-01/04 Gateway East, Singapore 189721, Singapore

This book is a heartfelt dedication to all patients and surgeons navigating the complexities of Total Laparoscopic Hysterectomy (TLH), particularly in the challenging realm of difficult bladder dissection.

Foreword

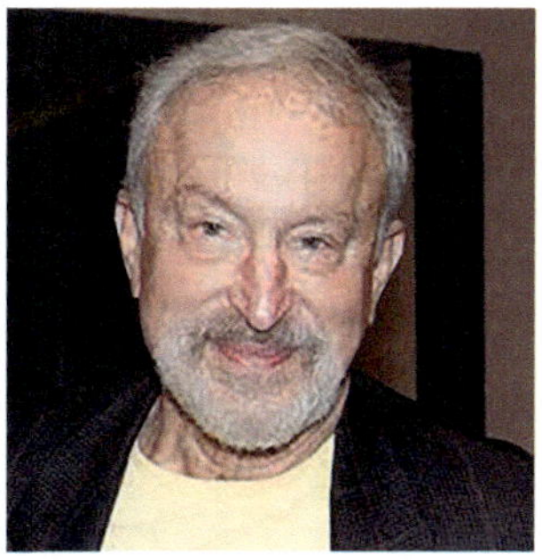

This new addition, the Canopy Concept, to the laparoscopic hysterectomy forum is really helpful. I like the term and the technique with obvious benefits to simplification of bladder dissection. We have come a long way since before the advent of video laparoscopy, when we had to do extensive operations using our eye attached to the scope optic. This new Canopy Concept continues our goal to eliminate laparotomy in complex total laparoscopic hysterectomy surgery. I always emphasized the posterior cul-de-sac dissection, but here in this book are papers and chapters emphasizing the anterior dissection. Both talk about what I always referred to as loose areolar issue between anterior rectum and post vagina and now this anteriorly bladder dissection from cervix, I like the term, cotton candy appearance and dissection, instead of loose areolar tissue. This dissection looks to be the core basic to creating a good canopy.

Continuingly, the dissections of the ureters is particularly of interest for all gynaecologists for a safe hysterectomy, as suggested, the use of ICG can make it easier. I disagree with transverse closure of the vaginal cuff and believe all vaginal cuffs should be closed vertically incorporating the utero sacral ligaments. That may be something to consider in the future.

In conclusion, all I can say is keep up the good work!

Dallas, Pennsylvania, USA | Harry Reich, MD, FACOG, FRCOG, FACS

Foreword

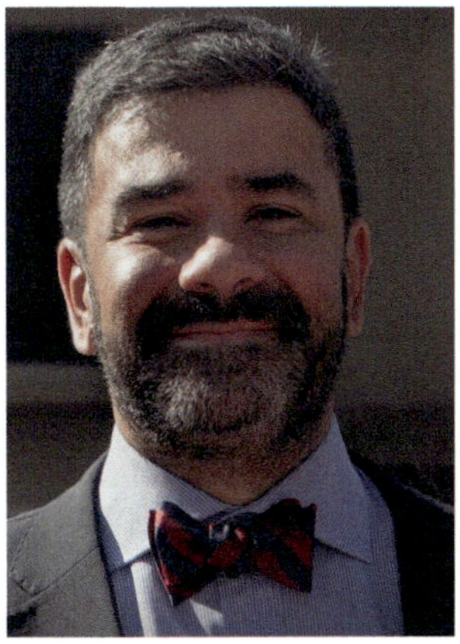

It is both an honor and a privilege to introduce TLH in Complex Total Laparoscopic Hysterectomy (TLH) with Newer Approaches in Bladder Dissection, authored by the esteemed Dr. Nutan Jain. Dr. Jain's reputation as a pioneer in laparoscopic surgery precedes her, and this volume further cements her legacy as a trailblazer in the field. This book will offer guidance on navigating the complex hysterectomy, with a specific focus on dissecting the anterior compartment, featuring the Comprehensive Canopy Concept: three-step technique. It also delves into the complexities of combining TLH with hernia and gall bladder procedures, offering invaluable guidance for managing such intricate scenarios.

Throughout her distinguished career, Dr. Jain has exemplified an unwavering dedication to advancing the frontiers of surgical innovation. Her relentless pursuit of excellence and exploration of novel techniques have garnered widespread recognition and respect within our medical community.

What distinguishes Dr. Jain's work is not only her technical prowess but also her commitment to improving outcomes. Grounded in a holistic approach to patient care, Dr. Jain ensures that surgical interventions are not only effective but also tailored to the unique individual needs.

I am confident that the knowledge imparted within these pages will equip healthcare providers with the necessary tools to address even the most challenging TLH cases, thereby enhancing clinical outcomes for patients. By sharing her expertise in managing complex scenarios, Dr. Jain empowers us to deliver the highest standard of care, thus advancing the field of complex laparoscopic surgery.

Reflecting on Dr. Jain's extraordinary journey, one cannot help but be inspired by her vision for the future of surgical practice. Driven by an unyielding commitment to excellence, Dr. Jain continues to push the boundaries, serving as a beacon of inspiration for colleagues and mentees alike.

I extend my deepest gratitude to Dr. Nutan Jain for inviting me to contribute to her work. It is my earnest belief that this book will serve as a source of knowledge and inspiration for medical professionals worldwide, propelling us towards a future where the art and science of laparoscopic surgery flourish unabated.

Unidad de Laparoscopia Ginecológica
Avanzada y Dolor Pélvico, Pereira, Colombia

Juan Diego Villegas-Echeverri

Foreword

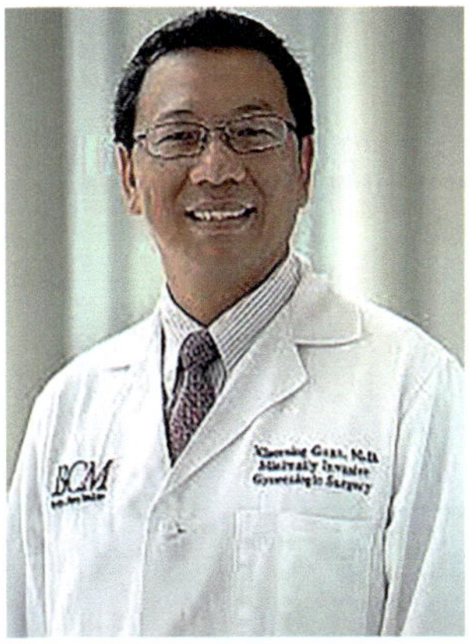

It is with great pleasure and respect that I write this foreword for Dr. Nutan Jain's upcoming book, *Complex Total Laparoscopic Hysterectomy (TLH) with Newer Approaches in Bladder Dissection*. Dr. Jain's work has been instrumental in advancing the field of laparoscopic surgery, and her expertise is evident throughout this comprehensive guide.

Laparoscopic surgery has revolutionized gynecologic procedures, offering patients less invasive options with quicker recovery times and fewer complications. Dr. Jain, with her extensive experience and innovative techniques, has continually pushed the boundaries of what is possible in this field. Her dedication to improving surgical outcomes and educating the next generation of surgeons is truly inspiring.

The content of this book includes pelvic anatomy, different approaches, various clinical case scenarios, and complications. It thoroughly covers all the complex TLH techniques for handling bladder dissection.

Bladder dissection presents significant challenges in complex cases such as those involving previous Cesarean sections or endometriosis. Navigating this part of the procedure while mitigating bladder complications is pivotal for all minimally invasive gynecologic surgeons (MIGS). This book delves into the complexities of TLH, providing detailed insights into the latest approaches in bladder dissection. Dr. Jain's meticulous attention to detail and clear, practical guidance make this an invaluable resource for both novice and experienced surgeons. Each chapter is a testament to her commitment to excellence and her passion for advancing surgical education.

I am confident that readers will find this book not only informative but also transformative in their surgical practice. Dr. Jain's contributions to gynecologic surgery are immense, and this publication reflects her outstanding expertise and unwavering dedication to the field.

I extend my heartfelt congratulations to Dr. Jain on this remarkable achievement and look forward to the positive impact it will undoubtedly have on the practice of laparoscopic surgery.

Warm regards,

Department of Obstetrics and Gynecology
Baylor College of Medicine, Houston, TX, USA

Xiaoming Guan

Foreword

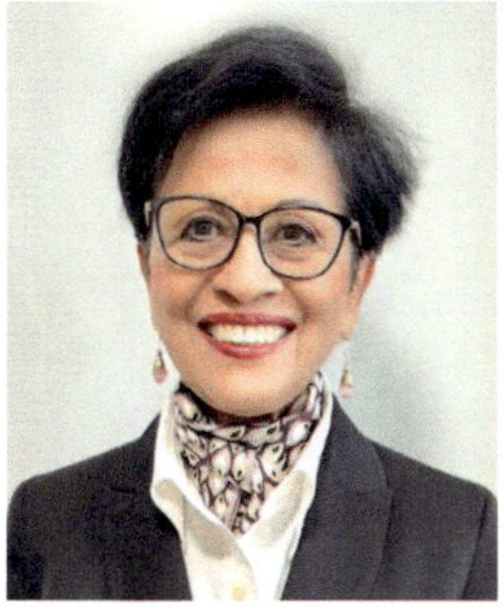

It is a distinct pleasure and privilege to pen a foreword for my esteemed colleague of 30 years, Dr. Nutan Jain, on the publication of her groundbreaking textbook. Her pioneering work in Minimally Invasive Gynecological Surgery has not only revolutionized practices in India but has also earned her recognition on the international stage, including in the United States.

Nutan's contributions extend beyond mere innovation; she has introduced groundbreaking surgical techniques that have become industry standards, such as the widely acclaimed "Jain Point." Her expertise in suturing techniques, particularly in challenging cases like Total Laparoscopic Hysterectomy (TLH) in the presence of fibroids and endometriosis, underscores her commitment to safe and effective surgery. Nutan's pedagogical approach, akin to methods used in fields like American football and aviation, emphasizes hands-on learning through systematic, reproducible steps, ensuring a thorough understanding of critical anatomical principles.

As a patient educator, Nutan goes beyond conventional teaching methods, employing personal demonstrations and video learning to disseminate knowledge effectively. Her Fellowship programs have attracted aspiring gynecologists from around the globe to her learning center in India, further cementing her status as a global leader in the field.

In her comprehensive textbook on Total Laparoscopic Hysterectomy, Nutan not only showcases her mastery of complex cases but also generously shares insights from skilled surgeons worldwide. I extend my heartfelt congratulations to Dr. Nutan Jain on this monumental achievement, which is sure to guide and inspire future generations of gynecological surgeons.

Well done, Nutan!

With warm regards,

Radha Syed, MD, FACOG

Society of Laparoscopic and Robotic Surgery
Staten Island, NY, USA
President, 2024

Foreword

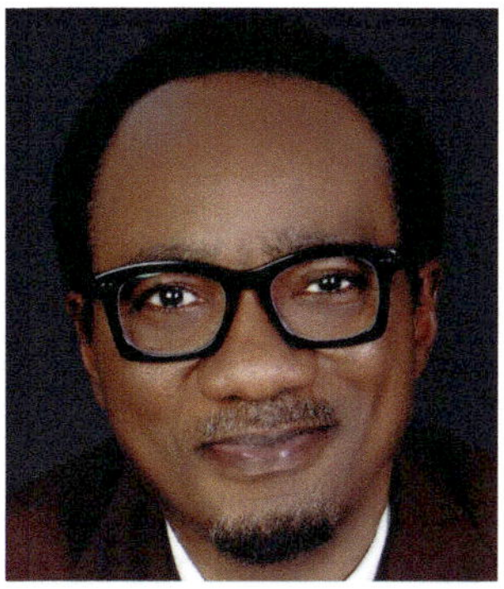

It is with pleasure that I write the forward of this unique textbook written by an authority in the field of laparoscopic surgery. I have known Dr. Nutan Jain for over 15 years as a brilliant minimal-access surgeon and prolific writer with a penchant for demystifying complex surgical conditions. We both play active leadership roles in the American Association of Gynecologic Laparoscopists (AAGL), where she currently serves as a Board member of the urogynecology/vaginal surgery special interest group.

As part of her contributions to knowledge, she introduced the Jain Point, named after her. It has gained widespread popularity and is used as an entry point during complex laparoscopic surgeries and also in situations where Palmer's Point is contraindicated.

Rapid technological and surgical advancements have been made in gynecological minimal-access surgery. Despite this, urologic complications, including bladder injury, remain a significant cause for concern. This textbook takes the reader on a journey to simplify Total Laparoscopic Hysterectomy in the most complex of situations of bladder adherence. Dr. Nutan Jain not only simplifies these complex procedures but also describes Canopy Concept for bladder dissection, reducing complication rates and shortening the procedure duration.

It is indeed a pleasant read.

AAGL Professional Education Committee Member
Medical Director, Gynaescope Specialist Hospital, Nigeria

Jude E. Okohue, MD (Africa)

Preface

Performing Total Laparoscopic Hysterectomy (TLH) in patients with a history of abdominal or pelvic surgery, especially those with dense adhesions from multiple caesarean sections or extensive endometriosis, presents unique challenges. These factors significantly impact the approach, technique, and outcomes of the procedure. Over the years, the global rates of caesarean sections have significantly increased and are projected to continue rising. Patients with previous surgeries pose a higher risk of intraoperative complications during TLH, particularly urinary tract injuries. In such cases, increased operative time, higher blood loss, and a greater likelihood of conversion to open surgery are common, along with an elevated risk of bladder injury exists.

In patients with previous caesarean sections and an adherent bladder, various approaches, both central and lateral, have been attempted to find a plane of bladder dissection, often with persistent difficulties. This challenge prompted us to explore alternative methods for managing the bladder during these hysterectomies. We began performing TLH with a posterior approach and eventually developed the Comprehensive Canopy Concept, which involves addressing the uterine artery before bladder dissection and simplifying the dissection in the utero-vesical space. Though this concept is not new has been by several researchers since very long, the only thing new is our enthusiasm and passion for pushing it further, as earlier it could never achieve the coveted place of being appreciated and accepted by all and kept going into oblivion.

When presenting this technique at conferences and live surgery workshops, particularly in patients with multiple previous surgeries, we initially faced significant opposition. Critics argued that this approach deviated from the conventional anatomical wisdom of performing bladder dissection before addressing the uterine artery. Despite witnessing its effectiveness, skeptics doubted its applicability in more challenging situations. This book aims to dispel such doubts as we have described the TLH approach with the Comprehensive Canopy Concept in virtually all complex situations. We have dedicated years to refining this method, and we urge you to set aside any preconceived notions and give it a try. I assure you that this approach will not only simplify your procedures but also transform your total laparoscopic hysterectomy (TLH) practice. Several authors have contributed their expertise to make this a valuable resource for managing complex TLH scenarios.

Apart from above techniques, in this book we have also included all recent advances like the use of ICG for better delineation of the ureters and use of ICG for Sentinel node mapping in Ca body uterus. A special section has been devoted to making the surgeons adept with the use of cystoscopy and other cystoscopy procedures relevant to complex hysterectomies. Chapter on anesthesia covers the modern technique of "ERAS" for faster recovery. A very relevant section of the book includes tackling the complications of TLH including the fistula repair and vault dehiscence repair. We have made every effort to make this book a one-stop solution for all queries related to complex TLH. Enjoy reading....

Muzaffarnagar, Uttar Pradesh, India Nutan Jain

Acknowledgement

As I sit to write the acknowledgement for this valuable book on such a complex topic, my heartfelt gratitude extends to my esteemed fellows: Dr. Sakshi Srivastava, Dr. Divyanee Gulati, Dr. Priyanka Sureddi and Dr. Suksham Sharma, and especially my co-director Dr. Vandana Jain. Our dedicated IT team comprises Mr. Pranay Chaudhary, Mr. Vishram Singh, Miss. Asha Rathi, Mr. Deepak Daksh, Mr. Subham Kashyap and Mr. Bhopal Singh. Their immense help and support throughout the creation of this book—from performing deft surgeries, capturing images, and editing videos to crafting the manuscript and ensuring its accuracy—have been invaluable. The commitment and high morale of the team maintained over the past year, along with the readiness of our patients to participate, have made it possible to share these images and videos in a comprehensive textbook cum atlas.

I would also like to extend a profuse thank you to the Springer team, especially Mr. Naren Aggarwal, Ms. Vandana Joshi, Mr. Ejaz Ahmed and Mr. Vishal Anand, for their unwavering support throughout the book's creation. Vandana, in particular, was a constant resource, addressing all our queries and needs during the process.

My heartfelt thanks to all the contributors, especially Dr. Ted Lee, Dr. Suketu Mansuria, Dr. Andrea Tinelli, Dr. Shailesh Puntambekar, Dr. Rooma Sinha, Dr. Pandit Palaskar, Dr. Hrshikesh Pandit, Dr. Shivam Vatsal, Dr. Prateek Gupta, Dr. Sidhartha Gupta and Dr. Aarushi Jain. Their timely submission of manuscripts and images has been instrumental in bringing this project to fruition.

Nothing is possible without a strong backbone. Thanks to my wonderful family for their unique help in the compilation of this book. In the end, I would like to thank my teachers and worthy colleagues who enabled me to reach this point in my career.

It is our collective effort that has resulted in this comprehensive textbook cum atlas, which we believe will serve as a valuable resource for endoscopic surgeons worldwide. Our aim and passion in creating this book is to provide a worthwhile addition to the existing literature and to enhance patient care through improved TLH techniques.

Contents

Editor and Contributors

About the Editor

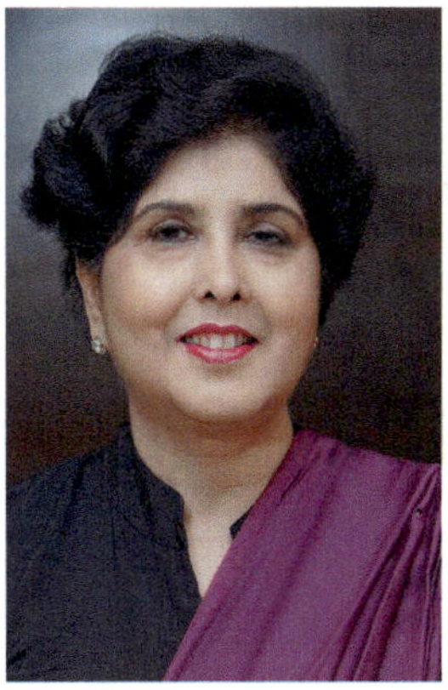

Nutan Jain an eminent figure in the field of obstetrics and gynecology, completed her MBBS and MD from GSVM Medical College, Kanpur, India. She pursued advanced training in laparoscopy at Texas Medi Tech University, USA, and laparo-hysteroscopy at the Royal Free Hospital, London. Under the mentorship of world-renowned pioneers in endoscopic surgery from the early 1990s, Dr. Jain honed her expertise in minimally invasive techniques.

Currently, Dr. Jain heads the gynecology, IVF, and laparoscopic surgery departments at Vardhman Hospital, Muzaffarnagar, India. Her clinical interests encompass laparoscopic hysterectomy, management of extensive endometriosis, pelvic floor disorders, laparoscopic myomectomy, infertility treatment, IVF, and hysteroscopy. Passionate about education, she has been running highly acclaimed fellowship programs for over two decades, shaping the next generation of specialists in her field.

A prolific contributor to medical literature, Dr. Jain has published numerous papers in peer-reviewed national and international journals and has delivered lectures at prestigious conferences worldwide. She is the author of several books, translated into Spanish and Chinese, extending her knowledge and innovations across the globe. Dr. Jain frequently demonstrates her surgical techniques through live surgeries at workshops, including those organized by the American Association of Gynecologic Laparoscopists (AAGL).

Dr. Jain's notable innovation, the "Jain Point," has significantly advanced the safety of laparoscopic entry for gynecologists and other minimally invasive surgeons, including general surgeons, urologists, oncologists, pediatricians, and bariatric surgeons. Her leadership roles in various international organizations of endoscopic surgery highlight her dedication to the advancement of the field and her impact on surgical practices worldwide.

Contributors

Rupa Bana Apollo Health City, Hyderabad, Telangana, India

Mihir Chitale Galaxy Care Hospital, Pune, Maharashtra, India

Kate Denny Minimally Invasive Gynecologic Surgery Fellow, Department of Obstetrics, Gynecology and Reproductive Sciences, Magee-Womens Hospital, University of Pittsburgh Medical Center, Pittsburgh, PA, USA

Divyanee Gulati Department of Obstetrics and Gynecology, Vardhman Trauma and Laparoscopy Centre Pvt. Ltd., Muzaffarnagar, Uttar Pradesh, India

Obstetrics and Gynaecology, GMC Patiala, Affiliated by Baba Farid University of Health Sciences, Patiala, Punjab, India

Gynaecology Endoscopy, Vardhman Trauma and Laparoscopy Centre Pvt. Ltd., Muzaffarnagar, Uttar Pradesh, India

Prateek Gupta City Nursing Home and Surgical Center, Bhiwani, Haryana, India

Siddharth Gupta Advanced Laparoscopy and Robotics, GEM Hospital Coimbatore, Coimbatore, Tamil Nadu, India

Sunil Gupta Jyoti Nursing Home, Muzaffarnagar, Uttar Pradesh, India

Aarushi Jain Anaesthesiology, University College of Medical Sciences, Affiliated by Delhi University, Delhi, India

Department of Anaesthesia, Vardhman Trauma and Laparoscopy Centre Pvt. Ltd., Muzaffarnagar, UP, India

Nutan Jain Obstetrics and Gynaecology, GSVM Medical College, Affiliated by Kanpur University, Kanpur, Uttar Pradesh, India

Department of Obstetrics and Gynecology, Vardhman Trauma and Laparoscopy Centre Pvt. Ltd., Muzaffarnagar, Uttar Pradesh, India

Parima Jain City Nursing Home and Surgical Center, Bhiwani, Haryana, India

Vandana Jain Obstetrics and Gynaecology, Kasturba Hospital, Affiliated by Delhi University, Delhi, India

Department of Obstetrics and Gynecology, Vardhman Trauma and Laparoscopy Centre Pvt. Ltd., Muzaffarnagar, Uttar Pradesh, India

Priyanka Jha Department of Anaesthesia, Muzaffarnagar Medical College, Muzaffarnagar, Uttar Pradesh, India

Ted Lee Division of Minimally Invasive Gynecologic Surgery, Surgical Innovation for Gynecology, Department of Obstetrics and Gynecology, New York University Grossman School of Medicine, New York, NY, USA

Kshitij Manerikar Galaxy Care Hospital, Pune, Maharashtra, India

Suketu Mansuria Gynecologic Minimally Invasive Surgery, Magee-Womens Hospital, University of Pittsburgh Medical Center, Pittsburgh, PA, USA

Pandit Palaskar Indian Association of Gynecological Endoscopists (IAGE), Gynecological Endoscopic Surgeon & IVF-ICSI Infertility Specialist, Endoworld Hospital, Chikalthana, Aurangabad, Maharashtra, India

Hrishikesh Pandit Pandit Hospital and 3D Laparoscopic Center, Ahmednagar, Maharashtra, India

Gaetano Panese Department of Obstetrics and Gynecology, and CERICSAL (CEntro di RIcerca Clinico SALentino), Veris delli Ponti Hospital, Lecce, Italy

Mangesh Panse Galaxy Care Hospital, Pune, Maharashtra, India

Madhavi Patil Galaxy Care Hospital, Pune, Maharashtra, India

Giovanni Pecorella Department of Gynecology, Obstetrics and Reproduction Medicine, Saarland University, Homburg, Germany

Aishwarya Puntambekar Galaxy Care Hospital, Pune, Maharashtra, India

Seema Puntambekar Galaxy Care Hospital, Pune, Maharashtra, India

Shailesh Puntambekar Galaxy Care Hospital, Pune, Maharashtra, India

Ravindra M. Sathe Galaxy Care Hospital, Pune, Maharashtra, India

Ambreen Shaikh Department of Obstetrics and Gynaecology, Seth G S Medical College and Kem Hospital, Mumbai, Maharashtra, India

Suksham Sharma Obstetrics and Gynecology, Government Medical College, Affiliated by Jammu University, Jammu, Jammu and Kashmir, India

Gynae Endoscopy, Vardhman Trauma and Laparoscopy Centre Pvt. Ltd., Muzaffarnagar, Uttar Pradesh, India

Rooma Sinha Gynecology, AHERF, Hyderabad, Telangana, India

Macquarie University, Sydney, NSW, Australia

Gynecological Robotic Surgery, Apollo GROUP of Hospitals, Hyderabad, Telangana, India

Apollo Health City, Hyderabad, Telangana, India

AGRS (Association of Gynecological Robotic Surgeons of India), Hyderabad, Telangana, India

ASGRS (Asian Society of Gynecological Robotic Surgeons), Singapore, Singapore

SERGS (Society of European Robotic Gynecological Surgeons), Waregem, Belgium

Sakshi Srivastava Department of Obstetrics and Gynecology, Vardhman Trauma and Laparoscopy Centre Pvt. Ltd., Muzaffarnagar, Uttar Pradesh, India

Obstetrics and Gynaecology, Rohilkhand Medical College and Hospital, Affiliated by Bareilly International University, Bareilly, Uttar Pradesh, India

Gynaecology Endoscopy, Vardhman Trauma and Laparoscopy Centre Pvt. Ltd., Muzaffarnagar, Uttar Pradesh, India

Rohilkhand Medical College and Hospital, Affiliated by Bareilly International University, Bareilly, India

Gynaecological Endoscopic, Vardhman Trauma and Laparoscopy Centre Pvt. Ltd., Muzaffarnagar, Uttar Pradesh, India

Priyanka Sureddi Gynaecology Endoscopy, Vardhman Trauma and Laparoscopy Centre Pvt. Ltd., Muzaffarnagar, Uttar Pradesh, India

Obstetrics and Gynecology, Seth GS Medical College and KEM Hospital, Affiliated by Maharashtra University of Health Sciences, Mumbai, Maharashtra, India

Amit Tajane Archit Hospital, Sangamner, Maharashtra, India

Andrea Tinelli Department of Obstetrics and Gynecology, and CERICSAL (CEntro di RIcerca Clinico SALentino), Veris delli Ponti Hospital, Lecce, Italy

Shivam Vatsal HOD Surgical Oncology, Metro Hospital, Faridabad, India

Madhura Waghmare Endoworld Hospital, Chikalthana, Aurangabad, Maharashtra, India

Hrishikesh Wagholika Waghollikar Hospital, Sangamner, Maharashtra, India

Alison M. Zeccola Minimally Invasive Gynecologic Surgery, Magee-Womens Hospital, University of Pittsburgh Medical Center, Pittsburgh, PA, USA

Prathmesh Zende Endoworld Hospital, Chikalthana, Aurangabad, Maharashtra, India

Part I

General

Retroperitoneal Anatomy

1

Pandit Palaskar, Prathmesh Zende,
and Madhura Waghmare

1.1 Introduction

The field of anatomy is a systematic study that encompasses observation, conception, and experimentation to gain insights into the workings of the human body. Surgery, on the other hand, represents the pragmatic application of this scientific knowledge to address diseases, excise tumors, alleviate symptoms, and enhance overall function and quality of life. As technology continues to advance, our capacity to visualize and intricately examine structures and organs has grown, leading to a deeper and more refined understanding [1].

Gynaecological malignancies span a wide clinical range, from localized tumors to those displaying aggressive behaviour within the pelvic region, and eventually advancing to extensive metastatic spread throughout the abdomen, lungs, thorax, and, occasionally, the brain. The journey of anatomical education, which commenced with cadaveric studies, has evolved into dynamic lessons conducted in real-time during surgical procedures. The educational evolution has transitioned from traditional open surgery to the modern approach of teaching anatomy through minimally invasive [1]. The latter, offering an amplified view of anatomical structures, stands as one of the most effective mediums for acquiring knowledge and advancing our comprehension of anatomy in the present era.

P. Palaskar (✉)
Indian Association of Gynecological Endoscopists (IAGE), Gynecological Endoscopic Surgeon & IVF-ICSI Infertility Specialist, Endoworld Hospital,
Chikalthana, Aurangabad, Maharashtra, India
e-mail: dr@panditpalaskar.com

P. Zende · M. Waghmare
Endoworld Hospital, Chikalthana, Aurangabad, Maharashtra, India

1.2 Retroperitoneal Anatomy

The peritoneum, an extensive and intricately organized serous membrane, is thin and transparent, making it the largest of its kind in the body. The section covering the abdominal wall is termed the parietal peritoneum, while the portion enveloping a viscus or organ is referred to as visceral peritoneum. Both types consist of a singular layer of simple, low-cuboidal epithelium known as mesothelium. A fine layer of serous fluid, approximately 50–100 mL, acts as a lubricant, separating and facilitating movement between the parietal and visceral layers of the peritoneum [2].

The posterior abdominal wall acts as the posterior boundary of the abdominal cavity, seamlessly connecting with the posterior thoracic wall from the diaphragmatic level upwards to the posterior pelvic wall downwards. It comprises the lumbar vertebrae, pelvic girdle, and the muscles of the posterior abdominal wall, including the quadratus lumborum, major and minor psoas muscles, iliacus, and the diaphragm, along with their corresponding fascia [3].

Within the abdominal cavity, the retroperitoneum forms a distinct segment, bounded anteriorly by the parietal peritoneum and posteriorly by the transversalis fascia [4].

Extending extensively from the pelvis to the diaphragm, this area encompasses a variety of organs and structures. Structures positioned behind the peritoneum are labeled retroperitoneal (Fig. 1.1).

The primary retroperitoneal organs include the adrenal glands, kidneys, ureters, abdominal aorta, inferior vena cava, and their branches. Conversely, secondary retroperitoneal organs, initially intraperitoneal, experience a positional change during embryological development. This shift occurs as a result of the regression of peritoneal tissue along the posterior wall of the abdominal cavity, causing the mesentery of these structures to fuse with the posterior abdominal wall. The secondary retroperitoneal organs include the ascending and descending colon, the duodenum (excluding the bulbous part or the first half of duodenum segment 1), and the pancreas [3].

N. Jain (ed.), *Complex Total Laparoscopic Hysterectomy (TLH) with Newer Approaches in Bladder Dissection*,
https://doi.org/10.1007/978-981-97-3226-5_1

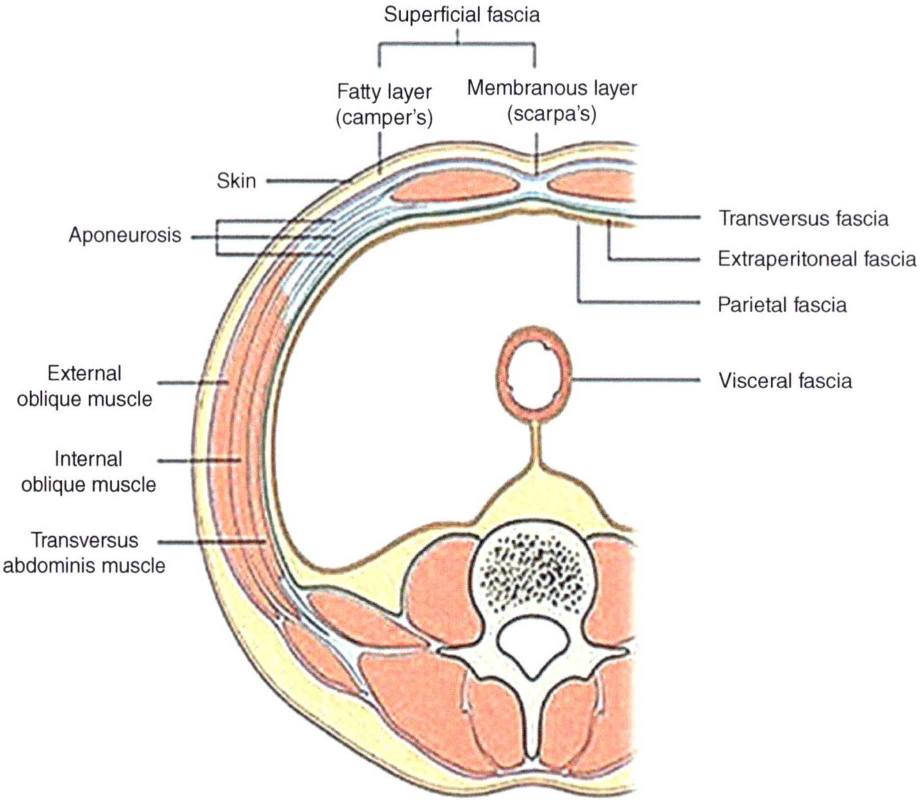

Fig. 1.1 Transverse section of the anterior abdominal wall; the extraperitoneal fascia containing fatty tissue beneath the parietal peritoneum rests against the posterior abdominal wall, known as the retroperitoneum [4]

1.3 The Retroperitoneal Zones

The retroperitoneal space is classified into three zones using anatomico-clinical criteria. This gross classification is beneficial for evaluating organs that might be simultaneously affected by disease or injury due to their close proximity, even if they belong to distinct functional systems [5]. The delineation of these zones, along with their boundaries and contents, is outlined as follows

Zone I (Central)
Upper: Diaphragmatic, esophageal, and aortic openings
Lower: Sacral promontories Lateral: Psoas muscles
Structures included: Abdominal aorta, inferior vena cava, pancreas, duodenum (partial)

Zone II (Lateral, Left and Right Flank)
Upper: Diaphragm
Lower: Iliac crests
Lateral: Psoas muscles
Structures included: Kidneys and their vessels, ureters and their abdominal portions, ascending and descending colon, hepatic and splenic flexure

Zone III (Pelvic)
Anterior: Space of Retzius
Posterior: Sacrum

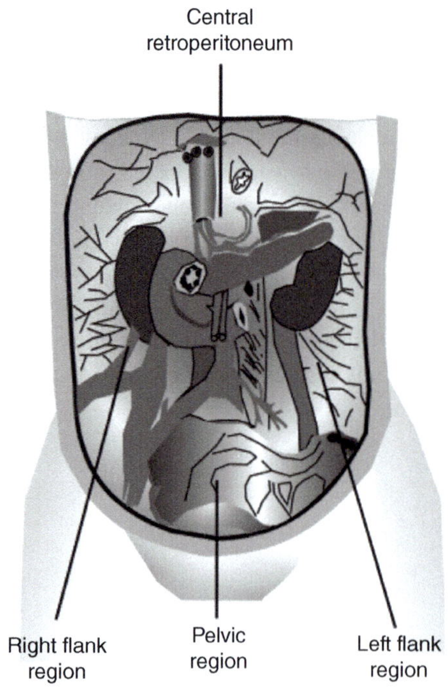

Fig. 1.2 Three zones of the retroperitoneum [6]. (From Ross and Lamperti [11]; with permission)

Lateral: Bony pelvis
Structures included: Entire pelvis, pelvic wall, rectosigmoid colon, iliac vessels, urogenital organs (partial) (Fig. 1.2)

1.4 Compartments of Retroperitoneal Space

The renal fascia delineates three compartments within the retroperitoneal space associated with the kidney.

- Anterior pararenal compartment
- Posterior pararenal compartment
- Perirenal compartment

1.5 Pelvic Vasculature

The sacral promontory, quite literally the pinnacle of the pelvis, serves as a critical anatomical landmark. Pathological conditions affecting the pelvis may extend into the abdomen and beyond, but their origin consistently resides below the sacral promontory. As the most prominent feature in the bony pelvis, the sacral promontory offers a stable reference point for various surgical procedures. It proves especially valuable as a fixed reference in cases where pelvic anatomy appears distorted or marked by scarring. Consequently, any orientation of pelvic structures should begin with identifying the sacral promontory. This anatomical landmark holds significance for several reasons.

At this particular level:

- The common iliac vessels divide into the internal and external iliac vessels.
- The ureter shifts from the lateral to the medial side, passing over the bifurcation of the iliac vessels.
- At this junction, the superior hypogastric nerve plexus, a parasympathetic network, converges to form the left and right hypogastric nerves. The nerve fibers of the plexus are discernible here and, when traced downward, give rise to the hypogastric nerves.

The sacral promontory marks the starting point for transperitoneal para-aortic lymph node dissection. With the sacral promontory as the reference point, meticulous dissection performed laterally to it reveals the pararectal retroperitoneal space. Another method to reach the same landmark involves initiating dissection medial to the infundibulopelvic ligament. This technique, known as the endometriotic approach or the medial approach, is used to access the retroperitoneal space [1].

1.5.1 Arteries

1.5.1.1 Abdominal Aorta

The thoracic aorta is often termed the abdominal aorta due to its passage through the diaphragm into the abdominal cavity. It positions itself anterior to the vertebral column at the posterior abdominal wall. At the L4-L5 vertebra level, the abdominal aorta bifurcates into the right and left common iliac arteries. Subsequently, the common iliac artery further divides into the external and internal iliac arteries at the pelvic brim. Within the pelvic retroperitoneal vasculature, critical structures include the ovarian artery, median sacral artery, external iliac artery, internal iliac artery, and their respective branches (Fig. 1.3).

The ovarian artery is positioned on the anterolateral surface of the abdominal aorta, typically at the L2 vertebra level, approximately 2 cm below the left renal vein. On the left side, it courses over the psoas major muscle and gains entry into the pelvic cavity by crossing the common iliac artery. On the right side, it initially travels over the anterior surface of the inferior vena cava, then descends alongside the

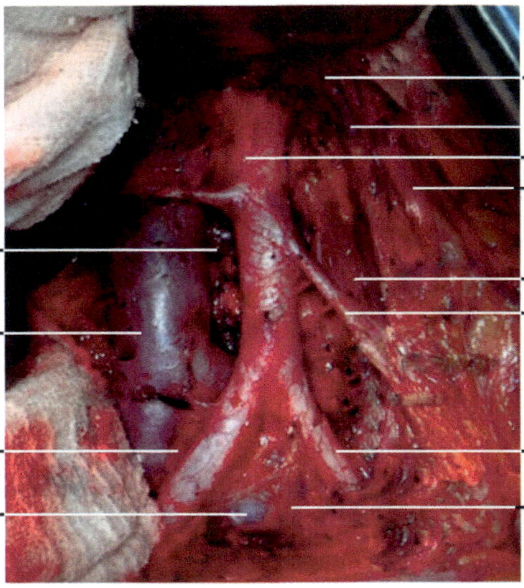

Fig. 1.3 The paraaortic region, aorta, and inferior vena cava following paraaortic lymphadenectomy

ascending colon, approximately 1 cm above the right ureter. It enters the pelvic cavity by crossing either over the common iliac artery or, occasionally, over the external iliac artery.

The median sacral artery is a continuation of the abdominal aorta, tracing the anterior surface of the sacrum and coccyx. It intersects with the left common iliac vein, requiring caution in hysteropexy and colpopexy procedures.

The common iliac artery, dividing into the external and internal iliac arteries, serves as the predominant point for the origin of polar renal arteries. Precise dissection is crucial in surgical interventions within this domain.

The external iliac artery The external iliac artery courses along the medial border of the psoas muscle, extending to the femoral ring below the inguinal ligament. Situated on the lateral border of the external iliac artery, the genitofemoral nerve holds relevance in pelvic lymphadenectomy. Serving as a crucial artery for the lower limb, it branches into the deep circumflex femoral artery and the inferior epigastric artery.

The internal iliac artery courses infero-medially beyond the pelvic brim and acts as the primary vascular supply for the pelvic cavity. It bifurcates into posterior and anterior trunks. The posterior trunk branches into the superior gluteal artery, lateral sacral artery, and iliolumbar artery. The anterior trunk's branches include the umbilical, uterine, superior and inferior vesical, vaginal, obturator, middle rectal, internal pudendal, and inferior gluteal arteries (Fig. 1.4).

The umbilical artery, an end artery of the internal iliac artery's anterior trunk, extends longitudinally to the abdominal wall, eventually transforming into the medial umbilical ligament. Traction on the umbilical artery during laparoscopic procedures serves as an indicator of the uterine artery's origin.

The uterine artery, arising from the anterior trunk, courses medially through the broad ligament (lig. latum uteri) [within the cardinal ligament (lig. transversum cervicis)]. It proceeds toward the isthmic portion of the uterus, supplying blood to the uterus and cervix. Notably, it crosses the ureter in close proximity to the uterus (Fig. 1.5).

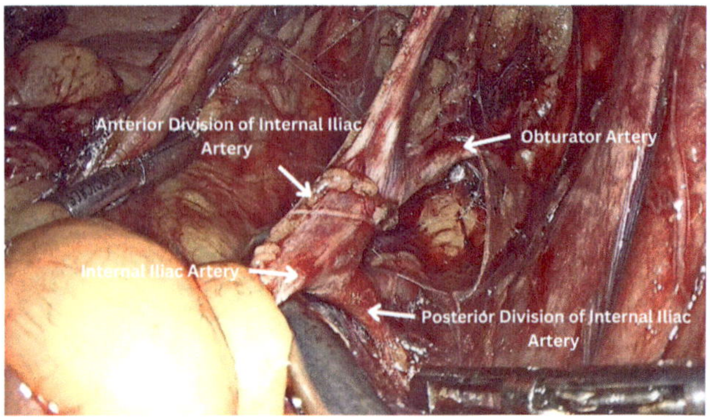

Fig. 1.4 Internal iliac Artery and its branches

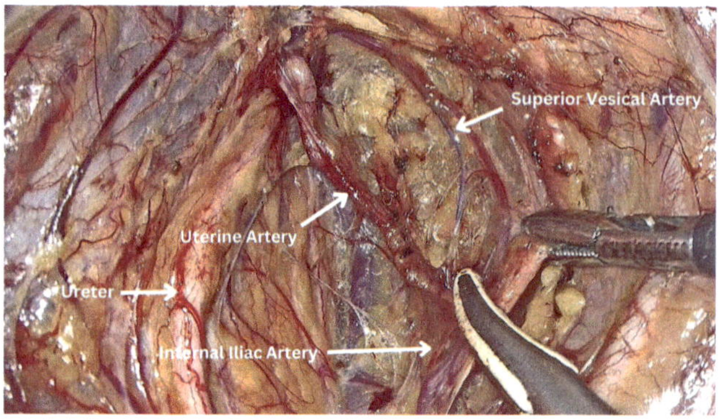

Fig. 1.5 **Anterior** division of internal iliac Artery and branches

1.5.2 Veins

The inferior vena cava (IVC) starts just below the L5 vertebra, aligning with the bifurcation of the common iliac arteries from the abdominal aorta. Below the umbilicus, it sits slightly behind the abdominal aorta. As it ascends, passing over the right psoas major muscle, it stays to the right of the aorta. Beyond the umbilicus, it moves closer to the front of the abdominal aorta.

The external iliac vein extends from the femoral vein above the inguinal ligament, running posteriorly to the external iliac artery.

The pubic vein acts as a vascular connection linking the external iliac/inferior epigastric and obturator veins. Hemorrhage from this vein is referred to as corona mortis and is situated on the posterior aspect of the pubic bone over the obturator fossa. During pelvic lymphadenectomy in gynecologic oncology practice, this area is dissected, and surgeons must exercise caution to prevent hemorrhage from this venous connection.

The internal iliac vein generally runs parallel to its corresponding branches of the internal iliac artery, receiving drainage from various anomalous and collateral veins.

The common iliac vein originates at the confluence point of the internal and external iliac veins, eventually joining its counterpart to form the inferior vena cava.

1.5.3 Nerves

The pelvic structures, such as the uterus, rectum, vagina, and urinary bladder, are innervated by the autonomic nervous system, comprising both motor and sensory sympathetic and parasympathetic nerves. The inferior hypogastric nerve (T10–L2) supplies the sympathetic nerves, while the parasympathetic fibers are contributed by the pelvic splanchnic nerve. These fibers converge to form the inferior hypogastric plexus, supplying both the uterus and the urinary bladder.

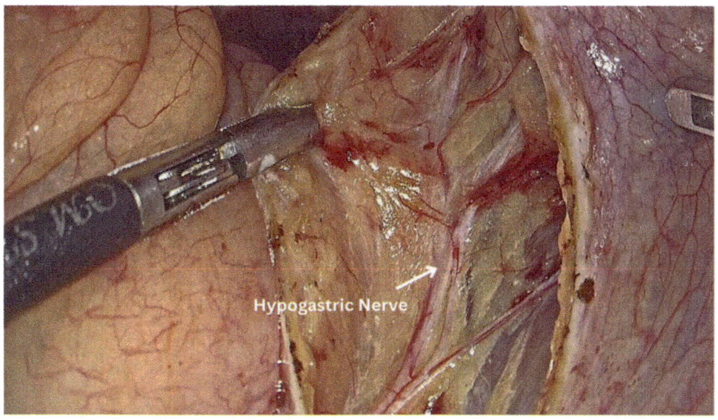

Fig. 1.6 Hypogastric nerve dissection

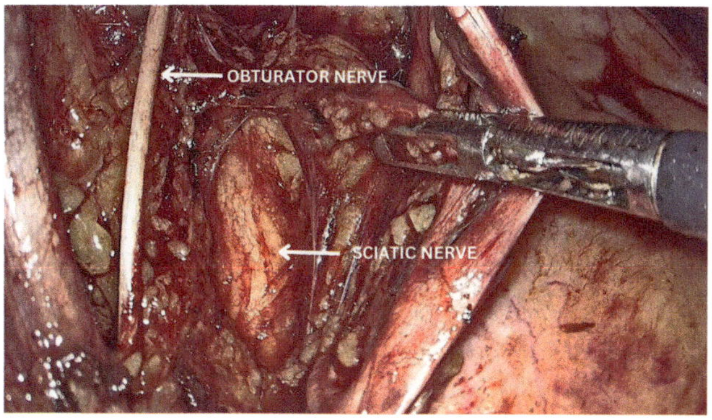

Fig. 1.7 Obturator nerve and Sciatic nerve

Detailed anatomy of the inferior hypogastric plexus has been extensively described by Fujii [7].

The pelvic splanchnic and inferior hypogastric nerves intersect to form a cross-shaped plexus. In nerve-sparing radical hysterectomy, the focus is on identifying the inferior hypogastric nerve and the plexus, selectively dividing the uterine branch, and safeguarding the bladder branches from the plexus. This approach aims to enhance the preservation of urinary bladder function post-surgery (Fig. 1.6).

1.5.4 Genitofemoral Nerve

The genitofemoral (L1-L2) nerve delineates the lateral boundary of pelvic lymph node dissection. It is situated on the anterior aspect of the Psoas major muscle, lateral to the External iliac artery, and passes beneath the inguinal ligament, medial to the anterior superior iliac spine.

Injury to this nerve can cause paresthesia over anterior and lateral thigh caused by excessive flexion of hip in lithotomy position or by pressure from retractor. Genitofemoral nerve can also be injured during pelvic lymphadenopathy.

1.5.5 Obturator Nerve

The obturator nerve originates from the L2-L3-L4 nerve roots and is situated between the external and internal iliac vessels. It serves as the lower boundary of pelvic lymph node dissection. Running parallel and posterior to the obturator nerve are the obturator vein and artery.

1.5.6 Sciatic Nerve

Sciatic nerve is the largest nerve of the body (L4L5, S1S2). It can be approached by iliolumbar space dissection and lies deep to obturator nerve (Fig. 1.7).

1.5.7 Ureter

The ureter, a muscular structure facilitating the transportation of urine from the kidney to the bladder, typically measures around 23–30 cm in length. Emerging from the narrowing of the renal pelvis at the kidney hilum, it descends inferiorly. After traversing the bifurcation of the common iliac arteries or the origin of the external iliac artery over the pelvic brim, the ureter follows the medial aspect of the psoas major muscle and runs adjacent to the posterior leaf of the broad ligament before reaching the urinary bladder. In its distal segment, the ureter is crossed anteriorly by the uterine artery. The terminal part of the distal ureter enters the bladder obliquely, connecting to the smooth muscle wall and providing sphincter-like action [3].

Anatomically, the ureter is divided into abdominal, pelvic, and intravesical segments. The abdominal portion follows the medial border of the psoas muscle fascia, guided by the genitofemoral nerve. Originating near the posterior aspect of the second part of the duodenum, the right ureter descends within the peritoneum adjacent to the ascending colon, passing lateral to the root of the small bowel mesentery and inferior vena cava beneath the ovarian vessels. It then curves posteriorly around the terminal ileum and cecum. Conversely, the left ureter descends along the lateral aspect of the abdominal aorta over the psoas muscle fascia, intersecting anteriorly with the left colic artery and ovarian vessels. During this trajectory, it runs parallel to the inferior mesenteric vein and travels posteriorly along the sigmoid colon.

As it enters the true pelvis, the ureter descends inferiorly to the ovarian vessels, following the posterior leaf of the broad ligament towards the bladder. It crosses the uterine artery and passes through the ureteric tunnel within the cardinal ligament, proceeding laterally to the antero-lateral vaginal fornix within the bladder pillar, eventually reaching the trigone of the bladder. The ureteral orifices are located on the postero-lateral aspect of the trigone, with the ureters spanning a 1.5–2 cm course within the bladder wall (Fig. 1.8).

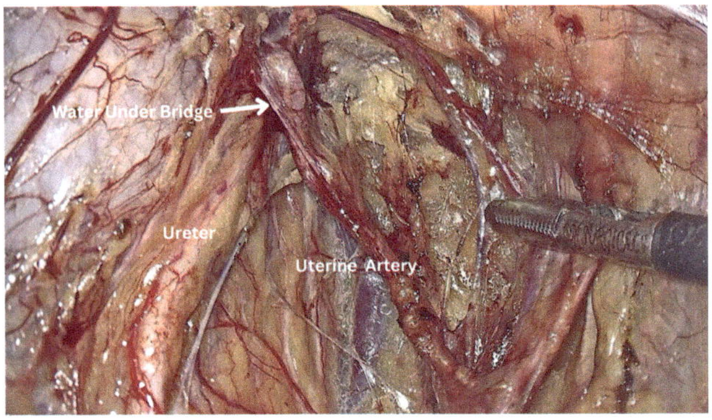

Fig. 1.8 Water under Bridge (Ureter courses under Uterine Artery)

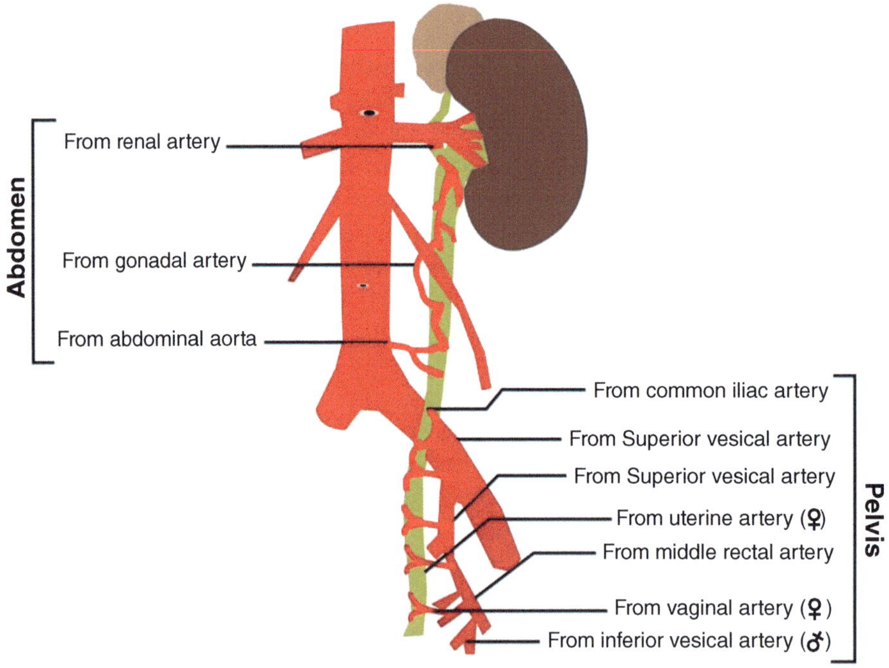

Fig. 1.9 Vascularization of ureter from the kidney to the bladder (left side), while dissecting the ureter traction should be applied towards the side of blood vessels [8]

The ureter does not have a single dedicated primary arterial vessel for its blood supply. Instead, it receives arterial branches from multiple sources, including the renal, ovarian, common iliac, internal iliac, uterine, superior gluteal, vaginal, middle rectal, inferior, and superior vesical arteries along its course from the renal pelvis to the bladder. These arterial branches interconnect with each other, creating a continuous longitudinal blood supply (Fig. 1.9).

1.6 Avascular Spaces in Pelvis

The term "spaces" denotes the regions delineated by at least two distinct fascial layers. Pelvic spaces are virtual spaces developed by dissection to separate or retract organs during dissection [9]. These spaces play a crucial role in the functioning of the urinary, reproductive, and gastrointestinal systems, and are indispensable in pelvic surgeries. They serve as significant anatomical landmarks in retroperitoneal and pelvic surgery. The existence of spaces is attributable to the derivation of pelvic viscera from various embryological structures. Retroperitoneal spaces are designated based on the proximity to adjacent organs, each possessing its unique significance. Conceptually, spaces can be likened to pyramids, with a broad base over the levator ani muscle and an apex directed toward the peritoneal cavity. Virtual spaces, though not naturally occurring, are created and easily developed through dissection to access vital underlying structures or to facilitate the separation or retraction of organs during surgery. Avascular spaces derive their names from nearby organs, with the roof formed by the peritoneal lining and the floor comprised of the levator ani muscles. The retroperitoneal spaces are classified as follows [9] (Fig. 1.10).

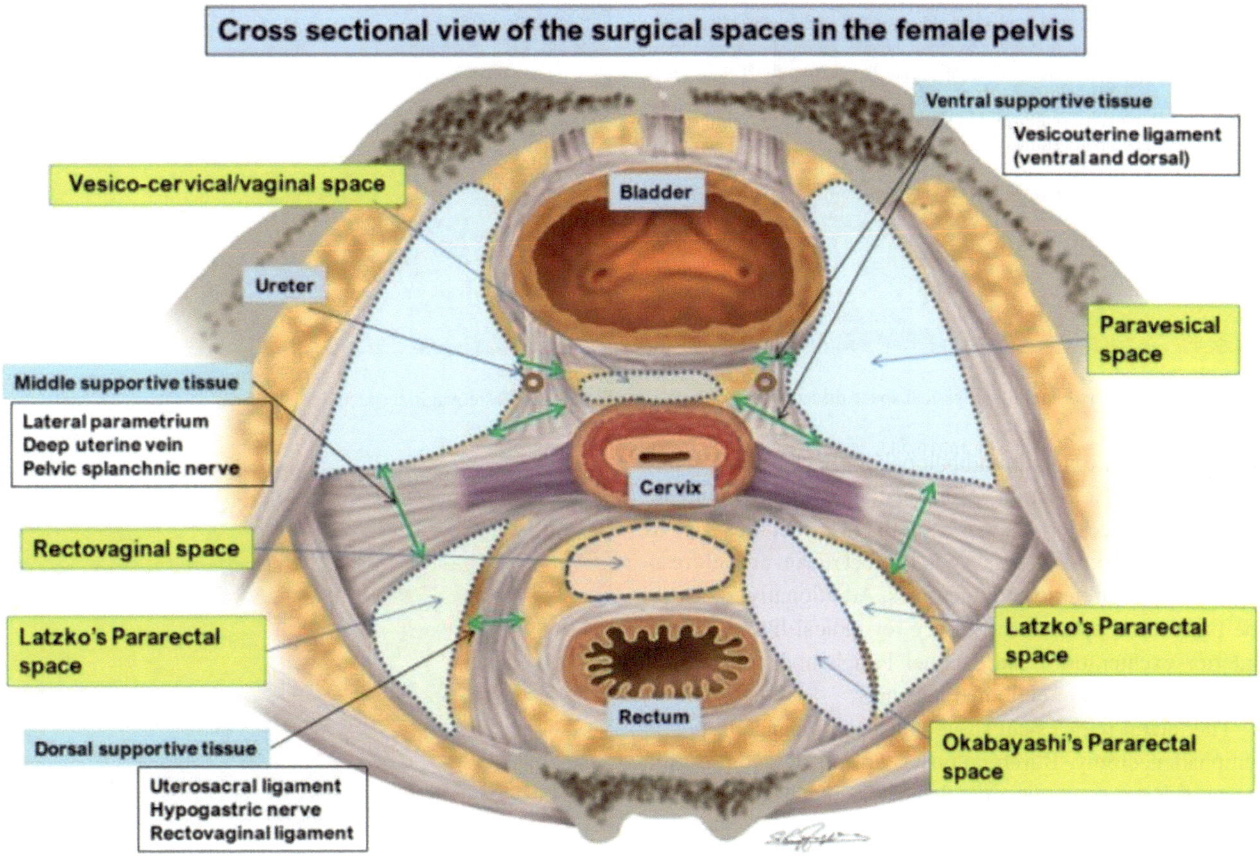

Fig. 1.10 Avascular spaces

1. **Median**
   (a) Retropubic (Retzius)
   (b) Vesicocervical (Vesicovaginal)
   (c) Rectovaginal
   (d) Presacral (Retrorectal)
2. **Lateral Spaces**
   (a) Paravesical
   (b) Pararectal

1.7 Paravesical Space

The paravesical space is a retroperitoneal area delineated ventrally by the superior pubic ramus and the arcuate line of the ilium, and dorsally by the cardinal ligament encompassing the parametrium and paracervix, as well as the uterine artery and vein [3] (Basic Clinical Retroperitoneal Anatomy for Pelvic Surgeons, 2018) (Fig. 1.11).

The medial boundary of the paravesical space comprises the vesico-uterine ligament, bladder, while the lateral boundary is defined by the obturator internus fascia/muscle and the external iliac artery/vein. The roof of the paravesical space is composed of the peritoneum of the anterior leaf of the broad ligament, while the floor is formed by the iliococcygeus muscle and the pubocervical fascia.

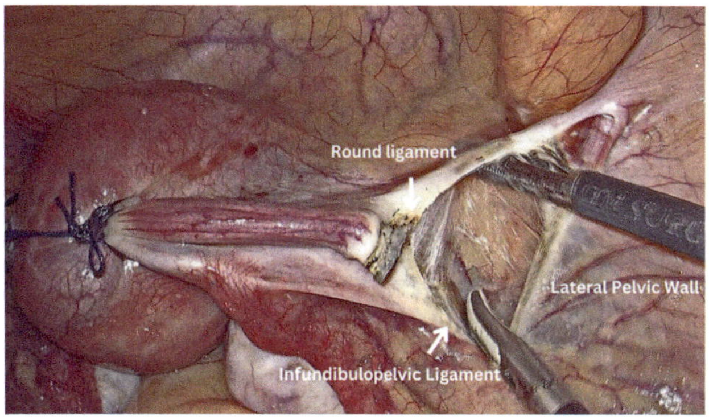

Fig. 1.11 Boundaries of pelvic triangle

The contents of the paravesical space include the umbilical artery, superior vesical artery, obturator neurovascular bundle, and lymphatic tissue. The obliterated umbilical artery divides this space into the lateral paravesical space (LPS) and the medial paravesical space (MPS).

Approaches to the paravesical space vary based on the surgical objective. In oncological procedures, dissection is per-

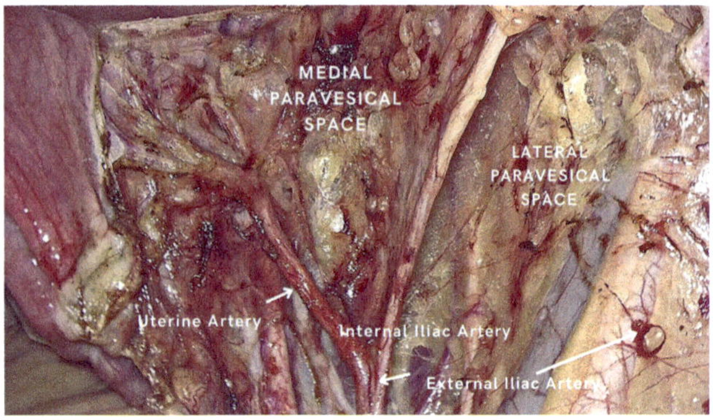

Fig. 1.12 Medial and lateral paravesical space dissection

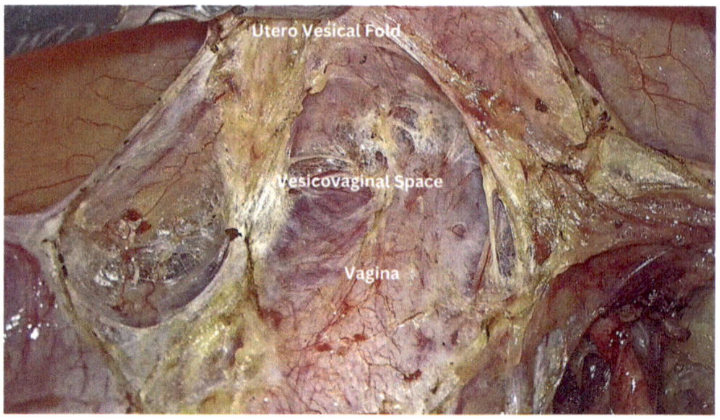

Fig. 1.13 Vesicovaginal space dissection

formed laterally to the infundibulopelvic (IP) ligament, while in benign cases, dissection occurs medially to the IP ligament. Paravesical space dissection is essential in procedures such as ureteric reanastomosis, paravaginal defect repair, and addressing bladder or ureteric endometriosis. Additionally, access to the paravesical space is necessary for radical hysterectomy, anterior exenteration, and sentinel lymph node procedures related to cervical or endometrial cancer.

The lateral paravesical space holds significance in pelvic lymphadenectomy, Burch colposuspension by avoiding the space of Retzius, paravaginal defect repair without entering the medial paravesical space, and pectopexy. In obstetrics, access to the paravesical space is crucial for procedures such as cesarean hysterectomy for placenta percreta to clip uterine arteries and laparoscopic cerclage using Whittle's surgical technique with a broad ligament window (Fig. 1.12).

1.8 Vesicocervical and Vesicovaginal Space

The vesicocervical space is defined by the bladder ventrally, the pubocervical fascia and upper portion of the cervix dorsally, the cranial segment of the vesicouterine ligament laterally, and the peritoneal reflection of the anterior cul-de-sac cranially.

1.9 Vesicovaginal Space

The trigone of bladder forms ventral boundary of vesicovaginal space and pubocervical fascia and vagina forms the dorsal boundary [10]. (Anatomy of the Vesicovaginal Fascia and Its Relation to Branches of the Inferior Hypogastric Plexus, 2022) Laterally, it is defined by the caudal portion of the vesicouterine ligament, while cranially, it is delineated by the peritoneal reflection between the dome of the bladder and the junction of the low uterine segment. The caudal boundary is marked by the junction of the proximal and middle thirds of the urethra.

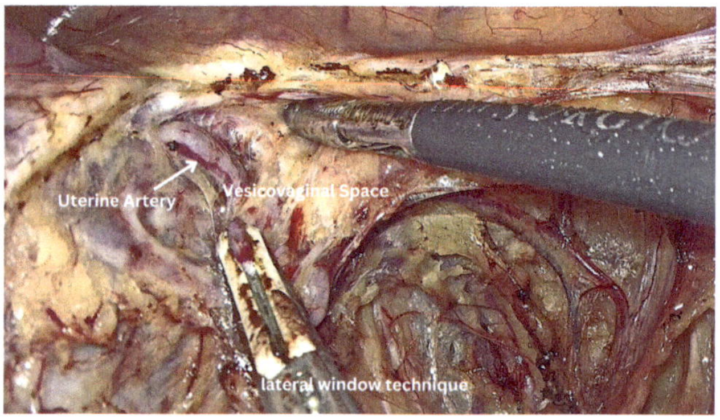

Fig. 1.14 Lateral window technique of bladder dissection

Vesicovaginal space-approach (Fig. 1.13)

- Medial approach
- Lateral approach

Vesicovaginal space dissection is needed urogynecological surgeries like VVF-UVF repair, SUI, transvaginal cystocele operation. In laparoscopic sacrocolpopexy or hysteropexy and also in Vaginal, abdominal, laparoscopic, robotic hysterectomy, nerve-sparing radical hysterectomy, and cases of bladder endometriosis involving deep infiltrating endometriosis (DIE), dissection of the vesicovaginal space is necessary. This dissection is also required for procedures such as vaginal cuff resection in cases of vaginal vault endometriosis or vaginal cuff recurrence following oncogynecological procedures, cesarean section, cesarean hysterectomy, or laparoscopic/robotic/open cerclage. Additionally, in situations like cesarean section scar ectopic pregnancy and the vaginal approach for cystocele repair or Shirodkar cerclage, access to the vesicovaginal space is essential (Fig. 1.14).

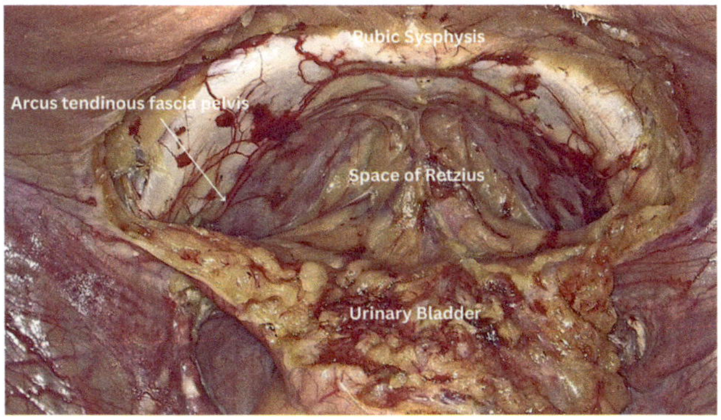

Fig. 1.15 Prevesical space dissection (space of Retzius)

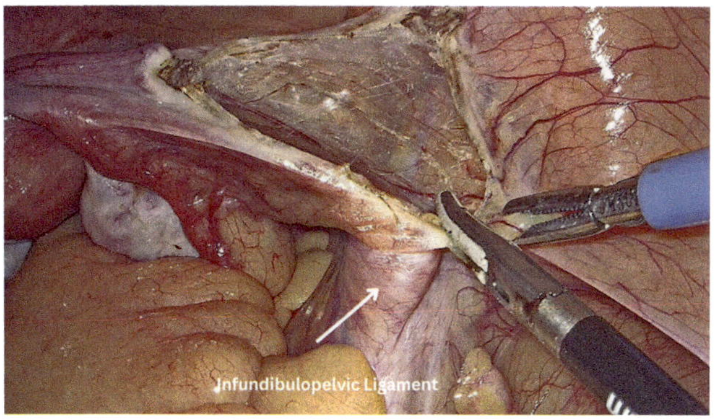

Fig. 1.16 Lateral approach to Retroperitoneum

1.10 Prevesical Space

The prevesical space, also recognized as the space of Retzius, is characterized by its boundaries: ventrally by the pubic symphysis, dorsally by the bladder, cranially by the transversalis fascia, and caudally by the urethra, bladder neck, and pubocervical fascia. Laterally, it is defined by the arcus tendinous fasciae pelvis, situated on the inner surface of the obturator internus and levator ani muscle. Access to the prevesical space can be attained by pulling the median umbilical ligament downward with traction and cutting (Min, n.d.)

Prevesical space is of importance for urogynecological surgeries like SUI procedures, i.e. Burch colposuspension, retropubic TVT, mesh removals, anterior vaginal compartment repairs and oncogynecological surgeries like Anterior exenteration & pelvic anterior peritonectomy and other gynaecological procedures like bladder endometriosis & ureteric reimplantation (Fig. 1.15).

1.11 Pararectal Space

The ventral boundary of pararectal space is formed by Cardinal ligament including the parametrium & paracervix and dorsal boundary by presacral fascia, sacrum.

It is bounded laterally by the internal iliac artery and medially by the Rectum. The cranial boundary is established by the peritoneum of the posterior leaf of the broad ligament, while the caudal boundary is delineated by the levator ani muscle.

Pararectal space can be accessed via either a medial or lateral approach. The lateral approach is situated lateral to the infundibulopelvic ligament, while the medial approach is positioned medial to the infundibulopelvic ligament. The ureter serves as the dividing line, creating the medial portion known as Okabayashi's space and the lateral portion known as Latzko's space. Opening the pararectal space can be achieved using the extraperitoneal approach (Fig. 1.16).

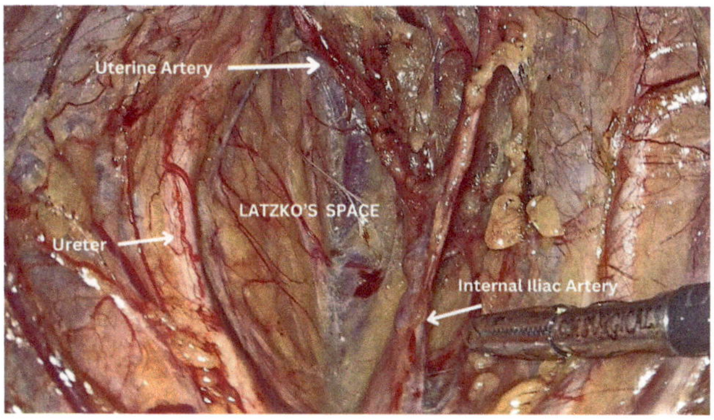

Fig. 1.17 Lateral pararectal space (Latzko's space) dissection

The lateral pararectal space, recognized as Latzko's space, is defined by specific anatomical landmarks. Its ventral boundary is constituted by the cardinal ligament, while posteriorly, it is demarcated by the presacral fascia along with the ventrolateral aspect of the sacrum. On its lateral aspect, it is bordered by the internal iliac artery, and medially, by the ureter and mesoureter. Of particular note, the uterine artery is the sole structure traversing Latzko's space laterally. This area is frequently explored during procedures such as pelvic lymphadenectomy and those requiring access to the pelvic splanchnic nerves and the inferior hypogastric plexus. The process of ligating the uterine artery at its origin and performing internal iliac artery ligation may involve manipulation within Latzko's space (Fig. 1.17).

The anatomical confines of Okabayashi's space are meticulously defined: ventrally, it is delineated by the cardinal ligament, while dorsally, it is demarcated by the presacral fascia and the sacrum. Laterally, it is bounded by the ureter and mesoureter, and medially, by the rectum [9]. This area is accessed by making an incision and subsequently opening the space between the posterior leaf of the broad ligament and the ureter, facilitating the lateralization of important structures such as the ureter, mesoureter, hypogastric nerve, and providing access to the uterosacral ligament. Within Okabayashi's space, two anatomical structures intersect: the lateral liga-

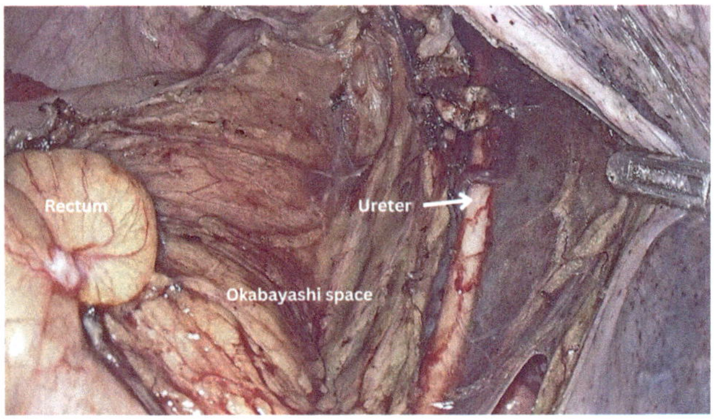

Fig. 1.18 Okabayashi space—medial pararectal space dissection

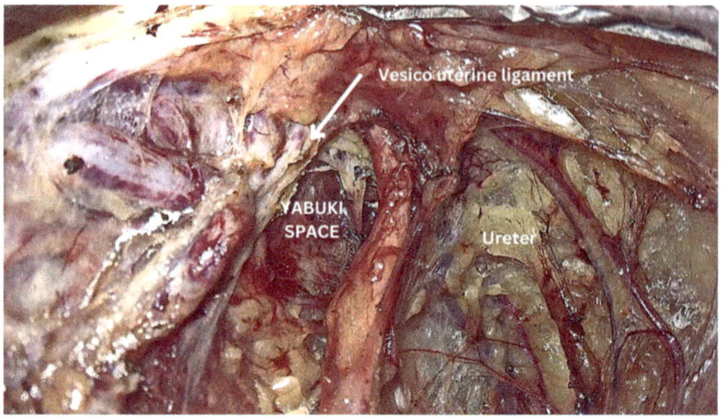

Fig. 1.19 Yabuki space dissection

ment of the rectum and the middle rectal artery. Surgical dissection within this space is warranted in procedures such as nerve-sparing deep endometriosis, nerve-sparing radical hysterectomy, identification and dissection of hypogastric nerves, laparoscopic uterosacral nerve ablation (LUNA), and in cases necessitating entry into the rectovaginal space laterally due to obliteration of the pouch of Douglas (Fig. 1.18).

The pararectal space is an essential area dissected not only in abdominal surgeries but also in various vaginal procedures, including the sacrospinous ligament fixation procedure, vaginal radical trachelectomy (Dargent's operation), vaginal radical hysterectomy (Shauta's operation), and laparoscopic-assisted radical vaginal hysterectomy.

1.11.1 Yabuki Space

Yabuki space, also known as the fourth place, was initially delineated in 2000 by Yoshihiko Yabuki. Positioned between the upper section of the vesicouterine ligament and the ureter, this space is of particular interest during nerve-sparing surgeries due to its housing of the pelvic splanchnic nerves involved in bladder innervation. Upon dissecting the upper part of the vesico-uterine ligament, the Yabuki space becomes accessible. Subsequent dissection and coagulation reveal the fourth space, leading towards the vesicoureteral junction (Fig. 1.19).

1.11.2 Rectovaginal Space

The boundaries of the rectovaginal space are delineated ventrally by the posterior vaginal wall, dorsally by the anterior rectal wall, and laterally by the uterosacral ligaments (at the cranial end) and the rectovaginal ligament (at the caudal end). Cranially, the peritoneal reflections of the pouch of Douglas define the space, while caudally, it is bounded by the levator ani muscle. Access to the rectovaginal space can be achieved through either a medial or lateral approach.

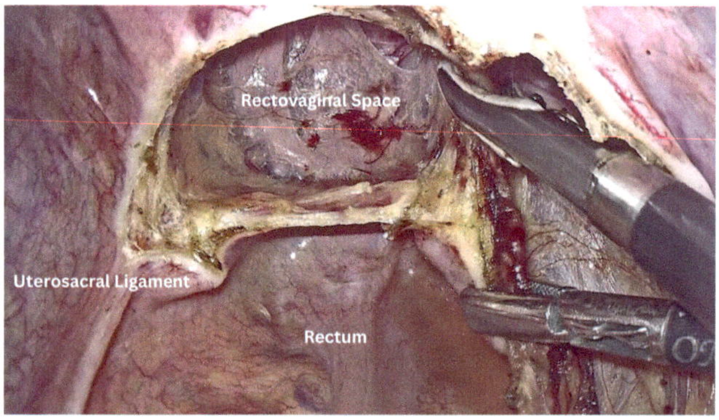

Fig. 1.20 Rectovaginal Space dissection

In the medial approach, the rectouterine pouch is incised, exposing Denonvillier's fascia. Alternatively, in the lateral approach, after opening both pararectal spaces, development of the rectovaginal space proceeds lateromedially, craniocaudally, and dorso-ventrally. During dissection, it is essential to adhere to the principle that fat belongs to the rectum.

The medial rectovaginal space is accessed in procedures such as sacrocolpopexy, uterosacral ligament suspension, radical hysterectomy, pelvic adhesions, deep endometriosis, and rectovaginal fistula repair. Conversely, the lateral approach to rectovaginal space dissection is employed in cases of endometriosis, posterior colpotomy, or V notes (Fig. 1.20).

1.11.3 Presacral Space (Retrorectal Space)

Boundaries -Ventrally by Mesorectal fascia/rectum, dorsally by sacral promontory and anterior aspect of sacrum.
Laterally -Right (right common iliac artery/right ureter), left (left common iliac vein/left ureter)
Cranially by peritoneal reflection of the rectosigmoid colon
Caudally by Pelvic floor
The presacral space can be accessed via a lateral approach by mobilizing the rectosigmoid from the left side to the right

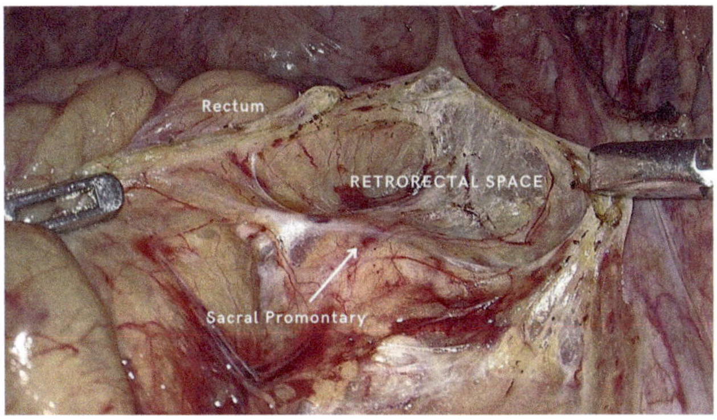

Fig. 1.21 Presacral space (Retrorectal space) dissection

side of the pelvis and vertically incising the peritoneum along the left sigmoid attachment to the posterior pelvis. This incision extends from the sacral promontory along the right common iliac artery

Presacral space dissection needed in cases like Excision of endometriosis (trans-mesorectal approach), presacral neurectomy

In urogynecological procedures like Laparoscopic sacrocolpopexy, Rectopexy, oncogynecological procedures like total mesorectal excision (Inter-fascial approach)- for ovarian cancer infiltrating the rectal wall, at the beginning of para-aortic lymphadenectomy and laparoscopic nerve-sparing complete excision of rectal endometriosis (Interfascial approach)

Lumbosacral space is bounded medially by External iliac artery & vein laterally by Psoas major muscle. It lies below obturator nerve

Lumbosacral space dissection is crucial in deep endometriosis involving sciatic nerve Sciatic nerve & pudendal nerve are exposed in neuropelveology –LION Procedures (Fig. 1.21).

Learning Points

- The retroperitoneal space is crucial, situated between the parietal peritoneum and the posterior abdominal wall. It encompasses various compartments, including centromedial, lateral, and pelvic zones.
- Retroperitoneal space is classified into three zones (I, II, III) based on anatomical and clinical criteria. Each zone has specific boundaries and includes different structures.
- The renal fascia delineates three compartments: anterior pararenal, posterior pararenal, and perirenal compartments.
- Sacral promontory is crucial for pelvic surgeries as it serves as a key landmark for navigating the abdominal aorta and its branches, which include the ovarian artery, median sacral artery, external iliac artery, and internal iliac artery, all of which play critical roles in surgical interventions within the pelvis.
- The ureter lacks a dedicated primary arterial supply and receives branches from various sources.
- Avascular spaces in the pelvis, are paravesical, prevesical, pararectal, and rectovaginal spaces.
- Pararectal space can be classified as medial (Okabayashi's space) or lateral (Latzko's space), ureter divides it into lateral and medial spaces.

Competing Interest The author declares no conflict of interest that are relevant to content of this chapter.

Ethical Approval Informed consent was obtained from individual participants and patients regarding publication and documentation without disclosing their identity.

References

1. Puntambekar S, Manchanda R. Surgical pelvic anatomy in gynecologic oncology. Int J Gynecol Obstet. 2018;143:86–92.
2. Kim S, Kim TU, Lee JW, et al. The perihepatic space: comprehensive anatomy and CT features of pathologic conditions. Radiographics. 2007;27(1):129–43.
3. Selçuk İ, Ersak B, Tatar İ, Güngör T, Huri E. Basic clinical retroperitoneal anatomy for pelvic surgeons. Turk J Obstet Gynecol. 2018;15(4):259.
4. Drake R, Vogl W, Mitchell AWM. Gray's anatomy for students. 3rd ed. Philadelphia: Churchill Livingstone/Elsevier; 2015.
5. Mirilas P, Skandalakis JE. Surgical anatomy of the retroperitoneal spaces part II: the architecture of the retroperitoneal space. Am Surg. 2010;76(1):33–42.
6. Schuenke M, Schulte E, Schumacher U, Johnson N. General anatomy and musculoskeletal system (THIEME atlas of anatomy). 3rd ed. New York: Thieme; 2020; 636 p. ISBN 9781626237186.
7. Fujii S. Anatomic identification of nerve-sparing radical hysterectomy: a step-by-step procedure. Gynecol Oncol. 2008;111(2 Suppl):S33–41. https://doi.org/10.1016/j.ygyno.2008.07.026. Epub 2008 Aug 27. PMID: 18752840.
8. Moore KL, Dalley AF, Agur AMR. Clinically oriented anatomy. 7th ed. Philadelphia: Wolters Kluwer Health/Lippincott Williams & Wilkins; 2014.
9. Kostov S. Avascular spaces of the female pelvis—clinical applications in obstetrics and gynecology. J Clin Med. 2020;9(5):1460. MDPI.
10. Stupart D, Pickles K, Briggs C. Anatomy of the vesicovaginal fascia and its relation to branches of the inferior hypogastric plexus. Clin Anat. 2022;35:855–60. https://doi.org/10.1002/ca.23858.
11. Ross LM, Lamperti ED, editors. Thieme atlas of anatomy. Neck and internal organs. New York: Thieme; 2006. p. 162.

2 To Avoid Trocar Injuries in Multiple Previous Surgeries-Jain Point

Nutan Jain, Sakshi Srivastava, and Divyanee Gulati

2.1 Introduction

Laparoscopic access in patients with multiple previous surgery poses various challenges due to altered anatomy and the presence of visceral and omental adhesions, thereby leading to vascular injuries in 0.1–6.4 per 1000 laparoscopies [1] and bowel injury in 0.03–0.65% of patients [2]. Consequently, the imperative to devise effective strategies to minimize trocar injuries becomes even more important, particularly in patients with a complex surgical history characterized by multiple previous scars.

For years, umbilical entry has been the most commonly used, although the crux of adhesions has been found to be at the umbilicus [3] (Fig. 2.1a, b). These adhesions are usually

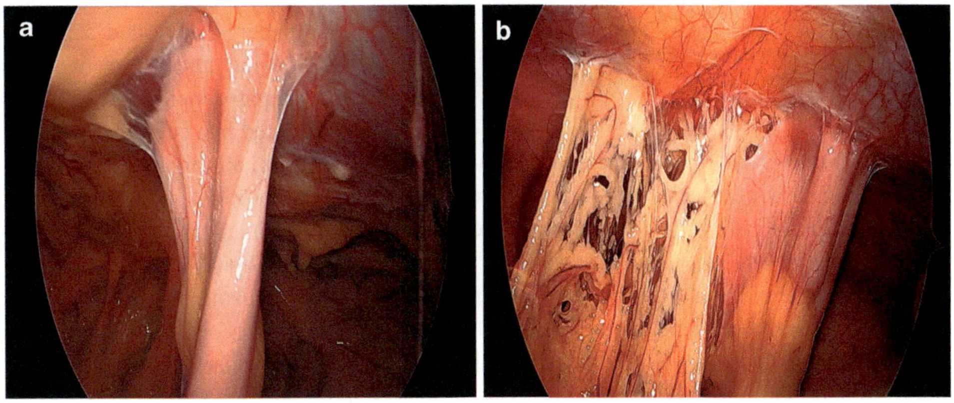

Fig. 2.1 **a** Bowel adhesions noted at umbilicus. **b** Bowel and omental adhesions noted at umbilicus

Supplementary Information The online version contains supplementary material available at https://doi.org/10.1007/978-981-97-3226-5_2. The videos can be accessed individually by clicking the DOI link in the accompanying figure caption or by scanning this link with the SN More Media App.

N. Jain (✉)
Obstetrics and Gynaecology, GSVM Medical College, Affiliated by Kanpur University, Kanpur, Uttar Pradesh, India

Department of Obstetrics and Gynecology, Vardhman Trauma and Laparoscopy Centre Pvt. Ltd., Muzaffarnagar, Uttar Pradesh, India

S. Srivastava
Department of Obstetrics and Gynecology, Vardhman Trauma and Laparoscopy Centre Pvt. Ltd., Muzaffarnagar, Uttar Pradesh, India

Obstetrics and Gynaecology, Rohilkhand Medical College and Hospital, Affiliated by Bareilly International University, Bareilly, Uttar Pradesh, India

D. Gulati
Department of Obstetrics and Gynecology, Vardhman Trauma and Laparoscopy Centre Pvt. Ltd., Muzaffarnagar, Uttar Pradesh, India

Obstetrics and Gynaecology, GMC Patiala, Affiliated by Baba Farid University of Health Sciences, Patiala, Punjab, India

N. Jain (ed.), *Complex Total Laparoscopic Hysterectomy (TLH) with Newer Approaches in Bladder Dissection*,
https://doi.org/10.1007/978-981-97-3226-5_2

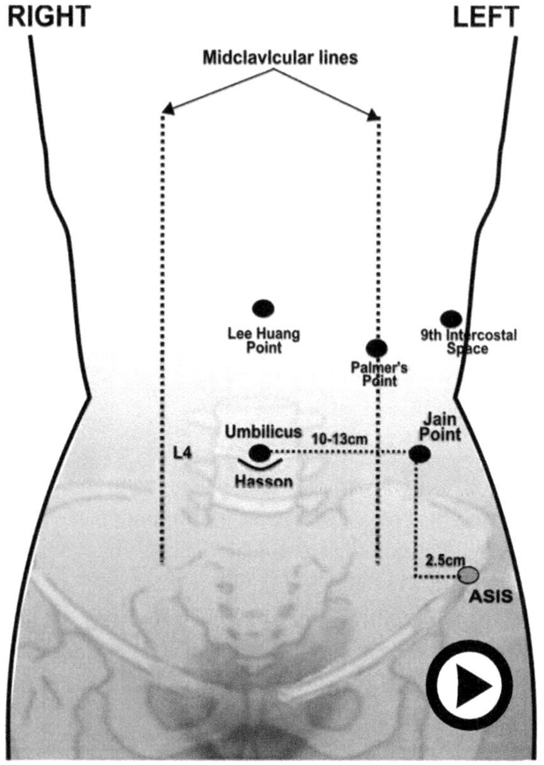

Fig. 2.2 Diagrammatic representation of Jain point (Video 2.2 Jain Point entry technique) (▶ https://doi.org/10.1007/000-c90)

omental, however in several cases of previous infectious pathologies, previous caesarean sections, previous ectopic pregnancy and laparotomy for several indications, lot of bowel adhesions have been noted as well.

To avoid umbilicus as primary entry and umbilical adhesions, other researchers kept moving upwards to devise a safe port for laparoscopic entry, like Palmers' point [4], Lee Huang point [5] and ninth intercoastal space [6]. But all these ports had contraindications of their own like hepatosplenomegaly, large upper quadrant masses, and upper abdominal scars [7]. We thought differently and made a port, Jain point, at the level of umbilicus but far laterally [8, 9] (Fig. 2.2). Till date it has no known contraindications and applicable in all contraindications of Palmer's point; and has been found to be safe in surgical scars in all quadrants of abdomen, and in situations where all other entry ports have limitations.

2.2 Rationale of Using Jain Point

We planned a primary port to avoid injuries during entry in patients with history of multiple previous surgeries, para-umbilical, 10–13 cm away from the umbilicus [10]. Jain point lies at the L4 level, where there are no viscera. The viscera on the left side, namely the stomach, spleen and kidneys, come maximum up to the level of T12, L1. Even if the spleen is enlarged; unless it is grossly enlarged because of some major pathology, it does not come down to L4. Lower down the sigmoid colon has physiological adherence to the pelvic brim. The anatomical location of the Jain point, at L4 level, allows for a wide nascent area on the left side, from L1 to the pelvic brim, devoid of vessels, viscera, adhesions and bowel (Fig. 2.3a, b) [11].

Irrespective of previous surgeries, Jain point has been found to be consistently free, avoiding trocar injuries with scars in upper (Fig. 2.4a, b), mid (Fig. 2.5a–d) or lower (Fig. 2.6a, b) quadrant of abdomen (Fig. 2.7a, b). Our published studies over a span of 12 years suggest that the Jain point entry was feasible in all 9549 patients who underwent gynaecological laparoscopic surgery at our advanced laparoscopic centre. Among these patients, at least one third of patients 2791 had a history of previous surgery, with 720 having undergone two or more (2–6) previous surgeries. Laparoscopic entry through the Jain point was safely executed by senior consultants, junior consultants, and fellows, with almost equal distribution across cases [12]. Ours being a multidisciplinary centre having combined gynae and general surgery cases and our general surgeon colleagues and urologists also favoured the Jain point for entry and continued using it as the camera or working port [13]. Across other sub specialities of minimally invasive surgeries, Jain point is being used by others also, as gastroenterologists, bariatric and onco surgeons.

The surface marking clearly defines the Jain point on a vertical line drawn 2.5 cm medial to the anterior superior iliac spine (ASIS), at the level of the umbilicus. It carries the advantage of a fixed and prominent bony landmark, the ASIS, ensuring accurate entry. Harry Reich, in his foreword for the book, "Non-Umbilical Laparoscopic Entry Ports", highlights that the Jain point, easily located by the ASIS, is the lowest of all three entry ports, and may be best for routine use [14].

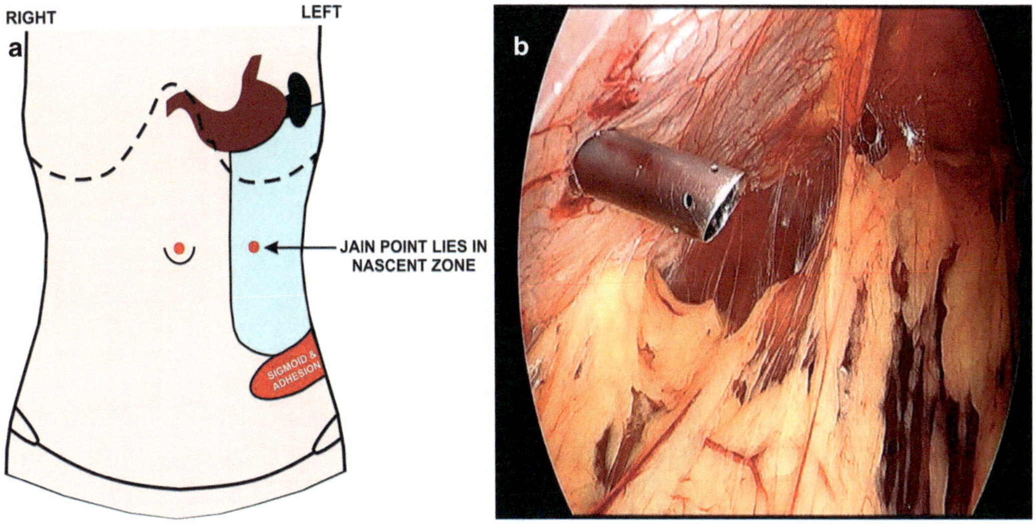

Fig. 2.3 **a** Rationale of Jain point. **b** Jain point free of any viscera, lying at L4 level

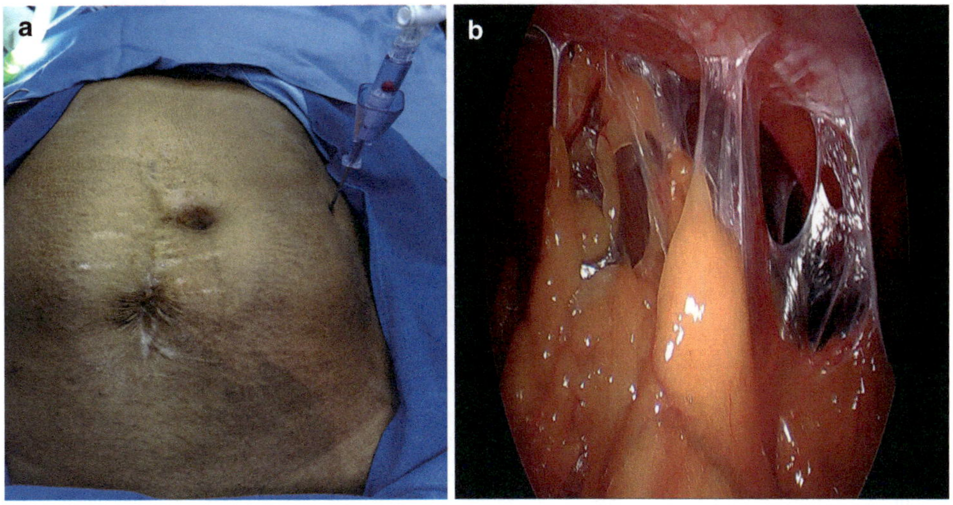

Fig. 2.4 **a** Jain point entry in a patient with upper abdomen scar. **b** Multiple bowel and omental adhesions in upper abdomen, avoided by Jain point entry

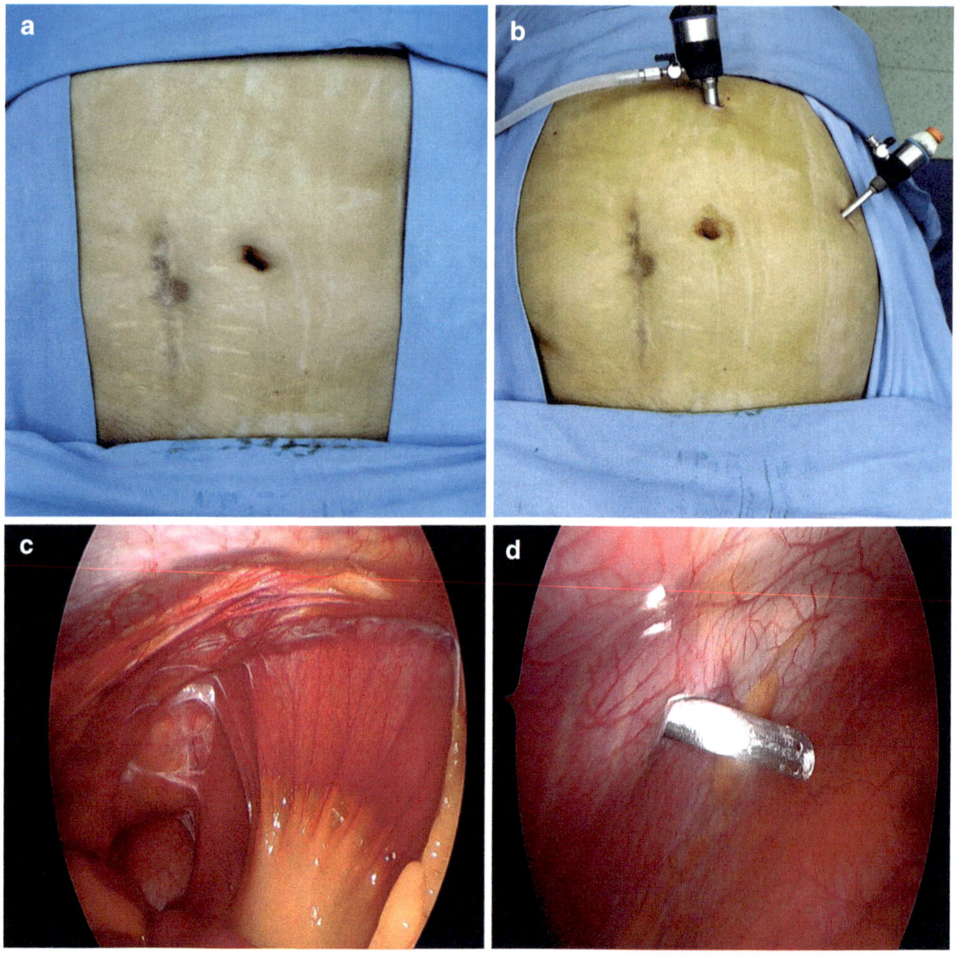

Fig. 2.5 **a** Patient with mid abdomen scar. **b** Jain point entry safe. **c** Bowel adhesions noted in that patient with history of laparotomy. **d** Jain point located on left side free of adhesions

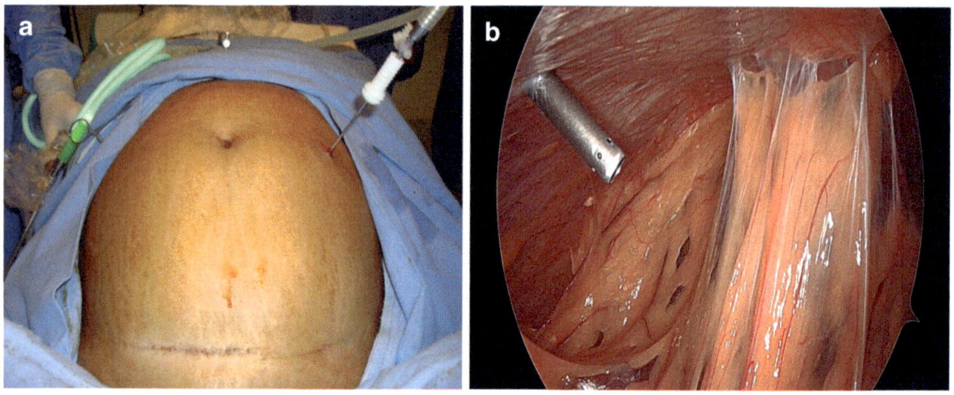

Fig. 2.6 **a** Jain point entry by veress needle in a patient with low transverse scar. **b** Dense omental adhesions noted in lower abdomen, with Jain point free

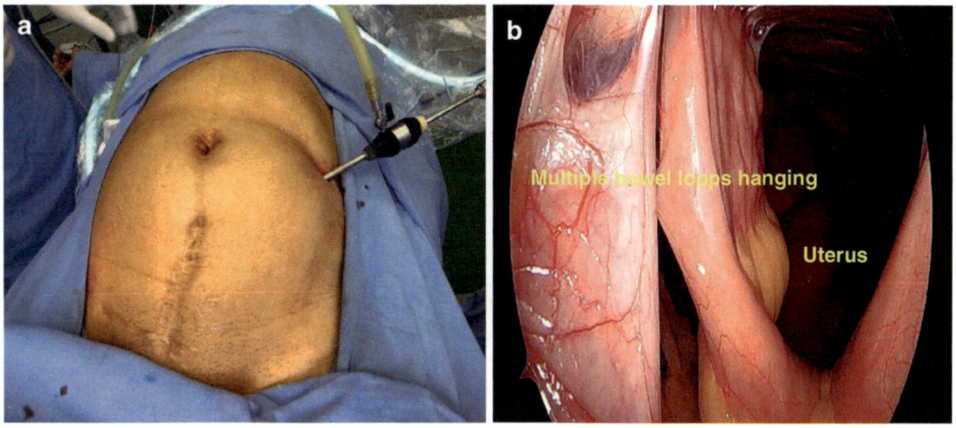

Fig. 2.7 **a** Jain point entry safe in low vertical scars. **b** Dense bowel adhesions noted in mid abdomen with Jain point free

2.3 Technique

The veress needle and subsequently 5 mm trocar are inserted in a vertical, perpendicular line at the Jain point. In our technique, we stress on the point that the abdomen need not be lifted during entry to avoid unequal forces, zigzag track and facilitating a simplified entry. Under the vision of 5 mm telescope, the 10 mm camera port is inserted, avoiding adhesions; and according to mandate of the case and the pelvic pathology. We have been using reusable pyramidal tip trocar for several years. But other surgeons can use the trocar according to their institutional norms, like the metal trocars, EndoTIP (Endoscopic Threaded Imaging Port) [15] and optical trocar systems [16]. Surgeons experienced in the technique of direct trocar entry have adopted the use of the Jain point without the need for prior Veress needle insertion [17]. Surgeons working in low resource setting can prefer reusable metal trocars, as we have found them safe in our series of close to ten thousand cases. Jain point entry is not only easy to learn but also applicable in versatile situations with large masses, in all ranges of BMI [18] and in pregnant patients [19].

Other all entry ports in the upper abdomen namely, Palmers' point, Lee Huang point and ninth intercoastal space are not safe in upper abdominal suspected adhesions; as in upper abdomen scars and in patients with history of infectious pathologies, like Fitz-Hugh Curtis syndrome (Fig. 2.8a, b) [20], and Koch's abdomen (Figs. 2.9a, b and 2.10a, b); leading to dense adhesions of liver, stomach, bowel and omentum. Hasson's open entry technique has been considered to be safe; however, it is unable to avoid type II bowel adhesions (Fig. 2.11a, b), where bowel loops are densely adherent to the anterior abdominal wall, making almost second layer of parietal peritoneum [21]. In multiple previous surgeries, Palmer's point has been routinely used but has certain limitations [22, 23]. Jain point can be used in upper abdomen scars (Figs. 2.12a, b and 2.13a, b), Kocher's incision and suspected adhesions in the upper quadrant (Fig. 2.14a, b). We widely reported our series of 106 cases proving the safety of Jain Point in upper abdominal scars [24]. It is feasible in all quadrants of abdomen and lies outside all possible surgical scars, therefore Jain point acts as a referee on a tennis court, sitting outside the surgical field, monitoring the movement of ball on either side of the court with equal agility. In situations with previous scars and drain sites at Jain point, mirror image (Fig. 2.15a, b) of Jain point on right side can be used for laparoscopic entry.

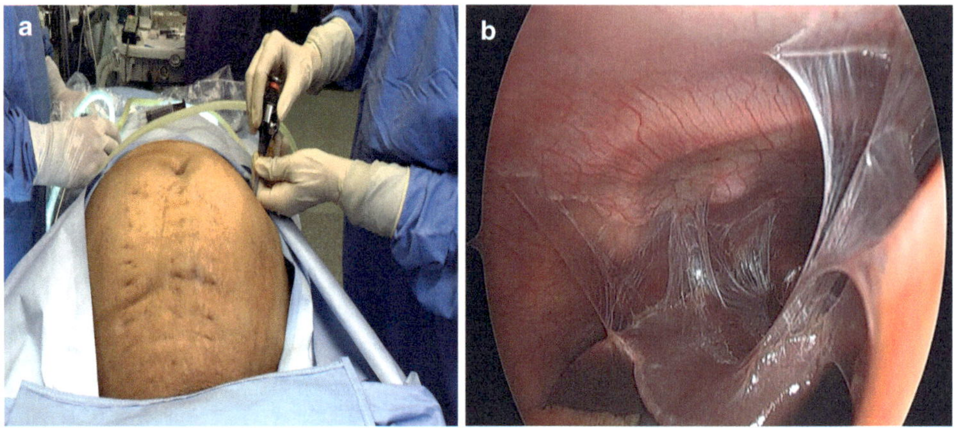

Fig. 2.8 **a** Trocar insertion at Jain point in a patient with multiple previous surgeries and history of pelvic inflammatory disease. **b** Adhesions of Fitz Hugh Curtis syndrome noted in upper quadrant

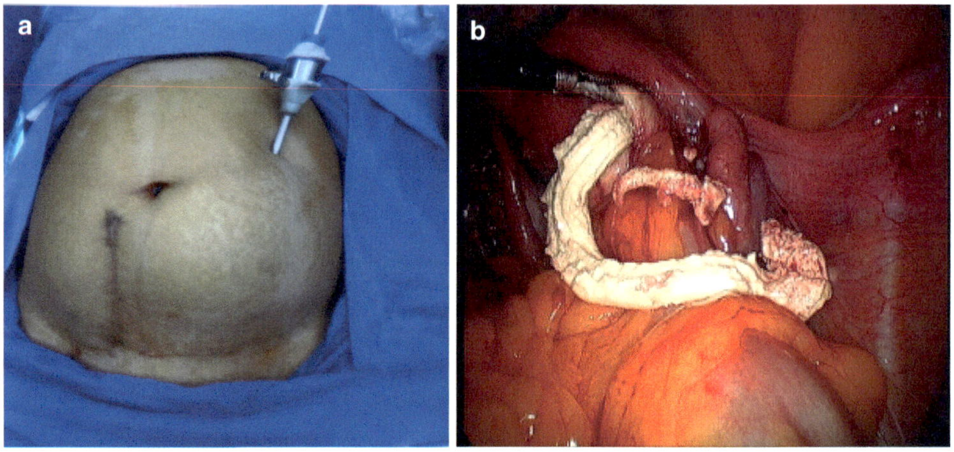

Fig. 2.9 **a** Jain point feasible in frozen pelvis with Genital Koch's. **b** Caseous material drained from ovary

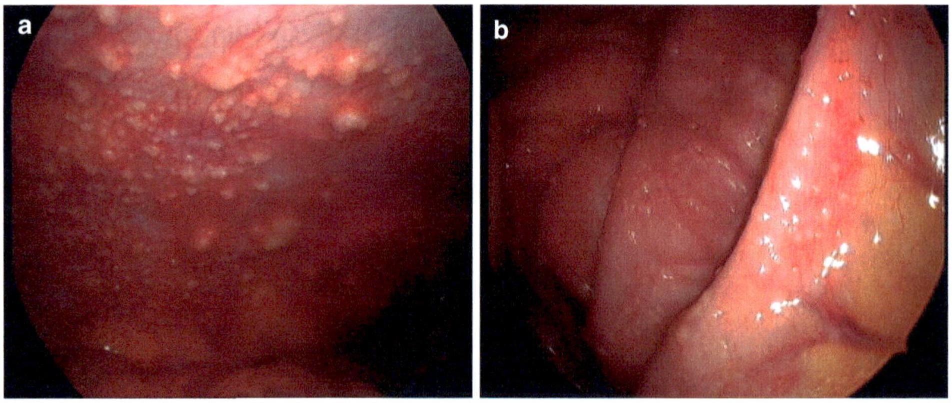

Fig. 2.10 **a** Jain point safe in a patient of Koch's with multiple caseomas on anterior abdominal wall. **b** Fluid filled vesicles noted over bowel loops also

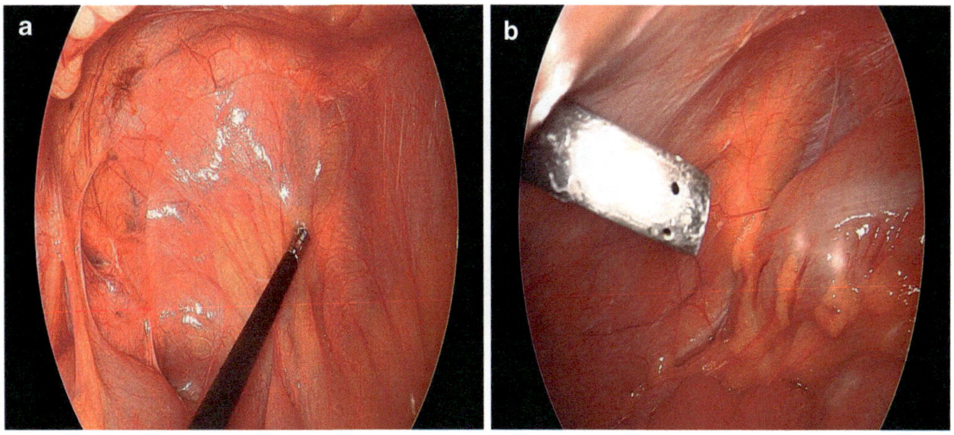

Fig. 2.11 **a** Type II bowel adhesions, with bowel loops forming the second layer of abdominal wall in mid abdomen, contraindicating Hasson's open entry technique. **b** Jain point was found to be free

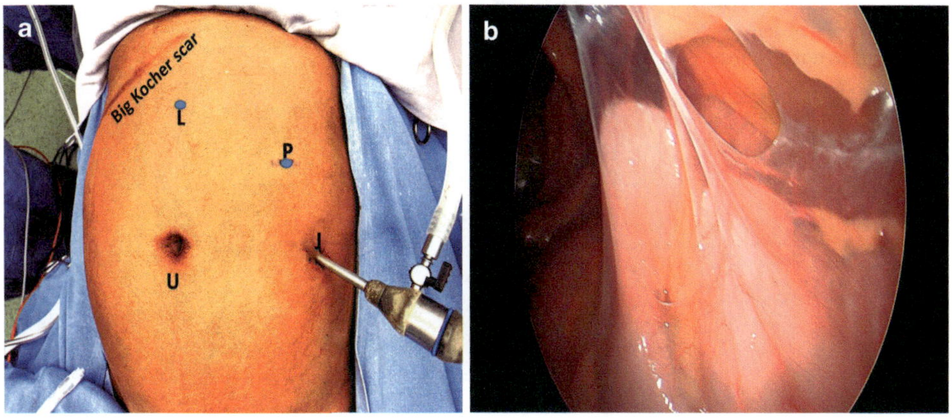

Fig. 2.12 **a** Jain point entry with reusable pyramidal tip metal trocar in a patient with upper abdominal Kocher's scar. **b** Dense bowel adhesions noted at Palmers point

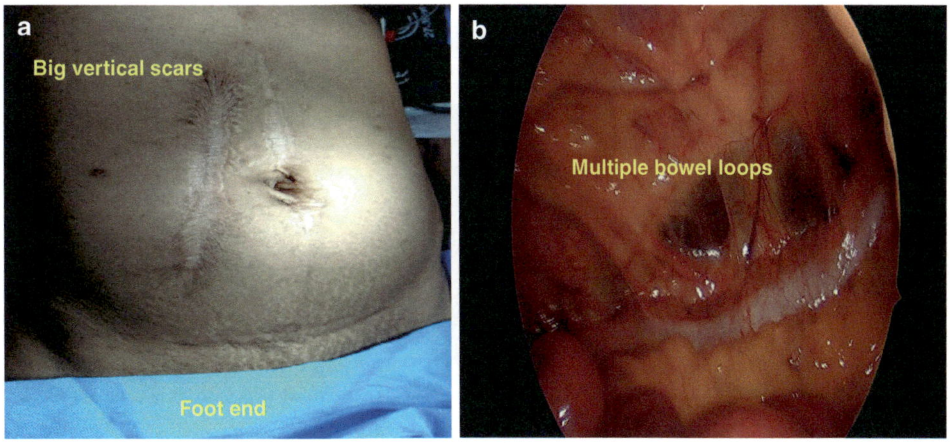

Fig. 2.13 **a** Jain point entry safe in big vertical scars. **b** Dense bowel adhesions noted in upper abdomen

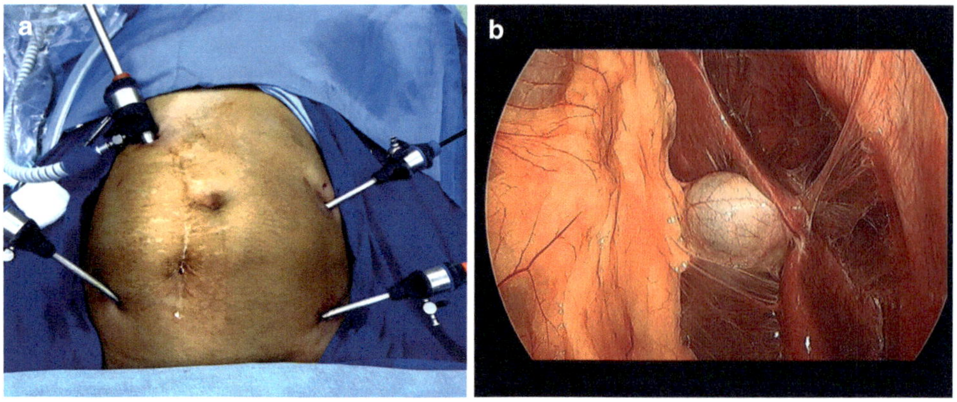

Fig. 2.14 **a** Jain point entry in a patient with long vertical scar and history of infection. **b** Dense post inflammatory adhesions in upper abdomen over liver, gall bladder and omentum

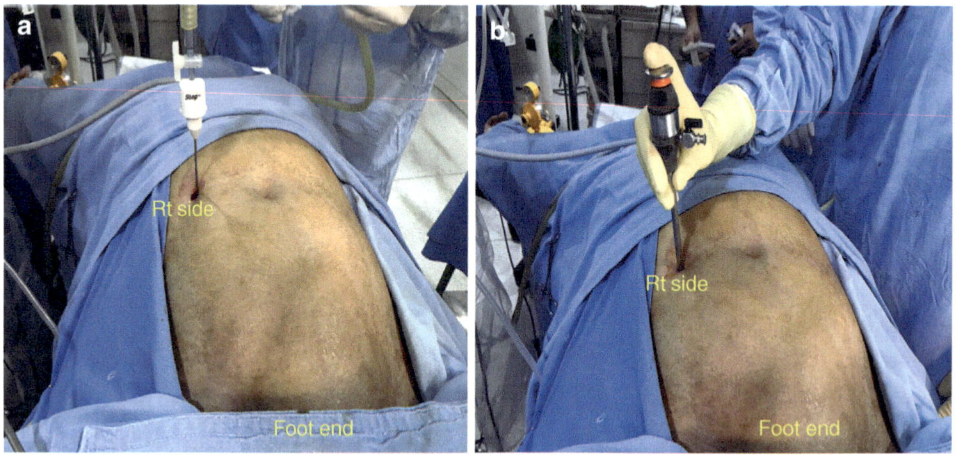

Fig. 2.15 **a** Veress insertion at mirror image of Jain Point. **b** Trocar insertion at mirror image of Jain point

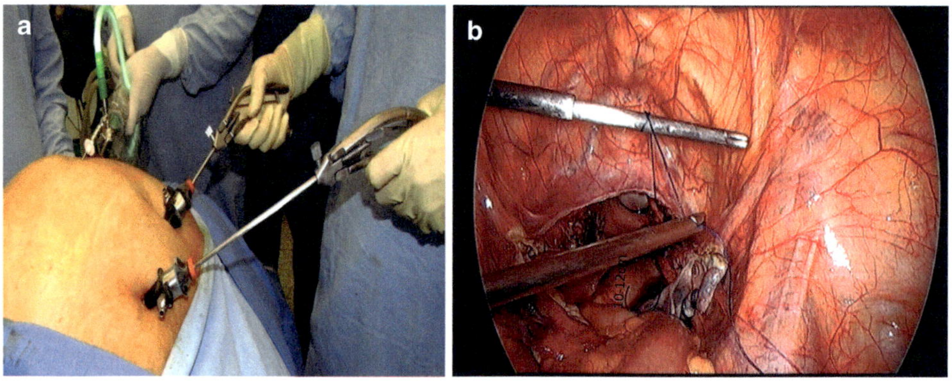

Fig. 2.16 **a** Jain point port continues as the main ipsilateral working port. **b** Laparoscopic view showing good ergonomic working

2.4 Ergonomics

Jain Point Port does not become redundant after initial entry rather it consistently serves as the primary ergonomic working port throughout the entirety of the surgery. In this context we can further add that Jain point is positioned at the mid-abdomen, extending to the depth of the pelvis and upper abdomen with equal ease, ensuring its continuous functionality in combined multidisciplinary surgeries (Fig. 2.16a, b).

2.5 Difference from Palmer's Point [25]

1. Palmer's point has been relied upon for almost 50 years, but as the number of previous surgeries have been escalating, several contraindications of Palmer's point have emerged, namely, bloated stomach, hepatosplenomegaly, upper quadrant scars, large upper quadrant masses and suspected post inflammatory adhesions. To tide over these, the Jain point emerged as an alternate entry port in these situations, which has no known contraindications till date.
2. Palmer's point is located by two surgical landmarks, subcostal margin and clavicle which lie in the unsterile arena; while Jain point is located by a single prominent bony landmark, the anterior superior iliac spine, which lies in the sterile surgical field.
3. In case of suspected adhesions at Palmer's point, entry from right side cannot be made due to risk of liver laceration; while Jain point can be used as mirror image on the right side.
4. In cases where laparoscopy is indicated in a pregnant patient, Palmer's point entry can be risky being closer to midline. Jain point lying far laterally is easily used as primary port in pregnant patients.
5. Palmer's point carries the risk of injury to bloated stomach, while Jain point entry had only 1 bowel complication in our series in a case with transverse scar at level of umbilicus coming up to Jain point, where bowel was plastered all over the abdomen, making other entry ports also not feasible.
6. Palmer's point entry is not applicable in big upper abdomen scars with densely plastered bowel, Jain point entry is feasible in such situations (Fig. 2.17a, b).
7. In patients with previous mesh ventral hernia repair, Palmer's point entry can be close to the mesh with risk of mesh perforation by trocar while Jain point lying away from the midline, stays away from the margin of mesh and can easily be used in such situations (Fig. 2.18).
8. In patients with history of infectious pathologies, Palmer's point entry is risky owing to adhesions in upper abdomen. Jain point entry can still be easily made as found in mid abdomen laterally it has been found to be adhesion free.

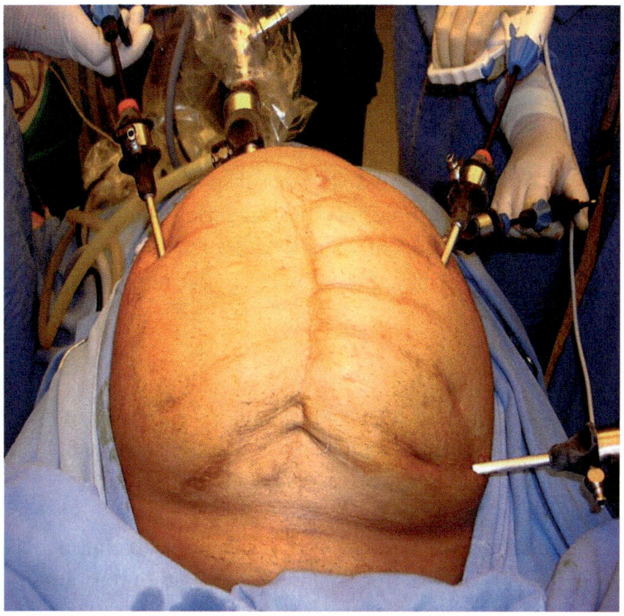

Fig. 2.18 Jain point entry in previous mesh hernia repair

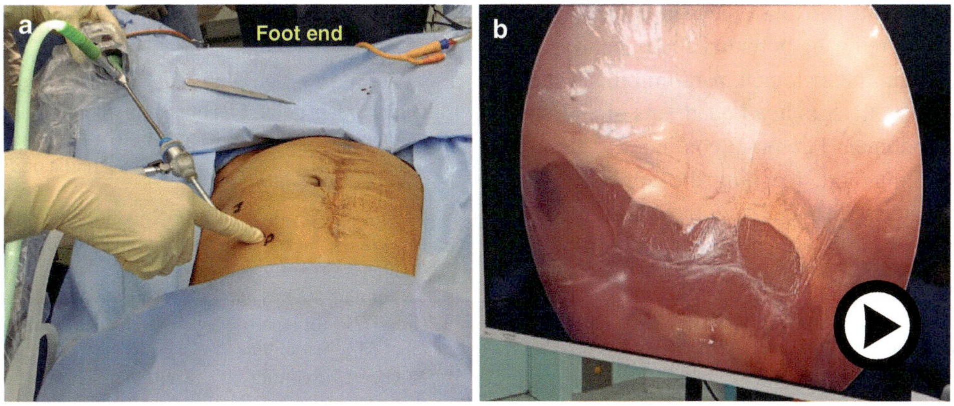

Fig. 2.17 **a** Finger pressing at Palmer's point in a patient with infectious pathology, entered through the Jain point port (Video 2.17a Jain Point entry technique in challenging situations) (▶ https://doi.org/10.1007/000-c8z). **b** Laparoscopic view showing bowel loops densely adherent at Palmer's point

9. Palmer's point entry has risk of injury to left kidney in thin patients; while Jain point having no underlying viscera eases the fear of visceral injury from novice minds, and has a short learning curve.
10. Palmer's point becomes redundant after entry, while Jain point continues as the main working port through the surgery.

2.6 Conclusion

Taking into account these four considerations—steering clear of central adhesions, avoiding interference with viscera, avoiding the contraindications of Palmer's point like upper abdominal scars, upper abdomen adhesions due to previous history of infectious pathologies; and continuous observation in large series reveal a lack of adhesions at the Jain point. The versatility of Jain point is evident in its successful application across various subspecialties and various scenarios with multiple previous surgeries, applicable with scars, in all quadrants of abdomen, large masses, and in varied BMI. After entry, it continues as the main ergonomic working port.

Learning Points

- Performing TLH in patients with a history of multiple previous surgeries requires a meticulous approach and detailed preoperative assessment, to avoid visceral injuries.
- Each patient's unique medical history, including the details of prior surgeries, should be taken into account to optimize overall patient safety and well-being.
- Safe entry is half the job done, so we utilize Jain point as the primary entry port; as strategic anatomical location contributes to a safer surgical entry, emphasizing the importance of careful port placement in achieving optimal outcomes and reducing potential complications.
- Jain point, lying in mid abdomen, para-umbilical, far laterally, is feasible with scars in all quadrants of abdomen.
- Lying in mid abdomen, Jain point continues as the main ergonomic working port, reaching the upper abdomen and lower abdomen with equal ease, facilitating its use in combined multidisciplinary surgeries, and ensuring a smoother surgical process.

Competing Interest The author declares no conflict of interest that are relevant to content of this chapter.

Ethical Approval Informed consent was obtained from individual participants and patients regarding publication and documentation without disclosing their identity.

References

1. King NR, Lin E, Yeh C, Wong JMK, Friedman J, Traylor J, Tsai S, Chaudhari A, Milad MP. Laparoscopic major vascular injuries in gynecologic surgery for benign indications: a systematic review. Obstet Gynecol. 2021;137(3):434–42. https://doi.org/10.1097/AOG.0000000000004280. PMID: 33543898.
2. Alkatout I. Complications of laparoscopy in connection with entry techniques. J Gynecol Surg. 2017;33(3):81–91. https://doi.org/10.1089/gyn.2016.0111. PMID: 28663686; PMCID: PMC5477171.
3. Varma R, Gupta JK. Laparoscopic entry techniques: clinical guideline, national survey, and medicolegal ramifications. Surg Endosc. 2008;22(12):2686–97. https://doi.org/10.1007/s00464-008-9871-6. Epub 2008 Apr 10. PMID: 18401653.
4. Palmer R. Safety in laparoscopy. J Reprod Med. 1974;13(1):1–5.
5. Lee CL, Huang KG, Jain S, Wang CJ, Yen CF, Soong YK. A new portal for gynecologic laparoscopy. J Am Assoc Gynecol Laparosc. 2001;8(1):147–50. https://doi.org/10.1016/s1074-3804(05)60565-8.
6. Lam KW, Pun TC. Left upper quadrant approach in gynecologic laparoscopic surgery using reusable instruments. J Am Assoc Gynecol Laparosc. 2002;9(2):199–203. https://doi.org/10.1016/s1074-3804(05)60132-6.
7. Taskforce for Abdominal Entry. Principles of safe laparoscopic entry. Eur J Obstet Gynecol Reprod Biol. 2016;201:179–88. https://doi.org/10.1016/j.ejogrb.2016.03.040.
8. Sharp HT. Overview of gynecologic laparoscopic surgery and non-umbilical entry sites. In: T Falcone, editor. Wolters Kluwers; 2019. p. 10. UpToDate.
9. Bedaiwy MA, Yong PJ, Farghaly TA, Abdelhafez FF, Tan J, Pope R, et al. The effect of age and body mass index on the surgical anatomy of supraumbilical port insertion: implications for laparoscopic and robotic surgery. Gynecol Obstet Investig. 2018;83(6):546–51. https://doi.org/10.1159/000488676.
10. Jain N, Sareen S, Kanawa S, Jain V, Gupta S, Mann S. Jain point: a new safe portal for laparoscopic entry in previous surgery cases. J Hum Reprod Sci. 2016;9(1):9–17. https://doi.org/10.4103/0974-1208.178637.
11. Jain N, Jain V, Chandi A, Srivastava S, Singh S, Vasundhara N. Jain point: an alternate laparoscopic non-umbilical first blind entry port to avoid vessel, viscera, adhesions and bowel (VVAB). Updat Surg. 2021;73(6):2321–9. https://doi.org/10.1007/s13304-021-01099-z.
12. Jain N., et al. Jain point: to avoid trocar injuries in multiple previous surgeries. Med Res Arch [S.l.] 2023;11(11). ISSN 2375–1924. Available at: https://esmed.org/MRA/mra/article/view/4734. Date accessed: 17 Jan 2024. https://doi.org/10.18103/mra.v11i11.4734.
13. Gupta S. Jain point: first blind entry port for laparoscopic cholecystectomy. Newsletter of Association of Surgeons of India - Asiindia.org. SCALPEL2022. https://asiindia.org/wpcontent/uploads/SCALPEL-2022-August.pdf
14. Reich H. Foreword. In: Jain N, editor. Nonumbilical laparoscopic entry ports. 1st ed. New Delhi: Jaypee Brothers Medical Publishers; 2020.
15. Ternamian AM, Deitel M. Endoscopic threaded imaging port (EndoTIP) for laparoscopy: experience with different body weights. Obes Surg. 1999;9:44–7.
16. Mettler L, Schmidt EH, Frank V, Semm K. Optical trocar systems: laparoscopic entry and its complications (a study of cases in Germany). Gynaecol Endosc. 1999;8:383–9.
17. Mulayim B, Aksoy O. J Gynecol Surg. 2020;36:37–9. https://doi.org/10.1089/gyn.2019.0077.

18. Jain N, Singh S, Mandal KK, et al. A retrospective study of a novel non-umbilical laparoscopic entry port in thin patients—Jain point. Gynecol Surg. 2020;17:13. https://doi.org/10.1186/s10397-020-01080-5.
19. Salcedo AMC, Guarin CB, et al. Glob Libr Women's Med. ISSN: 1756-2228. https://doi.org/10.3843/GLOWM.415713.
20. Basit H, Pop A, Malik A, Sharma S. Fitz-Hugh-Curtis syndrome. 2023 Jul 3. In: StatPearls [Internet]. Treasure Island: StatPearls Publishing; 2024 Jan–.
21. Hasson HM. Open laparoscopy as a method of access in laparoscopic surgery. Gynaecol Endosc. 1999;8:353–62. https://doi.org/10.1046/j.1365-2508.1999.00316.x.
22. Tulikangas RK, Nicklas A, Falcone T, Price LL. Anatomy of the left upper quadrant for cannula insertion. J Am Assoc Gynecol Laparosc. 2000;7:211–4.
23. Clark NV, Einarsson JI. 5. Laparoscopic entry techniques. In: Saridoğan E, Kilic GS, Ertan K, editors. Minimally invasive surgery in gynecological practice: practical examples in gynecology. Berlin, Boston: De Gruyter; 2020. p. 50–60. https://doi.org/10.1515/9783110535204-005.
24. Jain N, Jain V, Gupta S. Jain point: to study the efficacy and safety in previous upper abdominal scars. J Minim Invasive Gynecol. 2021;28(11): Supplement, S115. https://doi.org/10.1016/j.jmig.2021.09.179.
25. Nutan J, Sakshi S, Sri L, et al. Jain point laparoscopic entry in contraindications of Palmers point. Front Surg. 2022;9:928081. https://doi.org/10.3389/fsurg.2022.928081.

Laparoscopic Port Placement for TLH

3

Vandana Jain and Nutan Jain

Greatness doesn't demand perfection from the start,

but it does require you to start in order to achieve it.

3.1 Introduction

Laparoscopy, traditionally perceived as a surgical approach with a steep learning curve, finds its key to expediting mastery in the meticulous art of "Port Placement." The pathway to a swifter learning curve lies in correct port placements, a crucial step that holds the potential to mitigate numerous complications associated with laparoscopic procedures.

Unforeseen bowel injury or major vessel injury, although rare, are potential life-threatening complications that may arise during entry [1, 2]. The incidence of major complications following a laparoscopic procedure is estimated to be approximately 1.4 per 1000 procedures [3]. The incidence of port site complications following laparoscopic surgery is estimated to be around 21 per 100,000 cases [4]. This rate has demonstrated a proportional increase with the enlargement of the port site incision and trocar size [5, 6].

The intricacy of successful port placement depends on patient-specific variables such as BMI, abdominal fat distribution, the size of the pathology, and the patient's surgical history. This chapter deals with the details of port placement techniques tailored for diverse scenarios, encompassing the normal patient, the obese patient, individuals with a history of prior surgeries, and those presenting with sizable masses.

3.1.1 Body Mass Index (BMI)

Body Mass Index (BMI) serves as a numerical representation derived from an individual's weight and height. This calculated value is obtained by dividing the body mass by the square of the body height, expressed in units of kg/m^2. The formula combines the mass measured in kilograms (kg) with height in meters (m).

3.1.2 Classification of BMI

The classification of BMI offers a spectrum of health indicators, categorizing individuals into distinct ranges:

- Underweight: BMI under 18.5 kg/m^2
- Normal Weight: BMI ranging from 18.5 to 24.9 kg/m^2
- Overweight: BMI between 25 and 29.9 kg/m^2
- Obese: BMI of 30 or more kg/m^2

This classification not only provides a quantitative assessment of an individual's body composition but also serves as a valuable tool in gauging potential health risks associated with weight status.

V. Jain (✉)
Obstetrics and Gynaecology, Kasturba Hospital, Affiliated by Delhi University, Delhi, India

Department of Obstetrics and Gynecology, Vardhman Trauma and Laparoscopy Centre Pvt. Ltd, Muzaffarnagar, Uttar Pradesh, India

N. Jain
Department of Obstetrics and Gynecology, Vardhman Trauma and Laparoscopy Centre Pvt. Ltd, Muzaffarnagar, Uttar Pradesh, India

Obstetrics and Gynaecology, GSVM Medical College, Affiliated by Kanpur University, Kanpur, Uttar Pradesh, India

N. Jain (ed.), *Complex Total Laparoscopic Hysterectomy (TLH) with Newer Approaches in Bladder Dissection*,
https://doi.org/10.1007/978-981-97-3226-5_3

3.2 Entry Points (Fig. 3.1)

3.2.1 Umbilicus

Umbilical access is commonly utilized across various surgical specialties, yet it can pose challenges in patients with a history of prior surgeries resulting in periumbilical adhesions, in patients with periumbilical mesh placement, umbilical or ventral hernias, large pelvic masses, and during pregnancy. A systematic review indicates that the estimated risks for umbilical and/or anterior abdominal wall adhesions range from 0% to 5% for women without prior surgery, 20–30% for those with a previous transverse suprapubic laparotomy, and 50–65% for those with a previous midline laparotomy [7]. In such cases, non-umbilical access may be preferable [8]. We have proposed a non-umbilical entry port, the Jain point, which is feasible in patients with multiple previous surgeries, prior ventral hernia mesh repair, large pelvic masses, and during pregnancy.

3.2.2 Palmers Point

Minimally invasive surgery is an evolving field that demands surgeons to have ambidextrous skills and acquire new sets of motor skills, with a long and safe learning curve [9, 10]. The initial step in laparoscopy, the insertion of a primary port, is considered the most critical and potentially hazardous, as a significant portion of complications associated with laparoscopy arise even before the commencement of the intended procedure [3, 11, 12]. There is no single method proven to be the safest approach to access peritoneal cavity for all patients. Thus, a surgeon should be well versed with all kinds of entry. One of them is Palmer's point described by a French gynecologist, Raoul Palmer in 1974 in a paper titled "Safety in Laparoscopy" [13].

Raoul Palmer, well known in the field of laparoscopic surgery, in 1944, examined the pelvis of patients laparoscopically by positioning patients in the Trendelenburg position, facilitating the introduction of air into the pelvic cavity [14]. In 1947, Raoul advocated creation of pneumoperitoneum using a Veress needle as a crucial initial step for blind entry into the abdominal cavity [15]

Then in 1974, he introduced an alternative primary port located in the left upper quadrant for peritoneal entry, known as Palmer's point [13]. Thus Palmer changed laparoscopy from an occasionally performed technique to an absolutely indispensable method for acquiring invaluable diagnostic and therapeutic outcomes.

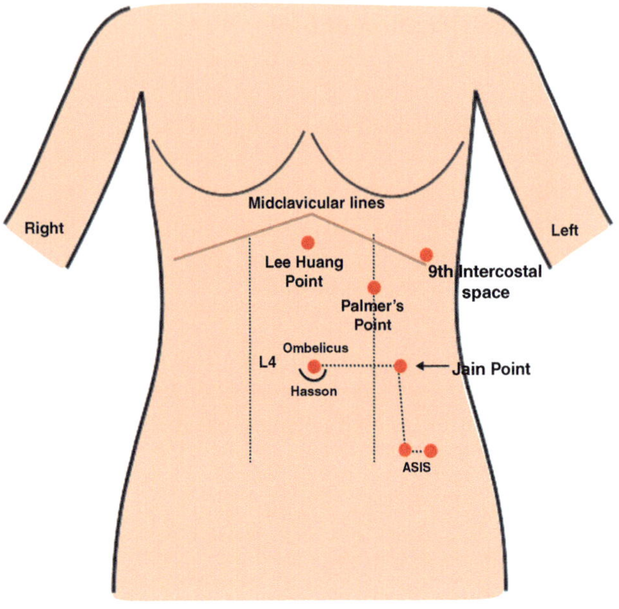

Fig. 3.1 Entry points

3.2.3 Technique

Patient is first placed in supine position and surgeon preferably stands on the left side of the patient with hand on left upper quadrant making skin taut between two fingers. Stab incision is given commonly using no. 11 blade. Veress needle inserted two fingers below the costal margin (3 cm) in mid clavicular line in 15° cephalad direction [6]. Pneumoperitoneum created and after insufflation, veress needle is removed and a 5-mm trocar is inserted into the peritoneal cavity using the same point. The laparoscope is then advanced, and intraabdominal placement is confirmed. Anterior abdominal wall adhesions are visualized and remaining ports placed according to convenience.

3.2.4 Hasson Technique

Since laparoscopy is relatively new, despite everything it excites discussion, especially as to the best method for making the pneumoperitoneum. The initial step in laparoscopic surgery is to build up a pneumoperitoneum, which is the most dangerous step [16–19] and most of the complications occur at this step, at times even becoming lethal at the rate of 0.05–0.2%. There are various diverse methods accessible to the specialist for it. However, clearly laparoscopic surgeries are not risk free. Access in the abdominal cavity is related with injuries to the gastrointestinal tract and significant vessels and 50% of these significant complications happen before initiation of the proposed actual surgical procedure. Champault et al. demonstrated that 83% of vascular injuries, 75% of bowel injuries, and 50% of local haemorrhagic injuries occurred during primary trocar insertion [20]. The incidence of these injuries may be elevated in patients with previous abdominal surgeries and suspected adhesions. Although there is no accord in regards to the best strategy for accessing the peritoneal cavity to make pneumoperitoneum, veress needle insertion is the most frequently used method by gynaecologists around the world. The dangers of visceral or vascular injury can be diminished by visualising the peritoneal cavity before any instrument is introduced. This technique is known as open laparoscopy. Open laparoscopy was first described by Dr. Harrith Hasson of Chicago, IL, who published this technique in the *American Journal of Obstetrics and Gynecology* in 1971 [20]. Thereafter, this procedure of open laparoscopy has turned out to be greatly acknowledged and is continually being modified to improve its performance. Open laparoscopy ports vary from standard closed ports. Most distinct is their absence of bladed or sharp trocars. Trocar used in open laparoscopy is blunt and consist of framework where abdominal fascia can be attached to the port by stay sutures, thus balancing and stabilizing the port to the patient. Hasson open laparoscopy port serves as an outstanding example of this framework [21].

3.2.5 Technique [22, 23]

For carrying out open laparoscopy, different techniques are available. Sharp dissection of abdominal wall layers is a common requirement for entry into the peritoneal cavity. The skin, deep fascia and parietal peritoneum of the anterior abdominal wall are in close proximity in the centre of the umbilicus. Hence, it is the preferred site for skin incision of Hasson technique. Most common technique is as follows –

- Both the surgeon and the assistant grasps the umbilical fold on each side by Allis forceps and stretch it anteriorly.
- Make a vertical incision in the centre of the umbilicus from the base of the umbilicus using scalpel.
- Skin on either side is retracted using two Langenbeck retractors to view the underlying subcutaneous fat which is then cut to expose the rectus sheath.
- The surgeon holds this rectus sheath on one side using Kocher's clamp. The same to be done on other side by the assistant. Now the rectus sheath is elevated anteriorly by pulling these two Kocher's clamp on each side and a vertical incision is given using scalpel. This incision excises the fascia and peritoneum and exposes the intra peritoneal cavity.
- If entry into the peritoneal cavity was not achieved previously, it can be elevated using any blunt artery forceps and then opened sharply.
- Confirm entrance into the intraperitoneal cavity using Metzenbaum scissors or any other thin blunt-tipped instrument.
- Stay sutures are given on either side of the fascia before placement of the trocar.
- At last, a blunt trocar (Hasson blunt tip trocar) is introduced through this incision and pneumoperitoneum created. Now introduce the camera to confirm the location and create other accessory ports.
- In case stay suture cannot be placed on fascia then it can be given on skin.
- In case of gas leakage purse string type of suture can be placed.
- In the presence of a bowel injury, extending the incision may be necessary. Subsequently, the damaged portion of the small bowel can be carefully exteriorized through the incision, repaired, and subsequently returned into the abdominal cavity.

3.2.6 Pitfalls of Hasson Technique

It may be very difficult in obese patients where the depth of subcutaneous fat is in few inches, so reaching the rectus sheath may also be difficult.

It can give rise to post-operative hernia from the site due to increase anterior abdominal pressure and inability to expose and suture closes the rectus sheath.

It cannot avoid type II bowel adhesions, characterized by the bowel forming adhesions that are inseparable from the abdominal wall.

3.2.7 Lee Huang Point

In 1993, Dr Chyi-Long Lee, a Gynae-endoscopic surgeon, and Dr Kuan-Gen Huang, a Gynae-oncologist, teamed up to upgrade the use of endoscopic surgery for treatment of gynecologic malignancies in Taiwan. Their main aim was to device a laparoscopic technique for para-aortic lymphadenectomy in advanced cervical cancer. Together they described the Lee–Huang point, which is the site of primary trocar insertion in the upper abdomen (in the midline), midway between the xiphoid process and the umbilicus [24]. Since then, the Lee–Huang point has been extensively used in various gynecological endoscopy procedures.

3.2.8 Jain Point

Jain Point, an anatomical reference point in laparoscopic entry, is easily identifiable amidst the surgical field, owing to

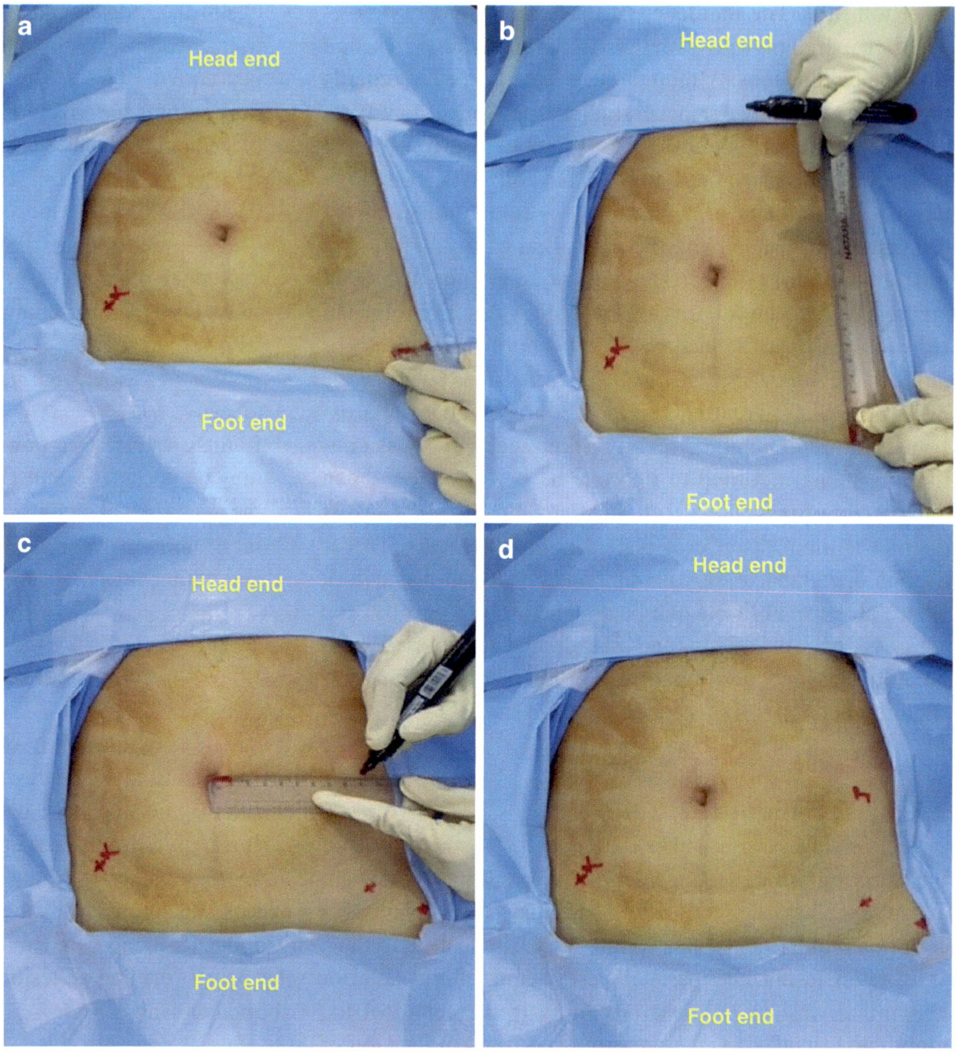

Fig. 3.2 **a–d** Surface marking of Jain point

its association with the prominent bony landmark—the anterior superior iliac spine (ASIS). The surface marking of Jain Point involves a meticulous process (Fig. 3.2a–d): To mark the Jain Point on the surface, start by identifying the ASIS (anterior superior iliac spine). Then, draw a vertical line 2.5 cm medial to the ASIS, extending upwards to the level of the umbilicus. Next, draw a horizontal line at the upper margin of the umbilicus. The intersection of these two lines precisely locates the Jain Point.

This entry point, situated at the level of the fourth lumbar vertebrae, is positioned approximately 10–13 cm lateral to the umbilicus. The specific location can vary based on the patient's BMI and body type, adding a nuanced dimension to the precision of port placement. Understanding and skill fully utilizing the Jain Point in laparoscopic procedures significantly contributes to the overall success and efficiency of the surgery.

3.2.9 But Why Jain Point?

The majority of complications in laparoscopy occur during primary access, particularly when the trocar penetrates the abdominal wall [25]. The incidence rates are 0.4 per 1000 cases for gastrointestinal injury and 0.2 per 1000 cases for major vascular injury [26]. Therefore, there is a need for a para-umbilical port.

In his recent article titled "Overview of Gynecological Laparoscopic Surgery and Non-umbilical Entry Site" published in UpToDate, Sharp [8] strongly advocates for non-umbilical entry in cases involving previous surgeries, large pelvic masses, extremes of body mass index (BMI), pregnancy, very lax abdomen, and umbilical hernia..

The Jain point offers an additional para-umbilical option for a safe entry port in laparoscopic surgeries, particularly in cases of previous surgeries, where Palmer's point may be contraindicated. Surgeons across various specialties, such as general surgery, urology, oncology, and bariatric surgery, can utilize the Jain point routinely. Additionally, the Jain point serves as the main ergonomic working port, while the Palmer's point port becomes redundant after the initial entry.

Cases with a history of previous surgeries often result in adhesions, which can pose challenges during laparoscopy. Typically, the first blind entry is made through the umbilicus, which is the most common site for surgical adhesions [27]. The incidence of intra-abdominal adhesions following laparotomy ranges from 30% to 90% [28]. Adhesions necessitate careful entry, particularly during Veress needle insertion and placement of the first port. The presence of adhesions and their associated complications has presented challenges for both the medical and legal communities in recent years [29].

The Jain point, situated away from visceral structures, minimizes complications related to previous surgeries, particularly in patients with suspected high adhesion scores (Type IIA adhesions) [30]. In contrast, Palmer's point is contraindicated in these cases due to potential omental and bowel adhesions affecting the upper abdomen. The versatility of the Jain point extends to patients across all BMI ranges, including those with low BMI [31] who have undergone previous surgery, whereas Palmer's point may pose limitations in low BMI patients due to its proximity to the left kidney [32]

3.3 Port Placement in Thin Patient (BMI 18.5) (Fig. 3.3)

Sharp stressed the importance of opting for non-umbilical entry in low-BMI patients [8]. This is because umbilical entry can expose thin patients to the anatomical vulnerability of structures such as the abdominal aorta, inferior vena cava, iliac vessels, or visceral vessels [33–36].

Using the Jain point entry method to create pneumoperitoneum, patients are advised to follow a low residue diet for 48 h prior to surgery. The stomach is emptied of secretions and air using an orogastric tube by an anesthetist after endotracheal intubation. The operating table is positioned horizontally. A small 1–2 mm incision is made just enough for the Veress needle's entry. Before insertion, there is no need to lift the abdominal wall as the point is away from major retroperitoneal vessels. Unlike umbilical entry, there is no need to change the direction of the Veress needle to 45°; it is simply inserted perpendicular to the abdominal wall in a vertical direction, regardless of the patient's BMI. The index finger is used as a guard on the Veress needle to prevent overshooting, adjusted according to the patient's abdominal wall thickness (Fig. 3.4a–c). As the needle passes through the abdomen, two distinct pops are heard: the first as it passes through the external oblique aponeurosis, and the second as it pierces the fused aponeurosis of the internal oblique and transverse abdominis muscles, followed by loss of resistance as the needle enters the peritoneal cavity. A saline drop test is performed, and the very initial intra-abdominal pressure (VIIP) is checked before starting insufflation [37]. Once adequate pneumoperitoneum is achieved, a 5 mm port is inserted (Fig. 3.5a, b). Further ports, including a 10 mm port if necessary, are inserted as required under the vision provided by the 5 mm port (Fig. 3.6a–e). The Jain point port becomes the main working port, with additional ipsilateral ports on the left side.

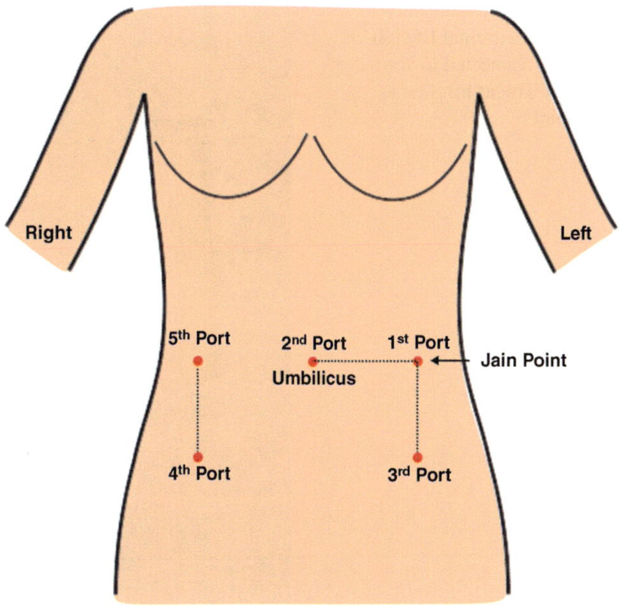

Fig. 3.3 Port placement of Jain Point in thin patient

The ideal distance between the upper and lower ports on the left side is approximately 10–12 cm (Fig. 3.7). This spacing ensures good logistics and efficacy [38], as demonstrated in animal models. Optimal efficacy is achieved with an ideal working angle between 45° and 60°, along with correct placement of ports. Similar efficacy is observed with the Jain point entry technique. This method ensures fatigue-free working during lengthy surgeries involving prolonged suturing in multiple myomas or cases with extensive adhesiolysis due to multiple surgeries. Mohapatra and Bhusan [39] have also reported the benefits of using the left lateral port as the main working port and entry port, offering dual benefits with good ergonomics (Fig 3.8a, b). Secondary ports are positioned accordingly (Fig. 3.9a–g). H.T Sharp [8] has recognized it as a suitable working port throughout the surgery, and other researchers have also acknowledged its ergonomic advantages as a working port.

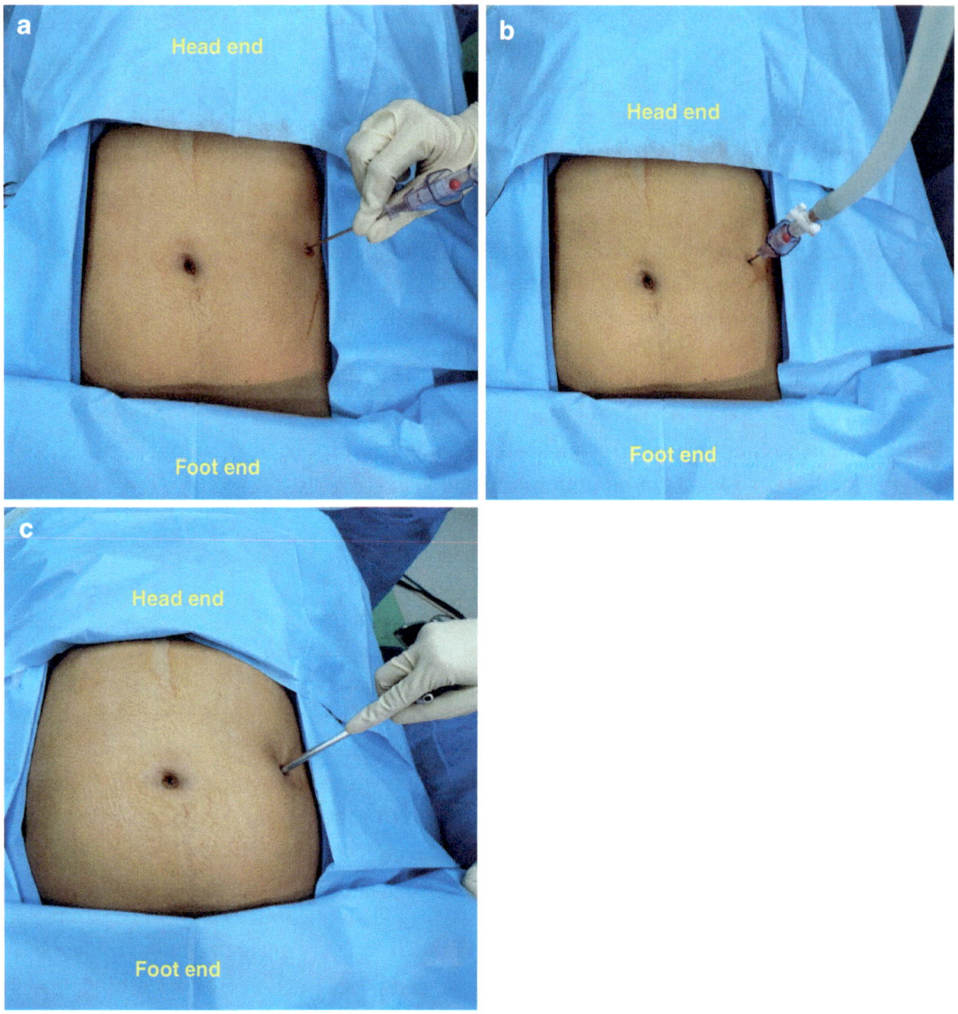

Fig. 3.4 **a** Veress needle at Jain point in normal BMI. **b** CO_2 pipe connected to veress needle. **c** Trocar inserted at Jain point

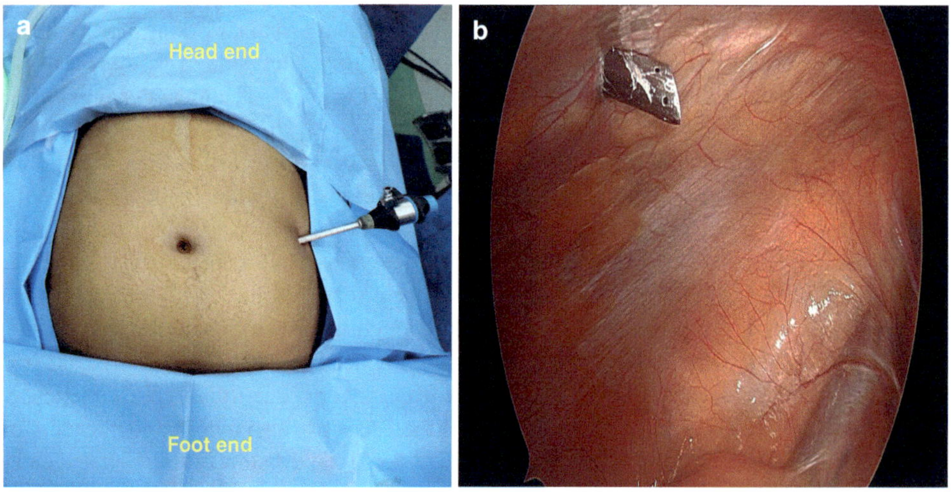

Fig. 3.5 **a**, **b** 5 mm trocar inserted at Jain point

There is no need to change the angulation of the Veress with the changing BMI or lift the abdominal wall [40, 41]. According to literature on Major Vessel Injuries (MVIs), thin patients are at a higher risk of aortic injury. This is because the variable relationship between the umbilicus and the aortic bifurcation presents technical challenges during blind entry through the umbilicus. With increasing BMI the umbilicus moves caudally in relation to the aortic bifurcation and is more

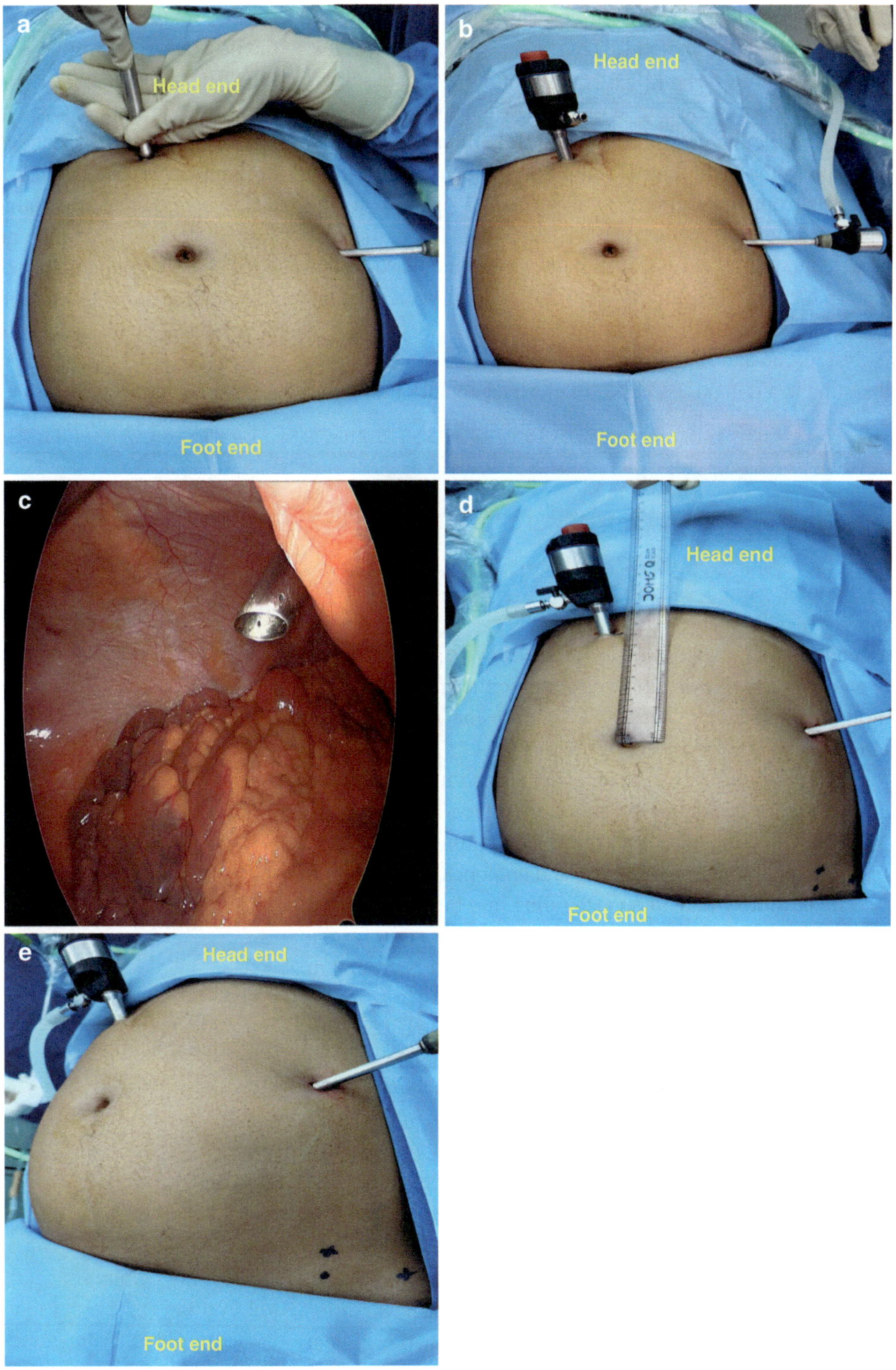

Fig. 3.6 **a** 10 mm trocar inserted. **b**, **c** 10 mm trocar inserted. **d** Under the vision of 5 mm port, supraumbilical 10 mm camera port inserted, very high up for large masses and pregnant uterus. **e** Marking ASIS

likely to lie directly above the aorta [42]. Even the aortic bifurcation can lie as low as the L5–S1 level [43]. For an average-built patient, the distance from the skin to the retroperitoneal vessels is typically 6 cm. However, a study has shown that during general anesthesia, with muscular relaxation, this distance can decrease to 2 cm [33, 35, 44]. Aortic injuries have been reported during Veress needle entry [45] or during primary trocar insertion. The primary concern is that retroperitoneal hematoma might go unnoticed since there is no free blood in the cavity. The delay in diagnosis or the dilemma of determining whether sudden hypotension is caused by CO_2 embolism or MVI [46, 47] can escalate morbidity or mortality rates.

Major vessel and visceral injury is more prevalent in thin or obese patients as noted by Hurd et al. [42] A prospective study by Narendran and Baggish [48] on 101 women undergoing laparoscopy measured distances from the entry trocar and perpendicular distance to the aortic bifurcation, oblique distance to the right and left common iliac vessels, oblique distance from the sub-umbilical peritoneal opening to the right and left common iliac vessels, etc. Their findings revealed a notable discrepancy in the perpendicular distance from the entry trocar to the aortic bifurcation, which varied with changes in BMI.

Narendran and Baggish [48] stated that laparoscopic trocar thrusting is a dynamic process. Even when counter traction is applied by lifting the abdomen, this force further diminishes the distance between the entry point and retroperitoneal vessels. This phenomenon is more noticeable in obese patients. However, thin patients typically have a relatively rigid anterior abdominal wall due to good muscle tone. Consequently, it becomes more challenging to lift their abdomen, potentially necessitating greater thrusting force and rendering them more vulnerable to injury to the major vessels. Jain point serves as good entry point in thin patients. The primary advantage of the Jain point lies in its anatomical positioning, as it prevents any direct contact with major retroperitoneal vessels. Positioned a minimum of 10 cm lateral to the bifurcation of the aorta, it effectively reduces the risk of inadvertent injury to these critical structures. Given that the entry into the peritoneal cavity is a crucial aspect of laparoscopy, it demands careful attention, particularly for upcoming surgeons.

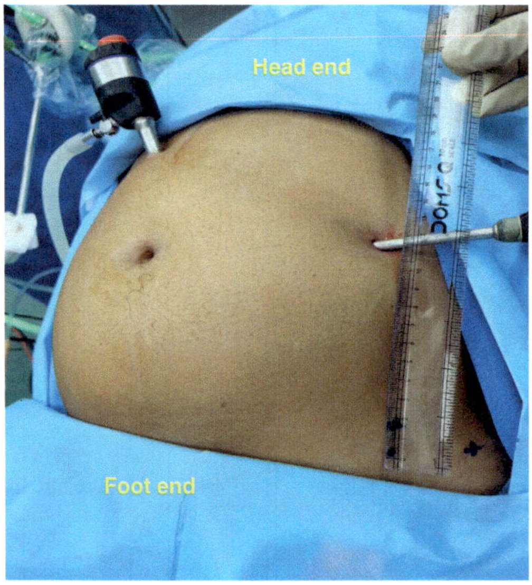

Fig. 3.7 Distance between the two ipsilateral ports is 10–12 cm for good ergonomic working

3.3.1 Points to Remember in Thin Patients

1. **Increased Risk of Injury to Vessels:**
   - Due to the heightened risk of injury to vessels, it's crucial to maintain awareness of the distance between the anterior abdominal wall, vessels, and viscera underneath.
2. **Constant Monitoring of Veress Needle Length:**
   - Vigilantly monitor the length of the Veress needle throughout the procedure, consistently using index finger to guard against unintentional advancement.
3. **Maintain a Vertical Angle to the Peritoneum:**
   - Keep the angle of the Veress needle vertical until reaching the peritoneum. Do not advance the needle any further beyond this point to minimize the risk of complications.

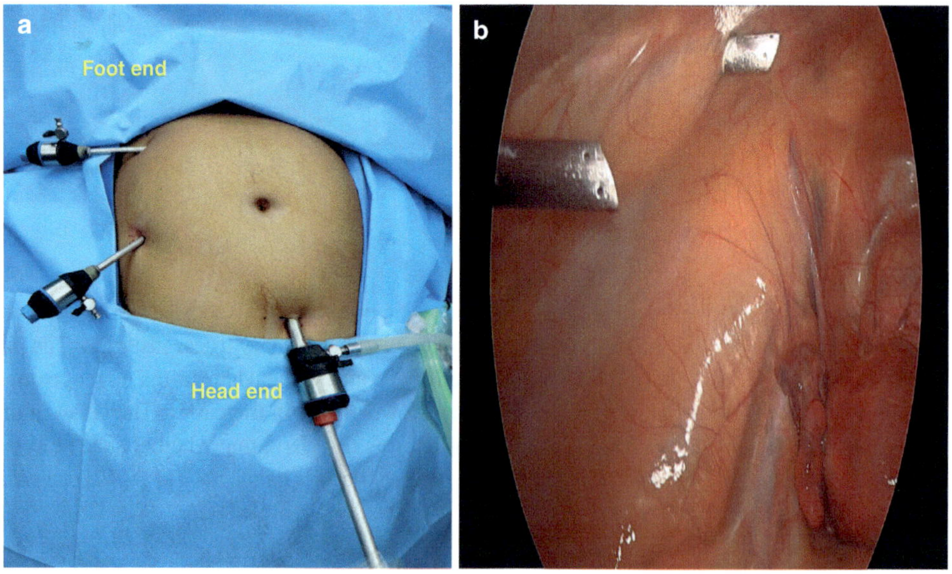

Fig. 3.8 **a**, b Ipsilateral working ports

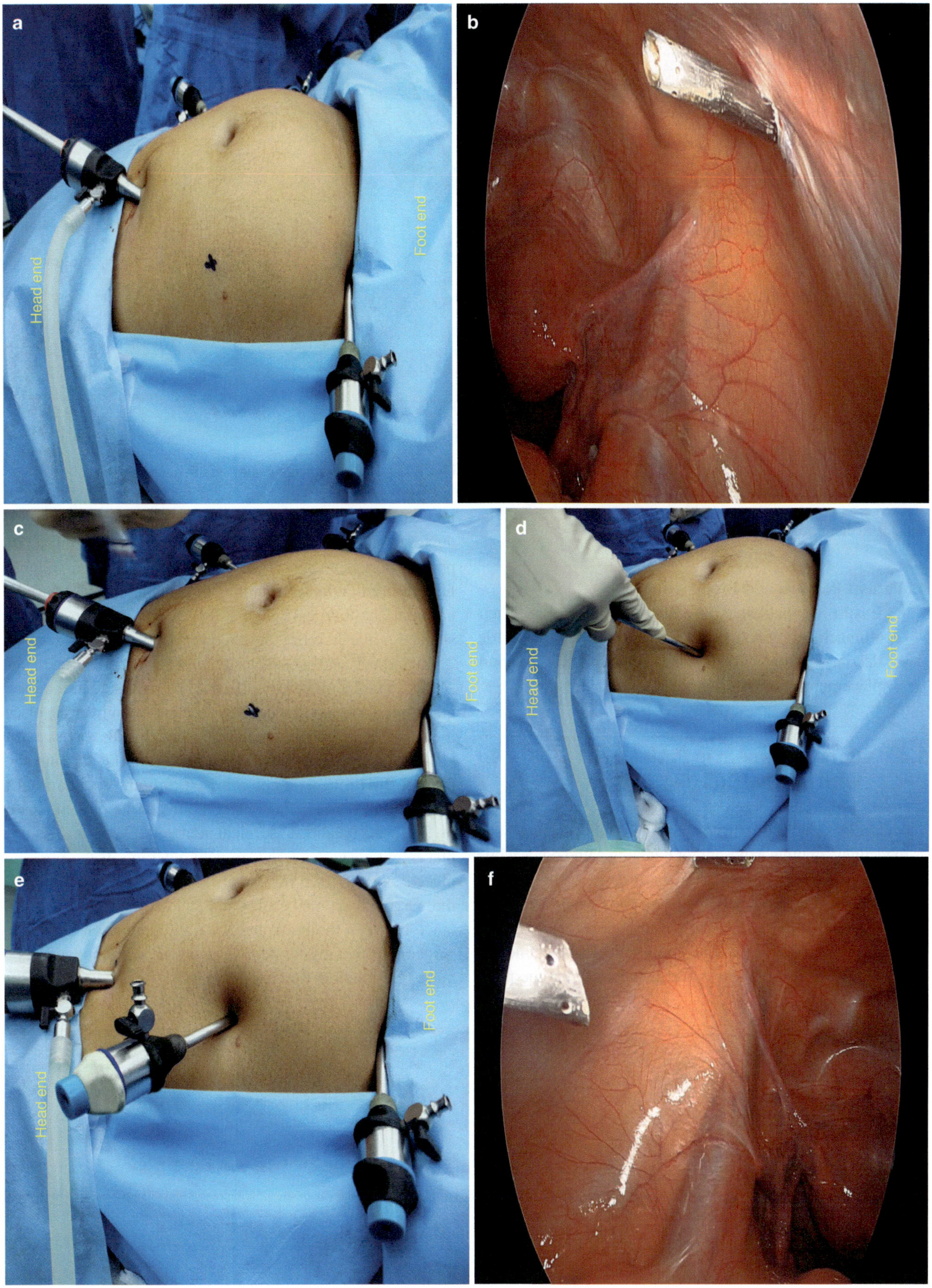

Fig. 3.9 **a**, **b** Trocar inserted on right lower port. **c** Marking right upper port. **d** Trocar inserted on right upper port. **e**, **f** 2 Port on right side. **g** Final port placement

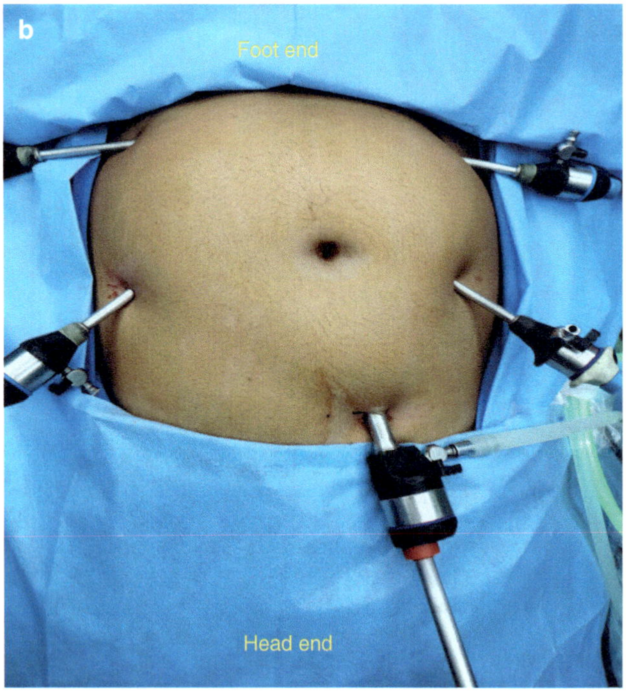

Fig. 3.9 (continued)

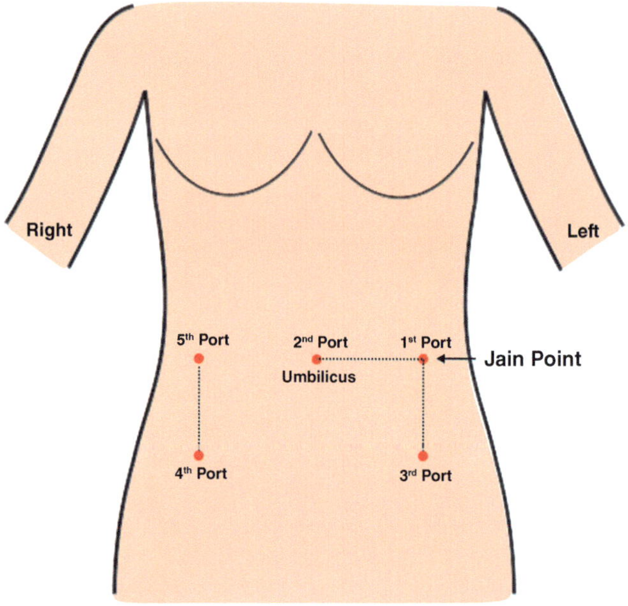

Fig. 3.10 Port placement of Jain point in normal BMI patient

4. **Patient Position and Preparation:**
   - Ensure the patient is in a supine position, and their stomach is empty, using a Ryles tube (RT) for gastric decompression by the anaesthetist before the port placement.

3.4 Port Placement in Patient with Normal BMI (Fig. 3.10)

Port placement in patients with a normal BMI is planned such as to facilitate optimal exposure for handling pathologies while prioritizing minimal cosmetic impact, especially in younger patients. The strategic arrangement of ports ensures discreet incisions, contributing to a visually pleasing outcome.

Initiating the procedure with the insertion of a Veress needle at the Jain Point, the first blind port is introduced at the para-umbilical level. Subsequent examination of the pelvis is conducted to confirm findings. The second port, serving as the primary port, is strategically positioned either through the umbilicus or infra-umbilically, aiming to maintain invisibility of the incision. The third port, with a diameter of 5 mm, is carefully situated at the Jain line in the lower quadrant, approximately 2.5 cm above and medial to the anterior superior iliac spine (ASIS). The fourth port is placed in the right side in the lower quadrant. If a fifth port is deemed necessary, it mirrors the placement of the Jain port but on the right side (Fig. 3.11a–g).

This nuanced approach to port placement in patients with normal BMI reflects a commitment to both procedural efficiency and the aesthetic considerations of the patient, ensuring a well-balanced surgical outcome. A correct port placement ensures a good surgical outcome. If the ports are placed as described we usually do not face complications, the surgery becomes easier and saves time. A correct distance between the ports and the right angulation also saves surgeon from fatigue. Also a standard technique makes it more reproducible for the beginners.

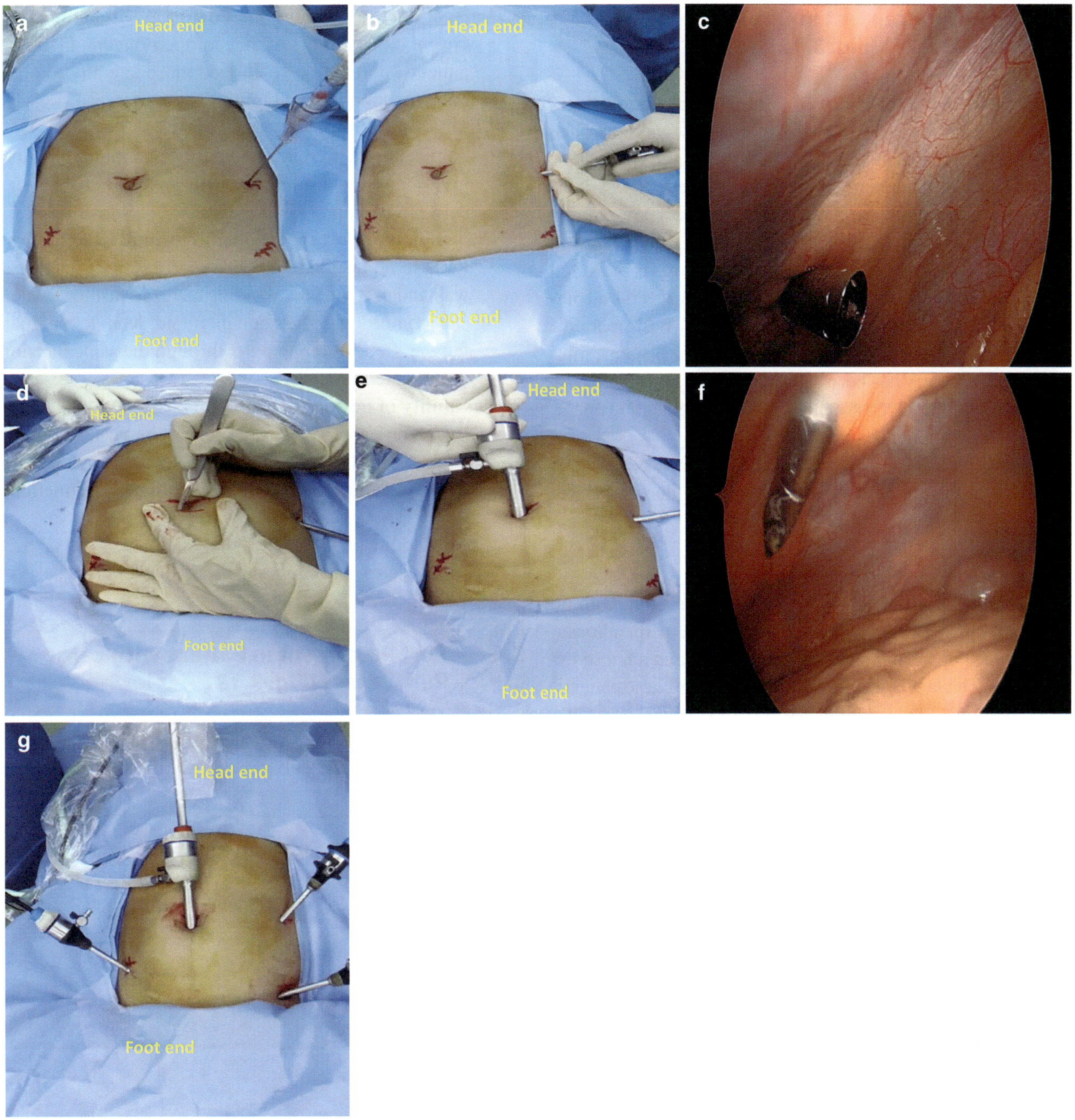

Fig. 3.11 **a** Veress needle insertion at Jain point. **b**, **c** Trocar insertion at Jain point. **d** Incision at umbilicus for telescope port. **e**, **f** 10 mm telescope at umbilicus. **g** Final port placement

3.5 Port Placement in Obese Patient (BMI > 24) (Fig. 3.12)

Obesity was traditionally viewed as a contraindication to laparoscopy due to the increased risk of associated conditions such as diabetes, hypertension, coronary artery disease, and venous thromboembolism. Laparoscopy can be done in obese/morbidly obese patients with due caution. Laparoscopy induces some physiological changes which may be exaggerated in obese which need to be understood. Laparoscopy is preferred over laparotomy in obese patients as it offers several advantages, including a shorter hospital stay, less post-operative pain, and fewer wound infections. Beyond these benefits, minimal access surgery has been shown to be safe and effective in obese patients; however, specific surgical strategies and operative techniques may need to be adopted [49]

Port placement in obese patients demands a well-planned approach to ensure both safety and efficacy during laparoscopic procedures:

1. **Veress Needle Insertion at Jain Point:**
   - The Veress needle is inserted at the Jain Point with no alteration in angle. Holding the needle perpendicular, three pops may be audible due to increased adipose tissue. The Jain Point, known for its safety in obese patients, minimizes the risk of injury to retroperitoneal vessels.
2. **Uniformity of Technique for Shorter Learning Curve:**
   - Maintaining a uniform technique not only contributes to procedural smoothness but also expedites the learning curve, enhancing overall proficiency.
3. **Tailored Port Placement Based on Patient Characteristics:**
   - Port placement considerations in obese patients hinge on factors such as height, abdominal fat distribution, and umbilicus position.
4. **Lateral Port Positioning for Pneumoperitoneum:**
   - Given the build-up of pneumoperitoneum in obese patients, ports to be positioned more laterally to optimize functionality and minimize interference.
5. **Minimum Distance Between Ports:**
   - To prevent interference and ensure seamless functioning, maintain a minimum distance of 10–12 cm between two ports on the same side (ipsilateral).
6. **Perpendicular Port Insertion for Optimal Ergonomics:**
   - Ports to be inserted perpendicularly to the abdominal wall and peritoneum, avoiding a zigzag fashion, which can compromise functionality and lead to surgeon fatigue. Repositioning ports through the same incision is warranted if needed.
7. **Possibility of an Additional Port:**
   - In certain cases, an extra port may be necessary, particularly on the right side at the mirror image of Jain Point, to handle excess fat and facilitate its retraction.

A correct working port placement not only makes the surgery shorter easier safer it also saves the surgeon from fatigue.

3.6 Port Placement in Patient with Large Pelvic Mass (Fig. 3.13)

Addressing contra indication for laparoscopic procedures in the presence of a large pelvic mass involves strategic port placement:

1. **High Jain Point for Veress Insertion:**
   - Optimal Veress needle insertion is done at a high Jain point, a variable location depending on the size of the

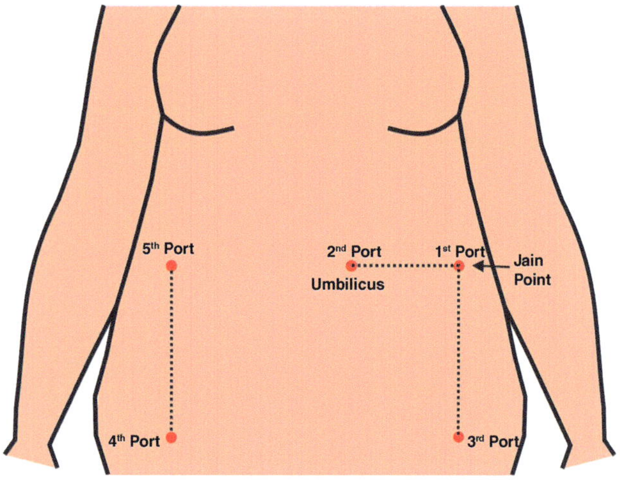

Fig. 3.12 Port placement of Jain point in obese BMI patient

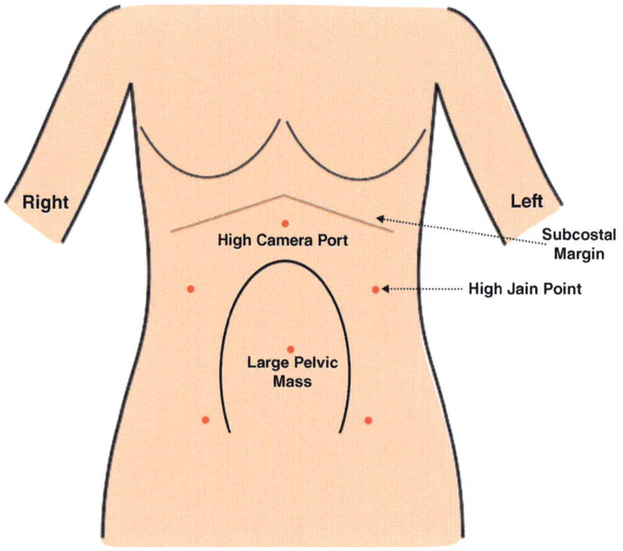

Fig. 3.13 Port placement in large pelvic mass

pathology. This can extend as high as one finger below the subcostal margin. The primary objective is to prevent inadvertent entry into the large mass or cyst.

2. **First Port (5 mm) at High Jain Point:**
   - Initiate port placement with a 5 mm port at the high Jain point. (High Jain point can go as high as one finger below the subcostal margin) [50]
3. **Second Port (10 mm) Placement:**
   - Depending on the pathology, position the 10 mm optical port as high as necessary, potentially reaching up to the epigastrium. This port is inserted under direct vision, of the High Jain Point port.
4. **Third Port Placement:**
   - Insert the third port in the left lower quadrant, 2.5 cm medial to the anterior superior iliac spine (ASIS).
5. **Fourth Port Placement:**
   - Position the fourth port in the right lower quadrant, 2.5 cm medial to the ASIS.

We can introduce one more port above the umbilicus considering the unique requirements posed by the large pelvic mass.

This strategic approach to port placement not only ensures a safe distance from the pelvic mass but also enables efficient visualization and manipulation of structures during the laparoscopic procedure.

3.6.1 Other Maneuver during Port Placement

- **Assistant- Manual Displacement with Hands:**
  - Hands can be utilized to gently displace the mass contralateral during the laparoscopic port placement, facilitating better visualization and access to targeted areas.
  - Place the ports Above & outside the mass

3.6.2 Patients with Hernia

- **Strategic Placement Above and Outside:**
  - When dealing with a hernia, it's crucial to strategically position ports above and outside the mesh to minimize interference with adhesions and optimize access.
- **Consideration of FIP (Fascial Introduction Point):**
  - When encountering a scarred abdomen or hernia, identifying an appropriate fascial Introduction Point (FIP) becomes essential. This strategic entry point helps navigate through scar tissue more effectively.
- **Challenges with Scarred Abdomen and Rising Surgery Rates:**
  - The prevalence of scarred abdomens and increasing surgery rates contribute to the challenges in laparoscopic procedures, emphasizing the need for meticulous planning and precise port placement.
- **Complications Related to Adhesions and Blind First Port:**
  - Complications often arise from adhesions in scarred abdomens, particularly when the first port placement is blind. Careful consideration of the anatomy and potential adhesions is crucial to minimize risks.

Learning Points
- Tailor port locations based on patient characteristics for efficient and safe procedures.
- Port placement depends on BMI/previous surgery/size of pathology
- In thin patients keep the distance of major vessels in mind, guard the needle with finger
- In obese patients keep the fat distribution in mind and avoid zig zag port insertion
- Large pelvic mass, primary entry port and rest of ports move vertically higher up depending on size of pathology
- In incisional hernia or previous mesh repair keep the first blind trocar outside the mesh
- In previous surgery cases Palmer's point or Jain Point can be used
- Jain point entry technique is simple and reproducible

Competing Interest The author declares no conflict of interest that are relevant to content of this chapter.

Ethical Approval Informed consent was obtained from individual participants and patients regarding publication and documentation without disclosing their identity.

References

1. Ahmad G, Duffy JM, Phillips K, Watson A. Laparoscopic entry techniques. Cochrane Database Syst Rev. 2008;2:CD006583.
2. Jansen FW, Kolkman W, Bakkum EA, de Kroon CD, Trimbos-Kemper TC, Trimbos JB. Complications of laparoscopy: an inquiry about closed- versus open-entry technique. Am J Obstet Gynecol. 2004;190:634–8.
3. Jansen FW, Kapiteyn K, Trimbos-Kemper T, Hermans J, Trimbos JB. Complications of laparoscopy a prospective multicentre observational study. Br J Obstet Gynaecol. 1997;104:595–600.
4. Aziz R. Practical manual of operative laparoscopy. New York: Springer-Verlag; 1992. p. 1–8.
5. Kadar N, Reich H, Liu CY, Manko GF, Gimpelson R. Incisional hernias after major laparoscopic gynecologic procedures. Am J Obstet Gynecol. 1993;168:1493.
6. Chiu CC, Lee WJ, Wang W, Wei PL, Huang MT. Prevention of trocar-wound hernia in laparoscopic bariatric operations. Obes Surg. 2006;16:913–8.
7. Varma R, Gupta JK. Laparoscopic entry techniques: clinical guideline, national survey, and medicolegal ramifications. Surg Endosc.

2008;22(12):2686–97. https://doi.org/10.1007/s00464-008-9871-6. Epub 2008 Apr 10. PMID: 18401653.
8. Sharp HT. Overview of gynecologic laparoscopic surgery and non-umbilical entry sites. In: T Falcone, editor. Wolters Kluwers; 2019. p. 10. UpToDate.
9. Deziel DJ. Avoiding laparoscopic complications. Int Surg. 1994;79:361–4.
10. Lekawa M, Shapiro S, Gordon LA, et al. The laparoscopic learning curve. Surg Laparosc Endosc. 1995;5:455–8.
11. Batemen BG, Kolp LA, Hoeger K. Complications of laparoscopy—operative or diagnostic. Fertil Steril. 1996;66:30–5.
12. Chandler JG, Corson SL, Way LW. Three spectra of laparoscopic entry access injuries. J Am Coll Surg. 2001;192:478–91.
13. Palmer R. Safety in laparoscopy. J Reprod Med. 1974;13(1):1–5.
14. Palmer R. Gynk. et Obstit.. 1949;48, 206.7.
15. Agarwala N, Liu CY. Safe entry techniques during laparoscopy: left upper quadrant entry using the ninth intercostal space–a review of 918 procedures. J Minim Invasive Gynecol. 2005;12(1):55–61.
16. Mac Cordick C, Lecuru F, Rizk E, et al. Morbidity in laparoscopic gynecological surgery: results of a prospective single-center study. Surg Endosc. 1999;13(1):57–61.
17. Yuzpe AA. Pneumoperitoneum needle and trocar injuries in laparoscopy. A survey on possible contributing factors and prevention. J Reprod Med. 1990;35(5):485–90.
18. Corson SL, Chandler JG, Way LW. Survey of laparoscopic entry injuries provoking litigation. J Am Assoc Gynecol Laparosc. 2001;8(3):341–7.
19. Chapron CM, Pierre F, Lacroix S, Querleu D, Lansac J, Dubuisson JB. Major vascular injuries during gynecologic laparoscopy. J Am Coll Surg. 1997;185(5):461–5.
20. Champault G, Cazacu F, Taffinder N. Serious trocar accidents in laparoscopic surgery: a French survey of 103,852 operations. Surg Laparosc Endosc. 1996;6(5):367–70.
21. Hasson HM. A modified instrument and method for laparoscopy. Am J Obstet Gynecol. 1971;110(6):886–7.
22. Hibner M, Desai N. Glob. Libr. Women's Med. 2008. ISSN: 1756–2228. https://doi.org/10.3843/GLOWM.10090.
23. Pickersgill A, Slade RJ, Falconer GF, Attwood S. Open laparoscopy: the way forward. Br J Obstet Gynaecol. 1999;106(11):1116–9.
24. Lai CH, Huang KG, Hong JH, et al. Randomized trial of surgical staging (extraperitoneal or laparoscopic) versus clinical staging in locally advanced cervical cancer. Gynecol Oncol. 2003;89:160–7.
25. Tinelli A, Malvasi A, Schneider AJ, Keckstein J, Hudelist G, Barbic M, et al. Primo accesso addominale in laparoscopia ginecologica: quale tecnica utilizzare? [First abdominal access in gynecological laparoscopy: which method to utilize?]. Minerva Ginecol. 2006;58(5):429–40. Italian.
26. Taskforce for Abdominal Entry. Principles of safe laparoscopic entry. Eur J Obstet Gynecol Reprod Biol. 2016;201:179–88. https://doi.org/10.1016/j.ejogrb.2016.03.040.
27. Jain N, Srivastava S, Bayya SLP, Jain V. Jain point laparoscopic entry in contraindications of Palmers point. Front Surg. 2022;9:928081. https://doi.org/10.3389/fsurg.2022.928081. PMID: 36439525; PMCID: PMC9696343.
28. Szomstein S, Lo Menzo E, Simpfendorfer C, Zundel N, Rosenthal RJ. Laparoscopic lysis of adhesions. World J Surg. 2006;30(4):535–40. https://doi.org/10.1007/s00268-005-7778-0.
29. Schreinemacher MH, ten Broek RP, Bakkum EA, van Goor H, Bouvy ND. Adhesion awareness: a national survey of surgeons. World J Surg. 2010;34(12):2805–12. https://doi.org/10.1007/s00268-010-0778-8.
30. Diamond MP. Reduction of de novo postsurgical adhesions by intraoperative precoating with sepracoat (HAL-C) solution: a prospective, randomized, blinded, placebo-controlled multicenter study. The Sepracoat Adhesion Study Group. Fertil Steril. 1998;69(6):1067–74. https://doi.org/10.1016/s0015-0282(98)00057-0.
31. Jain N, Sareen S, Kanawa S, Jain V, Gupta S, Mann S. Jain point: a new safe portal for laparoscopic entry in previous surgery cases. J Hum Reprod Sci. 2016;9(1):9–17. https://doi.org/10.4103/0974-1208.178637.
32. Giannios NM, Gulani V, Rohlck K, Flyckt RL, Weil SJ, Hurd WW. Left upper quadrant laparoscopic placement: effects of insertion angle and body mass index on distance to posterior peritoneum by magnetic resonance imaging. Am J Obstet Gynecol. 2009;201(5):522.e1–5. https://doi.org/10.1016/j.ajog.2009.07.017.
33. Roviaro GC, Varoli F, Saguatti L, Vergani C, Maciocco M, Scarduelli A. Major vascular injuries in laparoscopic surgery. Surg Endosc. 2002;16(8):1192–6. https://doi.org/10.1007/s00464-001-8238-.
34. Apelgren KN, Scheres DE. Aortic injury: a catastrophic complication of laparoscopic cholecystectomy. Surg Endosc. 1994;8:689–91.
35. Hanney RM, Carmalt HL, Merrett N, Tait N. Use of the Hasson cannula producing major vascular injury at laparoscopy. Surg Endosc. 1999;13(12):1238–40. https://doi.org/10.1007/pl00009630.
36. Krishnakumar S, Tambe P. Entry complications in laparoscopic surgery. J Gynecol Endosc Surg. 2009;1(1):4–11. https://doi.org/10.4103/0974-1216.51902.
37. Vilos GA. The ABCs of a safer laparoscopic entry. J Minim Invasive Gynecol. 2006;13:249–51.
38. Manasnayakorn S, Cuschieri A, Hanna GB. Ideal manipulation angle and instrument length in hand-assisted laparoscopic surgery. Surg Endosc. 2008;22(4):924–9. https://doi.org/10.1007/s00464-007-9520-5.
39. Mohapatra GSS, Bhusan B. Comparative study of different entry sites in laparoscopic surgery: which is safest? IOSR J Dent Med Sci. 2017;16:64–6. https://doi.org/10.9790/0853-1601086466.
40. Gupta J, Chu J. Safe laparoscopic entry in a thin patient. In: Coomarasamy A, Shafia M, Davila G, Chan K, editors. Gynecologic and obstetrics surgery: challenges and management options. New York: John Wiley and Sons, Ltd; 2016. Chapter 66. p. 199–203. https://doi.org/10.1002/9781118298565.ch66.
41. La Chapelle CF, Bemelman WA, Rademaker BM, van Barnveld TA, Jansen FW, On Behalf of the Dutch Multidisciplinary Guideline Development Group Minimally Invasive Surgery. A multidisciplinary evidence based guideline for minimally invasive surgery. Part 1. Entry techniques and the pneumoperitoneum. Gynecol Surg. 2012;9(3):271–82.
42. Hurd WW, Bude RO, DeLancey JO, Pearl ML. The relationship of the umbilicus to the aortic bifurcation: implications for laparoscopic technique. Obstet Gynecol. 1992;80(1):48–51.
43. Kurzel RB, Edinger DD Jr. Injury to the great vessels: a hazard of transabdominal endoscopy. South Med J. 1983;76(5):656–7. https://doi.org/10.1097/00007611-198305000-00032.
44. McDonald PT, Rich NM, Collins GJ Jr, Andersen CA, Kozloff L. Vascular trauma secondary to diagnostic and therapeutic procedures: laparoscopy. Am J Surg. 1978;135(5):651–5. https://doi.org/10.1016/0002-9610(78)90129-0.
45. Fruhwirth J, Koch G, Mischinger HJ, Werkgartner G, Tesch NP. Vascular complications in minimally invasive surgery. Surg Laparosc Endosc. 1997;7(3):251–4.
46. Seidman D, Nasserbakht F, Nezhat F, et al. Delayed recognition of iliac artery injury during laparoscopic surgery. Surg Endosc. 1996;10:1099–101. https://doi.org/10.1007/s004649900250.
47. Yanke BV, Horowitz M. Safety of the Veress needle in pediatric laparoscopy. J Endourol. 2007;21(7):695–7. https://doi.org/10.1089/end.2006.9950.

48. Narendran M, Baggish MS. Mean distance between primary trocar insertion site and major retroperitoneal vessels during routine laparoscopy. J Gynecol Surg. 2002;18(4):121–7. https://doi.org/10.1089/104240602762555920.
49. Afors K, Centini G, Murtada R, Castellano J, Meza C, Wattiez A. Obesity in laparoscopic surgery. Best Pract Res Clin Obstet Gynaecol. 2015;29(4):554–64. https://doi.org/10.1016/j.bpobgyn.2015.02.001. Epub 2015 Feb 17. PMID: 25770750.
50. Jain N, Jain V, Gupta S. 10225 High Jain point in large masses. J Minim Invasive Gynecol. 2023;30(6):343. https://doi.org/10.1016/j.jmig.2023.08.343.

Vault Closure

4

Vandana Jain and Nutan Jain

Unlocking potential requires many keys,
but persistence is the master key that opens the final door.

4.1 Introduction

Laparoscopy has become the chosen route of hysterectomy except for steps like removal of uterus and vault closure. Vault closure is a crucial step in TLH, which is a minimally invasive surgical procedure for removing the uterus. After the uterus is removed, the surgeon must close the vault, which is the upper part of the vagina where the uterus used to be. The closure is necessary to prevent complications such as infection and to provide support to the surrounding structures.

Reich et al. [1] first pioneered laparoscopic assisted vaginal hysterectomy (LAVH) in 1989 in patients who were ineligible for total vaginal hysterectomy, and successfully conducted total laparoscopic hysterectomy (TLH) in 1994. Reich the founder of LAVH and TLH proposed laparoscopic vault closure as a preventative measure against vault dehiscence during the 38th AAGL meeting in November 2009.

The creation of the vaginal cuff involves suturing the two edges of the vagina at the site where the colpotomy is performed. This is done by bringing the edges of the vagina together and including the uterosacral ligaments to provide support and prevent vault prolapse. To reduce vaginal cuff dehiscence, it is important to approximate the tissue meticulously. The closure needs to be tight but not strangulate the tissue, minimizing thermal energy usage during colpotomy and incorporation of healthy tissue in the suture line [2].

Here Are Some Key Points About Vault Closure in TLH

1. **Suturing Techniques**: Surgeons use various suturing techniques to close the vault laparoscopically. Common methods include the use of advanced energy devices for sealing and cutting tissues and then intracorporeal knot tying.
2. **Material Used:** Typically, absorbable sutures are used for vault closure. The choice of suture material depends on factors such as the patient's health, surgeon's preference, and the specific requirements of the procedure.
3. **Support and Strength:** Vault closure is not only about closing the incision but also providing sufficient support and strength to the vaginal cuff. This helps decreasing the risk of post operative complications such as dehiscence, vault prolapse and supports the healing process.
4. **Risk Management:** Surgeons carefully assess the condition of patient and consider any potential risk factors that might affect the success of vault closure. Proper closure is vital to reduce the risk of postoperative complications.

Supplementary Information The online version contains supplementary material available at https://doi.org/10.1007/978-981-97-3226-5_4. The videos can be accessed individually by clicking the DOI link in the accompanying figure caption or by scanning this link with the SN More Media App.

V. Jain (✉)
Obstetrics and Gynaecology, Kasturba Hospital, Affiliated by Delhi University, Delhi, India

Department of Obstetrics and Gynecology, Vardhman Trauma and Laparoscopy Centre Pvt. Ltd, Muzaffarnagar, Uttar Pradesh, India

N. Jain
Department of Obstetrics and Gynecology, Vardhman Trauma and Laparoscopy Centre Pvt. Ltd, Muzaffarnagar, Uttar Pradesh, India

Obstetrics and Gynaecology, GSVM Medical College, Affiliated by Kanpur University, Kanpur, Uttar Pradesh, India

N. Jain (ed.), *Complex Total Laparoscopic Hysterectomy (TLH) with Newer Approaches in Bladder Dissection*,
https://doi.org/10.1007/978-981-97-3226-5_4

5. **Postoperative Care:** Patients are typically given specific instructions for postoperative care, including restrictions on certain strenuous activities like sexual contact, to support proper healing of the vault.

Vault closure and its methods remain subject to debate due to the risk of post operative vault dehiscence. Vault prolapse is a known complication. The uterosacral ligaments at pericervical ring if not included during cuff closure predispose the patient to vault prolapse. Suture gets reabsorbed in nearly 3 months' time after which the type of cuff closure and sutures cannot be differentiated. The complications usually occur within 2 months of postoperative time. The use of delayed absorbable sutures is recommended. The risk factors that can compromise the vaginal cuff are sexual intercourse, chronic constipation, asthma, chronic obstructive pulmonary disease, and anything that can increase intra-abdominal pressure. Bleeding, hematoma and infection are the most common postoperative complications. Additionally, factors believed to influence wound healing include radiation therapy, age, pelvic organ prolapse, steroid use, immunocompromised conditions, and concurrent malignancy [3].

The role of suturing technique in postoperative vaginal cuff dehiscence [4] has been suggested, yet the ideal approach remains subject to debate. Various methods practiced by surgeons globally are described.

In minimally invasive hysterectomy, the vaginal cuff can be sutured using a variety of techniques. The choice of a specific method often depends on the surgeon's preference, patient characteristics, and the surgical situation. Here are some common types of vault closure:

4.2 Suturing Techniques

1. Continuous closure
   (a) Two layers
   (b) One layer
2. Interrupted sutures

Laparoscopy has a learning curve of which suturing is the step which requires maximum practice. Different techniques of vault suturing have been studied and tried. Vault suturing was earlier done by transvaginal route, then came extracorporeal followed by intracorporeal. Laparoscopy demands proficiency in intracorporeal suturing, which includes various techniques such as interrupted sutures, running sutures, and Figure-of-eight sutures

1. **Continuous closures single layer** (Fig. 4.1a–q)

At our centre we have been practising suturing using ipsilateral ports. We use 2 needle holders. The suture is loaded on the left needle holder and introduced through the lower port. Suture is held 2 cm away from the hub of the needle. The right needle holder is introduced from the upper port and needle is grasped at the junction of 2/3rd and 1/3rd. First bite is taken through, the utero sacral ligament and angle of the vault. We begin with right angle posterior lip and then anterior lip. The process involves using the right needle holder to create two loops over the left needle driver, followed by the left needle holder grasping the suture's tail and securing the knot.

In a continuous suture technique, the needle is inserted back through the tissue about 1 cm away from the initial bite, and this process repeats until reaching the angle of the wound. After reaching the angle on the other side the second knot is tied. The uterosacral are incorporated in the vault to prevent vault prolapse and provide adequate support post operatively.

2. **Continuous closure 2 layers** (Fig. 4.2a–q)

We at our centre suture the vault in 2 layers, ever since we started doing TLH almost three decades ago, this has given us almost negligible level of any vault prolapse. Incorporation of the utero sacral ligaments on both sides gives it a complete vault suspension. With two layers closure gives complete repair of the pubovesical and recto vaginal fascia which are incorporated adequately in the second layer. This type of closure which gives a complete pelvic floor repair goes a long way in giving secure anatomical support to the vault and prevent any post-operative vault prolapse.

After completing the first layer as described, we lock the left angle of the vault. We begin the second layer in a continuous fashion, embedding the first layer. Two layer closures ensures complete haemostasis and good support to the vault. Faster than interrupted sutures, may provide more uniform tension along the incision line.

3. **Interrupted closure**

In this method, the vaginal cuff is closed using individual sutures that are placed in a series of interrupted, separate stitches. To begin with angles are taken separately and 2 or 3 more stitches are required in between the angles to complete the closure. Allows precise control over the closure, and if one suture fails, it does not affect the entire closure and the angles are more secure.

4. **Running-Locking Sutures:**
   - **Description:** Similar to continuous sutures, but with additional locking stitches at intervals to secure the suture line. Its advantage is that it combines the speed of continuous sutures with the security of locking stitches.
5. **Figure of 8 Technique**

This technique of the Figure-of-eight suture is particularly useful for closing wounds under high tension. It's also employed to reinforce wounds closed with a continuous running suture. Similar to traditional hand suturing, Figure-of-eight sutures can be executed laparoscopically. The needle is inserted into the tissue at a 90° angle and exits clockwise, equidistant from the incision. Without tying a knot, the needle is re-inserted about 1 cm away on the same side of the incision as the first entry point, emerging near the initial bite, creating a square shape with an "X" connecting the angles. Finally, the knot is secured to complete the Figure-of-eight suture.

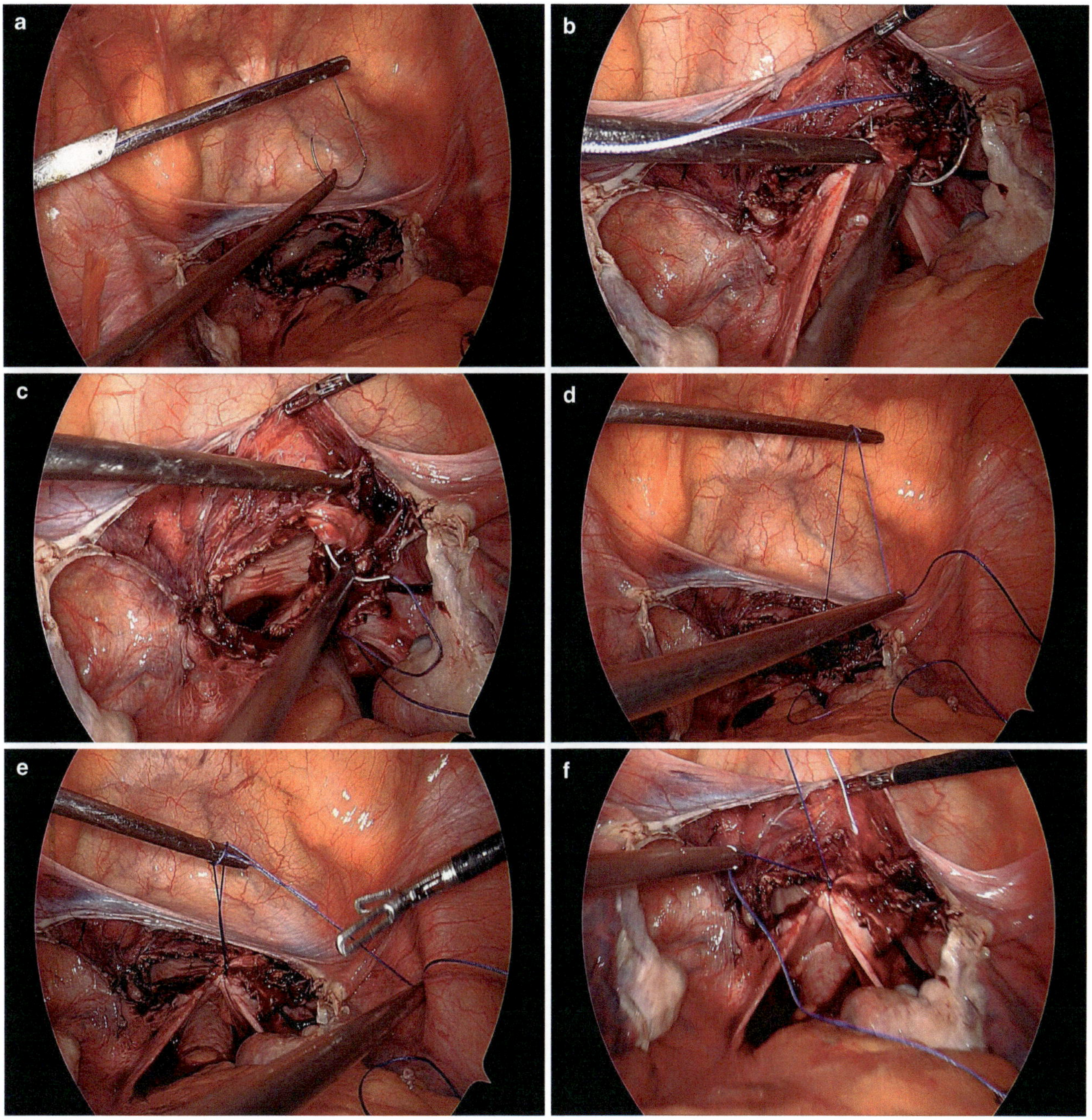

Fig. 4.1 **a** Holding the aligned needle. **b** Needle passed through posterior lip (right side). **c** Needle passed through anterior lip (right side). **d** Making an inverted "V" (Video.4.1d Vault closure technique) (▶ https://doi.org/10.1007/000-c91). **e** Making a knot. **f** Knot tied. **g** Needle passed through anterior and posterior lip (left side). **h** Making a loop. **i** Making an inverted "V". **j** Making a double loop. **k** Knot tied. **l** Both angles separately taken. **m** Suture rest of the vault. **n** Continuous suturing. **o** Needle passed through both lips. **p** Knot tied. **q** Vault closure completed

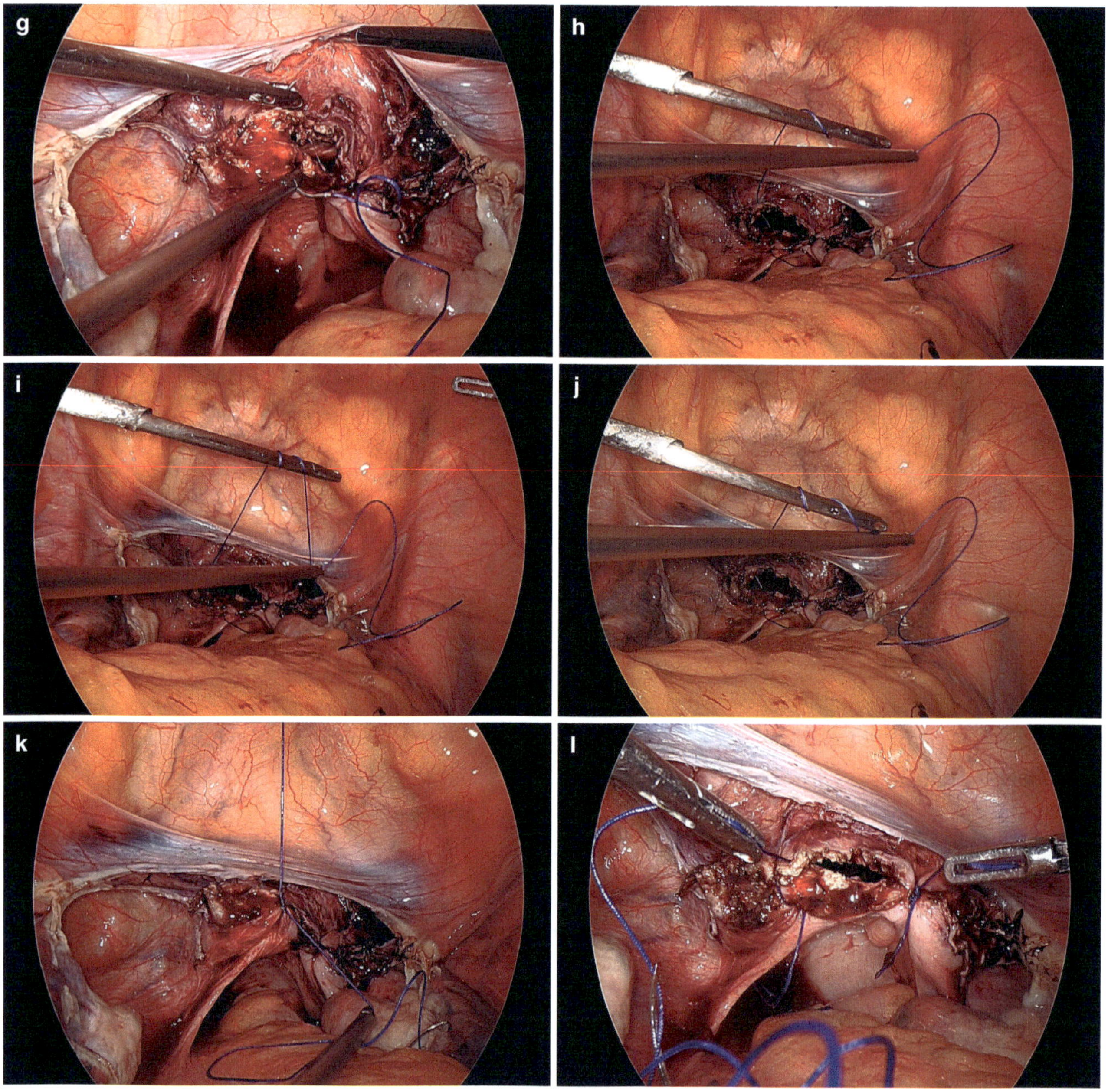

Fig. 4.1 (continued)

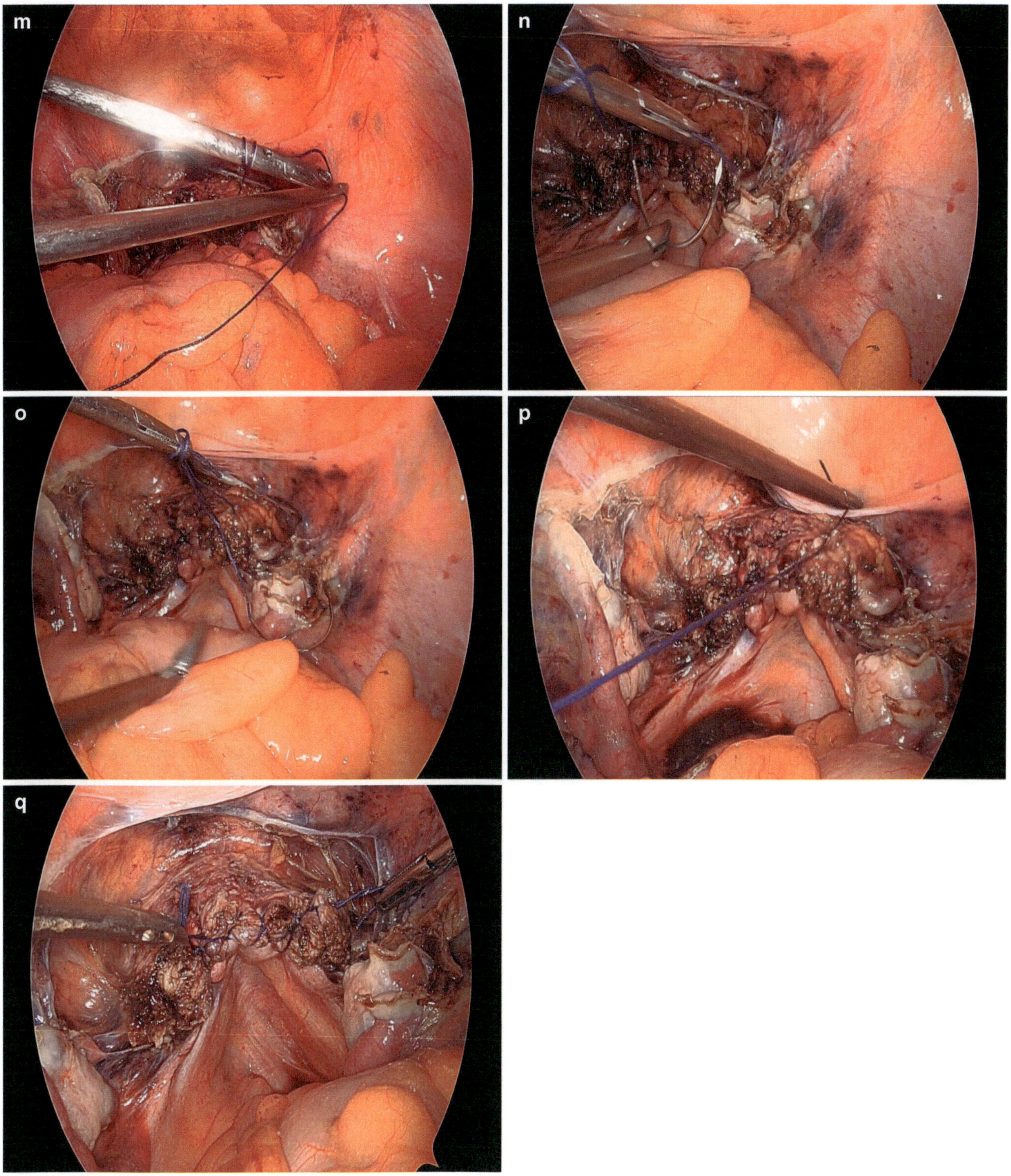

Fig. 4.2 (continued)

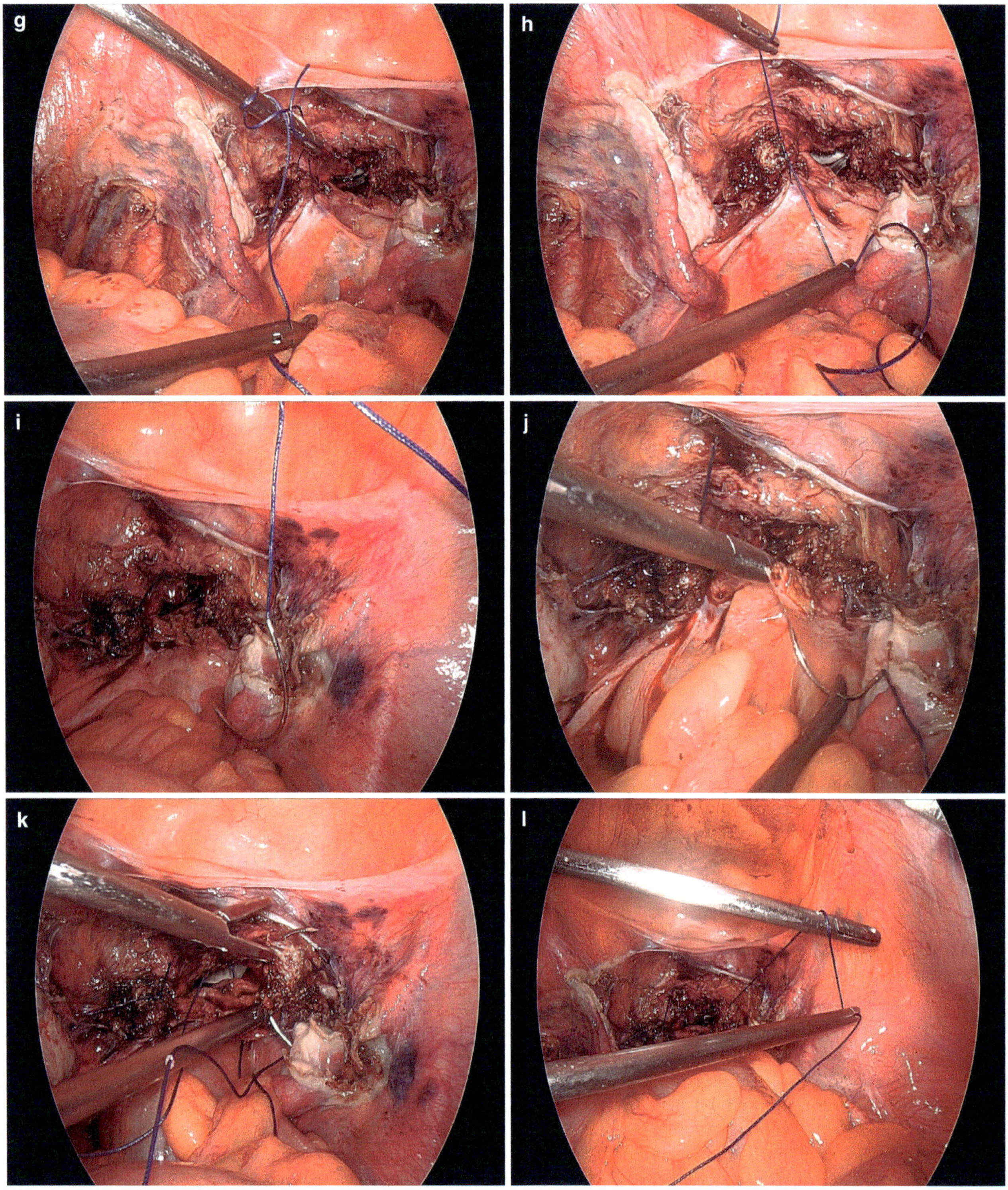

Fig. 4.2 (continued)

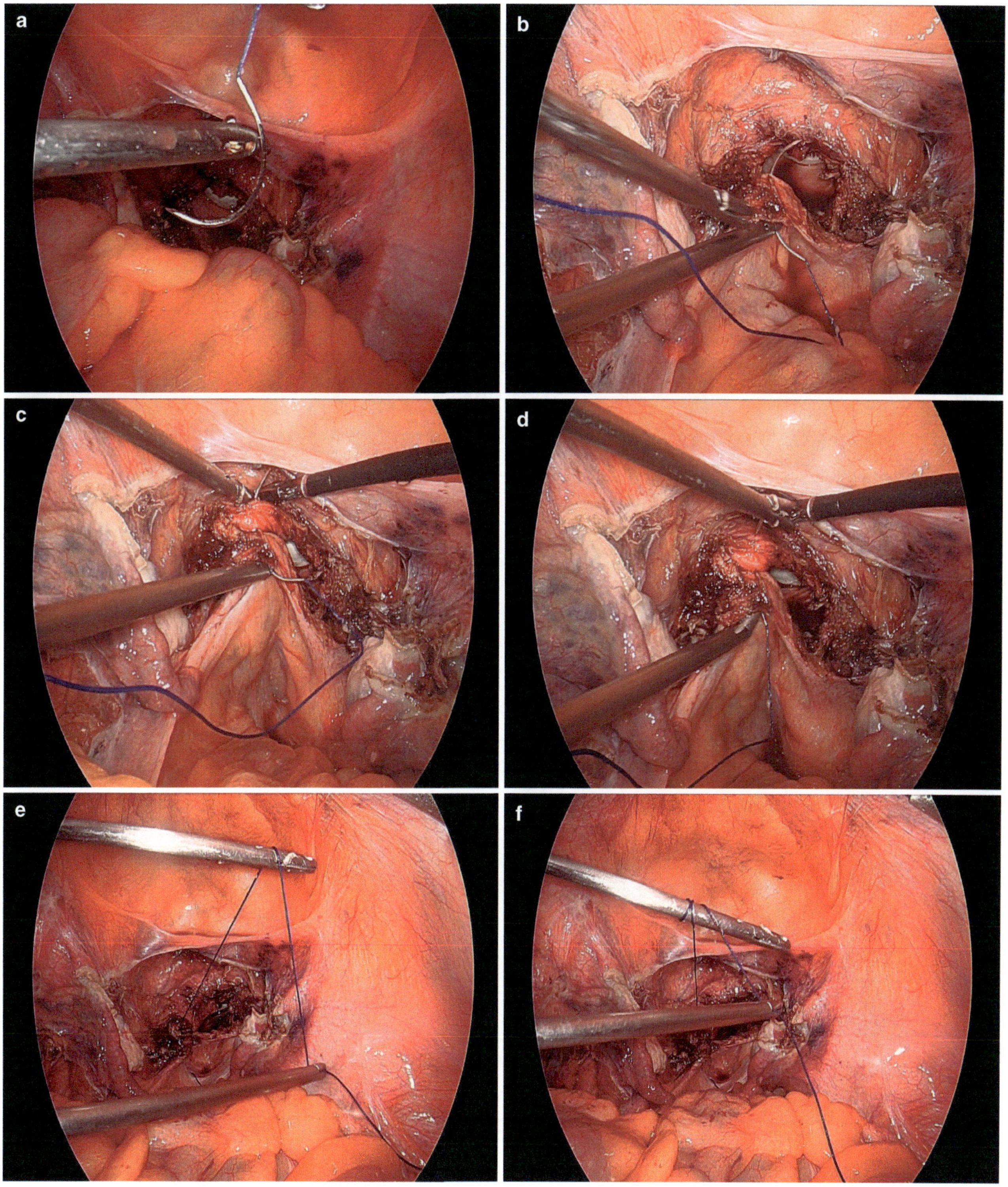

Fig. 4.2 **a** Holding the needle. **b** Needle passed through posterior lip from left angle. **c** Needle passed through both lips. **d** Needle taken out. **e** Making an inverted "V". **f** Making a loop. **g** Making a knot. **h** Knot tied from left side. **i** Hanging a needle. **j** Needle passed through posterior lip from right angle. **k** Needle passed through both lips from right angle. **l** Making a knot. **m** Making a loop. **n** Making another loop. **o** Making a knot. **p** Knot tied. **q** Vault closure completed

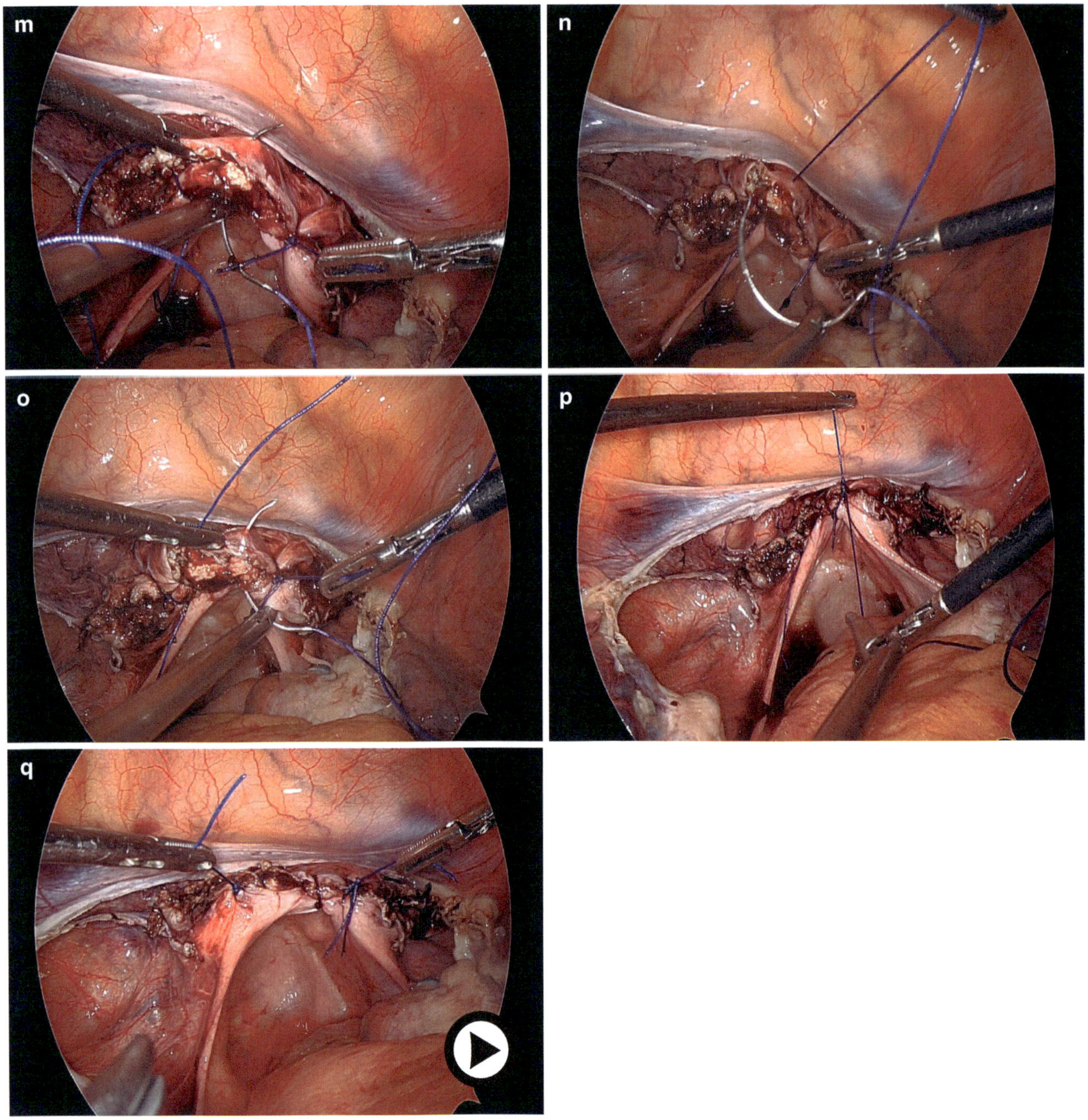

Fig. 4.1 (continued)

4.3 Choice of Suture Material

Suture material used is

1. VICRYL™ (POLYGLACTIN 910) Suture.
2. Barbed Sutures.
   - **Description:** Barbed or self-retaining sutures have small projections along their length, eliminating the need for knot tying.
   - **Advantages:** Can potentially reduce operative time and offer a more secure closure by maintaining proper tension at the suture.
   - **Disadvantages:** usage of barb suture increases the cost.

4.4 Barbed Versus Standard Suture

Dr. John Alcamo conceptualized the barbed suture in 1950, although its widespread use and manufacturing didn't occur until 2004. That year, the Quill Knotless Tissue Closure Device, developed by Angiotech Pharmaceuticals in Vancouver, British Columbia, received approval from the United States Food and Drug Administration. The three commercially available barbed sutures are

1. V-Loc™ Absorbable Wound Closure Device
2. The Quill Self-Retaining System
3. Stratafix™ (Ethicon Endosurgery, Somerville, New Jersey) [5]

Barbed sutures can be unidirectional or bidirectional. if the needle is at one end they are called unidirectional and if needle at both ends they are called bidirectional. Straight suture are converted into barb sutures by adding barbs and a needle with closure loop at the end [6]

Barbed sutures offer significant advantages over traditional ones. They enable tissue reapproximation without the need for surgical knots, addressing a common weak point in suture lines. Additionally, their use can reduce operative time, particularly beneficial in laparoscopic surgery where knot-tying can be challenging and time-consuming compared to open surgery [7, 8]. Moreover, barbed sutures have demonstrated a greater load to failure than traditional sutures, likely due to the distribution of force over a larger surface area provided by the barbs [9].

Greenberg and Einarsson pioneered the use of barbed sutures in laparoscopic gynecological surgery in 2008 [10]. Their initial cases involved the closure of the uterus during myomectomy and the vaginal cuff during hysterectomy. Subsequently, a significant study by Einarsson et al. in 2011 evaluated 138 laparoscopic myomectomies using bidirectional barbed sutures for uterine closure [11]. The study revealed reduced operative time and hospital stay duration without increasing intraoperative complications. This underscores the safety and added benefits of using barbed sutures in laparoscopic surgery for both surgeons and patients.

A comparative analysis was conducted to assess the operative time between cases using barbed sutures and those using conventional sutures [12–18]. Barbed suture closure of vaginal vault decreased the operative time by 15.6 min in comparison to conventional suture. (136.9 min vs. 151.7 min).

Vaginal cuff closure time was separately studied in 3 studies; the barbed suture groups took 5.4 min less time [19]

When comparing suture materials for the vaginal cuff, postoperative outcomes are also subject to debate. Previous studies suggest a potential decrease in intraoperative blood loss with the use of barbed sutures, although this finding was not consistently significant across studies. Some research indicates reduced postoperative vaginal bleeding, vaginal cuff cellulitis, and shorter hospital stays with barbed sutures compared to conventional sutures, but in many cases, the differences between the two groups were not statistically significant.

However, Seidhoff et al. [20] reported a significantly higher incidence of vaginal cuff cellulitis with barbed sutures. Despite this, overall postoperative complications did not show significant variation based on suture choice according to the literature. Vaginal cuff dehiscence (VCD) is among the most serious long-term complications postoperatively and was evaluated by all the studies. Seidhoff et al. and Rettenmaier [20, 21] reported a significantly decreased rate of dehiscence with barbed sutures, but few studies found a significant difference between the two groups. Because VCD is rare, it is challenging to demonstrate a decrease in its incidence. The heterogeneity of dehiscence rates and the abundance of non-significant results in the literature suggest that the use of barbed sutures may minimally change or leave unchanged the rate of VCD compared to standard suture materials.

While intraoperative outcomes seem similar for both barbed and traditional sutures, other factors should influence material selection, including cost. Barbed sutures carry a significantly higher material cost compared to traditional ones. However, this cost may be offset by the reduction in operating time (OT). Zeybek et al. [22] analyzed the costs of hysterectomy via laparoscopic and robotic routes in 2014, suggesting that decreased operative time can lead to reduced surgical expenses. Therefore, the shortened operative time associated with barbed sutures might balance out their higher material costs.

The use of barbed sutures over conventional has shown significant results in operative time and technicality with reduced postoperative complications [23] In a study done by Siedhoff et al., suture material used for vault closure was compared, which showed an increased rate of cellulitis and dehiscence up to 3.1% using braided sutures over monofilament. With the use of monofilament, the double knot technique needs expertise along with a secured angle has procured established advantages over braided sutures [20]

An additional consideration regarding barbed sutures warrants mention. Barb self-anchoring knotless suturing devices are commonly utilized for peritoneal closure. Proper handling of these sutures is paramount to prevent potential complications. Even with meticulous management, bowel adherence, injuries, or volvulus may arise [24]. Some studies have documented instances of subacute intestinal obstruction attributed to an elongated tail of the barbed suture. In such cases, after cutting and releasing the redundant tail of the barbed suture, the serosal and muscular defect was closed with two absorbable single knot sutures [25]. To avoid any chances of afore mentioned bowel complications it is suggested that extra one or two barb sutures bites be taken beyond the edge of the incision. And then to cut the barb sutures flush with the body tissue.

Regardless of the suture and technique employed, tissue handling plays a crucial role in vaginal cuff closure. Adequate bites of tissue at the serosal layer are essential. Bites should not be too shallow, as this may result in edges of the cuff that could bleed postoperatively. Additionally, bites should be taken separately in each layer, and the needle should be visible in the center after each bite. This technique ensures that the suture is properly placed within the tissue layer.

4.5 Review of Literature for Various Suturing Techniques

The selection of closure technique for the vaginal cuff receives less attention in minimally invasive hysterectomy compared to suture materials. Surgeon comfort and experience typically dictate the chosen technique for cuff closure. While the vaginal cuff suture technique may impact the rate of postoperative vaginal cuff dehiscence, the optimal technique has yet to be determined. O'Hanlan et al. [26] conducted a comprehensive retrospective cohort study involving 1924 patients to evaluate a standardized laparoscopic vaginal cuff closure technique.

The technique involved placing sutures five millimeters deep from the vaginal edge with a five-millimeter gap between sutures, including the uterosacral ligaments with the pubocervical fascia at the angles of the defect, and suturing the bladder peritoneum over the vaginal cuff edge. The cohort experienced a low rate of vaginal cuff complications [26] at 2.29%, with only 0.99% of patients requiring re-surgery for a complication associated with the vaginal cuff, indicating that this technique is associated with few vaginal cuff complications. However, there remains a deficiency of prospective trials comparing suture techniques. Three studies compared different intracorporeal suture techniques of the vaginal cuff in minimally invasive hysterectomy. Blikkendaal et al. [27] found no significant difference in the rates of VCD among different suture methods. Similarly, Tsafrir et al. [28] reported no cases of VCD in their study comparing various suture types. However, Landeen et al. [29] concluded a significant difference in VCD between different cuff closure techniques, suggesting that reinforcing sutures decreased the rate of dehiscence. Cuff closure with a single-layer continuous running suture and a single-layer continuous running suture with three reinforcing Figure-of-eight sutures was compared· Four cases of VCD were noted in their sample; three were in the non-reinforced arm of the trial. All four VCDs were in current smokers, but the relative risk of VCD in smokers in the non-reinforced group was 4.23 times higher than of VCD in smokers of the reinforced suture group. Thus it was suggested that reinforcing sutures decreased the rate of dehiscence. The advantage of these technical changes can be better demonstrated in future clinical trials using adequate sample size to detect differences in outcomes.

Overall, there isn't enough data to prove the superiority of any single cuff closure technique. Multiple techniques for vaginal cuff closure may be acceptable, but determining an ideal technique remains elusive. Surgeon preference, skill level, and clinical context influence the choice of technique. However, the current lack of literature on vaginal cuff closure techniques in minimally invasive hysterectomy underscores the need for large-scale trials with adequate sample sizes.

4.6 Conclusion

Vaginal cuff closure is a critical step in minimally invasive hysterectomy, with significant variability in techniques and suture choices among surgeons and institutions. While transvaginal suturing has traditionally been considered superior due to its ease and lower rates of vaginal cuff dehiscence, advancements such as the introduction of barbed sutures have shown promise in improving laparoscopic and robotic closure strength. Although some studies suggest that barbed sutures may offer advantages in postoperative outcomes and operative time, the benefits are not substantial, and the higher cost may offset the savings in operating room time. Further research, particularly larger randomized trials, is needed to evaluate suture techniques comprehensively, with a focus on the potential benefits of reinforcing sutures. In the realm of laparoscopic single-site surgery, the optimal technique for vaginal cuff closure remains unclear due to limited published trials. However, with advancements in technology and increased surgeon experience in minimally invasive techniques, intracorporeal vaginal cuff closure may eventually be considered as safe and effective as transvaginal closure. At our center, we have observed superior outcomes with intracorporeal closure, highlighting its potential as a preferred technique in minimally invasive hysterectomy.

Learning Points

- Vault closure in TLH is essential for preventing complications like vault dehiscence.
- Surgeons use various suturing techniques, including continuous, interrupted, and running-locking sutures.
- Barbed sutures offer benefits such as reduced operative time providing a constant tensile strength over the entire suture line.
- Technique selection depends on surgeon preference, patient characteristics, and surgical situation.
- Surgeon experience and skill are critical for successful vault closure and complication prevention.

Competing Interest The author declares no conflict of interest that are relevant to content of this chapter.

Ethical Approval Informed consent was obtained from individual participants and patients regarding publication and documentation without disclosing their identity.

References

1. Reich H, DiCaprio J, McGlynn F. Laparoscopic hysterectomy. J Gynecol Surg. 1989;5:213–6.
2. Kanti V, Verma V, Singh M, Vishwakarma S, Mittal N, Singh NP. A comparative analysis of nondescent vaginal hysterectomy, laparoscopy-assisted vaginal hysterectomy, and total laparoscopic hysterectomy for benign uterine diseases at a rural tertiary care center. Gynecol Minim Invasive Ther. 2022;11:164–70.
3. Radosa JC, Radosa MP, Zimmermann JS, Braun EM, Findeklee S, Wieczorek A, et al. Incidence of and risk factors for vaginal cuff dehiscence following total laparoscopic hysterectomy: a monocentric hospital analysis. Arch Gynecol Obstet. 2021;304:447–54.
4. Uccella S, Ghezzi F, Mariani A, Cromi A, Bogani G, Serati M, Bolis P. Vaginal cuff closure after minimally invasive hysterectomy: our experience and systematic review of the literature. Am J Obstet Gynecol. 2011;205(2):119.e1–12. https://doi.org/10.1016/j.ajog.2011.03.024. Epub 2011 Mar 22. PMID: 21620360.
5. Greenberg JA, Goldman RH. Barbed suture: a review of the technology and clinical uses in obstetrics and gynecology. Rev Obstet Gynecol. 2013;6(3–4):107–15. PMID: 24920976; PMCID: PMC4002186.
6. Iavazzo C, Mamais I, Gkegkes ID. The role of knotless barbed suture in gynecologic surgery: systematic review and meta-analysis. Surg Innov. 2015;22(5):528–39. https://doi.org/10.1177/1553350614554235. Epub 2014 Oct 15. PMID: 25320107.
7. Greenberg JA. The use of barbed sutures in obstetrics and gynecology. Rev Obstet Gynecol. 2010;3(3):82–91. PMID: 21364859; PMCID: PMC3046763.
8. Gözen AS, Arslan M, Schulze M, Rassweiler J. Comparison of laparoscopic closure of the bladder with barbed polyglyconate versus polyglactin suture material in the pig bladder model: an experimental in vitro study. J Endourol. 2012;26(6):732–6. https://doi.org/10.1089/end.2011.0194. Epub 2011 Oct 18. PMID: 22007838.
9. Arbaugh M, Case JB, Monnet E. Biomechanical comparison of glycomer 631 and glycomer 631 knotless for use in canine incisional gastropexy. Vet Surg. 2013;42(2):205–9. https://doi.org/10.1111/j.1532-950X.2012.01051.x. Epub 2012 Oct 23. PMID: 23094713.
10. Greenberg JA, Einarsson JI. The use of bidirectional barbed suture in laparoscopic myomectomy and total laparoscopic hysterectomy. J Minim Invasive Gynecol. 2008;15(5):621–3. https://doi.org/10.1016/j.jmig.2008.06.004. Epub 2008 Jul 10. PMID: 18619922.
11. Einarsson JI, Chavan NR, Suzuki Y, Jonsdottir G, Vellinga TT, Greenberg JA. Use of bidirectional barbed suture in laparoscopic myomectomy: evaluation of perioperative outcomes, safety, and efficacy. J Minim Invasive Gynecol. 2011;18(1):92–5. https://doi.org/10.1016/j.jmig.2010.10.003. Epub 2010 Nov 20. PMID: 21094097.
12. Nawfal AK, Eisenstein D, Theoharis E, Dahlman M, Wegienka G. Vaginal cuff closure during robotic-assisted total laparoscopic hysterectomy: comparing VICRYL™ (polyglactin 910) to barbed sutures. JSLS. 2012;16(4):525–9. https://doi.org/10.4293/108680812X13462882736772. PMID: 23484558; PMCID: PMC3558886.
13. Ardovino M, Castaldi MA, Fraternali F, Ardovino I, Mosca L, Colacurci N, Signoriello G, Cobellis L. Bidirectional barbed suture in total laparoscopic hysterectomy and lymph node dissection for endometrial cancer: technical evaluation and 1-year follow-up of 61 patients. J Laparoendosc Adv Surg Tech A. 2013;23(4):347–50. https://doi.org/10.1089/lap.2012.0079. PMID: 23573880.
14. Bassi A, Tulandi T. Evaluation of total laparoscopic hysterectomy with and without the use of barbed suture. J Obstet Gynaecol Can. 2013;35(8):718–22. https://doi.org/10.1016/S1701-2163(15)30862-8. PMID: 24007707.
15. Song T, Lee SH. Barbed suture vs traditional suture in single-port total laparoscopic hysterectomy. J Minim Invasive Gynecol. 2014;21(5):825–9. https://doi.org/10.1016/j.jmig.2014.03.012. Epub 2014 Mar 26. PMID: 24681166.
16. Medina BC, Giraldo CH, Riaño G, Hoyos LR, Otalora C. Barbed suture for vaginal cuff closure in laparoscopic hysterectomy. JSLS. 2014;18(1):83–8. https://doi.org/10.4293/108680813X13693422518795. PMID: 24680149; PMCID: PMC3939349.
17. Zhou Y, Guthrie G, Chuang A, Faro JP, Ali V. Unidirectional barbed suture versus interrupted VICRYL™ (polyglactin 910) suture in vaginal cuff healing during robotic-assisted laparoscopic hysterectomy. J Robot Surg. 2014;8(3):201–5. https://doi.org/10.1007/s11701-014-0451-6. Epub 2014 Mar 4. PMID: 27637678.
18. Cong L, Li C, Wei B, Zhan L, Wang W, Xu Y. V-Loc™ 180 suture in total laparoscopic hysterectomy: a retrospective study comparing

Polysorb to barbed suture used for vaginal cuff closure. Eur J Obstet Gynecol Reprod Biol. 2016;207:18–22. https://doi.org/10.1016/j.ejogrb.2016.09.012. Epub 2016 Oct 23. PMID: 27816737.
19. Kim JH, Byun SW, Song JY, Kim YH, Lee HJ, Park TC, Lee KH, Hur SY, Park JS, Lee SJ. Barbed versus conventional 2-layer continuous running sutures for laparoscopic vaginal cuff closure. Medicine (Baltimore). 2016;95(39):e4981. https://doi.org/10.1097/MD.0000000000004981. PMID: 27684850; PMCID: PMC5265943.
20. Siedhoff MT, Yunker AC, Steege JF. Decreased incidence of vaginal cuff dehiscence after laparoscopic closure with bidirectional barbed suture. J Minim Invasive Gynecol. 2011;18(2):218–23. https://doi.org/10.1016/j.jmig.2011.01.002. PMID: 21354068.
21. Rettenmaier MA, Abaid LN, Brown JV 3rd, Mendivil AA, Lopez KL, Goldstein BH. Dramatically reduced incidence of vaginal cuff dehiscence in gynecologic patients undergoing endoscopic closure with barbed sutures: a retrospective cohort study. Int J Surg. 2015;19:27–30. https://doi.org/10.1016/j.ijsu.2015.05.007. Epub 2015 May 14. PMID: 25980394.
22. Zeybek B, Oge T, Kılıç CH, Borahay MA, Kılıç GS. A financial analysis of operating room charges for robot-assisted gynaecologic surgery: efficiency strategies in the operating room for reducing the costs. J Turk Ger Gynecol Assoc. 2014;15(1):25–9. https://doi.org/10.5152/jtgga.jtgga.2014.79989. PMID: 24790513; PMCID: PMC4004300.
23. Croce E, Olmi S. Intracorporeal knot-tying and suturing techniques in laparoscopic surgery: technical details. JSLS. 2000;4(1):17–22. PMID: 10772523; PMCID: PMC3015354.
24. Köhler G, Mayer F, Lechner M, Bittner R. Small bowel obstruction after TAPP repair caused by a self-anchoring barbed suture device for peritoneal closure: case report and review of the literature. Hernia. 2015;19(3):389–94. https://doi.org/10.1007/s10029-014-1301-1. Epub 2014 Aug 12. PMID: 25112384.
25. Wang L, Maejima T, Fukahori S, Nishihara S, Yoshikawa D, Kono T. Bowel obstruction and perforation secondary to barbed suture after minimally invasive inguinal hernia repair: report of two cases and literature review. Surg Case Rep. 2021;7(1):161. https://doi.org/10.1186/s40792-021-01249-w. PMID: 34255201; PMCID: PMC8276904.
26. O'Hanlan KA, Emeney PL, Peters A, Sten MS, McCutcheon SP, Struck DM, Hoang JK. Analysis of a standardized technique for laparoscopic cuff closure following 1924 total laparoscopic hysterectomies. Minim Invasive Surg. 2016;2016:1372685. https://doi.org/10.1155/2016/1372685. Epub 2016 Aug 4. PMID: 27579179; PMCID: PMC4989084.
27. Blikkendaal MD, Twijnstra AR, Pacquee SC, Rhemrev JP, Smeets MJ, de Kroon CD, Jansen FW. Vaginal cuff dehiscence in laparoscopic hysterectomy: influence of various suturing methods of the vaginal vault. Gynecol Surg. 2012;9(4):393–400. https://doi.org/10.1007/s10397-012-0745-5. Epub 2012 May 3. PMID: 23144640; PMCID: PMC3491192.
28. Tsafrir Z, Palmer M, Dahlman M, Nawfal AK, Aoun J, Taylor A, Fisher J, Theoharis E, Eisenstein D. Long-term outcomes for different vaginal cuff closure techniques in robotic-assisted laparoscopic hysterectomy: a randomized controlled trial. Eur J Obstet Gynecol Reprod Biol. 2017;210:7–12. https://doi.org/10.1016/j.ejogrb.2016.11.018. Epub 2016 Nov 16. PMID: 27923167.
29. Landeen LB, Hultgren EM, Kapsch TM, Mallory PW. Vaginal cuff dehiscence: a randomized trial comparing robotic vaginal cuff closure methods. J Robot Surg. 2016;10(4):337–41. https://doi.org/10.1007/s11701-016-0604-x. Epub 2016 Jun 2. PMID: 27251474.

Enhanced Recovery After Surgery

5

Aarushi Jain and Priyanka Jha

5.1 Introduction

There have been remarkable advancements in the field of gynecological surgeries in the recent years with a primary focus on improving patient outcomes and accelerating the recovery process. One such development pertaining to this is the implementation of ERAS protocols [1].

Traditional components of perioperative care include bowel preparation, cessation of oral intake after midnight, liberal use of narcotics, patient-controlled analgesia, prolonged bowel and bed rest, the use of nasogastric tubes and drains, and gradual reintroduction of feeding. However, many of these commonly implemented interventions are not evidence-based, and their use frequently does not promote healing and recovery [2].

Initiated by Professor Henrik Kehlet in the 1990s [3], ERAS protocols are comprehensive, evidence based multimodal perioperative care pathways designed to minimize the surgical stress and achieve faster postoperative recovery, thereby facilitating a quicker return to normal routine activities [4–8]. These guidelines operate during the preoperative, intraoperative, postoperative and rehabilitation periods resulting in improved perioperative mortality and morbidity, reduced length of hospital stay, decreased complications and expedited recovery after major surgeries. The basis of implementation of ERAS protocols lies in the maintenance of patients' physiological and psychological response to surgical stress [9]. The various measures undertaken in these protocols aim at attenuating the stress response and keeping the internal milieu of the body well within the normal physiologic limits.

Initially implemented with colorectal surgeries [10], these protocols are now widely carried out in most major surgical procedures namely, thoracic [11], cardiac [12], urologic [13], vascular [14], orthopedic [15] and neurosurgeries [16]. These are now established as a global surgical quality improvement initiative that results in clinical improvements as well as cost benefits to the healthcare system [17]. The successful implementation of these protocols requires utmost coordination between the surgical, anesthetic and nursing personnel during the entire perioperative period.

5.2 Key Components of ERAS

Preoperative	Intraoperative	Postoperative
Patient education and counselling Alleviation of anxiety Optimisation of comorbidities Avoidance of prolonged perioperative fasting Smoking and alcohol cessation Antibiotic and VTE prophylaxis Avoidance of mechanical bowel preparation.	Minimally invasive surgical techniques Postoperative nausea and vomiting prophylaxis Multimodal non opioid analgesics Regional anesthesia techniques Normothermia Euvolemia Glycemic control Lung protective mechanical ventilation Early removal of tubes and drains	Early ambulation Early oral intake Use of multimodal non opioid analgesics

5.3 Preoperative Components

The preoperative period is crucial for proper assessment of the patient so as to whether the patient is stable to undergo the particular surgery [18]. The comorbidities such as diabetes mellitus, hypertension, COPD, CAD, anaemia, etc. are

A. Jain (✉)
Anaesthesiology, University College of Medical Sciences, Affiliated by Delhi University, Delhi, India

Department of Anaesthesia, Vardhman Trauma and Laparoscopy Centre Pvt. Ltd., Muzaffarnagar, UP, India

P. Jha
Department of Anaesthesia, Muzaffarnagar Medical College, Muzaffarnagar, Uttar Pradesh, India

N. Jain (ed.), *Complex Total Laparoscopic Hysterectomy (TLH) with Newer Approaches in Bladder Dissection*, https://doi.org/10.1007/978-981-97-3226-5_5

addressed and the patients are optimised accordingly prior to the surgery. This subsequently enables to choose the optimum surgical and anaesthetic technique and the postoperative care plan.

Another important aspect of ERAS protocols is patient education. A well informed patient displays lower anxiety levels during the perioperative period [19]. The patients and their family members should be informed about the risks associated with the surgical procedure, approximate length of hospital stay, postoperative ambulation, pain control, feeding and timing of catheter removal.

While the patients are traditionally required to remain NPO (nil per oral) 8 h prior to surgery, recent studies and meta-analysis show that allowing carbohydrate rich clear fluid upto 2 h prior to surgery prevents the body to enter the catabolic stress response [20, 21]. This, in turn, attenuates the postoperative insulin resistance, reduces nitrogen and protein losses, preserves skeletal muscle mass and decreases preoperative thirst, hunger and anxiety.

Preoperative mechanical bowel preparation has not shown to improve surgical outcomes [22]. In addition to patient dissatisfaction; its use has been associated with adverse surgical outcomes due to preoperative dehydration and electrolyte imbalance that can hamper postoperative recovery.

Cessation of smoking and alcohol intake is an important factor in determining the success of implementation of ERAS protocols [23, 24]. At least 1 month of abstinence from smoking and alcohol has shown to improve patient outcomes.

Another very important preoperative consideration is the deep venous thrombosis (DVT) prophylaxis. Venous thromboembolism (VTE) carries a significant morbidity and mortality in surgical patients, therefore, it becomes pertinent to provide adequate prophylaxis to mitigate this serious complication in the postoperative period [25]. The various measures include mechanical devices such as elastic stockings, compression devices and use of anticoagulants. Patients with high risk of VTE, as identified by using the modified Caprini score (Table 5.1) [26, 27], should receive dual prophylaxis i.e. mechanical as well as chemoprophylaxis with low molecular weight heparin or unfractionated heparin [28, 29]. (Table 5.2) [30].

Table 5.1 Modified Caprini risk assessment for minimally invasive gynecologic surgery

1 point	2 points	3 points	5 points
Age 41–60 y	Age 61–74 y	Age ≥75 y	Stroke (<1 mo)
Minor surgery	Major open surgery (>45 min)	History of VTE	Hip, pelvis, or leg fracture
BMI ≥40 kg/m^{2a}	Minimally invasive surgery (≥180 min)[a]	Family history of VTE	Acute spinal cord injury (< 1 mo)
Swollen legs	Malignancy	Factor V Leiden	Elective arthroplasty
Varicose veins	Bed rest (>72 h)	Prothrombin 2021A	
Pregnancy or postpartum	Immobilizing plaster cast	Lupus anticoagulant	
History of unexplained or recurrent spontaneous abortion	Central venous access	Anticardiolipin antibodies	
Oral contraceptives or hormone replacement	Arthroscopic surgery	Elevated serum homocysteine	
Sepsis (<1 mo)		Heparin-induced thrombocytopenia	
Severe lung disease, including pneumonia (<1 mo)		Other congenital or acquired thrombophilia	
Abnormal pulmonary function			
Acute myocardial infarction			
Congestive heart failure (<1 mo)			
History of inflammatory bowel disease			

BMI body mass index, *VTE* venous thromboembolism
[a]Modifications

Table 5.2 Venous thromboembolism prophylaxis recommendations for minimally invasive gynecologic surgery

Patient category	Preop	Intraop	Postop	Extended postop
Benign indications VTE or hereditary thrombophilia history	5000 units UFH SC given upto 2 h before induction of anaesthesia[a]	SCDs	SCDs Early ambulation 5000 units UFH SC every 8 h or 40 mg LMWH SC daily beginning 8 h from preop dose of UFH	Frequent ambulation 40 mg LMWH SC daily or prophylactic dose DOAC for 28 d
No history of VTE or hereditary thrombophilia and not on hormonal therapy	None	SCDs	SCDs Early ambulation	Frequent ambulation
On hormonal therapy	5000 units UFH SC given upto 2 h before induction of anaesthesia[a]		SCDs Early ambulation 5000 units UFH SC every 8 h 40 mg LMWH SC daily beginning 8 h from preop dose of UFH	Frequent ambulation
Malignant indications 1. mCaprini score[b] of ≥7 or	5000 units UFH SC given up to 2 h before induction of anesthesia[a]	SCDs	SCDs	Frequent ambulation
2. (2) mCaprini score[b] of 5–6 and high grade histology, stage III/IV disease, or		Early ambulation		40 mg LMWH SC daily or
3. Lymphadenectomy (SLN biopsy excluded)		5000 units UFH SC every 8 h or 40 mg LMWH SC daily beginning 8 h from preop dose of UFH		Prophylactic dose DOAC for 28 d
Not meeting criteria (1) or (2) above	5000 units UFH SC given up to 2 h before induction of anesthesia[a]	SCDs	SCDs Early ambulation 5000 units UFH SC every 8 h 40 mg LMWH SC daily beginning 8 h from preop dose of UFH	Frequent ambulation

DOAC direct oral anticoagulant (e.g., apixaban 2.5 mg orally twice daily), *Intraop* intraoperative, *LMWH* low molecular weight heparin, *Preop* preoperative, *Postop* postoperative, *SC* subcutaneously, *SCDs* sequential compression devices, *SLN* sentinel lymph node, *UFH* unfractionated heparin, *VTE* venous thromboembolism

[a]LMWH in the form of enoxaparin 40 mg SC given 2–4 h before induction of anesthesia and every 24 h thereafter is an alternative

[b]Modified Caprini score using a BMI of ≥40 kg/m^2 instead of 25 kg/m^2 and surgical time of 180 min instead of 45 min

5.4 Intraoperative Components

The choice of surgical technique and the conduct of anaesthesia are the key determinants of a successful ERAS program in the intraoperative period.

Choosing minimally invasive surgical techniques over open surgery has shown to give superior postoperative recovery by decreasing intraoperative blood loss and reduced analgesic requirements. Laparoscopic surgery is associated with lower level of inflammatory and immunomodulatory response to surgery as compared to open surgery [31, 32]. A study conducted by Lin et al. concluded that laparoscopic surgery allows earlier ambulation and better postoperative outcomes as compared to open surgery [33].

Proper antimicrobial prophylaxis is crucial to prevent surgical site infection and subsequent morbidity in the patients. First generation cephalosporins should be administered within 1 h prior to incision. Addition of anaerobic coverage is recommended in case of anticipated bowel handling or pelvic surgery [34, 35]. A second dose of antibiotic is considered for surgeries lasting longer than 4 h or if the blood loss is more than 1500 ml.

Anaesthetic management plays a pivotal role in the implementation of ERAS protocols. The goal is to use short acting medications having minimal postoperative hangover and favourable antiemetic profile [36]. Inhalational agents such as sevoflurane and desflurane are preferred as these have shorter wash out times, thereby resulting in faster recovery. Anaesthesia can be maintained using total intravenous techniques (TIVA) whereby targeted controlled infusions of short acting drugs such as propofol, remifentanil and dexmedetomidine are used, thereby eliminating the use of inhalational agents. Regional anaesthesia techniques such as peripheral nerve blocks, port site infiltration, epidural catheters are used wherever feasible. These techniques alone or in combination with intravenous analgesics, not only decrease the intraoperative volatile anaesthetics requirement but also provide prolonged postoperative analgesia and mitigate the use of opioid analgesics [37, 38]. Opioids are avoided due to their undesired side effects which includes nausea and vomiting, pruritus, ileus and increased sedation. Opioid free anaesthesia and analgesia helps in mitigating the issues of opioid addiction and tolerance which is a growing menace worldwide. Practicing the same over the years, we have not faced these burning issues in our clinical practice for the past 4 decades.

Postoperative nausea and vomiting (PONV) is the most incapacitating and undesired side effect of anaesthesia resulting in prolonged hospital stay as well as patient dissatisfaction. Combination antiemeic therapy using a $5HT_3$ antagonist with droperidol or dexamethasone effectively decreases the incidence of PONV [39]. Use of nitrous oxide should be avoided wherever possible.

Employing lung protective mechanical ventilation with tidal volume 6–8 ml/kg and positive end expiratory pressure of 6–8 cm H_2O have been shown to reduce pulmonary complications [40]. Applying lung recruitment maneuvers before extubation help in combating the basal atelectasis which occurs as a result of steep trendlenberg position, a prerequisite for gynaecological endoscopic procedures. All these measures tend to prevent the intraoperative and postoperative hypoxia, facilitating smooth extubation and recovery and good pulmonary function in the postoperative period.

Maintenance of intravascular volume status is crucial. The goal is to maintain a state of euvolemia and minimising excess salt and water. Excessive fluid administration results in intestinal edema, postoperative ileus, delayed return of bowel function and increased pulmonary complications [41]. Fluid requirements are maintained with 1–3 ml/kg/h infusion of balanced salt solution in low risk patients undergoing low risk surgery [42]. However, during major surgeries, goal directed fluid therapy (GDFT) is used whereby fluid requirements of the patient are individualised using a cardiac output monitor [43]. It avoids hypovolemia as well as postoperative oxygen debt.

Intraoperative hypothermia should be avoided at all times. It severely impairs wound healing, increases blood loss, stress response and oxygen consumption thereby predisposing to adverse cardiac events [44]. Temperature monitoring devices should be used and temperature should be maintained using fluid warmers, forced warmed air devices and underbody warming mattresses.

Glycemic control is a vital component of ERAS protocols. Perioperative hyperglycemia is associated with increased risk of infections and cardiovascular morbidity and mortality postoperatively in diabetic as well as non diabetic patients [45, 46, 47]. Therefore, it becomes pertinent to maintain blood glucose levels well within the recommended limits, i.e. under 200 mg/dl in order to prevent the above mentioned adverse events. Owing to high prevalence of diabetes mellitus in surgical patients, preoperative screening of the patients for diabetes also becomes crucial.

The use of drains, catheters and nasogastric tubes not only increases the risk of infections but are also a main reason for patient discomfort and pain in postoperative period [48]. The use of nasogastric tubes have been shown to predispose the patients to pulmonary aspiration, eventually leading to postoperative pneumonia [49, 50]. Hence, the use of peritoneal drains, subcutaneous drains and nasogastric tubes should be avoided after abdominal surgery as per the recent ERAS guidelines [17].

5.5 Postoperative Components

Postoperative period plays the most critical role in expediting the recovery of post surgical patient. The interventions during this period focus on early mobilisation of the patient, early enteral nutrition and use of opioid free analgesics.

Early ambulation improves respiratory function and oxygen delivery to tissues thereby facilitating faster recovery. It also reduces the risk of thromboembolic complications [51, 52]. Patients should be encouraged to be out of bed within 24 h of surgery.

Adequate nutrition is important to enhance wound healing, decrease infection and maintain muscle strength for mobilisation. Early enteral feeding decreases the incidence of ileus and postoperative intravenous fluid administration [53, 54].

Postoperative pain after major surgery hinders respiration and ambulation. It, therefore becomes important to provide for good pain control measures in the postoperative period. Opioid free multimodal analgesics such as acetaminophen, NSAIDS, dexamethasone, gabapentins, local anaesthetic infiltration, regional blocks such as transverse abdominis plane block, epidural analgesia, should be used as per the requirements [55].

Learning Points

- The successful implementation of ERAS protocols requires a multidisciplinary approach along with the support and coordination of doctors, nurses, paramedical staff and the patient itself. Having adequate personnel to implement the system and proper communication between the team members is crucial.
- As ERAS continues to shape the landscape of perioperative care, its application in gynaecological surgeries serves as a beacon of progress.

- Systematic audit is beneficial in improving the outcome through feedbacks which helps in identifying the fallacies, improving the compliance and successful adaptation of these evidence based protocols.

Competing Interest The author declares no conflict of interest that are relevant to content of this chapter.

Ethical Approval Informed consent was obtained from individual participants and patients regarding publication and documentation without disclosing their identity.

References

1. Abdelrazik AN, Sanad AS. Implementation of enhanced recovery after surgery in gynecological operations: a randomized controlled trial. Ain-Shams J Anesthesiol. 2020;12:70. https://doi.org/10.1186/s42077-020-00116-4.
2. Kalogera E, Dowdy SC. Enhanced recovery pathway in gynecologic surgery: improving outcomes through evidence-based medicine. Obstet Gynecol Clin N Am. 2016;43:551–73.
3. Kehlet H. Multimodal approach to control postoperative pathophysiology and rehabilitation. Br J Anaesth. 1997;78(5):606–17. https://doi.org/10.1093/bja/78.5.606. PMID: 9175983.
4. Wilmore DW, Kehlet H. Management of patients in fast track surgery. BMJ. 2001;322(7284):473–6. https://doi.org/10.1136/bmj.322.7284.473. PMID: 11222424; PMCID: PMC1119685.
5. Kehlet H, Wilmore DW. Multimodal strategies to improve surgical outcome. Am J Surg. 2002;183(6):630–41. https://doi.org/10.1016/s0002-9610(02)00866-8. PMID: 12095591.
6. Kehlet H, Dahl JB. Anaesthesia, surgery, and challenges in postoperative recovery. Lancet. 2003;362(9399):1921–8. https://doi.org/10.1016/S0140-6736(03)14966-5. PMID: 14667752.
7. Arumainayagam N, McGrath J, Jefferson KP, Gillatt DA. Introduction of an enhanced recovery protocol for radical cystectomy. BJU Int. 2008;101(6):698–701. https://doi.org/10.1111/j.1464-410X.2007.07319.x. Epub 2008 Jan 8. PMID: 18190646.
8. Kehlet H, Mogensen T. Hospital stay of 2 days after open sigmoidectomy with a multimodal rehabilitation programme. Br J Surg. 1999;86(2):227–30. https://doi.org/10.1046/j.1365--2168.1999.01023.x. PMID: 10100792.
9. Tippireddy S, Ghatol D. Anesthetic management for enhanced recovery after major surgery (ERAS). 2023 Jan 29. In: StatPearls [Internet]. Treasure Island (FL): StatPearls Publishing; 2023 Jan–. PMID: 34662081.
10. Wind J, Polle SW, Fung Kon Jin PH, Dejong CH, von Meyenfeldt MF, Ubbink DT, Gouma DJ, Bemelman WA, Laparoscopy and/or Fast Track Multimodal Management Versus Standard Care (LAFA) Study Group, Enhanced Recovery after Surgery (ERAS) Group. Systematic review of enhanced recovery programmes in colonic surgery. Br J Surg. 2006;93(7):800–9. https://doi.org/10.1002/bjs.5384. PMID: 16775831.
11. Tovar EA, Roethe RA, Weissig MD, Lloyd RE, Patel GR. One-day admission for lung lobectomy: an incidental result of a clinical pathway. Ann Thorac Surg. 1998;65(3):803–6. PMID: 9527217.
12. Rafiq S, Steinbrüchel DA, Wanscher MJ, Andersen LW, Navne A, Lilleoer NB, Olsen PS. Multimodal analgesia versus traditional opiate based analgesia after cardiac surgery, a randomized controlled trial. J Cardiothorac Surg. 2014;9:52. https://doi.org/10.1186/1749-8090-9-52. PMID: 24650125; PMCID: PMC3975463.
13. Melnyk M, Casey RG, Black P, Koupparis AJ. Enhanced recovery after surgery (ERAS) protocols: time to change practice? Can Urol Assoc J. 2011;5(5):342–8. https://doi.org/10.5489/cuaj.11002. PMID: 22031616; PMCID: PMC3202008.
14. Podore PC, Throop EB. Infrarenal aortic surgery with a 3-day hospital stay: a report on success with a clinical pathway. J Vasc Surg. 1999;29(5):787–92. https://doi.org/10.1016/s0741-5214(99)70204-1. PMID: 10231628.
15. Tucker A, McCusker D, Gupta N, Bunn J, Murnaghan M. Orthopaedic enhanced recovery programme for elective hip and knee arthroplasty—could a regional programme be beneficial? Ulster Med J. 2016;85(2):86–91. PMID: 27601761; PMCID: PMC4920494.
16. Hagan KB, Bhavsar S, Raza SM, Arnold B, Arunkumar R, Dang A, Gottumukkala V, Popat K, Pratt G, Rahlfs T, Cata JP. Enhanced recovery after surgery for oncological craniotomies. J Clin Neurosci. 2016;24:10–6. https://doi.org/10.1016/j.jocn.2015.08.013. Epub 2015 Oct 21. PMID: 26474504.
17. Nelson G, Bakkum-Gamez J, Kalogera E, Glaser G, Altman A, Meyer LA, Taylor JS, Iniesta M, Lasala J, Mena G, Scott M, Gillis C, Elias K, Wijk L, Huang J, Nygren J, Ljungqvist O, Ramirez PT, Dowdy SC. Guidelines for perioperative care in gynecologic/oncology: Enhanced Recovery After Surgery (ERAS) Society recommendations-2019 update. Int J Gynecol Cancer. 2019;29(4):651–68. https://doi.org/10.1136/ijgc-2019-000356. Epub 2019 Mar 15. PMID: 30877144.
18. Renner J, Moikow L, Lorenzen U. "Enhanced recovery after surgery" (ERAS): Weniger ist mehr: Was ist aus anästhesiologischer Sicht zu beachten? [Enhanced recovery after surgery (ERAS): less is more: What must be considered from an anesthesiological perspective?]. Chirurg. 2021;92(5):421–7. German. https://doi.org/10.1007/s00104-021-01360-6. Epub 2021 Feb 11. PMID: 33570691.
19. Oliveira ZSB, Silveira MLMD, Gomes PP, Silva JSPD, Germano AR. Early recovery after surgery protocol in orthognathic surgery: a randomized, blind clinical study. Braz Oral Res. 2021;35:e87. https://doi.org/10.1590/1807-3107bor-2021.vol35.0087. PMID: 34378669.
20. Soop M, Nygren J, Thorell A, Weidenhielm L, Lundberg M, Hammarqvist F, Ljungqvist O. Preoperative oral carbohydrate treatment attenuates endogenous glucose release 3 days after surgery. Clin Nutr. 2004;23(4):733–41. https://doi.org/10.1016/j.clnu.2003.12.007. PMID: 15297112.
21. Hausel J, Nygren J, Lagerkranser M, Hellström PM, Hammarqvist F, Almström C, Lindh A, Thorell A, Ljungqvist O. A carbohydrate-rich drink reduces preoperative discomfort in elective surgery patients. Anesth Analg. 2001;93(5):1344–50. https://doi.org/10.1097/00000539-200111000-00063. PMID: 11682427.
22. Slim K, Vicaut E, Launay-Savary MV, Contant C, Chipponi J. Updated systematic review and meta-analysis of randomized clinical trials on the role of mechanical bowel preparation before colorectal surgery. Ann Surg. 2009;249(2):203–9. https://doi.org/10.1097/SLA.0b013e318193425a. PMID: 19212171.
23. Lindström D, Sadr Azodi O, Wladis A, Tønnesen H, Linder S, Nåsell H, Ponzer S, Adami J. Effects of a perioperative smoking cessation intervention on postoperative complications: a randomized trial. Ann Surg. 2008;248(5):739–45. https://doi.org/10.1097/SLA.0b013e3181889d0d. PMID: 18948800.
24. Burnham EL. Identification of risky alcohol consumption in the preoperative assessment: opportunity to diagnose and intervene. Anesthesiology. 2008;109(2):169–70. https://doi.org/10.1097/ALN.0b013e31817f587a. PMID: 18648224; PMCID: PMC5695867.
25. Bell BR, Bastien PE, Douketis JD, Thrombosis Canada. Prevention of venous thromboembolism in the Enhanced Recovery After Surgery (ERAS) setting: an evidence-based review. Can J Anaesth. 2015;62(2):194–202. https://doi.org/10.1007/s12630-014-0262-2. Epub 2014 Nov 13. PMID: 25391732.

26. Caprini JA. Thrombosis risk assessment as a guide to quality patient care. Dis Mon. 2005;51(2–3):70–8. https://doi.org/10.1016/j.disamonth.2005.02.003. PMID: 15900257.
27. Caprini JA, Arcelus JI, Hasty JH, Tamhane AC, Fabrega F. Clinical assessment of venous thromboembolic risk in surgical patients. Semin Thromb Hemost. 1991;17(Suppl 3):304–12. PMID: 1754886.
28. Committee on Practice Bulletins--Gynecology, American College of Obstetricians and Gynecologists. ACOG Practice Bulletin No. 84: Prevention of deep vein thrombosis and pulmonary embolism. Obstet Gynecol. 2007;110(2 Pt 1):429–40. https://doi.org/10.1097/01.AOG.0000263919.23437.15. Erratum in: Obstet Gynecol. 2016 Jan;127(1):166. PMID: 17666620.
29. Gould MK, Garcia DA, Wren SM, Karanicolas PJ, Arcelus JI, Heit JA, Samama CM. Prevention of VTE in nonorthopedic surgical patients: antithrombotic therapy and prevention of thrombosis, 9th ed: American College of Chest Physicians Evidence-Based Clinical Practice Guidelines. Chest. 2012;141(2 Suppl):e227S–77S. https://doi.org/10.1378/chest.11-2297. Erratum in: Chest. 2012 May;141(5):1369. PMID: 22315263; PMCID: PMC3278061.
30. Stone R, Carey E, Fader AN, Fitzgerald J, Hammons L, Nensi A, Park AJ, Ricci S, Rosenfield R, Scheib S, Weston E. Enhanced recovery and surgical optimization protocol for minimally invasive gynecologic surgery: an AAGL white paper. J Minim Invasive Gynecol. 2021;28(2):179–203. https://doi.org/10.1016/j.jmig.2020.08.006. Epub 2020 Aug 20. PMID: 32827721.
31. Obermair A, Janda M, Baker J, Kondalsamy-Chennakesavan S, Brand A, Hogg R, Jobling TW, Land R, Manolitsas T, Nascimento M, Neesham D, Nicklin JL, Oehler MK, Otton G, Perrin L, Salfinger S, Hammond I, Leung Y, Sykes P, Ngan H, Garrett A, Laney M, Ng TY, Tam K, Chan K, Wrede DH, Pather S, Simcock B, Farrell R, Robertson G, Walker G, McCartney A, Gebski V. Improved surgical safety after laparoscopic compared to open surgery for apparent early stage endometrial cancer: results from a randomised controlled trial. Eur J Cancer. 2012;48(8):1147–53. https://doi.org/10.1016/j.ejca.2012.02.055. PMID: 22548907.
32. Walker JL, Piedmonte MR, Spirtos NM, Eisenkop SM, Schlaerth JB, Mannel RS, Spiegel G, Barakat R, Pearl ML, Sharma SK. Laparoscopy compared with laparotomy for comprehensive surgical staging of uterine cancer: Gynecologic Oncology Group Study LAP2. J Clin Oncol. 2009;27(32):5331.
33. Lin JH, Whelan RL, Sakellarios NE, Cekic V, Forde KA, Bank J, Feingold DL. Prospective study of ambulation after open and laparoscopic colorectal resection. Surg Innov. 2009;16(1):16–20. https://doi.org/10.1177/1553350608330478. Epub 2009 Jan 4. PMID: 19124446.
34. Bratzler DW, Dellinger EP, Olsen KM, Perl TM, Auwaerter PG, Bolon MK, Fish DN, Napolitano LM, Sawyer RG, Slain D, Steinberg JP. Clinical practice guidelines for antimicrobial prophylaxis in surgery. Surg Infect. 2013;14(1):73–156.
35. Alexander JW, Solomkin JS, Edwards MJ. Updated recommendations for control of surgical site infections. Ann Surg. 2011;253(6):1082–93. https://doi.org/10.1097/SLA.0b013e31821175f8. PMID: 21587113.
36. White PF, Kehlet H, Neal JM, Schricker T, Carr DB, Carli F, Fast-Track Surgery Study Group. The role of the anesthesiologist in fast-track surgery: from multimodal analgesia to perioperative medical care. Anesth Analg. 2007;104(6):1380–96, table of contents. https://doi.org/10.1213/01.ane.0000263034.96885.e1. PMID: 17513630.
37. Blaudszun G, Lysakowski C, Elia N, Tramèr MR. Effect of perioperative systemic α2 agonists on postoperative morphine consumption and pain intensity: systematic review and meta-analysis of randomized controlled trials. Anesthesiology. 2012;116(6):1312–22. https://doi.org/10.1097/ALN.0b013e31825681cb. PMID: 22546966.
38. Fragen RJ, Fitzgerald PC. Effect of dexmedetomidine on the minimum alveolar concentration (MAC) of sevoflurane in adults age 55 to 70 years. J Clin Anesth. 1999;11(6):466–70. https://doi.org/10.1016/s0952-8180(99)00081-1. PMID: 10526824.
39. Gan TJ, Diemunsch P, Habib AS, Kovac A, Kranke P, Meyer TA, Watcha M, Chung F, Angus S, Apfel CC, Bergese SD, Candiotti KA, Chan MT, Davis PJ, Hooper VD, Lagoo-Deenadayalan S, Myles P, Nezat G, Philip BK, Tramèr MR, Society for Ambulatory Anesthesia. Consensus guidelines for the management of postoperative nausea and vomiting. Anesth Analg. 2014;118(1):85–113. https://doi.org/10.1213/ANE.0000000000000002. Erratum in: Anesth Analg. 2014 Mar;118(3):689. Erratum in: Anesth Analg. 2015 Feb;120(2):494. PMID: 24356162.
40. Güldner A, Kiss T, Serpa Neto A, Hemmes SN, Canet J, Spieth PM, Rocco PR, Schultz MJ, Pelosi P, Gama de Abreu M. Intraoperative protective mechanical ventilation for prevention of postoperative pulmonary complications: a comprehensive review of the role of tidal volume, positive end-expiratory pressure, and lung recruitment maneuvers. Anesthesiology. 2015;123(3):692–713. https://doi.org/10.1097/ALN.0000000000000754. PMID: 26120769.
41. Jacob M, Chappell D, Rehm M. The 'third space'--fact or fiction? Best Pract Res Clin Anaesthesiol 2009;23(2):145–157. doi: https://doi.org/10.1016/j.bpa.2009.05.001. PMID: 19653435.
42. Chappell D, Jacob M, Hofmann-Kiefer K, Conzen P, Rehm M. A rational approach to perioperative fluid management. Anesthesiology. 2008;109(4):723–40. https://doi.org/10.1097/ALN.0b013e3181863117. PMID: 18813052.
43. Srinivasa S, Taylor MH, Singh PP, Yu TC, Soop M, Hill AG. Randomized clinical trial of goal-directed fluid therapy within an enhanced recovery protocol for elective colectomy. Br J Surg. 2013;100(1):66–74. https://doi.org/10.1002/bjs.8940. Epub 2012 Nov 6. PMID: 23132508.
44. Wong PF, Kumar S, Bohra A, Whetter D, Leaper DJ. Randomized clinical trial of perioperative systemic warming in major elective abdominal surgery. Br J Surg. 2007;94(4):421–6. https://doi.org/10.1002/bjs.5631. PMID: 17380549.
45. Steiner HL, Strand EA. Surgical-site infection in gynecologic surgery: pathophysiology and prevention. Am J Obstet Gynecol. 2017;217(2):121–8.
46. Mahdi H, Goodrich S, Lockhart D, DeBernardo R, Moslemi-Kebria M. Predictors of surgical site infection in women undergoing hysterectomy for benign gynecologic disease: a multicenter analysis using the national surgical quality improvement program data. J Minim Invasive Gynecol. 2014;21(5):901–9.
47. Martin ET, Kaye KS, Knott C, Nguyen H, Santarossa M, Evans R, Bertran E, Jaber L. Diabetes and risk of surgical site infection: a systematic review and meta-analysis. Infect Control Hosp Epidemiol. 2016;37(1):88–99.
48. Petrowsky H, Demartines N, Rousson V, Clavien PA. Evidence-based value of prophylactic drainage in gastrointestinal surgery: a systematic review and meta-analyses. Ann Surg. 2004;240(6):1074–84; discussion 1084–5. https://doi.org/10.1097/01.sla.0000146149.17411.c5. PMID: 15570212; PMCID: PMC1356522.
49. Cheatham ML, Chapman WC, Key SP, Sawyers JL. A meta-analysis of selective versus routine nasogastric decompression after elective laparotomy. Ann Surg. 1995;221(5):469–76; discussion 476–8. https://doi.org/10.1097/00000658-199505000-00004. PMID: 7748028; PMCID: PMC1234620.
50. Nelson R, Tse B, Edwards S. Systematic review of prophylactic nasogastric decompression after abdominal operations. J Br Surg. 2005;92(6):673–80.
51. Papaspyros S, Uppal S, Khan SA, Paul S, O'Regan DJ. Analysis of bedside entertainment services' effect on post cardiac surgery physical activity: a prospective, randomised clinical trial. Eur J

Cardiothorac Surg. 2008;34(5):1022–6. https://doi.org/10.1016/j.ejcts.2008.05.042. Epub 2008 Aug 15. PMID: 18706826.
52. Massey RL. A randomized trial of rocking-chair motion on the effect of postoperative ileus duration in patients with cancer recovering from abdominal surgery. Appl Nurs Res. 2010;23(2):59–64. https://doi.org/10.1016/j.apnr.2008.06.001. Epub 2009 Jan 15. PMID: 20420991.
53. Han-Geurts IJ, Hop WC, Kok NF, Lim A, Brouwer KJ, Jeekel J. Randomized clinical trial of the impact of early enteral feeding on postoperative ileus and recovery. Br J Surg. 2007;94(5):555–61. https://doi.org/10.1002/bjs.5753. PMID: 17443854.
54. Andersen HK, Lewis SJ, Thomas S. Early enteral nutrition within 24h of colorectal surgery versus later commencement of feeding for postoperative complications. Cochrane Database Syst Rev. 2006;(4):CD004080. https://doi.org/10.1002/14651858.CD004080.pub2. Update in: Cochrane Database Syst Rev. 2018 Oct 24;10:CD004080. PMID: 17054196.
55. Buvanendran A, Kroin JS. Multimodal analgesia for controlling acute postoperative pain. Curr Opin Anaesthesiol. 2009;22(5):588–93. https://doi.org/10.1097/ACO.0b013e328330373a. PMID: 19606021.

Part II

TLH by Different Approaches

Comprehensive Canopy Concept of Bladder Dissection 'The 3 Step Technique': An Approach to Total Laparoscopic Hysterectomy (TLH)

6

Nutan Jain, Sakshi Srivastava, and Priyanka Sureddi

6.1 Introduction

While gynaecologists have traditionally employed the lateral technique for bladder dissection in Total Laparoscopic Hysterectomy (TLH), recent meta-analyses and review papers from the last 5–6 years reveal that the incidence of bladder injuries has persisted [1]. Additionally, the prevalence of patients with ventrifixed uterus [2] identified as a surgical finding on the operating table, is on the rise due to the increased occurrence of caesarean sections [3] In response to the challenges posed by these adhesions, the Comprehensive Canopy Concept has been developed. This innovative technique, comprising three distinct steps, aims to address and improve outcomes in the presence of the most severe adhesions. This approach holds promise for enhancing the management of adhesions encountered during TLH, especially in cases with ventrifixed uterus and scarred utero vesical fold as a result of increased incidence of caesarean sections.

Total Laparoscopic Hysterectomy (TLH) is a minimally invasive surgical procedure promising faster recovery in all complex scenarios. With the rising rates of caesarean sections, gynaecologists are encountering an increasing number of patients with a history of caesarean sections. Bladder dissection is a crucial step in TLH, as it requires meticulous attention to detail to ensure a safe and effective procedure. We have developed our Comprehensive Canopy Concept, 'The 3 Step Technique' for bladder dissection during TLH, aiming to optimize visualization, minimize complications, and enhance surgical outcomes. With the increasing number of caesarean sections, we have been working persistently to pave our way to deal with extreme ventrifixed scarred uterus. We have diligently developed our Comprehensive Canopy Concept (Fig. 6.1a, b) to bladder dissection in total laparoscopic hysterectomy after patiently navigating through a spectrum of scarred uterus, aiming to enhance our capabilities in addressing these complex cases. We begin TLH by coagulating and cutting the left cornual structures in a sequential manner. After dealing with the left adnexa, our technique unfolds as described below.

Comprehensive Canopy Concept, 'The 3 Step Technique': Our systematic canopy approach to bladder dissection in total laparoscopic hysterectomy is clearly divided into three steps,

1. **Posterior approach of uterine artery section** (Fig. 6.2) [4–13]—The posterior leaf of broad ligament is transected widely from utero sacral ligaments to arcus torinus over the cephalad pushed manipulator cup, which is further pushed cephalad by the vaginal assistant at this step. This posterior approach exposes the uterine vein first, and then the uterine artery is exposed easily. The uterine artery pedicle is skeletonized, coagulated and cut with the

Supplementary Information The online version contains supplementary material available at https://doi.org/10.1007/978-981-97-3226-5_6. The videos can be accessed individually by clicking the DOI link in the accompanying figure caption or by scanning this link with the SN More Media App.

N. Jain (✉)
Obstetrics and Gynaecology, GSVM Medical College, Affiliated by Kanpur University, Kanpur, Uttar Pradesh, India

Department of Obstetrics and Gynecology, Vardhman Trauma and Laparoscopy Centre Pvt. Ltd., Muzaffarnagar, Uttar Pradesh, India

S. Srivastava
Obstetrics and Gynaecology, Rohilkhand Medical College and Hospital, Affiliated by Bareilly International University, Bareilly, Uttar Pradesh, India

Gynaecology Endoscopy, Vardhman Trauma and Laparoscopy Centre Pvt. Ltd., Muzaffarnagar, Uttar Pradesh, India

P. Sureddi
Gynaecology Endoscopy, Vardhman Trauma and Laparoscopy Centre Pvt. Ltd., Muzaffarnagar, Uttar Pradesh, India

Obstetrics and Gynaecology, Seth GS Medical College and KEM Hospital, Affiliated by Maharashtra University of Health Sciences, Mumbai, India

N. Jain (ed.), *Complex Total Laparoscopic Hysterectomy (TLH) with Newer Approaches in Bladder Dissection*,
https://doi.org/10.1007/978-981-97-3226-5_6

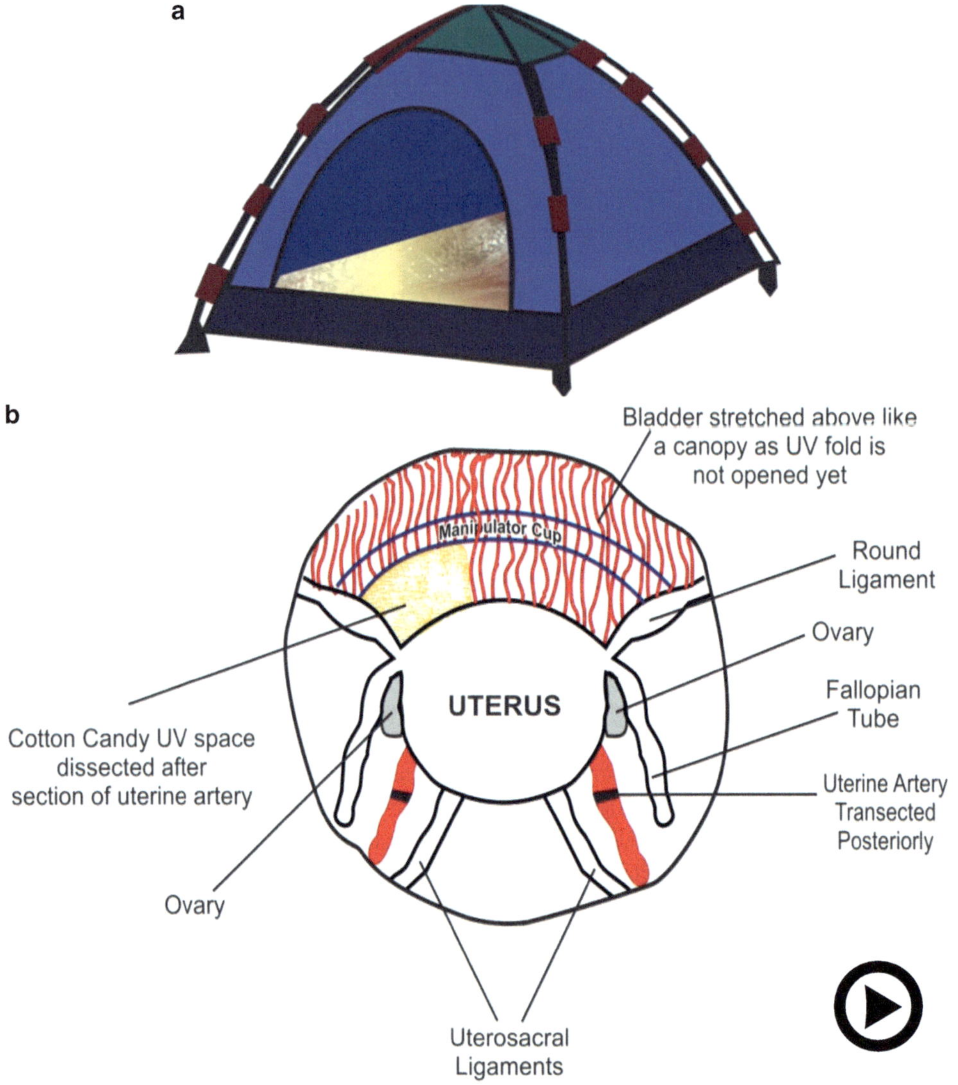

Fig. 6.1 **a** Canopy means that the bladder is stretched above and we create the cotton candy uterovesical space below (Video 6.1 Comprehensive Canopy Concept of Bladder Dissection in TLH) (▶ https://doi.org/10.1007/000-c92). **b** Diagrammatic Representation of Canopy Concept

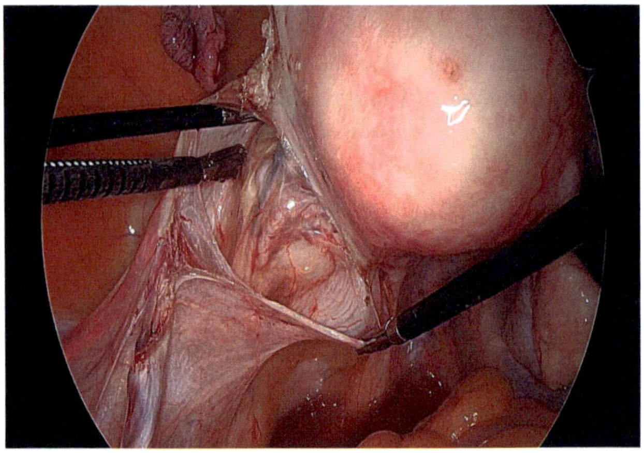

Fig. 6.2 The first step of Comprehensive Canopy Concept, 'The 3 Step Technique' is posterior approach of uterine artery section

help of ultrasonic energy, before developing the bladder flap and before any adhesiolysis in the anterior cul de sac.

The posterior approach works on three anatomical fundamental principles:

(a) The plane of the uterine artery is the same as bladder dissection (Fig. 6.3).
(b) The uterine artery holds the ureters to uterus, so early uterine artery sectioning cuts the transverse cervical ligament too, thereby facilitating lateral and inferior movement of the ureter, minimizing the risk of ureteric injury (Fig. 6.4).
(c) Bladder adherence is more on top at the body of uterus rather than at the level of cervical isthmus which is delineated by the manipulator cup, so dissection to reach the utero vesical cotton candy space is effortless, avascular & minimizes risk of bladder injury (Fig. 6.5).

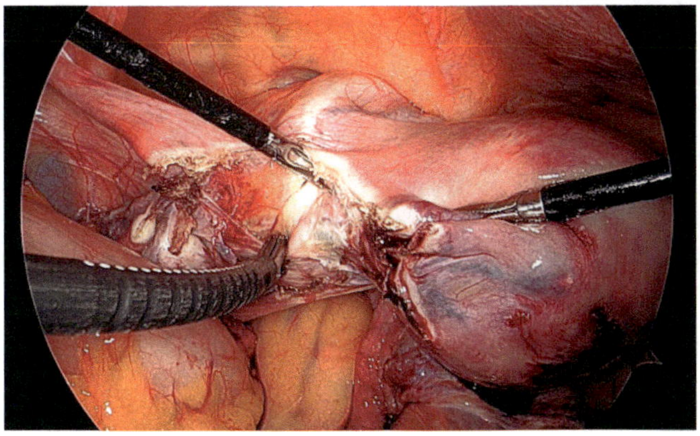

Fig. 6.3 The plane of uterine artery is same as bladder dissection

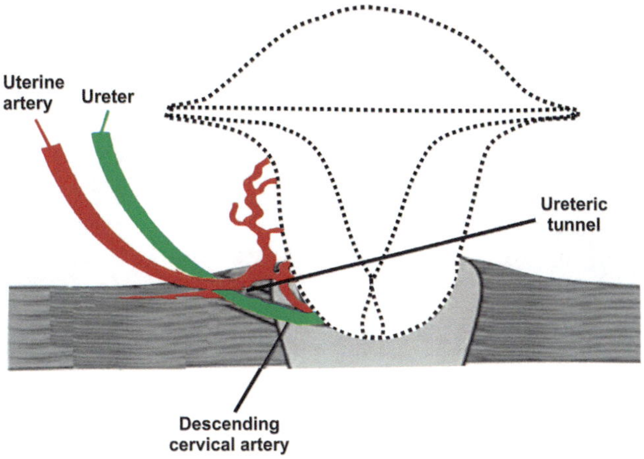

Fig. 6.4 The uterine artery holds the ureters to uterus, so early uterine artery sectioning cuts the transverse cervical ligament too, thereby facilitating lateral and inferior movement of the ureter, minimizing the risk of ureteric injury

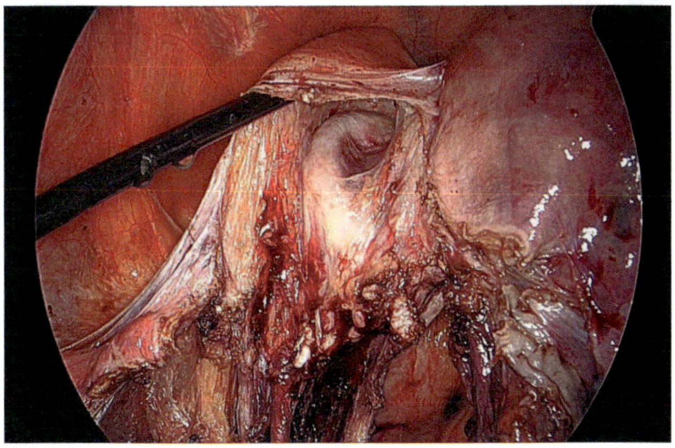

Fig. 6.5 Bladder adherence is more on top at the body of uterus rather than at the level of cervical isthmus which is delineated by manipulator cup

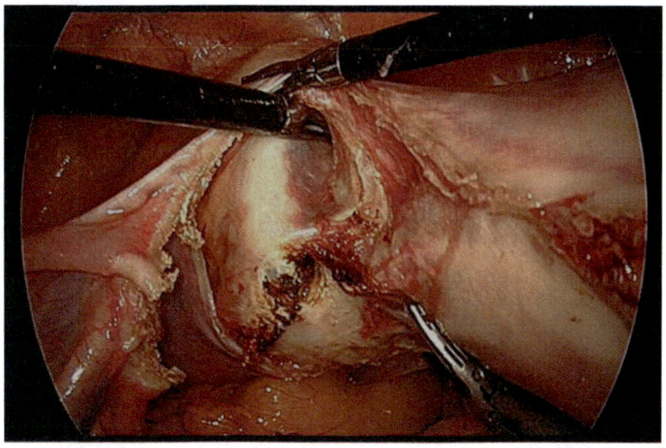

Fig. 6.6 The second step of 3 Step Technique is Canopy concept of bladder dissection

2. **Canopy Concept of bladder dissection** (Fig. 6.6) [14]
   - After sectioning of uterine artery over the cranially pushed manipulator cup, we dissect 1 cm anteromedial to the coagulated uterine artery and our atraumatic grasper is insinuated to find the plane of bladder dissection over the cephalad pushed manipulator cup. This dissection in the 1 cm, just area next to the cut pedicle of uterine artery is the most crucial step. It is pertinent not to give up soon, even in the face of densely adherent bladder, we need to persist at this point, continuing dissection until the shiny, glistening pubo-cervical fascia is exposed. Once we get the pubo-vesical cervical fascia the creation of bladder canopy becomes easy.
   - We navigate beneath the road block of bladder adhesions by using the underpass of cotton candy utero-vesical space which is demarcated by the manipulator cup (Fig. 6.7a, b). We keep dissecting in this avascular plane and the uterovesical space is dissected under the bladder canopy of adhesions until we reach the other end of the manipulator cup. This manoeuvre is facilitated by the cephalad push of the manipulator cup (Fig. 6.8) and the bladder is gently pushed downward beneath the manipulator cup, employing atraumatic graspers to ensure an avascular, effortless and precise procedure (Fig. 6.9).
   - Once the uterovesical space is opened completely (Fig. 6.10), then the stuck bladder flap at the top is cut, remaining close to the uterus to avoid any bladder injury. This allows for avascular effortless downward movement of the densely adherent bladder flap. In fact, the bladder simply walks down (Fig. 6.11).

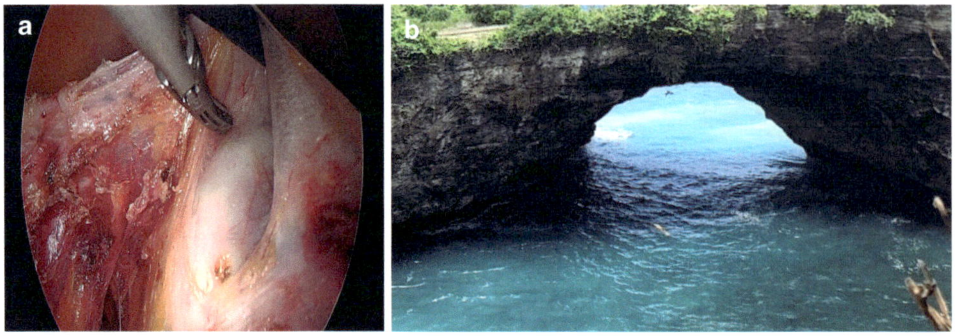

Fig. 6.7 **a**, **b** We navigate beneath the road block of bladder adhesions by using the underpass of cotton candy uterovesical space demarcated by the manipulator cup

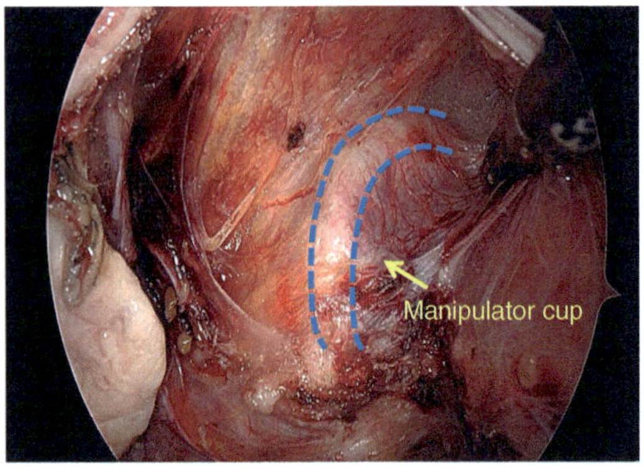

Fig. 6.8 The cup of the uterine manipulator is pushed cephalad by pelvic assistant, and the loosely adherent bladder at this level just walk down in an avascular manner

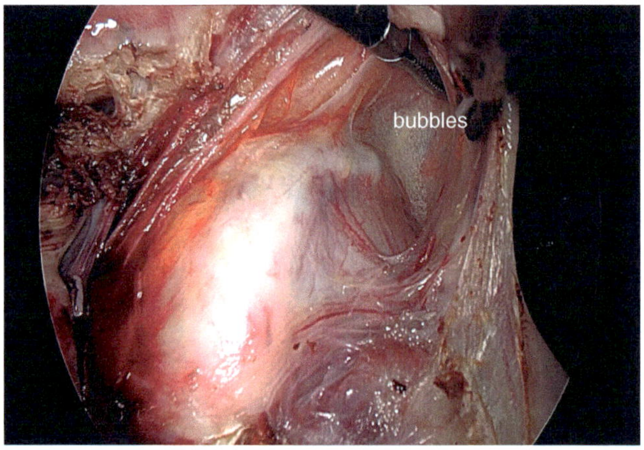

Fig. 6.10 Cotton candy uterovesical space

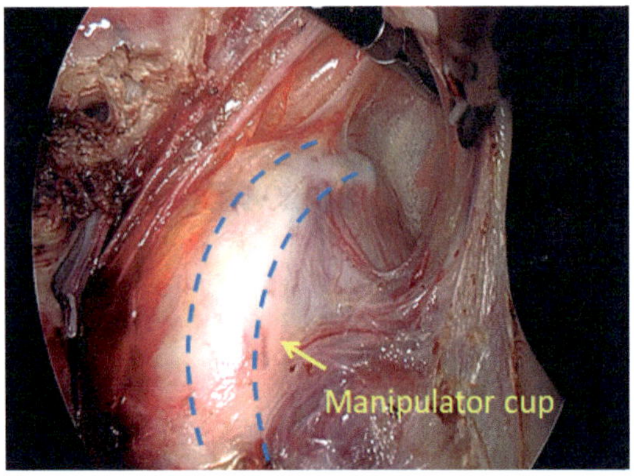

Fig. 6.9 Pneumoperitoneum seeps in the uterovesical space and opens up the cotton candy space making the dissection easier

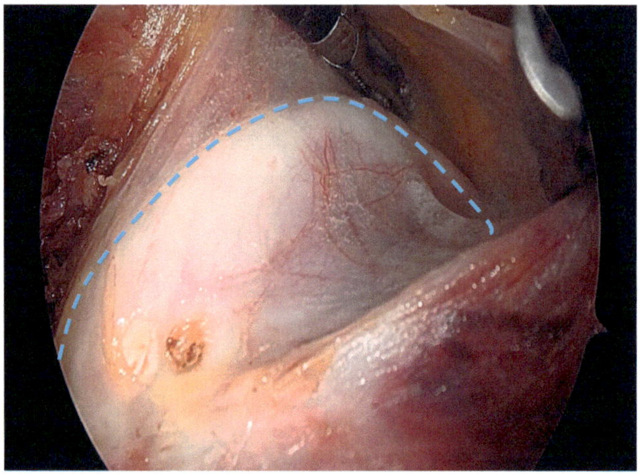

Fig. 6.11 Avascular effortless downwards movement of the bladder

3. **Anterior approach of contralateral uterine artery dissection** (Fig. 6.12)—This is third step in canopy approach, and that is why we call it as Comprehensive Canopy Concept, 'The 3 Step Technique'. As we realized that the avascular plane of bladder dissection can be further worked up till the contralateral round ligament. And, in doing so, the uterine artery and vein are exposed by the side of the manipulator cup. By few snips by grasper or better by ultrasonic device, we get beautiful skelotonization of uterine artery and vein which are coagulated & cut by the anterior approach.

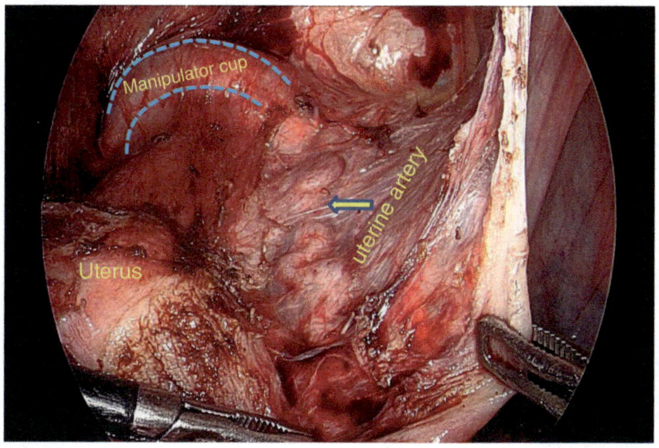

Fig. 6.12 The third step of comprehensive canopy concept is anterior approach of contralateral uterine artery dissection

- We keep dissecting beneath the established canopy until we reach the spirally winding right side uterine artery and vein, positioned adjacent to the manipulator cup rim.
- Once the contralateral (usually the right) uterine artery and vein are skeletonized completely, they are coagulated and cut with the help of ultrasonic energy. The uterine pedicle is cut beneath the edge of the manipulator cup, and is thus shaved off the manipulator cup rim.

Then the right-sided adnexa is coagulated and cut in a sequential manner. We perform a circumferential culdotomy with a monopolar hook. The colpotomy can be performed by ultrasonic energy also, but we will need a stainless-steel cup for that. The vault suspension is done and the vault is sutured in double layers using polygalactin sutures. We perform all types of TLH at our centre with this 3 step technique which is easily reproducible by the fellows and other consultants at our setup, making the TLH safe in daunting situations of previous caesarean section and ventrally fixed uterus. Our steps of total laparoscopic hysterectomy are portrayed through the following figures (Fig. 6.13a–t). So gradually we progressed from only posterior approach of uterine artery to making a bladder canopy and the third step of anterior approach of contralateral uterine artery dissection to complete the comprehensive canopy approach.

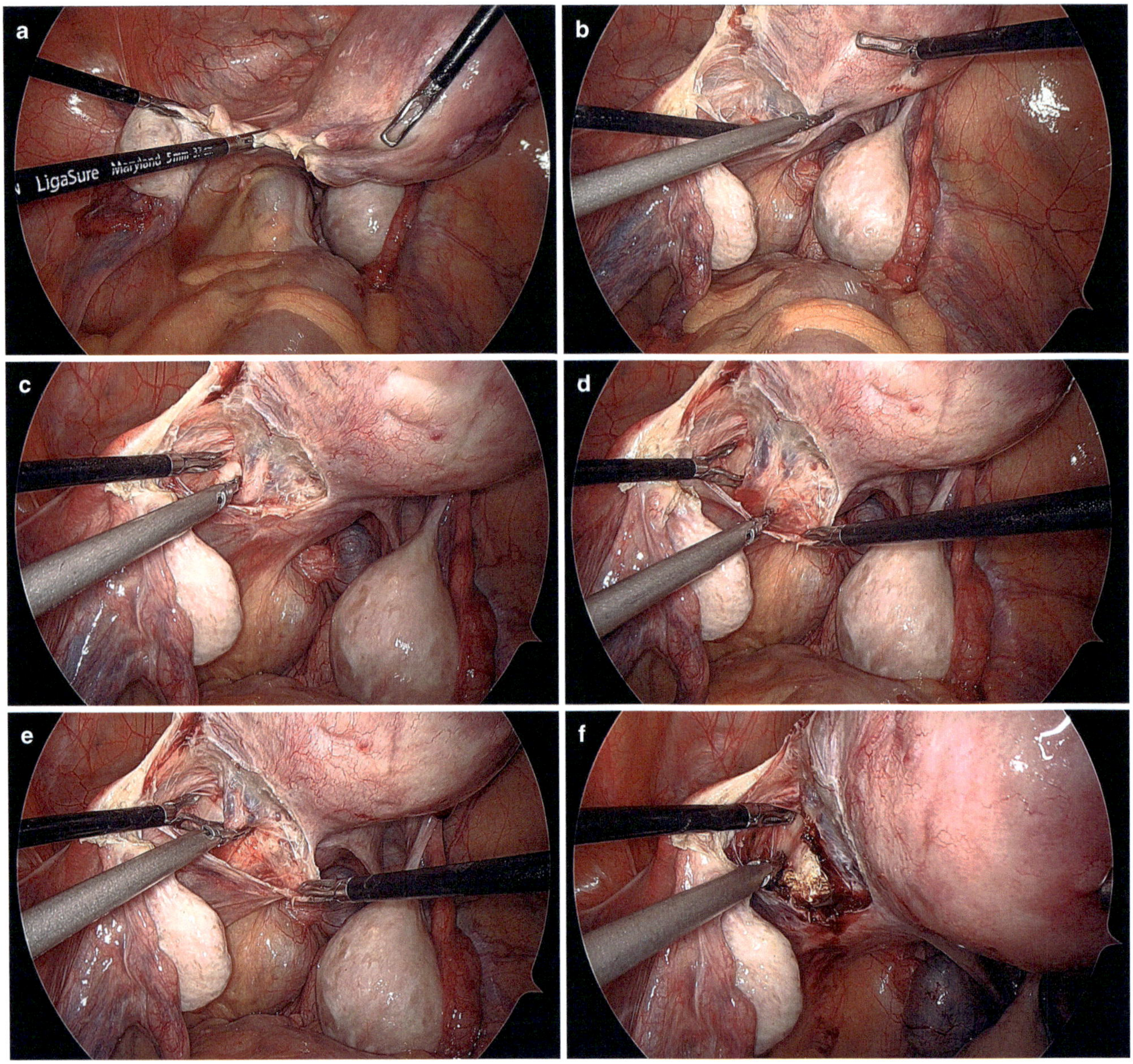

Fig. 6.13 **a** Coagulation and cutting of left adnexa. **b** Opening of posterior leaf of broad ligament. **c** Uterine vein followed by uterine artery starts showing up. **d** Skeletonization of left uterine artery pedicle. **e** Coagulation and transection of left uterine artery pedicle. **f** Dissection 1 cm anterior to coagulated uterine artery to find the plane of bladder dissection. **g** This plane is the key to a successful bladder dissection. **h** Dissection continues under the bladder canopy over the stretched out manipulator cup. **i** Cotton candy uterovesical space opens up easily as pneumoperitoneum seeps in. **j** Dissection continues under the canopy to open up the uterovesical space completely. **k** Once the uterovesical space opens up, the stuck bladder flap at the top is cut. **l** Further dissection done till we reach the right round ligament. **m** Anterior approach of contralateral uterine artery dissection. **n** Skeletonization of right uterine artery by anterior approach. **o** Coagulation and cutting of right uterine artery pedicle. **p** The cut uterine artery pedicle is shaved off the manipulator cup. **q** Right adnexa is coagulated and. **r** The bare manipulator cup is ready for colpotomy. **s** Circumferential culdotomy performed by monopolar hook. **t** Vault closure and suspension done in double layers using polyglactin sutures

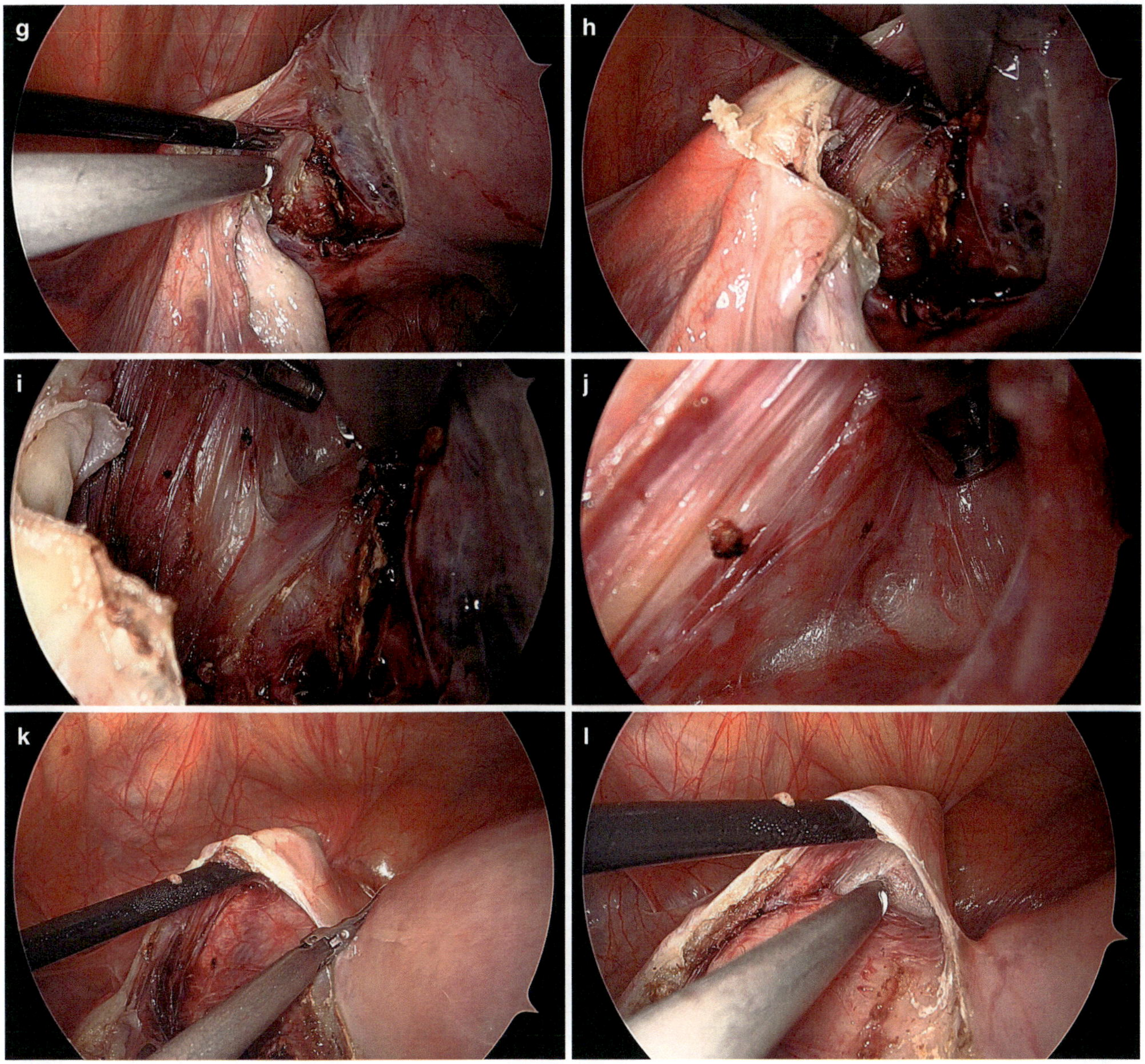

Fig. 6.13 (continued)

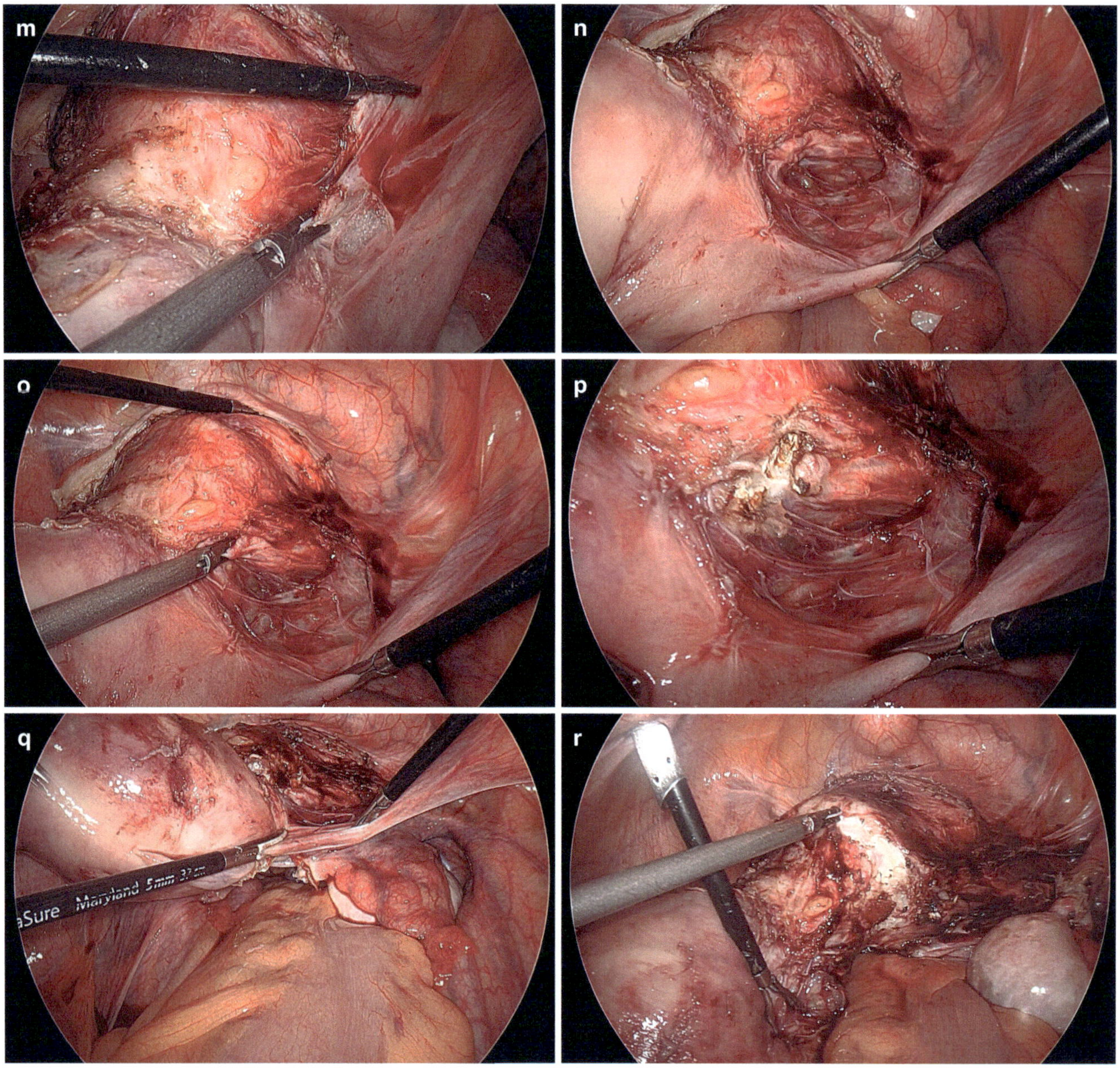

Fig. 6.13 (continued)

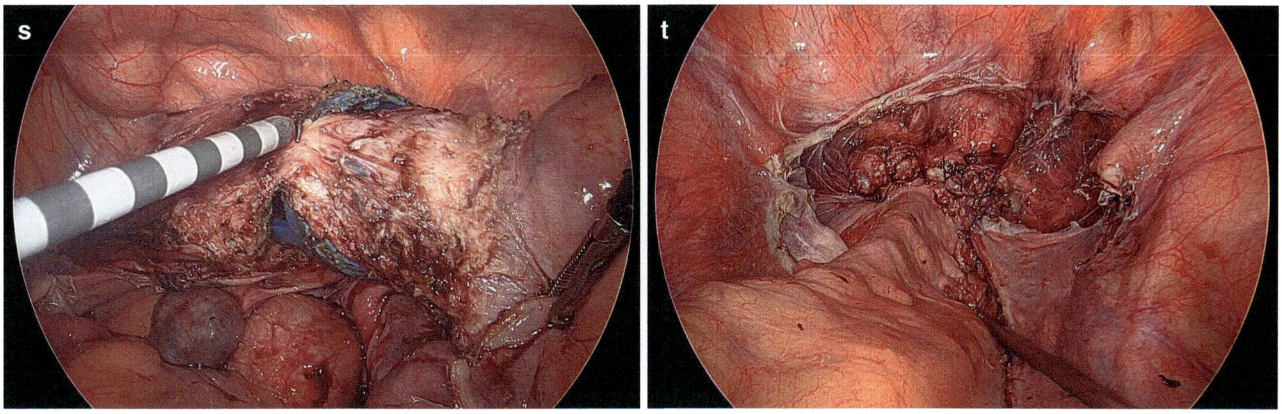

Fig. 6.13 (continued)

6.2 Role of Uterine Manipulator

The role of uterine manipulator as described in our 3 step technique is paramount. Uterine manipulator inserted in the beginning of surgery plays a pivotal role in TLH by providing the manipulation of uterus, creating the correct amount of tissue tension for better visualization, identification of the vaginal fornices, sealing of the vagina during a hysterectomy and facilitating precise surgical manoeuvres. The posterior approach of uterine artery ligation is begun on the rim of the manipulator cup. We use stout platform provided by the broad rim of the cup to open up the retroperitonium posteriorly, skeletonize and section the uterine artery. The cephalad push by the assistant during the maneuver of dissecting out the pubo-vesico cervical fascia, becomes well defined in a much easier manner over the cup. Once the plane is defined, a further cephalad push on the manipulator cup pushes the bladder down effortlessly. Similarly doing the anterior approach of contralateral uterine artery ligation becomes much easy over the rim of the manipulator cup. So in the Comprehensive Canopy Concept, role of good manipulator cannot be further emphasized. Hence, every surgical units need to patronize one or two types of uterine manipulators, with which the team gets comfortable. This also takes into consideration the disposable components or totally re-usable manipulator. In several units, disposable components may not be cost effective. Luckily over a span of three decades of the advent of the laparoscopic hysterectomy, a wide array of manipulators are available with specific features and the surgical units choose upon a manipulator which suits their specific needs, best.

6.3 Conclusion

We present our Comprehensive Canopy Concept, 'The 3 Step Technique' for bladder dissection in total laparoscopic hysterectomy; which starts with one side uterine artery dissection by posterior approach before the bladder dissection, navigate in the cotton candy space beneath the stretched-out bladder canopy of adhesions and finish the contralateral uterine artery section by anterior approach. In a way it is an endeavour to complete TLH safely in one single sweep, starting from one side usually the left. This systematic approach to Total Laparoscopic Hysterectomy (TLH), employing a series of these manoeuvres, is designed to facilitate easy bladder dissection in an avascular plane with a single sweep. The primary goal is to minimize the risk of bladder and ureteric injuries [15], underscoring our commitment to enhancing the safety of TLH procedures.

Learning Points

- Identification of key structures before proceeding with the dissection is must.
- Exposing and skeletonizing the uterine artery with the easier posterior approach ensures haemostasis throughout the dissection.
- The plane of uterine artery is the same as bladder dissection, so insinuating grasper adjacent to the cut pedicle of uterine artery opens up the uterovesical space.
- Immediate 1–2 cm area anterior and medial to cut uterine artery pedicle is most important to continue dissection till we reach the shiny glistering pubo-vesicle cervical fascia. This step is the key to gaining access to vesico-cervical cotton candy space.

- Bladder flap is adherent to the body of uterus and free at the level of cervical isthmus so navigating the cotton candy uterovesical space below the densely adherent bladder canopy, helps in avascular effortless downward movement of the bladder; preventing bladder and ureteric injury.
- Anterior approach to uterine ligation includes continuous dissection upto the round ligament in the cotton candy utero vesical space skeletonizes the uterine artery and vein very easily on the contralateral side.

Competing Interest The author declares no conflict of interest that are relevant to content of this chapter.

Ethical Approval Informed consent was obtained from individual participants and patients regarding publication and documentation without disclosing their identity.

References

1. Jelovsek JE, Chiung C, Chen G, Roberts SL, Paraiso MF, Falcone T. Incidence of lower urinary tract injury at the time of total laparoscopic hysterectomy. JSLS. 2007;11(4):422–7. PMID: 18237504; PMCID: PMC3015849.
2. Rao T, Kade S. Ventrofixed uterus: unfreezing the uterus in 6 standardized steps. J Gynecol Surg. 2023;39(5):220–1. https://doi.org/10.1089/gyn.2023.0041. Epub 2023 Oct 3. PMID: 37817874; PMCID: PMC10561766.
3. Angolile CM, Max BL, Mushemba J, Mashauri HL. Global increased cesarean section rates and public health implications: a call to action. Health Sci Rep. 2023;6(5):e1274. https://doi.org/10.1002/hsr2.1274. PMID: 37216058; PMCID: PMC10196217.
4. Sinha R, Sundaram M, Lakhotia S, Hedge A, Kadam P. Total laparoscopic hysterectomy in women with previous cesarean sections. J Minim Invasive Gynecol. 2010;17(4):513–7. https://doi.org/10.1016/j.jmig.2010.03.018. PMID: 20621012.
5. Nezhat C, Grace LA, Razavi GM, Mihailide C, Bamford H. Reverse vesicouterine fold dissection for laparoscopic hysterectomy after prior cesarean deliveries. Obstet Gynecol. 2016;128(3):629–33. https://doi.org/10.1097/AOG.0000000000001593.
6. Marwah V, et al. Total laparoscopic hysterectomy with bilateral salpingectomy with sutures using posterior approach for uterine artery ligation. J Minim Invasive Gynecol. 2016;23(S1):S252.
7. Chamsy DJ, Lee T. Posterior approach to uterine artery ligation for anterior cul-de-sac obliteration. J Minim Invasive Gynecol. 2012;19(6):S10.
8. Jain N. Posterior approach for uterine artery ligation in TLH (tackling the uterine artery first before bladder dissection). J Minim Invasive Gynecol. 2022;29(11):S135–6.
9. Srivastava S, Jain N, Jain V, Jain S. Posterior approach: a new approach for dealing uterine artery first, before the bladder dissection in TLH. Presented in European Society for Gynaecological Endoscopy (ESGE), October 2–5, 2022, Lisbon, Portugal.
10. Musgrove F. Abdominal total hysterectomy: a new technique: the posterior approach. Proc R Soc Med. 1955;48(9):692.
11. Frank M. Abdominal total hysterectomy. A new technique: the posterior approach. JAMA. 1957;165(10):1350–1. https://doi.org/10.1001/jama.1957.02980280124026.
12. Li D, Zhang Y, Cao J, Shi L. Application of the posterior approach technique in laparoscopic radical hysterectomy for cervical cancer. J Cancer Sci Clin Oncol. 2019;6(1):101.
13. Fiori C, Patel NR, Namaky DD. Posterior approach to uterine artery ligation. J Minim Invasive Gynecol. 2019;26:S98–S231.
14. Jain N. Canopy concept of difficult bladder dissection in TLH. Presented in The Society of Laparoscopic & Robotic Surgeons (SLS), October 4–7, 2023, at Lake Buena Vista, Florida, USA.
15. Ostrzenski A, Ostrzenska KM. Bladder injury during laparoscopic surgery. Obstet Gynecol Surv. 1998;53(3):175–80. https://doi.org/10.1097/00006254-199803000-00023. PMID: 9513988.

Lateral Approach for Bladder Dissection

7

Alison M. Zeccola and Suketu Mansuria

7.1 Introduction

When performing a laparoscopic hysterectomy, surgeons may encounter dense adhesions between the bladder and the lower uterine segment. Cesarean delivery is the most common risk factor for formation of these dense adhesions. In the United States, rates of cesarean delivery increased to 60% from 20.7% in 1996 to 32.9% in 2009. Since 2009, the cesarean delivery rate in the US has been relatively stable at 31–32%. In general, this rate varies but may be higher in other countries. This accounts for a significant number of births, and many women require subsequent hysterectomy for numerous indications after their child bearing is complete [1]

Studies show that cesarean delivery is a significant risk factor for genitourinary tract (GU) injury at time of hysterectomy. Rooney et al. (2005) published a case-control study examining relationship between history of prior cesarean and GU injury during subsequent hysterectomy and found that cesarean delivery is an independent risk factor for GU injury (OR 2.04). Their study also found a greater risk of cystotomy in a laparoscopic versus abdominal approach (OR 7.5 vs 1.26) in this patient population (Rooney). Therefore, having a systematic approach to the difficult, scarred bladder flap is crucial in order to avoid genitourinary tract injury [2].

We propose a three-step approach to the difficult bladder dissection. In order to illustrate each step, we present a case of a patient with 2 prior cesarean deliveries undergoing total laparoscopic hysterectomy for benign indications. The uterus was completely adherent to the anterior abdominal wall with dense scarring of the anterior cul de sac (Fig. 7.1).

In general, it is important to perform the straightforward steps of the hysterectomy first, and we recommend leaving the bladder flap for the last part of the case, as securing the blood supply and restoring normal anatomy will aid in dissection.

7.1.1 Step 1: Secure the Blood Supply

We secure the four major vascular pedicles of the uterus prior to proceeding with bladder flap dissection. Typically, the upper pedicles with the ovarian blood supply are accessible and should be secured first. In this case, the utero-ovarian (UO) ligaments have been coagulated and transected bilaterally (Fig. 7.2).

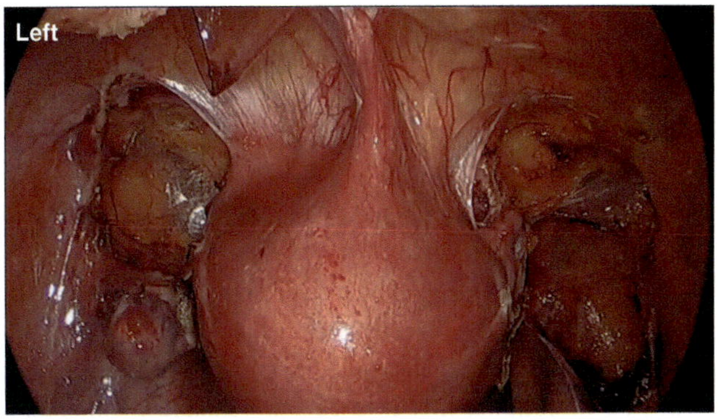

Fig. 7.1 Uterus densely adherent to anterior abdominal wall after 2 cesarean deliveries

Supplementary Information The online version contains supplementary material available at https://doi.org/10.1007/978-981-97-3226-5_7. The videos can be accessed individually by clicking the DOI link in the accompanying figure caption or by scanning this link with the SN More Media App.

A. M. Zeccola
Minimally Invasive Gynecologic Surgery, Magee-Womens Hospital, University of Pittsburgh Medical Center, Pittsburgh, PA, USA

S. Mansuria (✉)
Gynecologic Minimally Invasive Surgery, Magee-Womens Hospital, University of Pittsburgh Medical Center, Pittsburgh, PA, USA
e-mail: manssm@upmc.edu

N. Jain (ed.), *Complex Total Laparoscopic Hysterectomy (TLH) with Newer Approaches in Bladder Dissection*,
https://doi.org/10.1007/978-981-97-3226-5_7

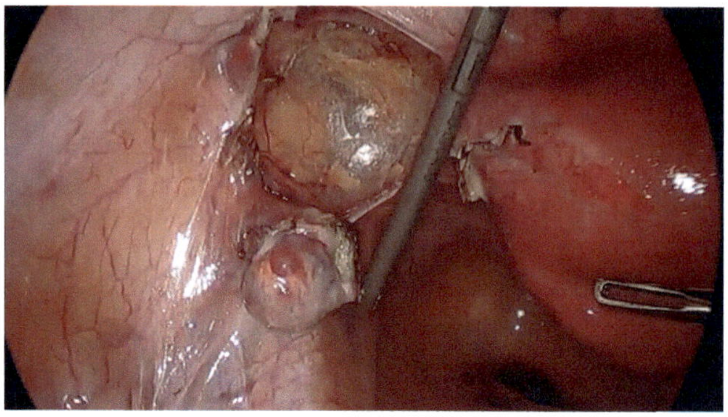

Fig. 7.2 Upper vascular pedicles—Utero-ovarian ligaments coagulated and transected

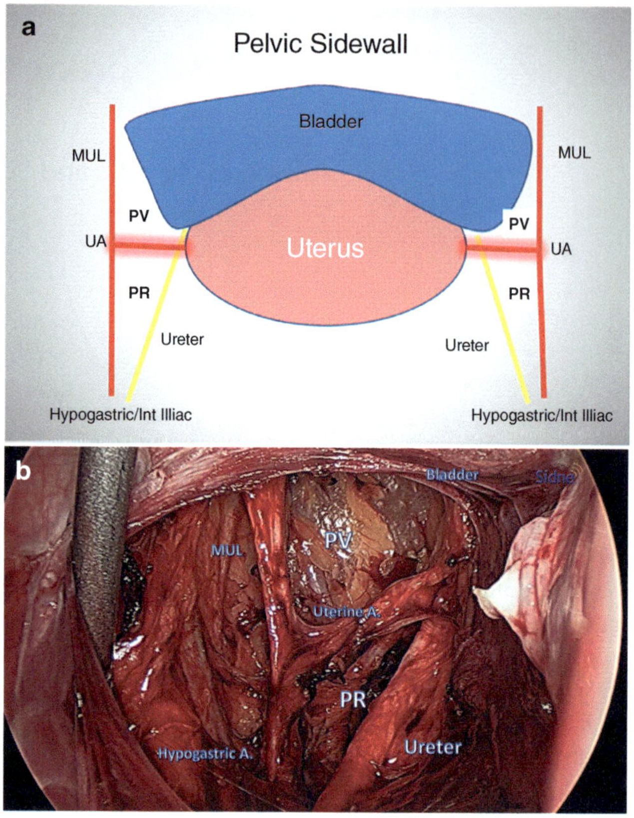

Fig. 7.3 **a** Diagram of paravesical (PV) and pararectal (PR) retroperitoneal spaces. **b** Dissection of paravesical (PV) and pararectal (PR) retroperitoneal spaces. MUL medial umbilical ligament, PV paravesical space, PR pararectal space, UA uterine artery

Next, we recommend securing the lower pedicles of the uterine arteries bilaterally. When the bladder is severely scarred, it is typically pulled towards the location where the uterine artery is traditionally controlled—at the level of the internal os. In these cases, we recommend controlling the uterine artery at its origin off of the hypogastric or internal iliac artery prior to approaching the adherent bladder flap. By controlling the uterine artery out laterally at its origin off the hypogastric artery, unintentional thermal injury to the scarred bladder is avoided and the uterus is devascularized. Securing the blood supply minimizes blood loss during the difficult bladder dissection; thereby improving visualization and reducing the risk of inadvertent bladder injury.

In order to find the uterine artery at it is origin off the hypogastric artery, it is important to know and develop the avascular spaces of the retroperitoneum. Here we discuss our approach to developing the paravesical and pararectal spaces. Both spaces are triangular and share a common border of the uterine artery. The paravesical space has a medial border of the bladder, lateral border of the medial umbilical ligament (MUL) and inferior border of the uterine artery. The pararectal space has a medial border of the ureter, lateral border of the hypogastric artery and superior border of the uterine artery (Fig. 7.3a, b).

There are three approaches to perform this dissection: lateral, posterior and anterior. The lateral approach is most familiar to gynecologists. This involves making a peritoneal incision from the round ligament parallel to the infundibulopelvic ligament (IP). The assistant then pulls the posterior leaf of the broad ligament both medially and posteriorly, allowing the surgeon to identify the ureter along the posterior leaf of the broad ligament (Figs. 7.4 and 7.5).

The pararectal space is just lateral to the ureter (Fig. 7.6). This avascular space is developed further with blunt dissection by spreading two instruments in the areolar tissue in opposing directions; first in a cephalo-caudad manner and then in a lateral to medial vector. The uterine artery is the border between the pararectal and paravesical space, so the same blunt dissection technique is then used anterior to the uterine artery to develop the paravesical space (Fig. 7.7).

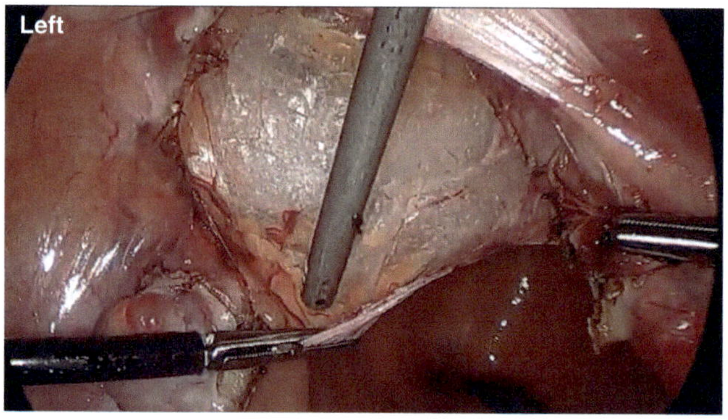

Fig. 7.4 Lateral approach to retroperitoneal dissection on the left side of the pelvis

Given the anatomic relationship of these retroperitoneal spaces, once one component is identified, such as the ureter, gentle dissection can help find the other structures easily (ie. dissection lateral to the ureter will develop the pararectal space and identify the hypogastric artery). Once these avascular surgical spaces are delineated, we can see the uterine

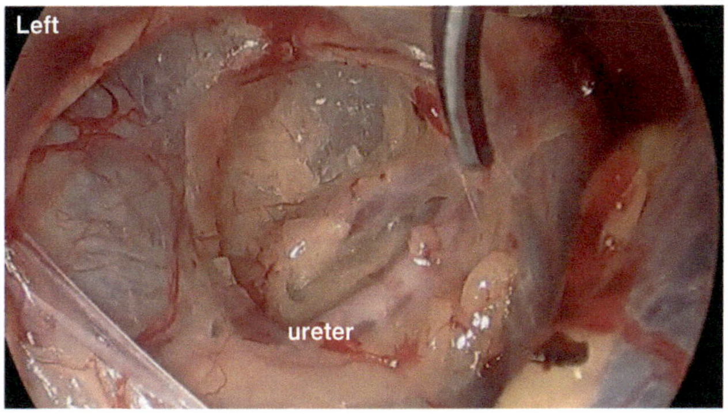

Fig. 7.5 Ureter located retroperitoneally on posterior leaf of broad ligament on the left side of the pelvis

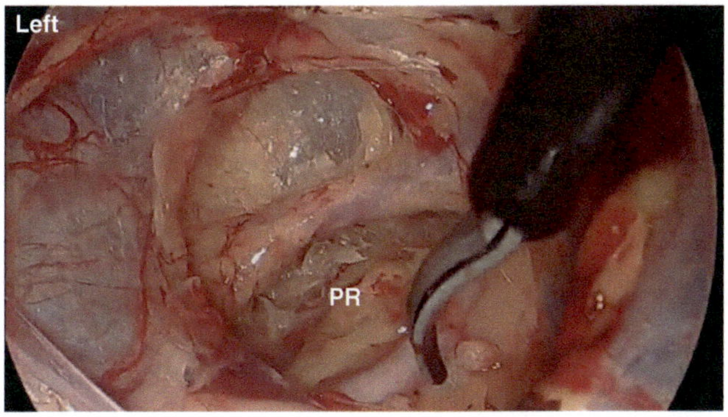

Fig. 7.6 Pararectal space

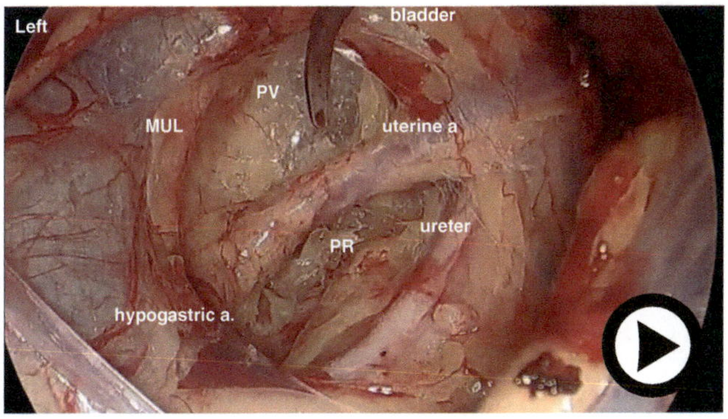

Fig. 7.7 Paravesical Space, with uterine artery (UA) and ureter (U)—'Water under the bridge' (Video 7.7 Uterine Artery ligation in Lateral approach of bladder dissection) (▶ https://doi.org/10.1007/000-c94)

artery coursing over the ureter in the classic 'water under the bridge' fashion.

Now that the uterine artery is isolated, a window is made posteriorly to skeletonize it before it is coagulated. Care is taken to gently retract the ureter medially away from the electrosurgical device to minimize the risk of thermal injury (Fig. 7.8). The same procedure is performed on the contralateral side, at which point all 4 blood supplies are secured (Fig. 7.9).

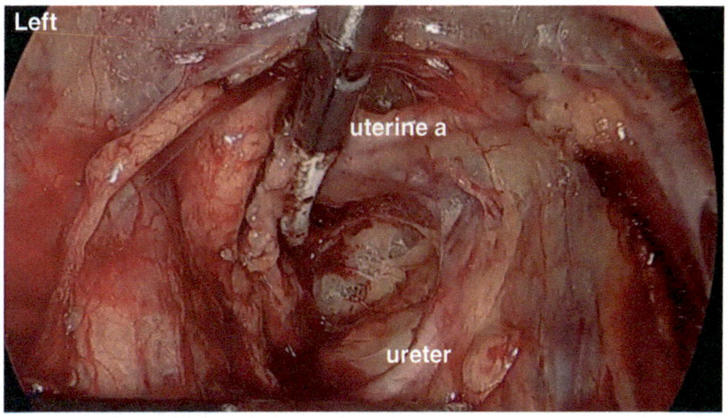

Fig. 7.8 Uterine artery secured at its origin off the Hypogastric artery with ureter gently retracted medially

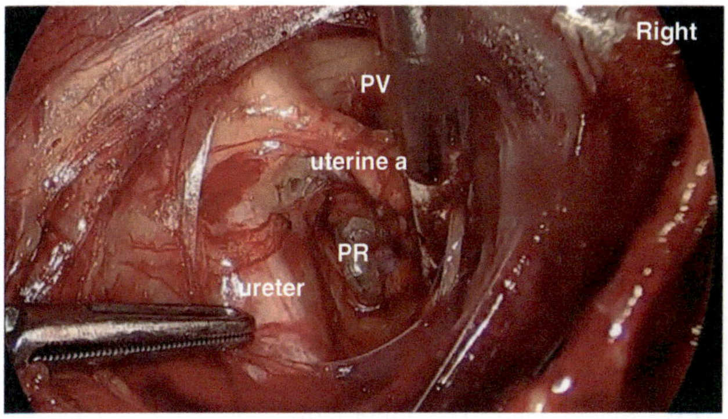

Fig. 7.9 Securing the uterine off its origin on the right side

A posterior approach can be utilized to find these avascular retroperitoneal spaces by making a peritoneal incision inferior to the infundibulopelvic ligament and superior to the ureter, when the ureter can easily be visualized transperitoneally. This incision then gives access to the retroperitoneum of the pelvic sidewall and the dissection commences in a similar fashion to the lateral approach (ie. identify the ureter along the posterior leaf of the broad ligament, etc.). An anterior approach can be performed to find these retroperitoneal spaces, as well. This is most useful in the case of distorted anatomy or obliterated posterior cul de sac. This involves identifying the medial umbilical ligament, the terminal branch of the hypogastric artery, along the anterior abdominal wall. Once it is identified, a peritoneal incision is made over it and it is skeletonized in a retrograde fashion until the origin of the uterine artery is reached. When utilizing this approach, you will often encounter the superior vesicle artery coursing towards the bladder before identifying the uterine artery. Once the uterine artery is identified, the paravesical and pararectal spaces can then be developed as described above, and the uterine artery can be secured at its origin. In regards to which approach to take, typically the anatomy and pathology will dictate which approach is easiest to access and safest.

7.1.2 Step 2: Delineate Borders of the Bladder

Next, we need to delineate the borders of the bladder to ensure we do not inadvertently injure it during dissection. This can be done through two techniques. We recommend backfilling the bladder to identify its borders. This can be done by using the suction irrigator or a syringe to instill 300-400 cc of fluid into the bladder. The foley's catheter can then be clamped to keep the bladder inflated and easily visible for the dissection (Fig. 7.10). It is not uncommon to need to fill and deflate the bladder multiple times through the case to delineate its borders during dissection. Alternatively, a uterine sound can be used by gently placing it through the urethra to probe the borders of the bladder under laparoscopic visualization.

7.1.3 Step 3: Initiate Dissection Laterally and Inferiorly

Once the blood supply is secured and the bladder is backfilled, we can begin the bladder flap dissection. In general, we work on the dissection from known to unknown territory in order to restore normal anatomy.

We recommend proceeding with a low lateral technique for the scarred bladder flap. After cesarean deliveries, the bladder is scarred to the uterus centrally on the lower uterine segment at the area of the hysterotomy. We aim to find the virgin plane lateral and inferior (ie. low lateral technique) to the adhesions along the colpotomy cup to facilitate the remainder of the dissection (Fig. 7.11a, b). By beginning the dissection in this virgin, unscarred tissue plane, the surgeon is able to identify the proper plane for dissection before tackling the area of scarring and thereby avoid injury to the bladder [3]. In order to find the appropriate plane for dissection, we deflate the bladder partially and use gentle blunt dissection at the region just anterior to the ascending uterine vessels at the level of the colpotomy cup to find the endopelvic fascia (Fig. 7.12). Once this plane (ie. the endopelvic fascia) is found, we gently tunnel our instrument with blunt dissection along the cup to further develop the plane (Fig. 7.13). Since this is a virgin tissue plane, it should develop very eas-

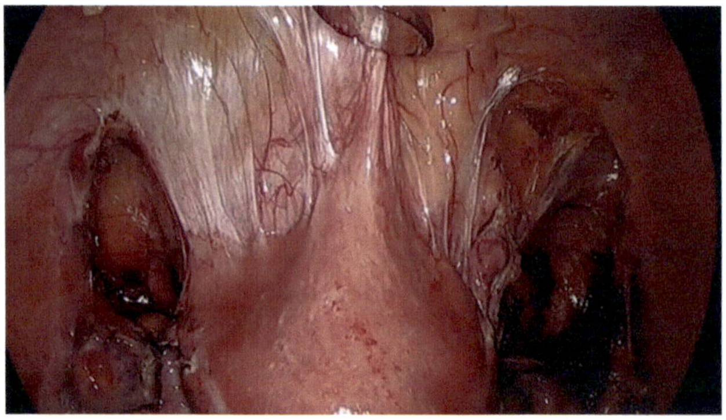

Fig. 7.10 Bladder inflated with 300–400 cc fluid

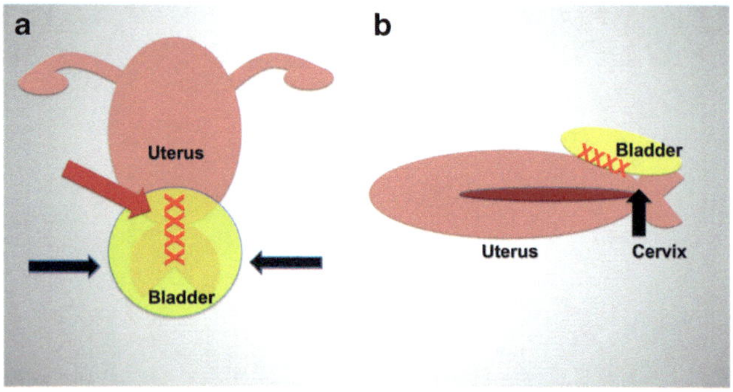

Fig. 7.11 Illustration of adhesion between bladder and lower uterine segment after cesarean delivery (**a**) anterior view (**b**) cross section/lateral view. The black arrow indicates the proper plane for dissection and the red XXXX indicates the scar between the bladder and the lower uterine segment

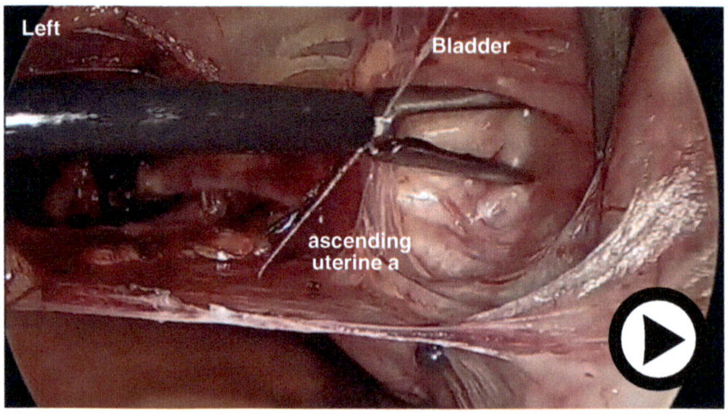

Fig. 7.12 Low lateral technique for bladder dissection with bladder partially decompressed—dissecting anteriorly to ascending uterine vessels on the left side to identify endopelvic fascia at the colpotomy cup on the left side (Video 7.12 Lateral approach of bladder dissection) (▶ https://doi.org/10.1007/000-c93)

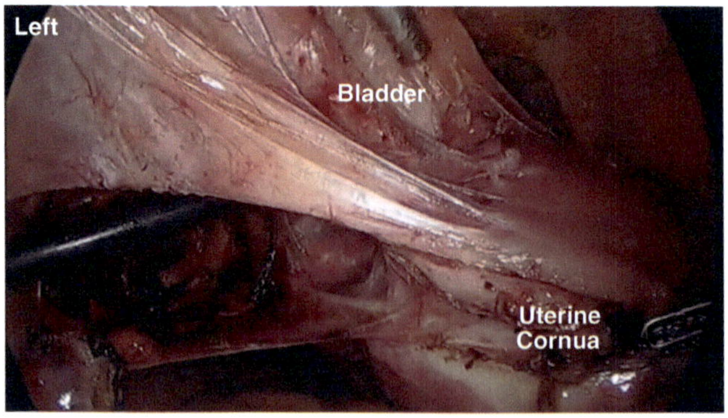

Fig. 7.13 Dissection tunneled on the endopelvic fascia in virgin plane along the colpotomy cup

ily with blunt dissection. If resistance is encountered, the surgeon should refocus their dissection more inferiorly (ie. lower). Once we have identified the appropriate dissection plane and the bladder adhesions are isolated, we can start taking down these adhesions with a combination of both sharp and blunt dissection (Figs. 7.14, 7.15 and 7.16).

The tunnel created along the endopelvic fascia below the adhesion can be utilized throughout the dissection to retract the bladder inferiorly, provide countertraction, and delineate the adhesive band. Once again, backfilling the bladder is an important tool for delineating the borders of the bladder and providing the surgeon with easy visual cues for differentiating bladder from adhesive bands. These visual cues will guide the surgeon's dissection and allow them to incise the adhesive bands off the endopelvic fascia without injuring the bladder (Fig. 7.17).

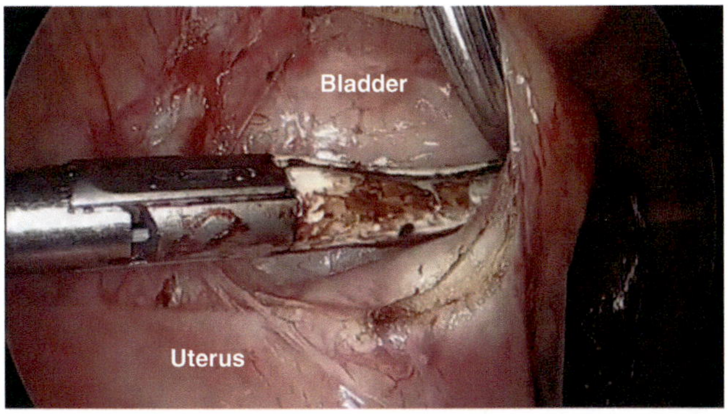

Fig. 7.14 Blunt/Sharp dissection to separate the adhesion

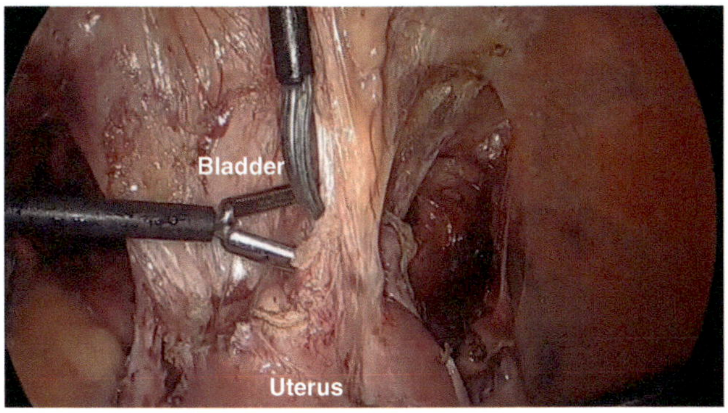

Fig. 7.15 Blunt/Sharp dissection to separate the adhesion

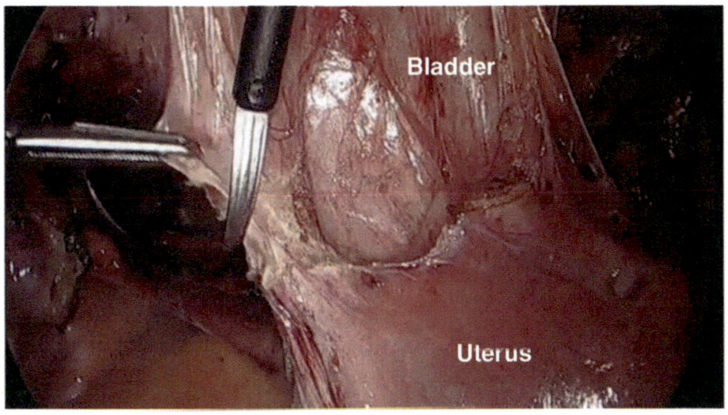

Fig. 7.16 Blunt/Sharp dissection to separate the adhesion

First, the vesicouterine peritoneum is incised and then subsequent layers of adhesions are transected. The adhesions are taken down from lateral to mid-line (*ie.* known to unknown) on both sides. Uterine manipulation is vital to provide counter traction to facilitate smooth dissection. We take down the adhesive bands in thin layers, alternating between right and left sides until the entire band is taken down (Fig. 7.18). Once the bladder adhesion is lysed, we can proceed with the rest of the hysterectomy in the usual fashion.

Learning Points

- Uterine artery ligation at origin helps to minimize blood loss and enhance visibility, especially in patients with prior cesarean deliveries.
- Techniques like bladder backfilling aid in precise bladder dissection, preventing unintended bladder injury during surgery.

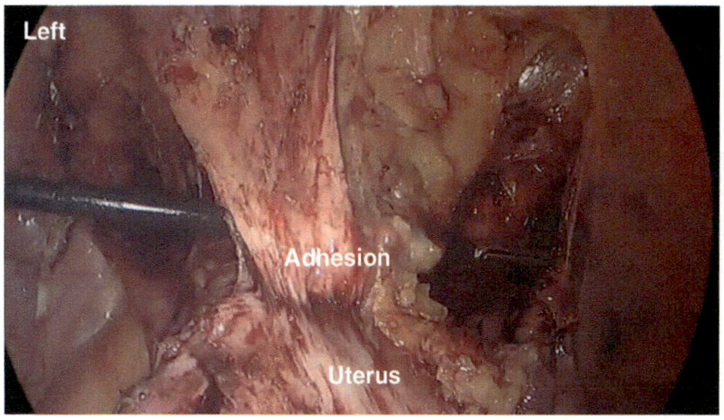

Fig. 7.17 Instrument tunneled along colpotomy cup providing anterior traction

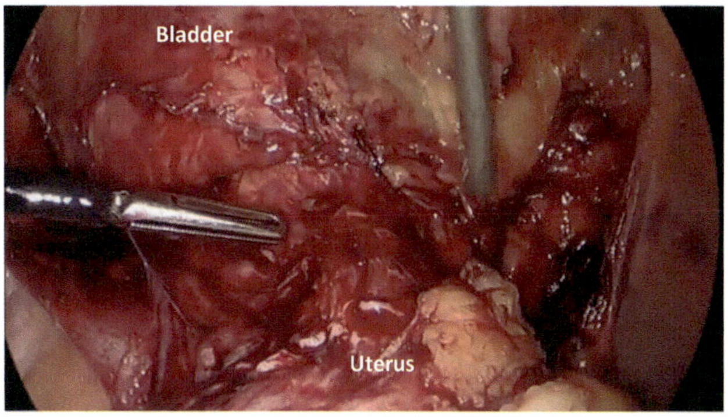

Fig. 7.18 Adhesion completely taken down with bladder dissected off the lower uterine segment

- Beginning dissection laterally and inferiorly helps identify a safe tissue plane, reducing bladder injury risks and ensuring smoother surgical progress.
- Visual cues from bladder backfilling assist in distinguishing bladder tissue from adhesions, guiding surgeons in safe incision practices.
- Adopting a systematic approach to bladder adhesiolysis, including thin-layer dissection and alternating sides, maintains surgical precision and minimizes risks to adjacent structures, ensuring successful hysterectomy outcomes.

Competing Interest The author declares no conflict of interest that are relevant to content of this chapter.

Ethical Approval Informed consent was obtained from individual participants and patients regarding publication and documentation without disclosing their identity.

References

1. Osterman MJK. Changes in primary and repeat cesarean delivery: United States, 2016–2021. Vital statistics rapid release; no 21. Hyattsville: National Center for Health Statistics; July 2022. https://doi.org/10.15620/cdc:117432.
2. Rooney CM, Crawford AT, Vassallo BJ, Kleeman SD, Karram MM. Is previous cesarean section a risk for incidental cystotomy at the time of hysterectomy? A case-controlled study. Am J Obstet Gynecol. 2005;193(6):2041–4. https://doi.org/10.1016/j.ajog.2005.07.090. PMID: 16325612.
3. Mansuria S. Development of the scarred and difficult bladder flap. SurgeryU by AAGL 2017 Jun 30. Available from: surgeryu.aagl.org/view?m=zkaPLYmGi. Accessed 11 Oct 2023.

8 Posterior Approach for Uterine Artery Ligation

Ted Lee and Kate Denny

8.1 Introduction

One of the most common scenarios encountered in performing a total laparoscopic hysterectomy is adhesions from prior cesarean deliveries [1, 2]. These adhesions which obliterate the anterior cul de sac cause significant challenges to completing the procedure. Normal anatomy and tissue planes are obscured, complicating dissection and in some cases precluding the use of a uterine manipulator if the cervix is deviated anteriorly behind the pubic bone. These challenges may increase the risk of urinary tract injury and blood loss specifically from bladder or uterine serosal adhesions.

We describe our anatomic based strategy to address these issues called "the posterior approach," which is excellent for patients with extensive and dense uterine adhesions to the bladder and anterior abdominal wall. This approach involves ligation of the ascending branch of the uterine artery without fully developing bladder flap, enabling the surgeon to identify anatomy and secure the blood supply prior to dissecting the adhesions, decreasing the risk of injury and blood loss.

8.1.1 Dissection Techniques

In general, for safe and effective dissection, we recommend performing the easy task first, and dissecting from known to unknown. This strategy usually avoids direct confrontation with the pathology, echoing the technique for the posterior approach in which we dissect the anterior cul de sac adhesions last. Throughout any dissection, frequently identify the surrounding anatomy to continually reestablish relevant landmarks and regain perspective.

8.1.2 Optimizing Visualization and Landmarks

We perform a Hasson open technique for most patients but will chose a Palmer's point entry if extensive abdominal adhesions are expected as in the patient with a prior vertical midline incision or subfascial umbilical mesh. Various non-umbilical entry techniques are available including the Jain point entry [3].

After entry, if the uterine adhesions to the abdominal wall extend above halfway between the pubic symphysis and umbilicus, we use a subxiphoid port as the visual trocar and the umbilical port as a midline operative port. This enables visual and operative access to the bilateral pelvis without the obstruction of the adhesions.

The use of a uterine manipulator with a colpotomizer cup is important to accentuate the vaginal fornices, allowing for identification of the vesicovaginal plane below the level of dense bladder adhesions. If a manipulator cannot be placed due to the position of the cervix, we use a Briesky retractor placed in the anterior vaginal fornix, as described below.

Finally, upon initial abdominal survey and intermittently throughout the dissection, we back fill the bladder to identify its borders. Using the suction irrigator tip, we instill normal saline into the foley catheter and either suction the fluid to decompress the bladder or clamp the Foley for continued delineation during dissection.

T. Lee (✉)
Division of Minimally Invasive Gynecologic Surgery, Surgical Innovation for Gynecology, Department of Obstetrics and Gynecology, New York University Grossman School of Medicine, New York, NY, USA
e-mail: leextt@upmc.edu

K. Denny
Minimally Invasive Gynecologic Surgery Fellow, Department of Obstetrics, Gynecology and Reproductive Sciences, Magee-Womens Hospital, University of Pittsburgh Medical Center, Pittsburgh, PA, USA

N. Jain (ed.), *Complex Total Laparoscopic Hysterectomy (TLH) with Newer Approaches in Bladder Dissection*,
https://doi.org/10.1007/978-981-97-3226-5_8

8.2 Surgical Steps of the Posterior Approach

8.2.1 Part 1: Securing the Blood Supply

First begin by securing the blood supply before addressing the adhesions.

8.2.1.1 Case I

See Figs. 8.1, 8.2, 8.3, 8.4 and 8.5.

8.2.1.2 Case 2

See Figs. 8.6, 8.7, 8.8, 8.9, 8.10, 8.11, 8.12 and 8.13.

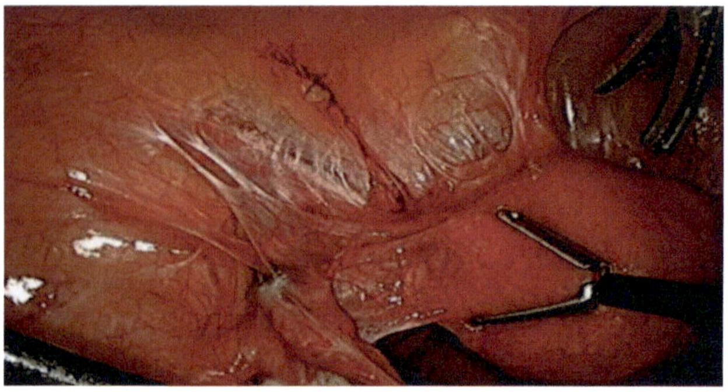

Fig. 8.1 As you can see, the patient has dense bladder adhesions obliterating the anterior cul de sac from several prior cesarean deliveries

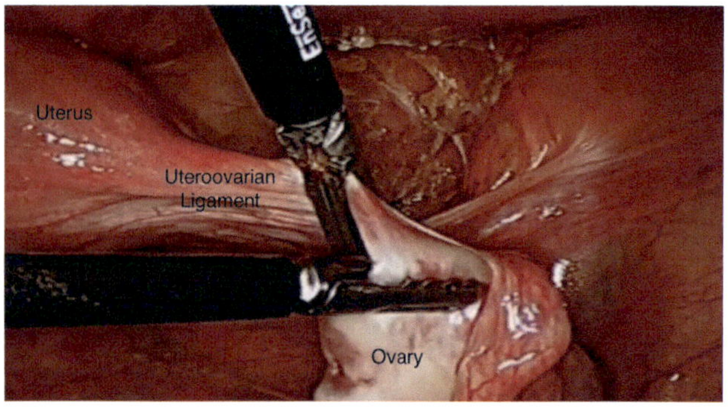

Fig. 8.2 Secure the cornual pedicles

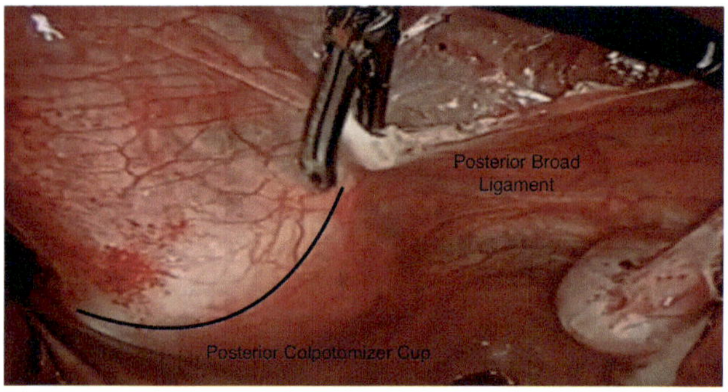

Fig. 8.3 March along the posterior leaf of the broad ligament toward the colpotomizer cup

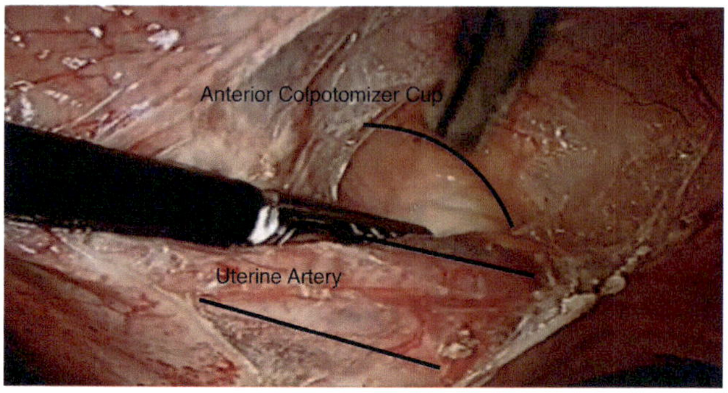

Fig. 8.4 Once you have identified the uterine artery, feel for the colpotomizer cup anteriorly. Identify the vesicovaginal plane. Find the natural tissue plane between the bladder and vagina. This is present even in dense adhesions

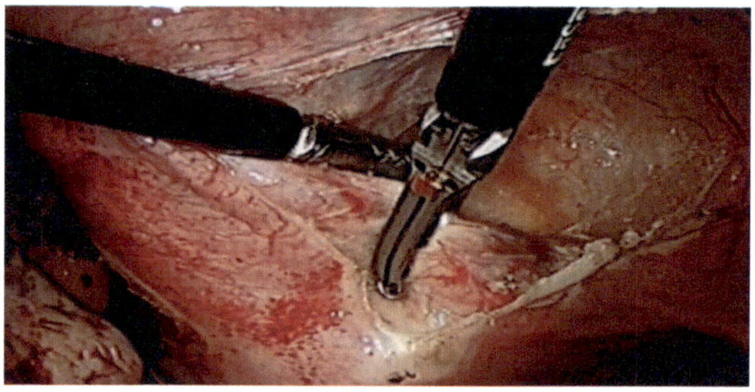

Fig. 8.5 Retract the bladder and adhesions superiorly and seal the ascending uterine artery and ligate, making sure to be above the level of the colpotomizer cup to avoid the ureter

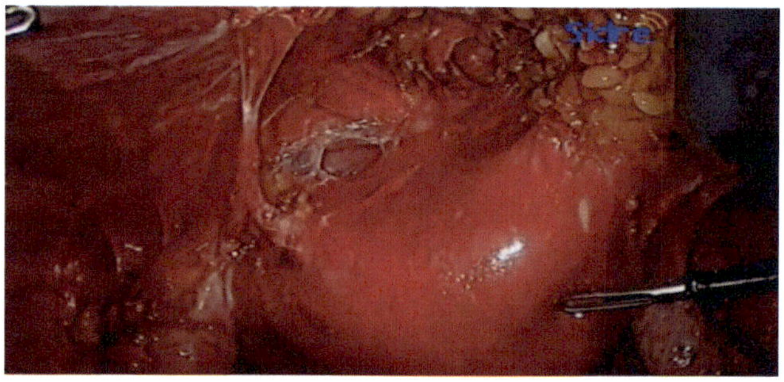

Fig. 8.6 The patient has dense uterine adhesions to the abdominal wall

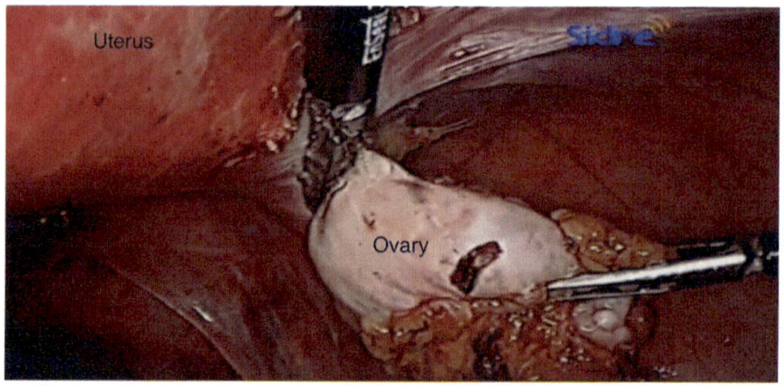

Fig. 8.7 Secure the utero-ovarian ligament

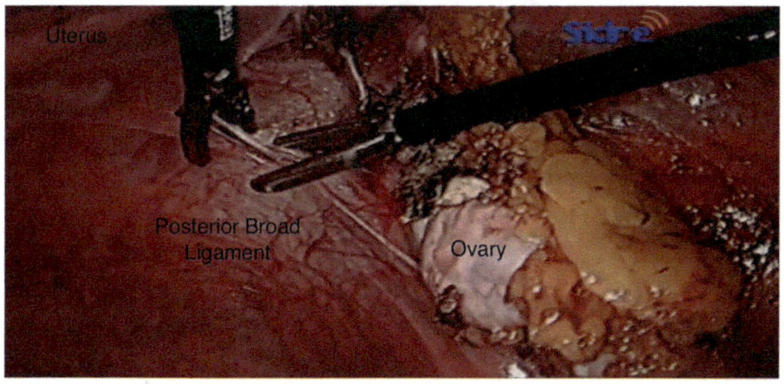

Fig. 8.8 Slide along the posterior leaf of the broad ligament toward the colpotomizer cup. Identify ureter before and during this step

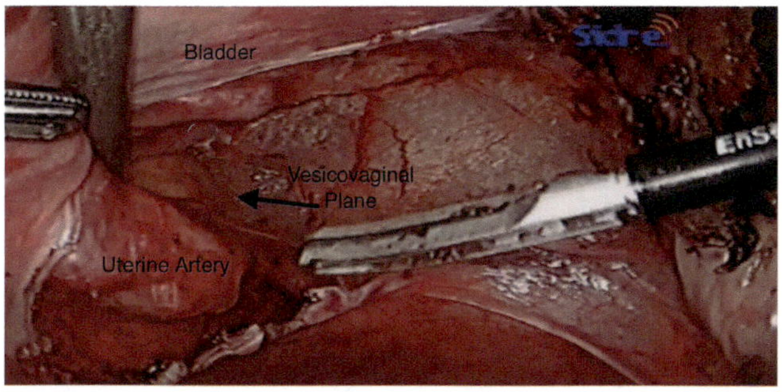

Fig. 8.9 Make sure the uterus is in an anteverted position and identify the ascending uterine artery and identify the vesicovaginal plane with the suction displacing the bladder anteriorly

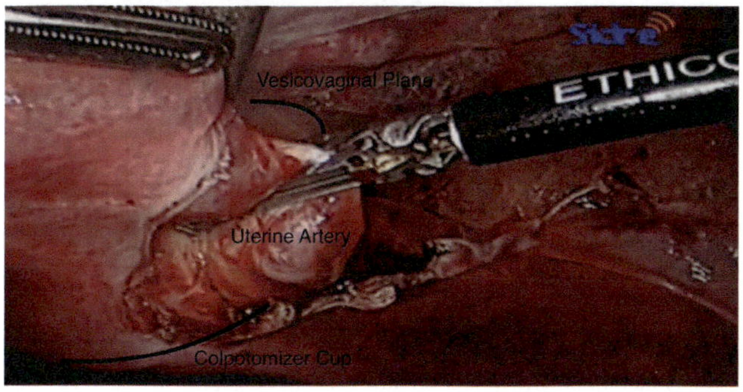

Fig. 8.10 Seal the uterine artery below the level of the adhesions and above the edge of the colpotomizer cup

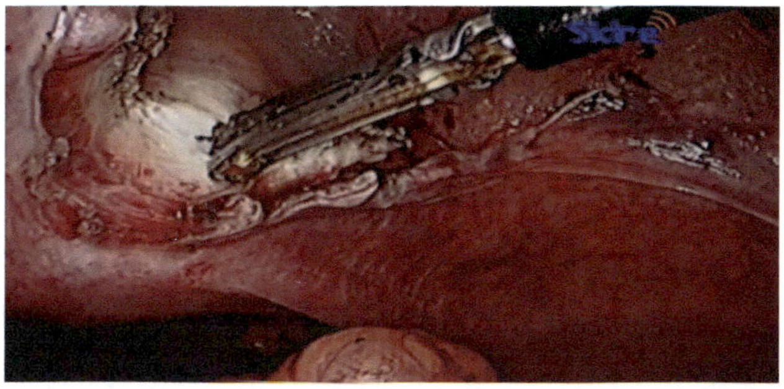

Fig. 8.11 Seal the uterine artery below the level of the adhesions and above the edge of the colpotomizer cup

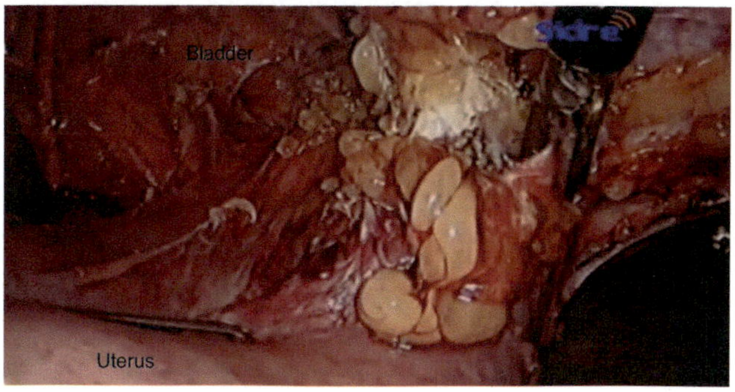

Fig. 8.12 Separate the uterus from the anterior abdominal wall. As the uterine blood supply is already secure, bleeding from the adhesions is decreased

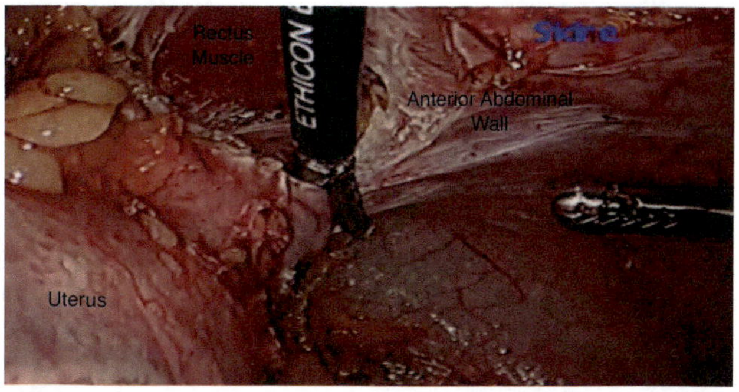

Fig. 8.13 Separate the uterus from the anterior abdominal wall. As the uterine blood supply is already secure, bleeding from the adhesions is decreased

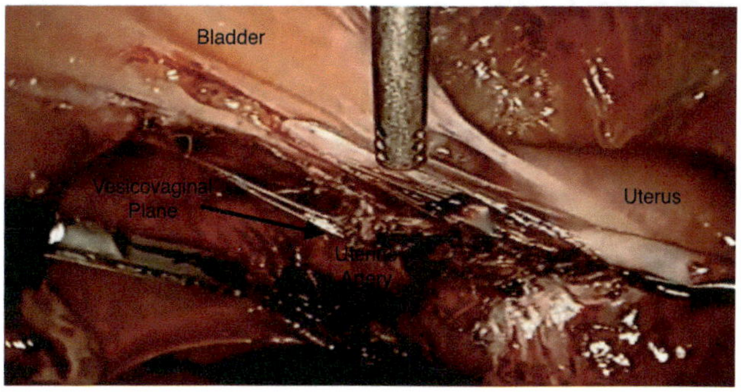

Fig. 8.14 Once the blood supply is secured and the vesicovaginal space identified under the adhesions, we develop the bladder flap by creating a tunnel under the adhesions

8.2.2 Part 2: Developing the Bladder Flap and Bladder Tunnel

See Fig. 8.14.

8.3 Vesicovaginal Dissection

See Figs. 8.15, 8.16, 8.17 and 8.18.

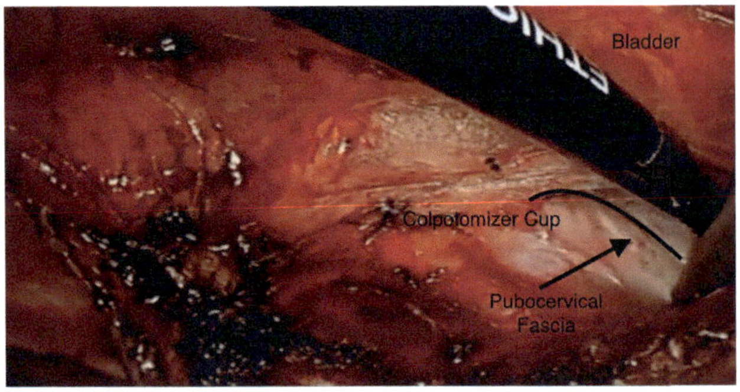

Fig. 8.15 Keeping the fatty tissue with the bladder, identify the white pubocervical fascia over the colpotomizer cup. Using blunt dissection, tunnel across the colpotomizer cup

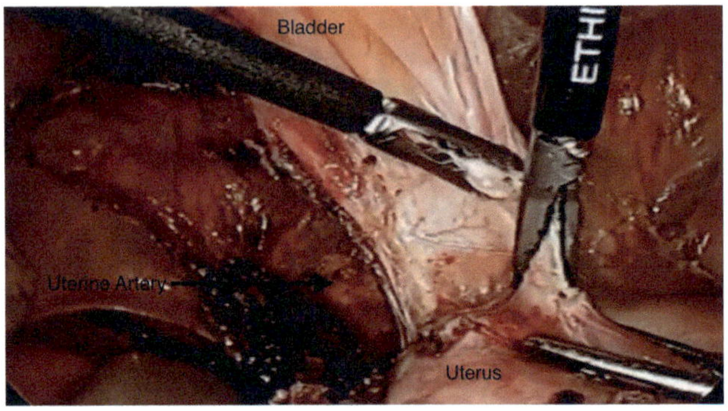

Fig. 8.16 Dissect close to the uterus to prevent residual uterine tissue

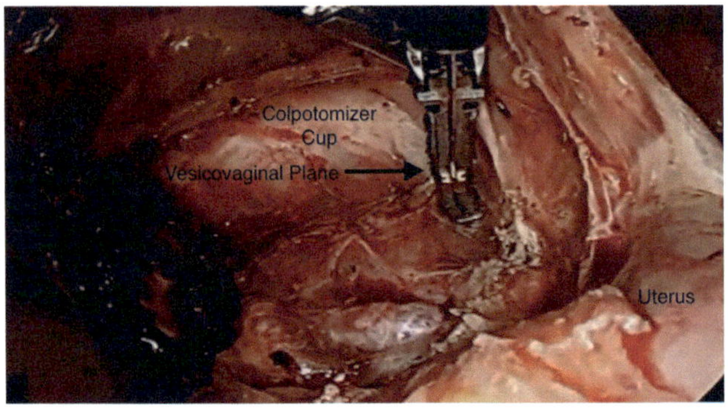

Fig. 8.17 Use blunt dissection as an interrogation tool that separate the looser adhesions. Separate the dense adhesions sharply or with energy

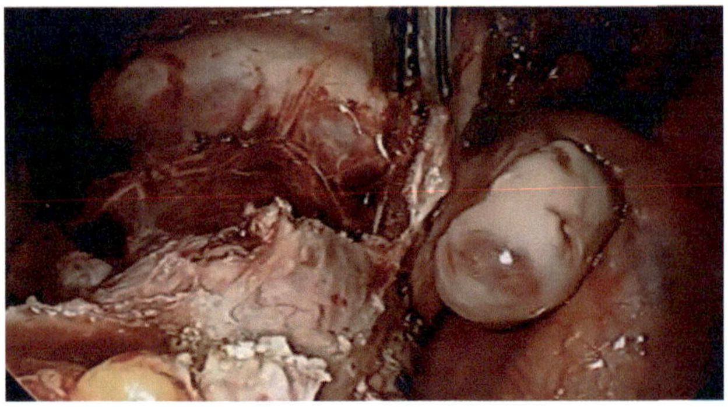

Fig. 8.18 Use blunt dissection as an interrogation tool that separate the looser adhesions. Separate the dense adhesions sharply or with energy

8.3.1 Using a Briesky Retractor

See Figs. 8.19 and 8.20.

8.3.2 Creating the Bladder Tunnel

In this patient with a didelphis uterus and a double cervix, the vesicovaginal space is less easily identified (Figs. 8.21, 8.22 and 8.23).

8.3.3 Diagnosing a Bladder Injury

Even with the perfect dissection technique, cystotomy may not be avoidable due to extremely dense adhesions [3]. However, a bladder injury is easy to identify and repair.

An injury is diagnosed if the Foley bag fills with air, or a cystotomy is visualized during cystoscopy or while backfilling the bladder.

Once the injury is diagnosed, identifying the location of the injury is important. We recommend the use of stents to delineate the uretero orifaces and trigone, and maintaining the stents during repair as to not incorporate the ureters (Fig. 8.24).

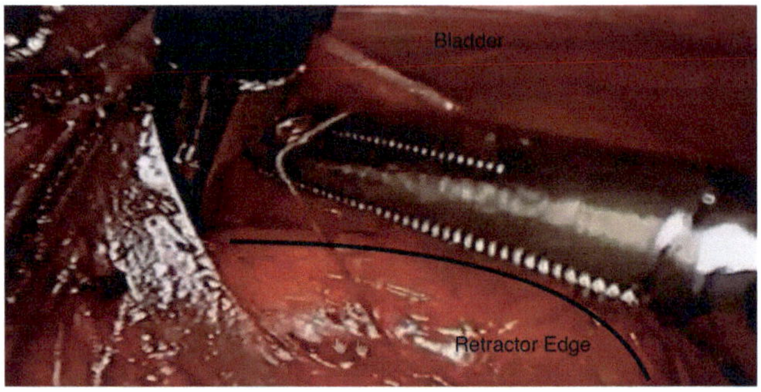

Fig. 8.19 In this patient with a prior ablation and cesarean scar adhesions, placement with a manipulator was not possible. We use a Briesky retractor to create the bladder flap tunnel. Place the retractor in the anterior fornix as the landmark of the vesicovaginal plane. Once the right tissue plane is identified, retract the bladder anteriorly and continue to bluntly dissect medially along the plane to create a tunnel

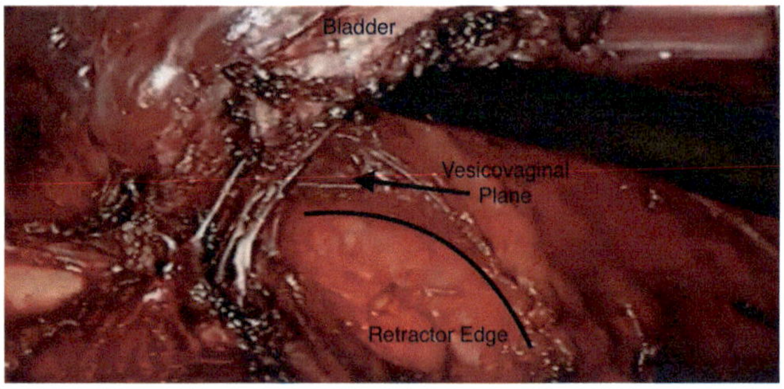

Fig. 8.20 Finding the right plane is important and the dissection will progress easily. If the tunnel is not easily developed, re-identification is necessary

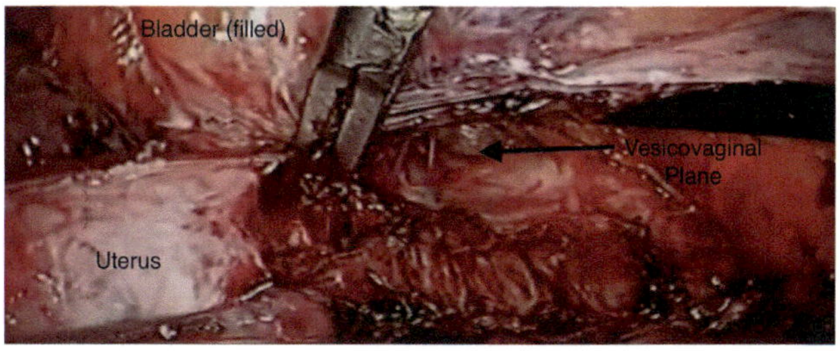

Fig. 8.21 Staying close to the uterus and displacing the bladder anteriorly helps to separate the key anatomy. Here the bladder is backfilled with fluid for easier identification

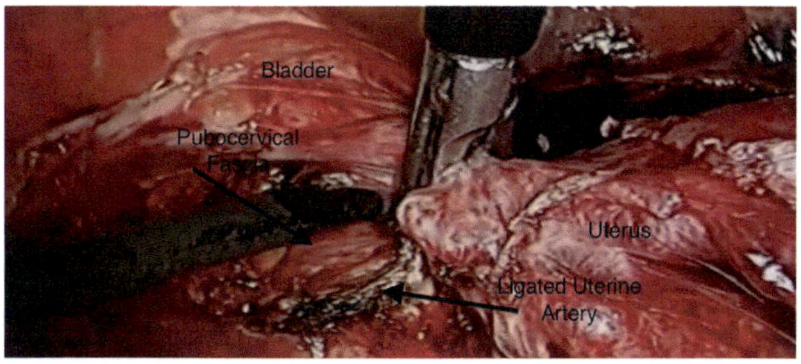

Fig. 8.22 Blunt and sharp dissection are continued along the tunnel from the opposite side to "connect the dots"

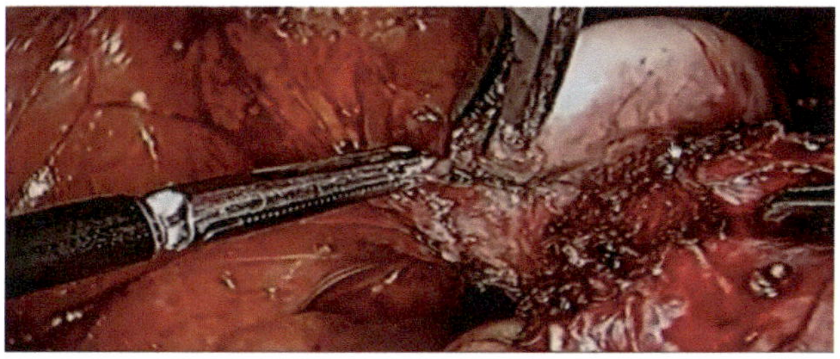

Fig. 8.23 Blunt and sharp dissection are continued along the tunnel from the opposite side to "connect the dots"

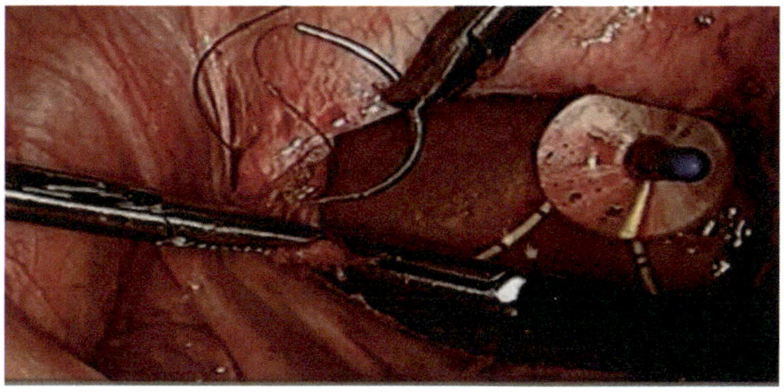

Fig. 8.24 Below the foley balloon is visible in the bladder along with stents to identify the ureterus

We repair a cystotomy similarly to our colpotomy closure, using extracorporeally tied angle stitches with 3-0 PDS, pulled through the lateral trocars and maintained on tension as shown above. We close the cystotomy in 2 layers with a 90-day absorbable 3-0 v-lock suture [4, 5]. We ensure the repair is airtight by instilling NS.

Finally, the Foley catheter is kept in place for 10 days and removed after obtaining a satisfactory cystogram.

8.4 Conclusion

In conclusion, the surgical challenges of an obliterated cul de sac and its associated risks may be mitigated by using the "posterior approach" in conjunction with our surgical principles of dissection and visualization.

Learning Points

- 1. Use of "Posterior Approach" as a strategic response to challenges posed by anterior cul-de-sac adhesions, due to previous history of cesarean section leading to extensive and dense uterine adhesions to the bladder and anterior abdominal wall.
- Initiate surgery by securing the uterine artery's blood supply, prioritizing ligation of the ascending uterine artery to reduce the risk of bleeding during adhesion dissection.
- Emphasize the use of tools like uterine manipulators or Briesky retractors to enhance visualization of anatomical landmarks and propose a systematic entry approach based on patient-specific factors.
- Despite surgical expertise, dissection of dense adhesions may still result in accidental injury to the bladder. Prompt recognition of injury and repair is necessary.
- Advocate the principle of dissecting from known to unknown for safe and effective surgery, encouraging frequent identification of surrounding anatomy to maintain perspective.

Competing Interest The author declares no conflict of interest that are relevant to content of this chapter.

Ethical Approval Informed consent was obtained from individual participants and patients regarding publication and documentation without disclosing their identity.

References

1. Fortin CN, Saed GM, Diamond MP. Predisposing factors to post-operative adhesions development. Hum Repord Update. 2015;21(4):536–51.
2. Awonuga AO, Fletcher NM, Saed GM, Diamond MP. Postoperative adhesion development following cesarean and open intra-abdominal gynecological operations: a review. Reprod Sci. 2011;18(12):1166–85.
3. Jain N, Jain V, Chandi A, Srivastava S, Singh S, Vasundhara N. Jain point: an alternate laparoscopic non-umbilical first blind entry port to avoid vessel, viscera, adhesions and bowel (VVAB). Updat Surg. 2021;73(6):2321–9. https://doi.org/10.1007/s13304-021-01099-z. Epub 2021 Jun 13. PMID: 34121164; PMCID: PMC8606393.
4. Selivianskaia A, Bradley S, Morozov V. Best practices for repair of iatrogenic bladder injury, AJOG Glob Rep. 2022, 2, 100062.
5. Chamsy D, King C, Lee T. The use of barbed suture for bladder and bowel repair. J Minim Invasive Gynecol. 2015;22(4):648–52.

Part III

TLH in Different Clinical Case Scenario

9 Total Laparoscopic Hysterectomy (TLH) in Ventrifixed Uterus by the Comprehensive Canopy Technique, '3 Step Technique'

Nutan Jain, Vandana Jain, and Sakshi Srivastava

9.1 Introduction

Rising rates of caesarean delivery worldwide has resulted in increasing numbers of pregnant women with a caesarean section (CS) scars [1]. The propensity for encountering a ventrifixed uterus is increasingly observed among laparoscopic procedures, pointing to two primary factors. One factor is a deviation from the classic standard technique of cesarean section [2], and the other is an increased rate of caesarean sections. Latest available data (2010–2018) from 154 countries shows that 21.1% of women gave birth by cesarean worldwide, with 42.8% in Latin America. Projections showed that by 2030, 28.5% of women worldwide will give birth by CS with 63.4% in Eastern Asia [3]. This high cesarean rate predisposes the utero-vesicle fold to be tampered with, posing a daunting challenge during TLH [4].

Supplementary Information The online version contains supplementary material available at https://doi.org/10.1007/978-981-97-3226-5_9. The videos can be accessed individually by clicking the DOI link in the accompanying figure caption or by scanning this link with the SN More Media App.

N. Jain (✉)
Obstetrics and Gynaecology, GSVM Medical College, Affiliated by Kanpur University, Kanpur, Uttar Pradesh, India

Department of Obstetrics and Gynecology, Vardhman Trauma and Laparoscopy Centre Pvt. Ltd., Muzaffarnagar, Uttar Pradesh, India

V. Jain
Department of Obstetrics and Gynecology, Vardhman Trauma and Laparoscopy Centre Pvt. Ltd., Muzaffarnagar, Uttar Pradesh, India

Obstetrics and Gynaecology, Kasturba Hospital, Affiliated by Delhi University, Delhi, India

S. Srivastava
Obstetrics and Gynecology, Rohilkhand Medical College and Hospital, Affiliated by Bareilly International University, Bareilly, Uttar Pradesh, India

Gynaecology Endoscopy, Vardhman Trauma and Laparoscopy Centre Pvt. Ltd., Muzaffarnagar, Uttar Pradesh, India

The increasing prevalence of caesarean sections has contributed to a decline in maternal mortality rates and obstetric fistula occurrences. However, it has also resulted in the emergence of scarred utero-vesical folds (Figs. 9.1a, b and 9.2a, b), posing challenges for surgeons in cases with a history of multiple previous caesarean sections. The adoption of the Misgav-ladach technique [5] in the early 1990s, characterized by single-layer closure and the omission of closure of peritoneal layers (both visceral and parietal), gained popularity for its efficiency in reducing surgical time [6]. This shift in approach emphasized speed in completing caesareans within a competitive environment, deviating from a dedicated surgical focus [7].

9.1.1 Causes of Ventrifixed Uterus

1. **Insufficient hemostasis in C-sections:** Increased incidence of ventrifixed uterus is associated with insufficient attention given to hemostasis during cesarean sections [8].
2. **Impact of peritoneal layer closure:** The absence of peritoneal layer closure leads to direct opposition between the cesarean scar and the abdominal wall musculature, resulting in severe adhesions of the uterus [8] due to increased work load.
3. **Challenges in teaching institutions:** Common performance of C-sections by residents in high volume teaching institutions contribute to complications; owing to inadequate closure, incomplete peritoneal lavage, and fatigue [8].

Manifestations of ventrifixed uterus vary from severe adhesions resembling a ***stamp on envelope or a lizard on a wall*** stretched out with blurred borders against abdominal wall; to less severe cases presenting as adherent uterus in a band- like fashion, or partially stuck on one side with other side free [8] (Fig. 9.3a–f).

The evolution of caesarean techniques from vertical to lower uterine scars had been smooth until the emergence of

N. Jain (ed.), *Complex Total Laparoscopic Hysterectomy (TLH) with Newer Approaches in Bladder Dissection*, https://doi.org/10.1007/978-981-97-3226-5_9

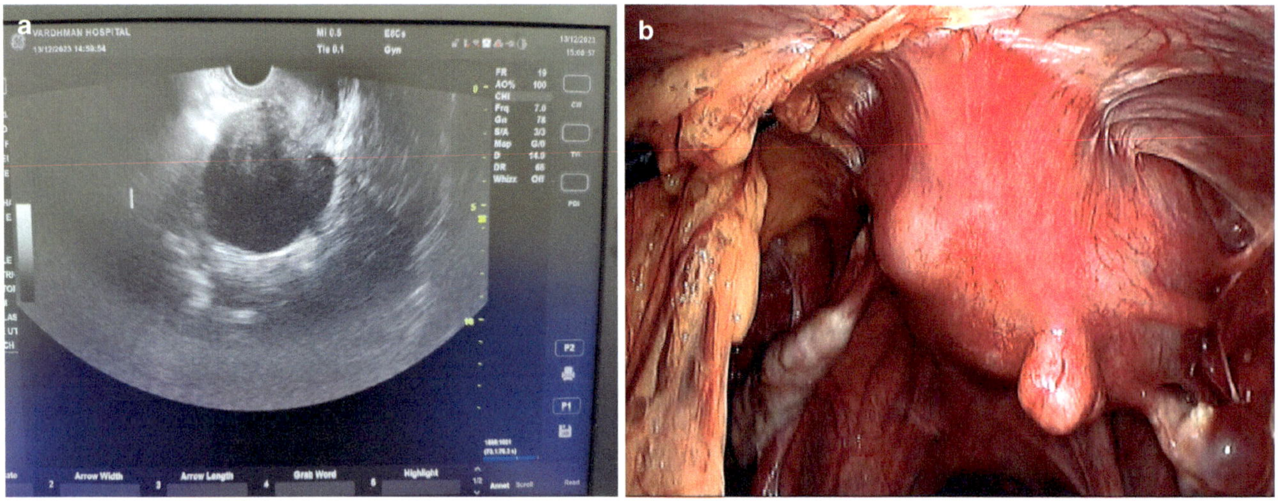

Fig. 9.1 Uterus stuck like a lizard on abdominal wall. **a** Ultrasound picture. **b** Laparoscopic view

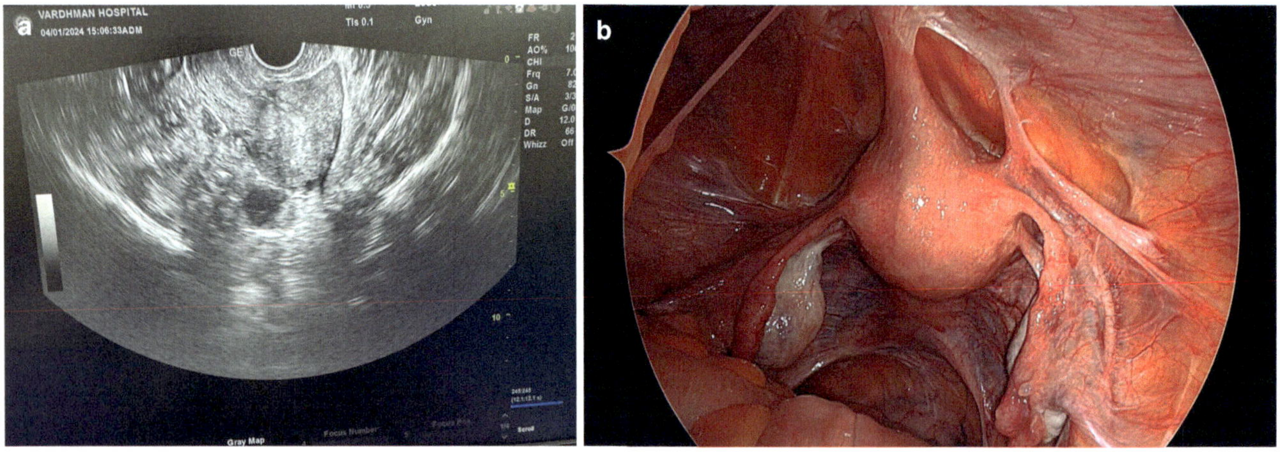

Fig. 9.2 Ventifixed uterus. **a** Ultrasound picture showing beaking. **b** Laparoscopic view

issues such as scar defects [9], caesarean scar pregnancies [10], ventrifixed uterus [11], placenta accreta and percreta [12] syndromes. Our setup has maintained a conservative approach, adhering to multiple-layer closure of the caesarean bed and closure of both visceral and parietal peritoneum. We have remained largely free of these unwanted post-surgical occurrences. Causes of niche formation and reduced residual myometrial thickness (RMT) may be incomplete closure of myometrium after single layer closure and counteracting forces due to the adhesions between uterus and anterior abdominal wall in retroflexed uterus (Fig. 9.4a–c).

9.1.2 Case Studies

1. **2Close study** [13]: The study conducted by Stegwee et al. focused on the "2Close study," which is a randomized controlled trial involving participants from multiple medical centers. The research aimed to compare the long-term performance of two different closure techniques (single-layer and double-layer closure) in repeat cesarean sections. The primary parameter examined was the residual myometrium thickness (RMT) at the cesarean scar site, a crucial factor indicating uterine wall integrity.

9.1.2.1 Key Findings

(a) **Closure Technique Impact:** The study revealed that the double-layer closure technique resulted in a thicker RMT compared to single-layer closure after cesarean section.
(b) **Association with Niche Formation**: A potential association was identified between RMT thickness and the development of a niche at the cesarean scar site. A niche represents an interruption in the myometrium due to incomplete healing.
(c) **Clinical Implications:** Thin RMT and the presence of a niche were linked to gynecological symptoms, compli-

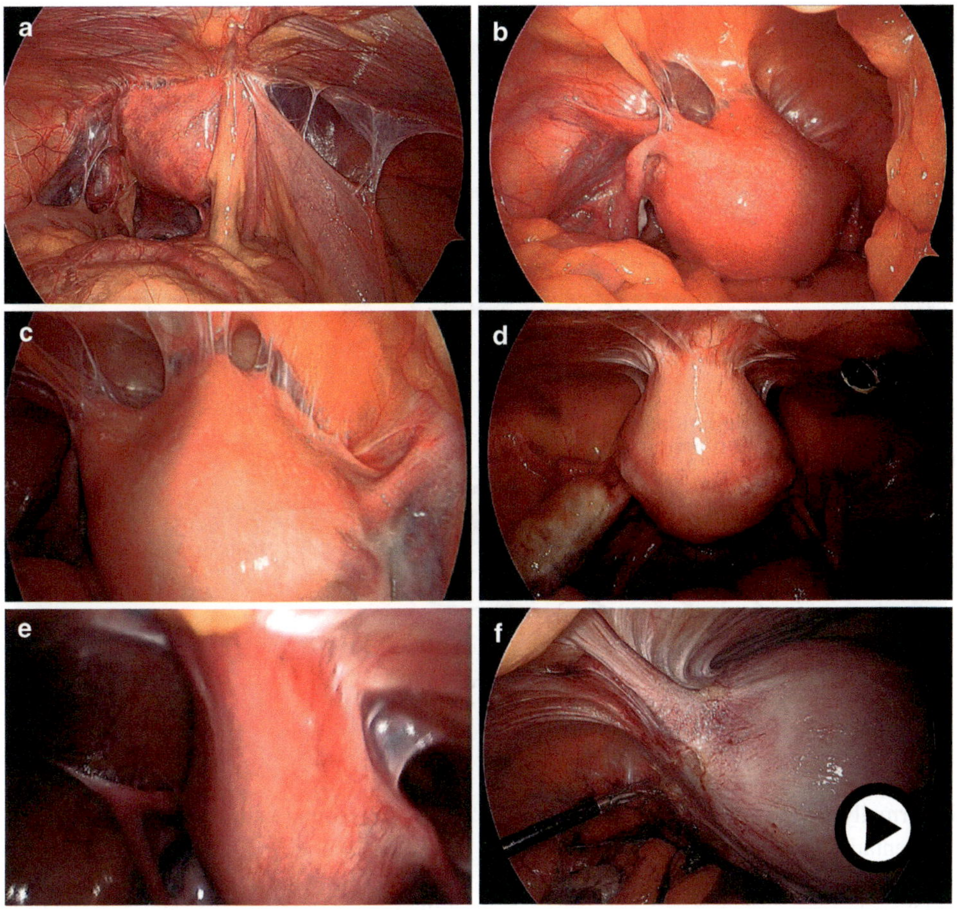

Fig. 9.3 **a** Ventrifixed uterus with dense bowel adhesions. **b** Adherent uterus to anterior abdominal wall. **c** Bladder adherence more on the top at the level of caesarean scar. **d** Uterus hanging like a lantern (Video 9.3d TLH with Ventrifixed uterus) (▶ https://doi.org/10.1007/000-c95). **e** Uterus densely stuck high up. **f** Uterus stuck to the anterior abdominal wall more on the left side

cations in subsequent pregnancies, deliveries, and potential subfertility.

(d) **Positive Health Implications:** Opting for the double-layer closure technique may have positive implications for women's health after cesarean section, potentially reducing the risk of complications associated with niche development and less challenges in repeat caesareans.

The study implies that the choice of closure technique during cesarean sections can influence RMT and may impact the development of a niche and ventrifixed uterus, raising concerns related to surgical safety.

The "2Close study" underscores the importance of closure technique selection in cesarean sections, highlighting potential benefits for women's health and emphasizing the need for further dedicated, multicenter trials to assess long-term performance in repeat cesareans.

2. The study by Lyell DJ [14] et al. investigates the impact of parietal peritoneal closure during primary cesarean delivery on adhesion formation. Conducting a prospective cohort analysis, the study found that parietal peritoneal closure was significantly associated with a *fivefold reduction* in all adhesions and a *threefold reduction* in dense adhesions. Surgeons assessed adhesion severity and location, immediately post-surgery. The study controlled for various variables, including prior infection and patient demographics. Results suggest that the common practice of not closing the parietal peritoneum during cesarean delivery should be reconsidered, emphasizing the need for further research to understand the long-term implications of different surgical techniques in cesarean deliveries, as their study highlighted omission of peritoneal layer closure as a significant factor in adherence.

9.1.3 Niche or Isthmocele

The caesarean scar defect, also known as a niche or isthmocele, is a potential space or indentation in the uterine scar that forms after a caesarean section [15].

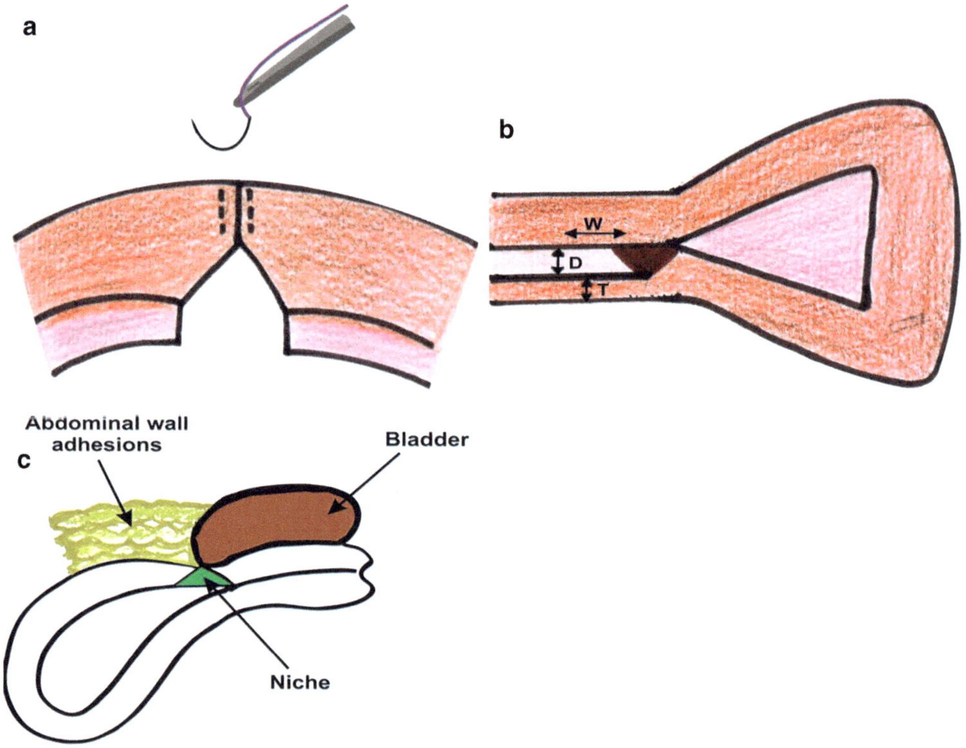

Fig. 9.4 **a** Incomplete closure of myometrial defect after single layer closure increases niche formation and reduces the residual myometrial thickness (RMT). **b**. D and W is the depth and width of niche (cesarean scar defect). Decreased myometrial thickness shown by T denotes poor scar integrity. **c**. Counteracting forces due to the adhesions between uterus and anterior abdominal wall in a retroflexed uterus may increase niche formation. Illustration by Dr Priyanka Sureddi

This entity is formally defined by the European Niche Taskforce as an "indentation in the uterine myometrium of at least 2 mm at the site of the caesarean scar assessed by trans vaginal ultrasound." [16]

Keeping the increasing incidence of a niche and its implications in modern day gynaecologic laparoscopic surgery, it looks pertinent to describe the sonographic appearance of the same. More & more gynaecologic laparoscopic surgeons need to acquire the skill of diagnosing caesarean scar defect (CSD) themselves in office.

9.1.3.1 Ultrasound Findings Related to a Caesarean Scar Defect (Uterine Niche)

1. Abnormal Uterine Contour.
2. A visible depression or indentation in the uterine wall at the scar site.
3. A cystic structure or hypo echoic area on ultrasound represents a fluid-filled space at the caesarean scar, indicating a potential defect in the uterine wall (Fig. 9.5).
4. Thinning in the muscular layer of the uterus (myometrium) at the scar site.
5. Measurement of the thickness of residual myometrium at the scar site. Thinner myometrium is associated with a higher risk of niche development and related complications.
6. Doppler ultrasound can show increased blood flow or vascularity in the region of the scar, associated with compromised healing of the scar.

These ultrasound findings collectively contribute to the identification and characterization of a caesarean scar defect [17]. It is essential for healthcare professionals, particularly skilled sonographers and clinicians to interpret these findings accurately. While ultrasound is valuable for diagnosing niche, the clinical significance varies, and management decisions depend on individual patient factors and symptoms.

9.1.4 Impact of Ventrifixed Uterus on TLH [18]

Ventrifixed uterus can be diagnosed pre operatively by careful history, examination and ultrasonography.

9.1.5 Symptoms

The problem of ventrifixed uterus could be anticipated by the following symptoms in the preoperative counselling which are continued postmenstrual spotting, dysmenorrhea, chronic pelvic pain, and dyspareunia; apart from the gynecological indication of TLH.

9.1.6 Clinical Examination

Per-Speculum On speculum examination, the cervix may not be visualized and it may be seen with great difficulty

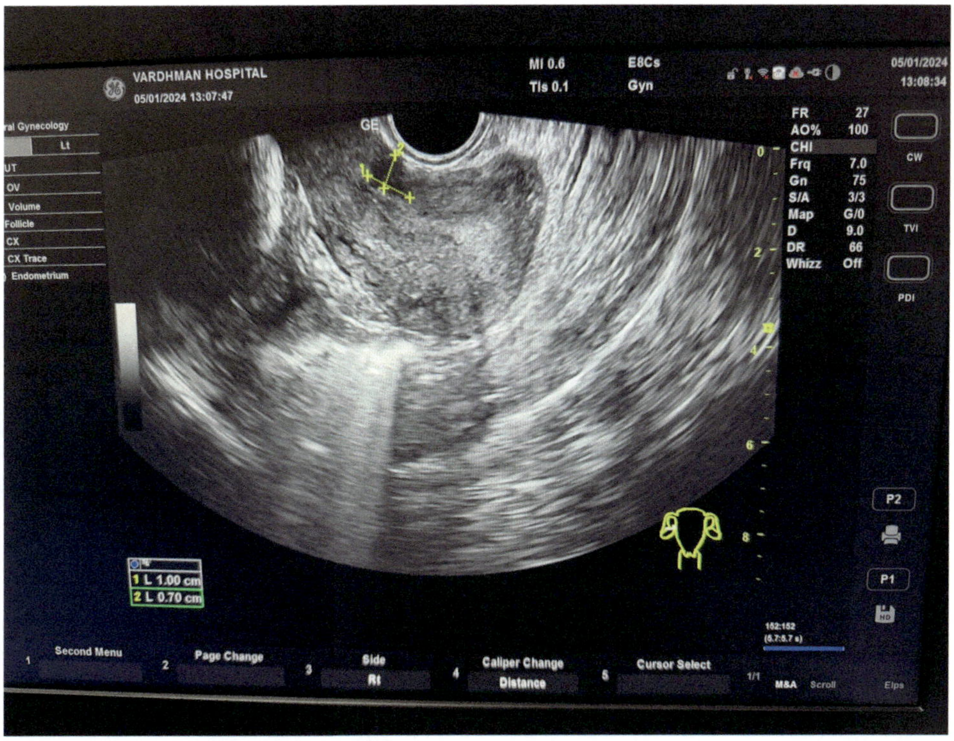

Fig. 9.5 Ultrasound picture showing niche

with the help of an anterior vaginal wall retractor, as the cervix remains behind the pubic symphysis with a stretched posterior wall. Traction on the cervix, with some difficulty, does not bring the cervix fully into view but pulls the lower abdominal wall inwards i.e., *the retraction sign*. The cervix is displaced anteriorly behind the symphysis pubis so it may not be possible or difficult to insert a uterine manipulator to perform TLH, in extreme forms of ventrifixed uterus.

Pre-operative Examination under EUA [19] Seth et al. described a useful sign to detect uterine adhesions. Adhesions between the utero cervical junction, bladder, and lower anterior abdominal wall cause retraction of the abdominal wall on application of cervical traction; which is done by grasping the cervical lip, inserting a uterine sound, and causing retroversion. This maneuver displays this important sign, showing the area of the uterine adherence on the abdominal wall. Cervical elongation is also a useful sign on sonography, which may have resulted due to a pull in the opposite direction from natural gravity and the adherent area.

9.1.7 Imaging for Ventrifixed Uterus

Ultrasonography Sonographic criteria which are most commonly the first warning signal that the uterus may be ventrifixed.

1. Elongated cervix 4.5–6 cm (Fig. 9.6a)
2. **Beaking sign**; the anterior wall of uterus show a spur like continuation to the anterior abdominal wall (Fig. 9.6b).
3. The uterus cannot be imaged with normal anterior & posterior margin. It looks, oblong, rhomboid like a mushroom, difficult to image on sonography (Fig. 9.6c).
4. Applying downward pressure on the abdomen towards the TVS probe markedly helps in presenting the uterus to be imaged in a better manner.
5. At the cervical uterine junction we see the dark colour collections or band like between the bladder and uterus.
6. Adenexa may be visualized high up not exactly by the side of the uterus, difficult to visualize depending on their adherence to anterior abdominal wall.
7. Trans abdominal ultrasound demonstration of absence of viscera slide movement on deep inspiration at the site of attachment between the uterus and anterior abdominal wall.

CT Scan Does not add anything more what can be seen on routine TVS and abdominal sonography.

MRI The anterior wall of the uterus is adherent to the anterior abdominal wall, as evidenced by obliteration of the fat plane. MRI further reveals that the uterine cervix is elongated facing the upper third of the posterior vaginal wall and located posterior to the bladder, with the absence of fat between the cervix and bladder suggesting the presence of adhesions.

Considering the increased incidence of causative factors for ventrifixed uterus, a comprehensive diagnostic approach becomes crucial. Ultrasonography (USG) diagnosis, as per ISUOG [20] guidelines, coupled with clinical examination provides essential insights. A higher position of the cervix and potential receding behind the pubic symphysis on exam-

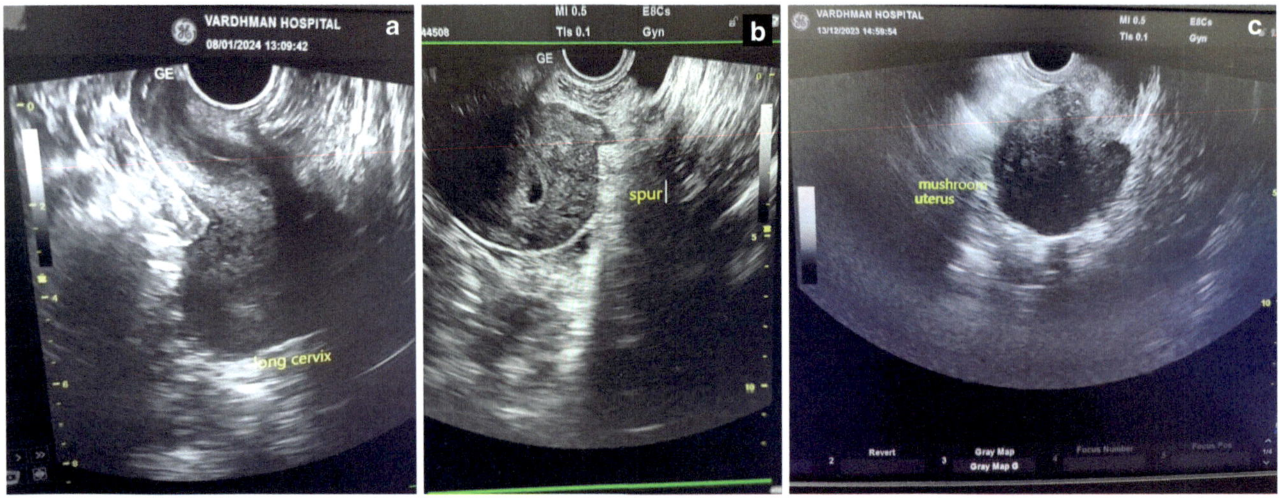

Fig. 9.6 **a** USG picture showing Long cervix. **b** USG picture showing spur like beaking. **c** USG picture showing mushroom uterus

ination raises suspicion of ventrifixed uterus. Thorough assessment and preparation by the surgical team become imperative, considering the severity of dense adhesions and adnexal involvement.

9.1.8 Surgical Approach in Ventrifixed Uterus

9.1.8.1 Points to Be Remembered Pre-Operatively

1. Always catheterize patients of TLH, but if there is ventrifixed uterus it is also good to have a surgical bougie on table, which may become handy in delineating the margins of the bladder in challenging situations.
2. We can also connect the CO2 tubing to the Foley's catheter which can help in cystosuffalation during surgery, which fills up bladder demarcating its anatomic boundaries. It also empties within no time, making it easier compared to saline instillation in urinary bladder.

Comprehensive Canopy Concept, 'The 3 Step Technique' As our surgical technique is evolving to a canopy based concept; we find it increasingly easier to navigate the uterovesical plane using this newer approach. In this technique we do not make any attempt to do the adhesiolysis of bladder or uterus from the anterior abdominal wall, instead we overcome the road block of bladder adhesions by working underneath the stretched out bladder canopy.

9.1.8.2 Laparoscopic Port Placements in TLH with Ventrifixed Uterus

Safe entry is half the battle won, so depending upon the size and mandate of the case we approach with carefully chosen laparoscopic ports.

1. **Jain Point—**For cases anticipating a ventrifixed uterus or multiple previous surgeries, the first blind laparoscopic access is performed through the Jain Point [21], the para-umbilical left lateral port, to avoid direct entry into potential adhesions, as could occur with primary umbilical entry.
2. **Supraumbilical Port—**A supraumbilical 10 mm port with a 30° scope is strategically placed. This port is dedicated to the camera and is managed by a separate assistant. The higher placement of this port is chosen for its potential to enhance the surgical field during laparoscopy. We prefer the supra-umbilical port in challenging situations, as per the belief that in laparoscopy there is no surgical field, we create our own field by CO_2 pneumoperitoneum, and so the higher we go, bigger the surgical field. The idea of sticking to the umbilical entry is hazardous for the patient and surgeon by not having adequate space for moving the instruments and exposure for safe execution of surgical steps in complex situations. Here it is pertinent to discuss the value of a well-trained assistant at the vaginal end, who can apply the manipulator and push the manipulator cup at various steps of much needed cephalad movement of the cervical isthmus.
3. **Other Ports—**The first assistant, positioned opposite the main surgeon, utilizes two ports. These are placed in standard para-umbilical and lower positions, typically 2.5 cm medial and above the ASIS. The specific positions may be adjusted based on uterine size, previous scars, and adhesions encountered within the surgical field. Port placement strategy is adapted to the unique requirements of each case.

These cases are previous caesarean sections, so firstly all adhesiolysis of bowel and omentum in the pouch of douglas is carried out. Adherent and ventrifixed uterus is not disturbed and we directly proceed to tackling the adenexa. We first start with ovaries, which are usually conserved, unless diseased. The adnexal pedicles are dissected with either ultrasonic energy or with a vessel sealer. Next is the fallopian tube and round ligament. Important steps of our technique start after transection of round ligament. One more pedicle after the round ligament is sectioned, as this opens up the broad ligament easily. We, then go by the posterior approach of uterine artery ligation.

Initial Appearance, we find a uterus which is stuck to anterior abdominal wall (Fig. 9.7a, b) We inject dilute vasopressin in large amounts with 1 ampoule in 400 normal saline. This helps in opening up the dissection planes and haemostasis. We start with the adhesiolysis, cutting & coagulation of the left adenexa (Fig. 9.8a, b).

Step 1—After cutting & coagulation of the round ligament, we open the posterior leaf of broad ligament widely almost till the **arcus torinus**. As we open up the retroperitoneal space, first the uterine vein appears in its entire splendor, appearing as a blue clearly seen vessel over the manipulator cup (Fig. 9.9a, b). Some more careful snips for avascular dissection in this space exposes the spirally winding uterine artery also. Care is taken for gentle dissection, avoiding bleeding, so that both artery and vein are fully exposed, skeletonized, coagulated and cut (Fig. 9.10). This maneuver is duly assisted by pushing the manipulator cup with steady cephalad pressure. We usually tackle the uterine pedicles with ultrasonic energy as it is a good dissector and helps in skeletonizing the uterine pedicle. Then coagulation and section is also easily accomplished. Till the uterine pedicles are done we do not disturb the bladder flap or contemplate any anterior dissection. We begin from the sectioned end of the left sided uterine artery, which when transected also cuts along with it the transverse cervical ligament and opens up the plane of bladder dissection.

Step 2: Creating the bladder canopy- The immediate 1 cm segment adjacent and anterior to the cut uterine artery pedicle (Fig. 9.11) is the most important point for dissection to expose the shiny glistening pubo-vesico cervical fascia and to start creating the bladder canopy. We need to persist at this point till we get the shiny glistening pubo-vesico cervical fascia. This step is the key to making a successful bladder canopy by getting access to the vesico vaginal space (Fig. 9.12a–e).

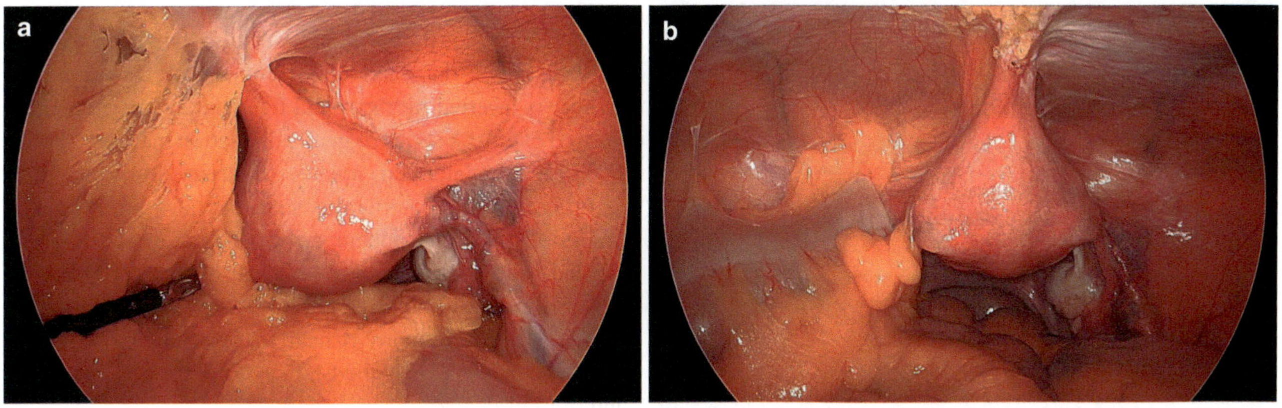

Fig. 9.7 **a** Dense omental adhesions with ventrifixed uterus. **b** Ventrifixed uterus with left adnexa covered with bowel adhesion

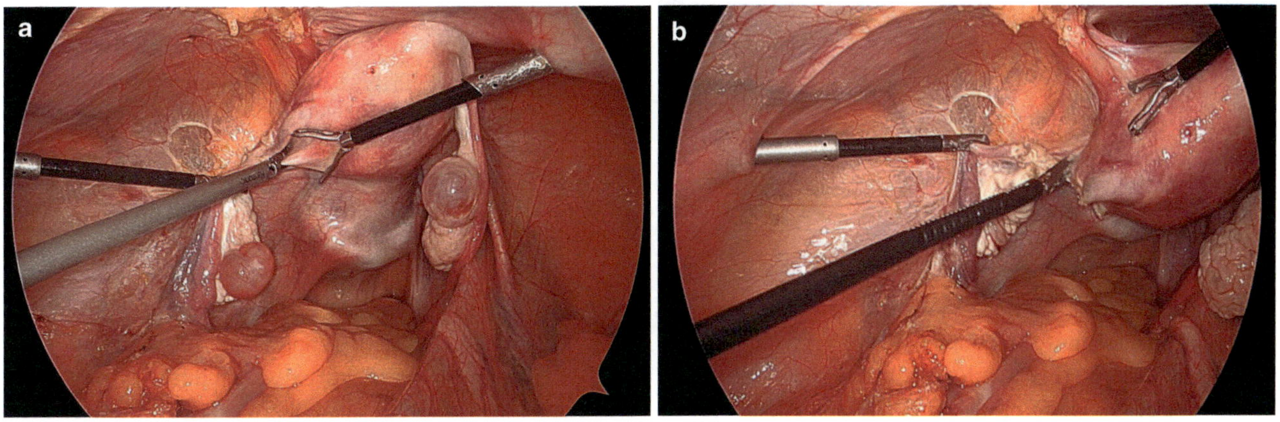

Fig. 9.8 **a** Left ovarian ligament coagulated. **b** Left round ligament coagulated

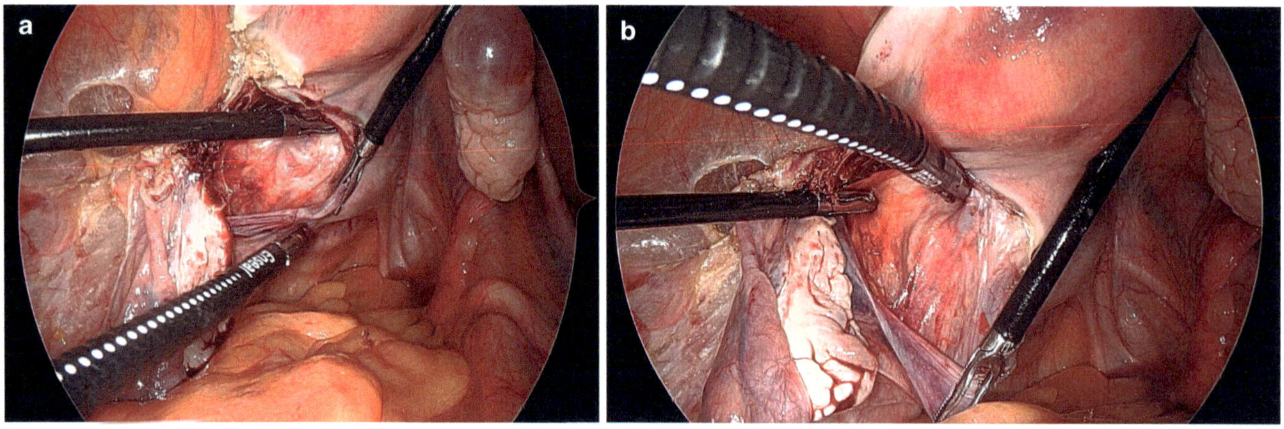

Fig. 9.9 **a** Opening up the posterior leaf of broad ligament to expose the left uterine artery. **b** uterine vein and artery skeletonized

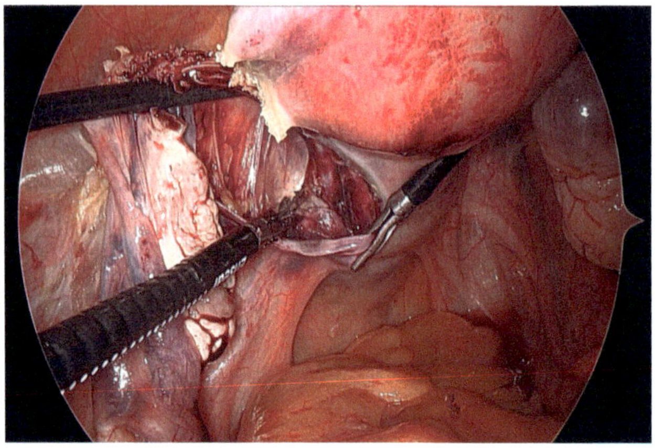

Fig. 9.10 Left uterine artery coagulated and transected

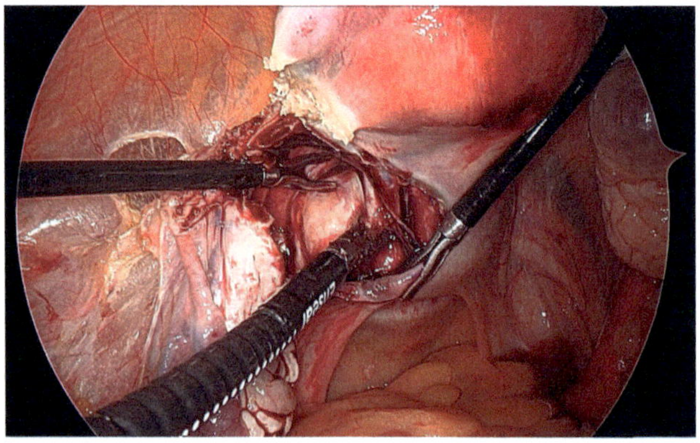

Fig. 9.11 Dissection in 1 cm area adjacent and anterior to left coagulated Uterine artery to expose the pubovesical fascia

Once we see the pearly glistening pubo-vesico cervical fascia, a more cephalad traction is given over the manipulator cup and the utero vesical space starts showing up. We gradually became more proficient in achieving this step, by the dictum "follow the bubbles". As the cotton candy plane starts appearing, it can be easily opened up and bladder walks down with combination of cephalad push of manipulator cup and atraumatic grasper working in cotton candy space. The surgical dictum is to persist at this step till the bubbles of cotton candy space become evident and a stretched bladder canopy is formed above.

Step 3: Anterior dissection of uterine artery- We now cut the utero vesical fold of peritoneum and we move forward to do the last step of our Comprehensive Canopy Concept, which is the anterior dissection of the uterine artery by the side of the manipulator cup. For it an atraumatic grasper is inserted till the round ligament and peritoneum is excised over it. A series of gentle dissection maneuver by the side of manipulator cup exposes the uterine artery.

In a ventrifixed uterus this step may also be difficult at times due to extreme adherence of uterus. We can use a bougie and show the limits of the bladder in between phases of dissection and difficulty, and best is to persistently try to dissect cotton candy utero vesical plane under the stretched bladder canopy. This is the best key to unlocking the frozen anterior cul-de-sac.

Once the canopy is fully created and is stretched over the underlying dissected utero vesicle space delineated by the manipulator cup, next step is to cut away the utero vesical fold of peritoneum close to the uterus, so that, after it is transected the flap goes flush with the abdominal wall and uterus and cervical isthmus easily falls down (Fig. 9.13a–c).

Many times we may need to come from the contralateral side as well for the right sided uterine artery; all this depends on the level of ventrifixation. So if this is the case, contralateral adnexal pedicles are dealt first, and posterior leaf of broad ligament is opened up and uterine artery skelotonization is done by the posterior approach.

But if we are proceeding easily from left side itself, then, we may find the right sided uterine artery from anterior approach itself by the side of the manipulator cup with more skilled, purposeful grasper strokes parallel to the uterine

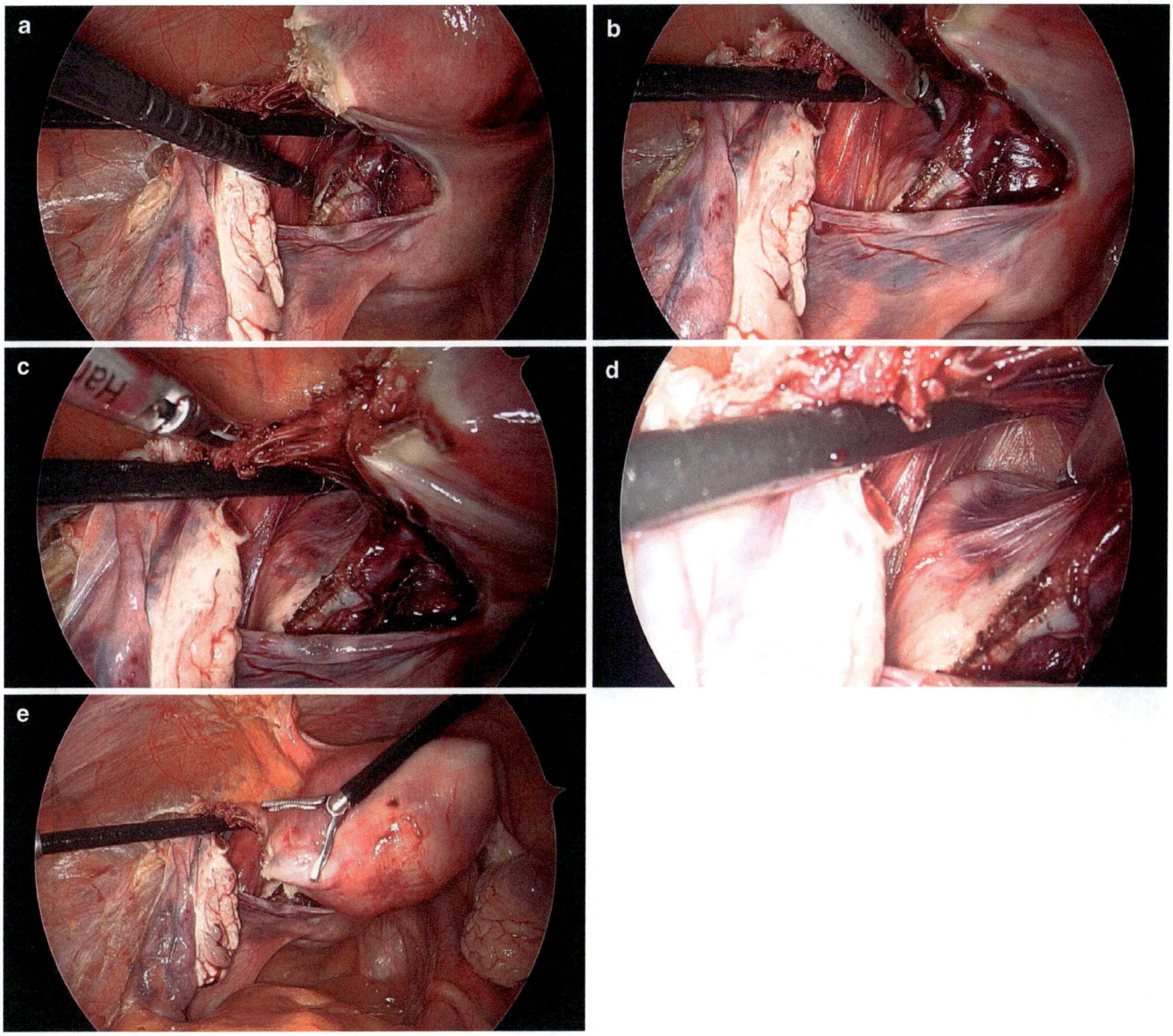

Fig. 9.12 **a** Making of bladder canopy to dissect uterovesical space. **b** Finding the uterovesical plane. **c**, **d** Cotton candy uterovesical space. **e** Dissection in UV space completed under the stretched bladder canopy; bladder is still completely adherent at the top

pedicle, opening it up in an avascular manner and the uterine pedicle is transected. Either way posterior or anterior approach, the uterine artery of the right side is transected (Fig. 9.14a–d). We then proceed to the culdotomy, which is done by monopolar hook (Fig. 9.15a, b). Double layer closure of vault and vault suspension is done with VICRYL™ (polyglactin 910) 1–0 (Fig. 9.16a–c).

Learning Points

- There is growing evidence that double layer closure of caesarean scar gives better healing.
- Visceral and parietal peritoneal closure gives decreased adhesions at caesarean scar and to abdominal wall.
- Pre-operative diagnosis of ventrifixed uterus can be made by clinical suspicion, history of abdominal pain, per vaginal and per speculum examination. Sonographic criteria are well established. Clinically elucidating retraction sign under anaesthesia is paramount in diagnosing and deft management of ventrifixed uterus.
- Comprehensive Canopy Concept, 'The 3 Step Technique' of bladder dissection without any attempt to separate the uterus from abdomen wall, is an attempt to navigate the dense bladder adhesions under the stretched bladder canopy, an endeavour to reduce bladder injury.

Competing Interest The author declares no conflict of interest that are relevant to content of this chapter.

Ethical Approval Informed consent was obtained from individual participants and patients regarding publication and documentation without disclosing their identity.

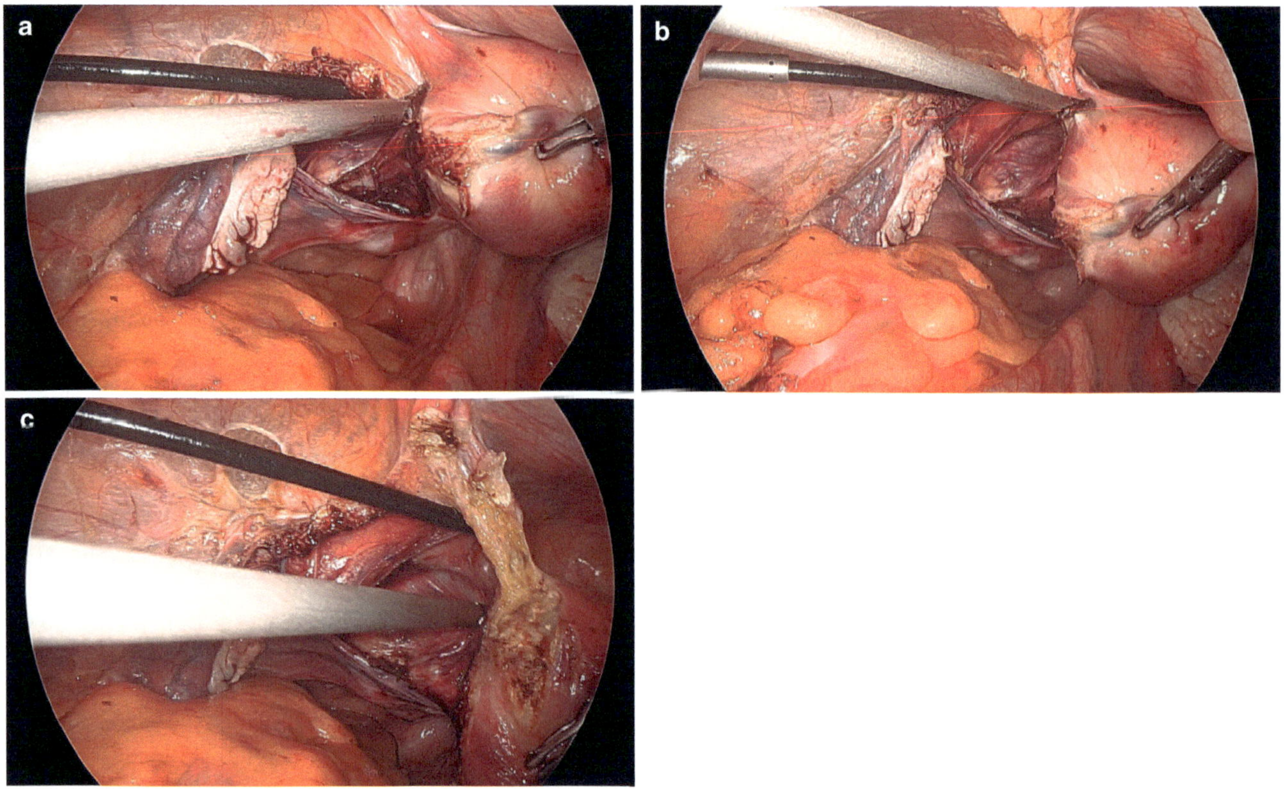

Fig. 9.13 **a** Cutting the uterovesical fold of peritoneum after completing the dissection of bladder canopy and opening of uterovesical space. **b** Cutting the uterovesical fold. **c** cutting the bladder flap which was separated by working in cotton candy uterovesical space

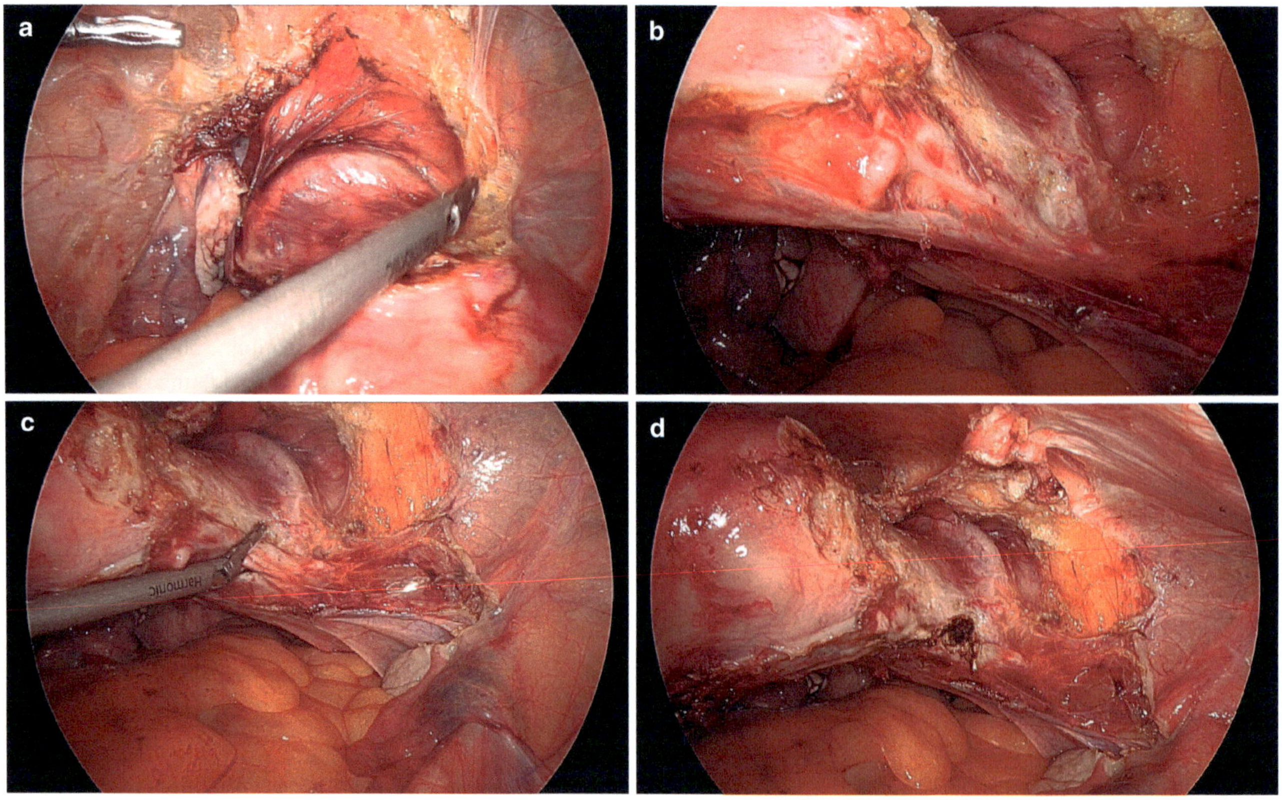

Fig. 9.14 **a** Dissection continued upto right round ligament. **b** Right uterine artery fully exposed by anterior approach. **c** Coagulating the uterine artery pedicle. **d** Uterine artery coagulated and transected off the manipulator cup rim

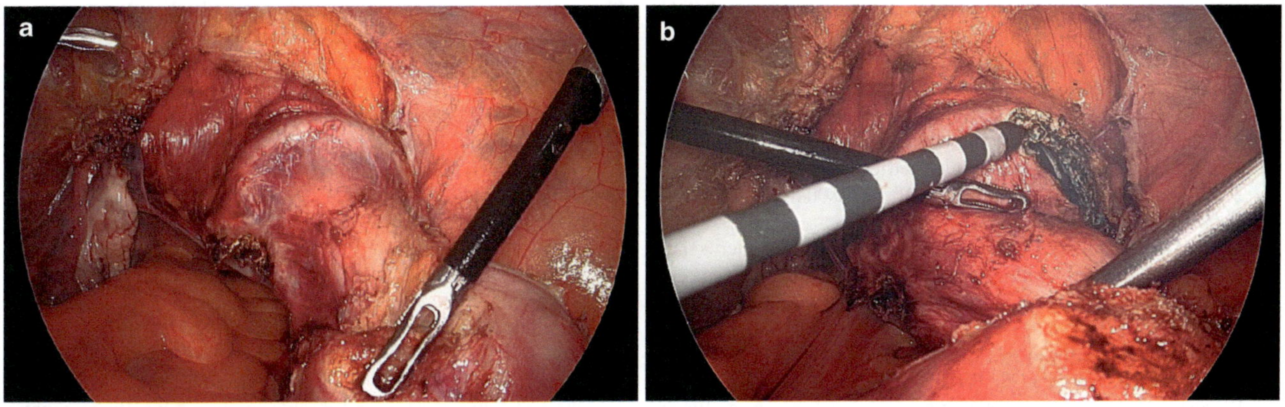

Fig. 9.15 **a**: Manipulator cup fully exposed for colpotomy. **b**: Circumferential culdotomy done by monopolar hook

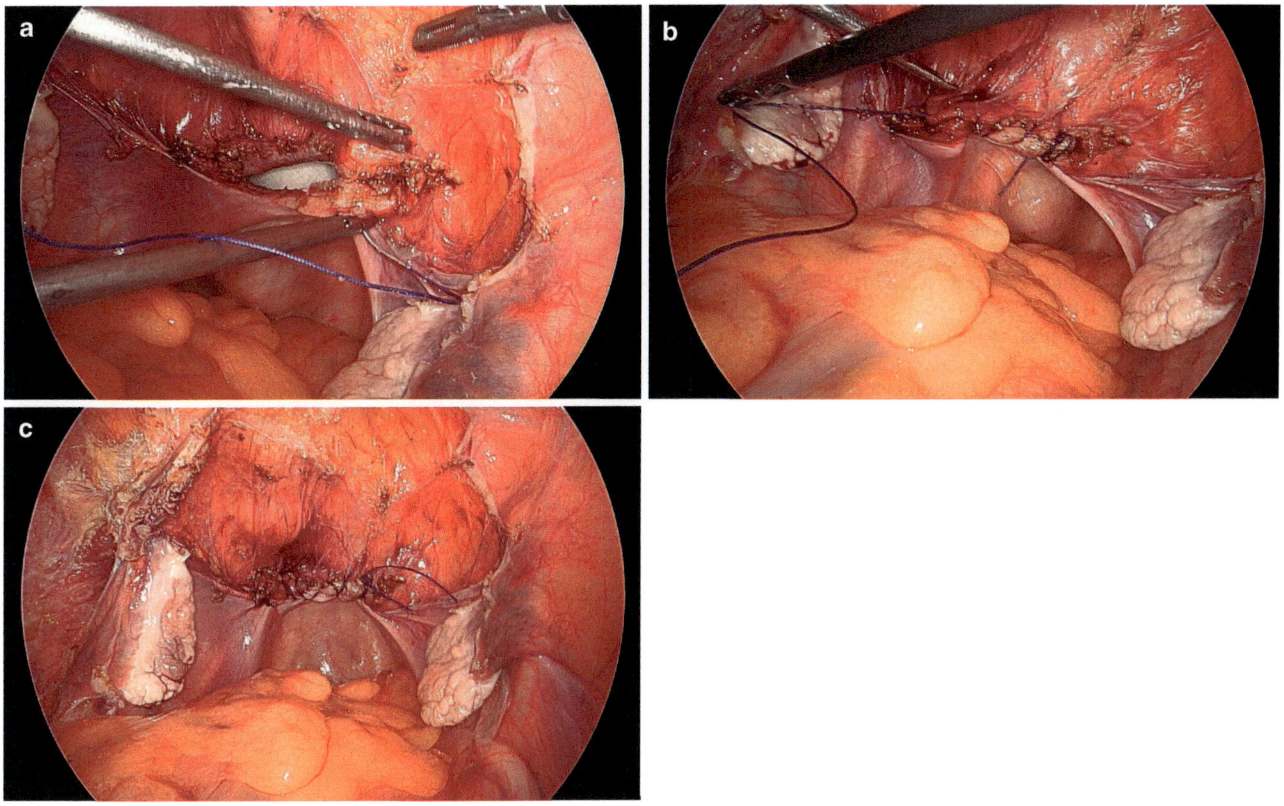

Fig. 9.16 **a** Needle passed through uterosacral ligament and anterior & posterior vault edges for suspension. **b** First layer of vault closure completed. **c** Final picture showing completed vault closure and suspension

References

1. RCOG - National Collaborating Centre for Women's and Children's Health. Caesarean section (NICE clinical guideline 132). London: Royal College of Obstetricians and Gynaccologists (RCOG) Press; 2011. p. 180–95.
2. Hofmeyr JG, Novikova N, Mathai M, Shah A. Techniques for cesarean section. Am J Obstet Gynecol. 2009;201(5):431–44. https://doi.org/10.1016/j.ajog.2009.03.018. PMID: 19879392.
3. Betran AP, Ye J, Moller AB, Souza JP, Zhang J. Trends and projections of caesarean section rates: global and regional estimates. BMJ Glob Health. 2021;6(6):e005671. https://doi.org/10.1136/bmjgh-2021-005671. PMID: 34130991; PMCID: PMC8208001.
4. Sinha R, Sundaram M, Lakhotia S, Hedge A, Kadam P. Total laparoscopic hysterectomy in women with previous cesarean sections. J Minim Invasive Gynecol. 2010;17(4):513–7. https://doi.org/10.1016/j.jmig.2010.03.018. PMID: 20621012.
5. Katsulov A, Nedialkov K, Koleva Z, Iankov M, Tashkov B, Iotov T, Kirov K, Genov M, Rusinov P, Doncheva Z, Grŭncharov I. Joel-Cohen (Misgav Ladach)-metod— nova operativna tekhnika pri tsezarovo sechenie i ginekologichna laparotomiia [The Joel-Cohen (Misgav Ladach) method—a new surgical technic for cesarean section and gynecological laparotomy]. Akush Ginekol (Sofiia). 2000;39(1):10–3. Bulgarian. PMID: 10826327.
6. Stegwee SI, Jordans I, van der Voet LF, van de Ven PM, Ket J, Lambalk CB, de Groot C, Hehenkamp W, Huirne J. Uterine caesarean closure techniques affect ultrasound findings and mater-

nal outcomes: a systematic review and meta-analysis. BJOG. 2018;125(9):1097–108. https://doi.org/10.1111/1471-0528.15048. Epub 2018 Jan 30. Erratum in: BJOG. 2019 Feb;126(3):431. PMID: 29215795.

7. Hudić I, Bujold E, Fatušić Z, Skokić F, Latifagić A, Kapidžić M, Fatušić J. The Misgav-Ladach method of cesarean section: a step forward in operative technique in obstetrics. Arch Gynecol Obstet. 2012;286(5):1141–6. https://doi.org/10.1007/s00404-012-2448-6. Epub 2012 Jul 3. PMID: 22752598.
8. Levin D, Tulandi T. Dense adhesions between the uterus and anterior abdominal wall: a unique complication of cesarean delivery. Gynecol Surg. 2011;8:415–6. https://doi.org/10.1007/s10397-010-0633-9.
9. Armstrong F, Mulligan K, Dermott RM, Bartels HC, Carroll S, Robson M, Corcoran S, Parland PM, Brien DO, Brophy D, Brennan DJ. Cesarean scar niche: an evolving concern in clinical practice. Int J Gynaecol Obstet. 2023;161(2):356–66. https://doi.org/10.1002/ijgo.14509. Epub 2022 Nov 21. PMID: 36317541.
10. Pędraszewski P, Wlaźlak E, Panek W, Surkont G. Cesarean scar pregnancy—a new challenge for obstetricians. J Ultrason. 2018;18(72):56–62. https://doi.org/10.15557/JoU.2018.0009. Epub 2018 Mar 30. PMID: 29844942; PMCID: PMC5911720.
11. Rao T, Kade S. Ventrofixed uterus: unfreezing the uterus in 6 standardized steps. J Gynecol Surg. 2023;39(5):220–1. https://doi.org/10.1089/gyn.2023.0041. Epub 2023 Oct 3. PMID: 37817874; PMCID: PMC10561766.
12. Morlando M, Collins S. Placenta accreta spectrum disorders: challenges, risks, and management strategies. Int J Women's Health. 2020;12:1033–45. https://doi.org/10.2147/IJWH.S224191. PMID: 33204176; PMCID: PMC7667500.
13. Stegwee SI, Jordans IPM, van der Voet LF, Bongers MY, de Groot CJM, et al. Single- versus double-layer closure of the caesarean (uterine) scar in the prevention of gynaecological symptoms in relation to niche development—the 2Close study: a multicentre randomised controlled trial. BMC Pregnancy Childbirth. 2019;19(1):85. https://doi.org/10.1186/s12884-019-2221-y. PMID: 30832681; PMCID: PMC6399840.
14. Lyell DJ, Caughey AB, Hu E, Daniels K. Peritoneal closure at primary cesarean delivery and adhesions. Obstet Gynecol. 2005;106(2):275–80. https://doi.org/10.1097/01.AOG.0000171120.81732.4c. PMID: 16055575.
15. Vervoort AJ, Uittenbogaard LB, Hehenkamp WJ, Brölmann HA, Mol BW, Huirne JA. Why do niches develop in caesarean uterine scars? Hypotheses on the aetiology of niche development. Hum Reprod. 2015;30(12):2695–702. https://doi.org/10.1093/humrep/dev240. Epub 2015 Sep 25. PMID: 26409016; PMCID: PMC4643529.
16. Jordans IPM, de Leeuw RA, Stegwee SI, et al. Sonographic examination of uterine niche in non-pregnant women: a modified Delphi procedure. Ultrasound Obstet Gynecol. 2019;53(1):107–15. https://doi.org/10.1002/uog.19049.
17. Rodgers SK, Kirby CL, Smith RJ, Horrow MM. Imaging after cesarean delivery: acute and chronic complications. Radiographics. 2012;32(6):1693–712. https://doi.org/10.1148/rg.326125516. PMID: 23065165.
18. El-Shawarby SA, Salim R, Lavery S, Saridogan E. Uterine adherence to anterior abdominal wall after caesarean section. BJOG. 2011;118(9):1133–5. https://doi.org/10.1111/j.1471--0528.2011.02965.x. Epub 2011 Apr 12. PMID: 21481158.
19. Sheth SS. Clinical and sonographic signs to diagnose uterocervical adhesions to the abdominal wall following caesarean section. BJOG 2012;119(1):116; author reply 117. https://doi.org/10.1111/j.1471-0528.2011.03185.x. PMID: 22168615.
20. Jordans IPM, Verberkt C, De Leeuw RA, Bilardo CM, Van Den Bosch T, Bourne T, Brölmann HAM, Dueholm M, Hehenkamp WJK, Jastrow N, Jurkovic D, Kaelin Agten A, Mashiach R, Naji O, Pajkrt E, Timmerman D, Vikhareva O, Van Der Voet LF, Huirne JAF. Definition and sonographic reporting system for Cesarean scar pregnancy in early gestation: modified Delphi method. Ultrasound Obstet Gynecol. 2022;59(4):437–49. https://doi.org/10.1002/uog.24815. PMID: 34779085; PMCID: PMC9322566.
21. Jain N, et al. Jain point: to avoid trocar injuries in multiple previous surgeries. Med Res Arch [S.l.]. 2023;11(11). ISSN 2375-1924. Available at: https://esmed.org/MRA/mra/article/view/4734. Date accessed: 17 Jan 2024. https://doi.org/10.18103/mra.v11i11.4734.

Total Laparoscopic Hysterectomy (TLH) in Extensive Endometriosis

10

Nutan Jain, Sakshi Srivastava, and Divyanee Gulati

10.1 Introduction

Total Laparoscopic Hysterectomy (TLH) is a complex surgical intervention for managing extensive endometriosis, marked by extensive fibrosis [1]. Adhesions [2] are often noted all around the uterus and obliterating the pouch of Douglas. If it is compounded by previous caesarean deliveries [3], it makes the adhesions worse as the anterior pouch also gets obliterated [4]. This chapter delves into the laparoscopic canopy guided posterior to contralateral uterine artery section, aimed at enhancing the safety and efficacy of TLH in the context of extensive endometriosis. From preoperative strategies to postoperative care, the chapter covers crucial aspects contributing to successful outcomes in the surgical management of such complex cases.

Supplementary Information The online version contains supplementary material available at https://doi.org/10.1007/978-981-97-3226-5_10. The videos can be accessed individually by clicking the DOI link in the accompanying figure caption or by scanning this link with the SN More Media App.

N. Jain (✉)
Obstetrics and Gynaecology, GSVM Medical College, Affiliated by Kanpur University, Kanpur, Uttar Pradesh, India

Department of Obstetrics and Gynecology, Vardhman Trauma and Laparoscopy Centre Pvt. Ltd., Muzaffarnagar, Uttar Pradesh, India

S. Srivastava
Obstetrics and Gynaecology, Rohilkhand Medical College and Hospital, Affiliated by Bareilly International University, Bareilly, Uttar Pradesh, India

Gynaecology Endoscopy, Vardhman Trauma and Laparoscopy Centre Pvt. Ltd., Muzaffarnagar, Uttar Pradesh, India

D. Gulati
Gynaecology Endoscopy, Vardhman Trauma and Laparoscopy Centre Pvt. Ltd., Muzaffarnagar, Uttar Pradesh, India

Obstetrics and Gynaecology, GMC Patiala, Affiliated by Baba Farid University of Health Sciences, Patiala, Punjab, India

10.2 Preoperative Workup in Cases of Endometriosis

Detailed preoperative workup is warranted before posting such extensive endometriosis cases for surgery, considering the disease extent, prior surgeries, and patient preferences.

- We take a detailed history regarding her symptoms of heavy bleeding, severity of dysmenorrhoea, dyspareunia, dysuria and dyschezia.
- Then we do a per speculum examination to look for any bluish vaginal nodule.
- We then do a per vaginal examination to assess the uterus size, mobility, degree of flexion, any adnexal endometriotic cysts and specially focus on the size and extent of rectovaginal nodules.
- Next step is to do a KUB scan to look for kidney size and any renal pelvis dilatation, giving evidence of ureteric endometriosis.
- Further we do a full bladder ultrasound to rule out any bladder nodule.
- Then we ask her to empty the bladder and we do a transvaginal scan, assess any adenomyosis, adenomyomas location, endometriotic cysts and the size and location of rectovaginal nodules, if any, and their distance from the anal verge.
- We also do MRI to further precise our findings. This is done to decide the extent of bowel endometriosis and formulate the further course of management.
- **Management plan**—The management of the rectal nodule is done in accordance with the pre-operative findings, ENZIAN scoring [5] MRI [6] and ultrasound [7]; which gives an idea about the extent of invasion of the rectum layers by the nodule [8].
  - If the nodule is less than 3 cm and does not go beyond one third of the muscularis, it is kept for shaving [9].

N. Jain (ed.), *Complex Total Laparoscopic Hysterectomy (TLH) with Newer Approaches in Bladder Dissection*,
https://doi.org/10.1007/978-981-97-3226-5_10

- If the nodule is bigger than 3 cm and penetrates the deeper layers of the muscularis, a disc excision is carried out [10].
- If the nodule is involving more than two thirds of the circumference of the rectum and is also invading the rectal mucosa, rectal resection anastomosis is carried out with the help of colorectal team [11].
- If the patient has significant and extensive disease involving ovaries, we do a thorough preoperative counselling [12]. We counsel the patient and her husband and clearly ask their choice about the ovarian removal or conservation, telling them the pros and cons of ovarian removal. We let them know the benefits of conservation with a little risk of recurrence. This way the patient and her husband make an informed choice whether they want to face the risk of recurrence, which could be about 21.5% after 2 years and 40–50% in the next 5 years [13]; or be completely sure that after the ovaries and rectovaginal nodules have been removed, the patient could remain disease and symptom free. Preoperatively, we keep the patient on liquid diet and clear her bowels with laxatives and then post her for surgery.

10.3 Use of ICG to Prevent Ureteric Injury

To make the procedure safer for avoidance of ureteric injury [14], we inject diluted ICG by ureteric catheters [15] during cystoscopy. (Fig. 10.1) ICG is prepared in the operating room by dissolving 25 mg of sterile amorphous Indocyanine green (ICG) in 10 ml of distilled water (concentration of 2.5 mg/ml). 2 ml of this is taken and further diluted in 10 ml of distilled water. A 5F ureteral catheter is cystoscopically inserted into the mid ureters and 5 ml of the diluted ICG is injected retrograde into the lumen of each ureter. We need special camera system to pick up the near infrared images of the fluorescent green dye which has been injected in the ureter [16]. In our set up we use camera systems which have the benefit of on lay mode. In this mode we keep getting the routine laparoscopic picture in 4k modality and over it, the fluorescent green path of the ureter is super imposed. This makes it extremely handy in scenarios of frozen pelvis [17] and parametrial endometriosis [18], where the extensive fibrotic disease is almost encircling the entire path of ureter.

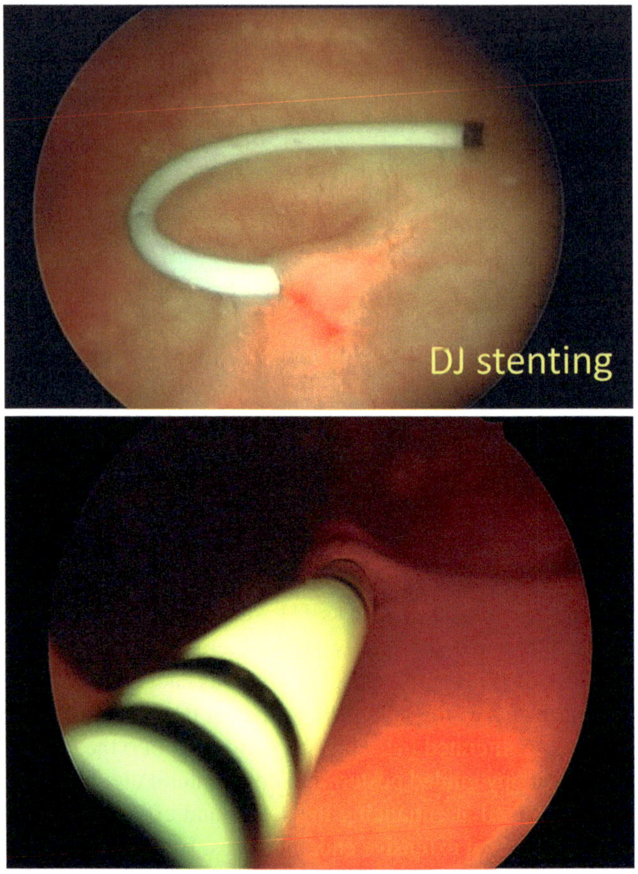

Fig. 10.1 ICG injected through Ureteric catheter

10.4 Surgical Approach in Eendometriosis

- **Vasopressin injection**—When we start the laparoscopic part of TLH in a case of stage IV endometriosis (Fig. 10.2), we first inject diluted vasopressin 1 amp in 400 ml normal saline (Fig. 10.3). This gives a very safe concentration of vasopressin [19] which helps the surgeon in two ways;
  (a) Firstly by doing vasoconstriction and decreasing the blood loss,
  (b) Secondly by creating a handy plane of cleavage by the principle of hydro dissection [20]. We always inject large amounts of vasopressin to get good easy avascular plane of cleavage.
- We then start dissection at the left pelvic brim (Fig. 10.4) at the physiological adherence of sigmoid colon to the lateral pelvic wall. Due to extensive adhesions, we use ultrasonic energy having less thermal spread [21], as the

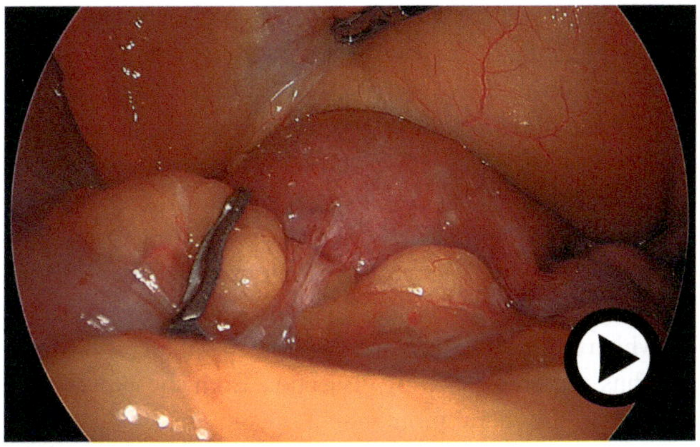

Fig. 10.2 Uterus densely retroverted, fixed in pouch of douglas with rectosigmoid stuck over the posterior surface of uterus (Video 10.2 TLH with Severe Endometriosis) (▶ https://doi.org/10.1007/000-c96)

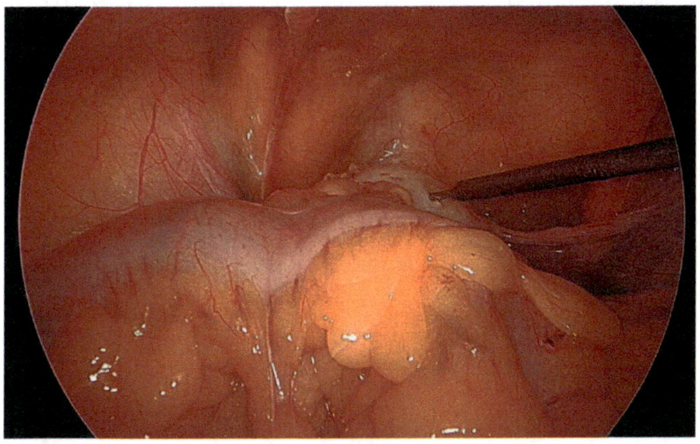

Fig. 10.3 Diluted vasopressin injected over the uterus

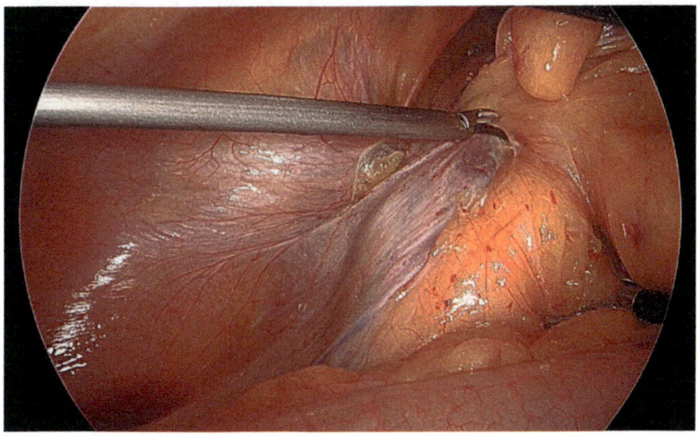

Fig. 10.4 Adhesiolysis started from left pelvic brim

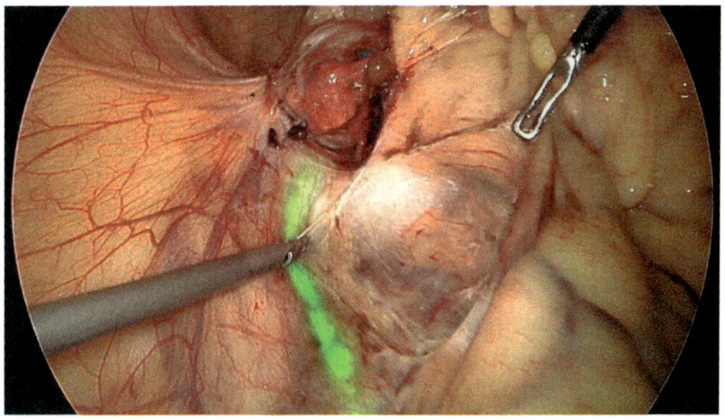

Fig. 10.5 Left ureterolysis started from pelvic brim toward the sacral promontory

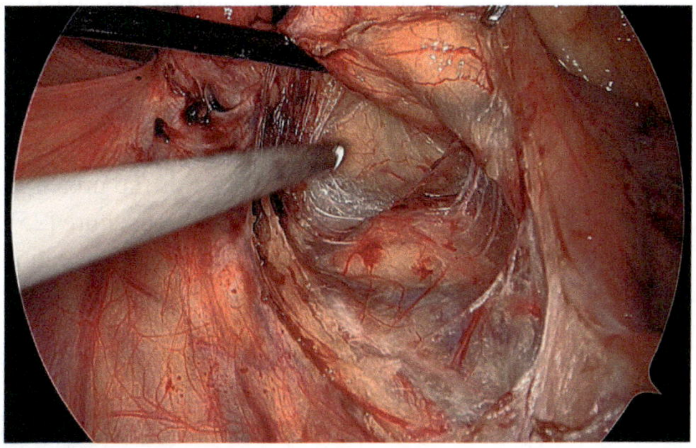

Fig. 10.6 Presacral fascia exposed on the left side

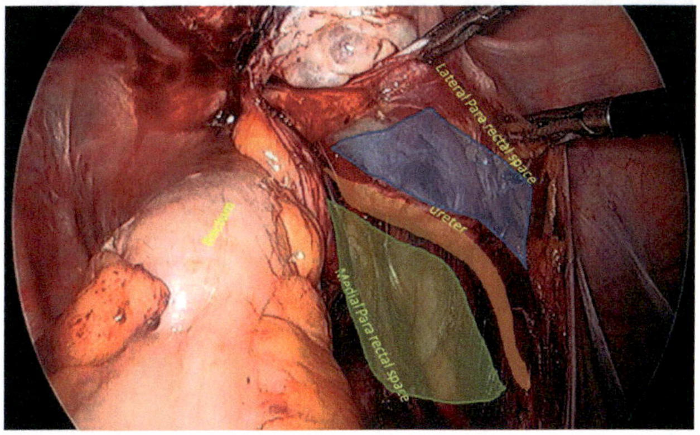

Fig. 10.7 Ureterolysis done to expose the medial and lateral pararectal spaces

dissector and energy source. We work over the pelvic brim (Figs. 10.5 and 10.6) towards the sacral promontory and expose the pre sacral fascia.

- We keep working towards the rectum and open up the medial and lateral para-rectal spaces (Fig. 10.7) [22]. This is accomplished by starting the dissection for exposure of the ureter. We inject ICG into the ureters beforehand, so it becomes very easy to localise the ureter and dissect it out to get entry into the medial para-rectal space. The assistant and surgeon work closely together in good coordination. Even in the worst possible adhesion scenario, instillation of ICG easily opens up these spaces without risk of ureteric injury. Very special care needs to be given to avoid thermal and mechanical injuries to the ureter [23]. We usually put a rectal probe to divert the rectum to the contralateral side and put a stretch on the rectum to delineate the boundary of rectum, further exposing the medial para-rectal space. Ureter makes the lateral boundary of this space so exposure and lateral retraction over the ureter, further opens up the medial para-rectal space.

- The other important structures in the medial para-rectal space is the **inferior hypogastric plexus** [24]. (Fig. 10.8) In order to expose the hypogastric plexus, we start our dissection as stated earlier over the pelvic brim. We palpate the sacral promontory and open up the pre-sacral fascia, advance further and make our way to the waldeyer's fascia.
- After the initial ureterolysis at the level of pelvic brim and opening up of medial para-rectal space, we proceed to the antegrade dissection of the left adnexa to be able to carry out the further dissection in the rectovaginal space (Figs. 10.9 and 10.10) Once the medial para-rectal space has been developed till the utero sacral ligaments (Fig. 10.11), then we identify the inferior hypogastric plexus and push it further laterally towards the ureter. In this way, we are able to do a nerve sparing procedure [25], thus avoiding difficulties in urine voiding and defecation [26] which can arise in the post-operative phase.
- After we push the ureter and the inferior hypo gastric plexus laterally, we reach the level of utero sacral ligaments. From there, we curve inwards in a coma shaped manner and direct the dissection towards the rectovaginal space. (Figs. 10.12, 10.13 and 10.14) This predictive anatomy [27], knowing exactly what structure come one after the other, helps in a smooth dissection. The dissection in the rectovaginal space is eased out by the presence of the rectal probe and stout ante-version of the uterus (Fig. 10.15) which is done by the help of uterine manipulator [28].
- Thus the entire step of dissection from the pelvic brim over to the sacral promontory, opening up of the medial para-rectal space, pushing laterally of the ureter and inferior hypogastric plexus, till reaching the mid of the recto-vaginal space is done on one side; and then we proceed to the right side, doing exactly the same steps as were done on the left side (Fig. 10.16, 10.17, 10.18, 10.19, 10.20, 10.21, 10.22, 10.23, 10.24, 10.25, 10.26 and 10.27). So at the end of the dissection on both the side we get the appearance of an ***hour glass*** (Fig. 10.28) [29]; where the uterus and the rectum are the two components of the hourglass and in the middle are the adhesions of severe endometriosis and rectovaginal nodules. We open up the

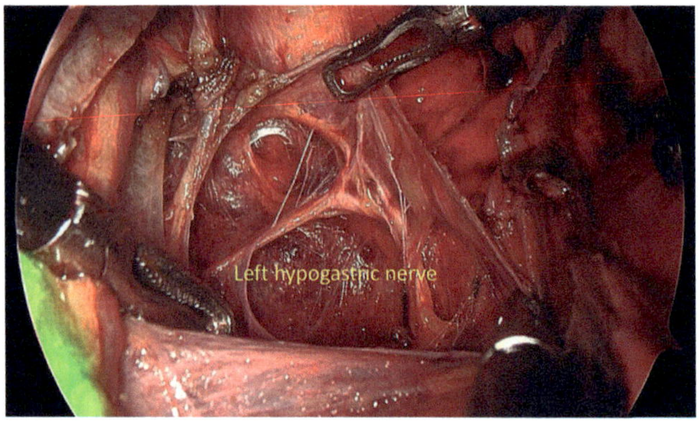

Fig. 10.8 Tracing the hypogastric nerve at the beginning of the surgery to ensure a nerve sparing procedure

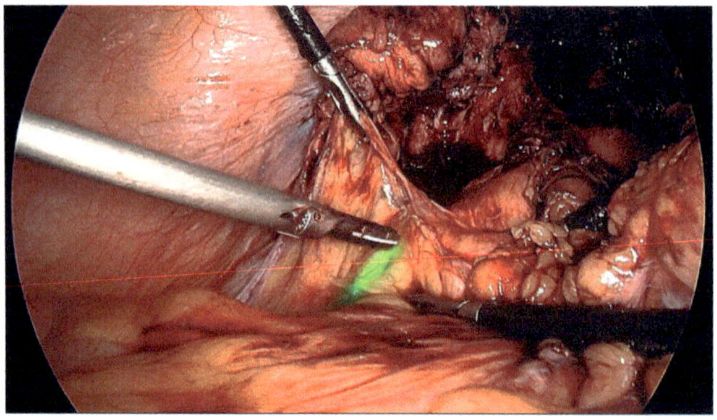

Fig. 10.9 After the initial ureterolysis at the level of pelvic brim and opening up of medial pararectal space, dissection proceeds further to reach the rectovaginal space

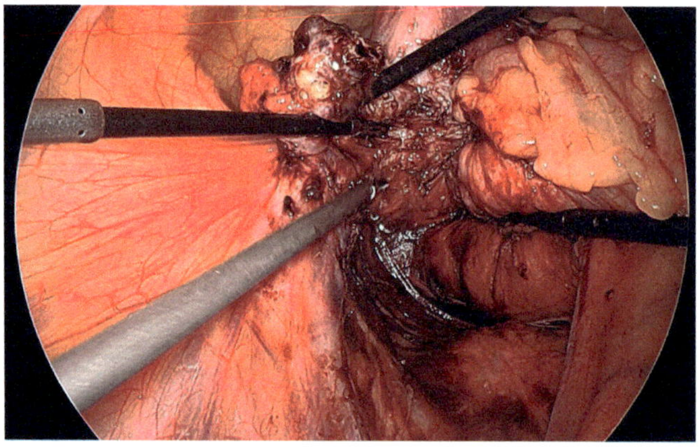

Fig. 10.10 Antegrade dissection of the left adnexa done to further open up the rectovaginal space

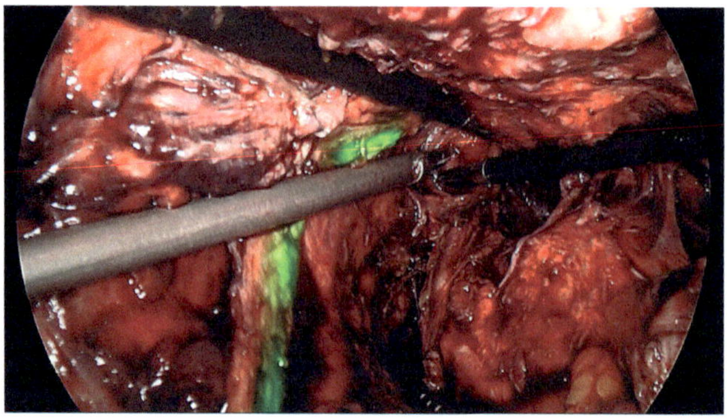

Fig. 10.11 Left side ureterolysis done upto the uterosacral ligaments

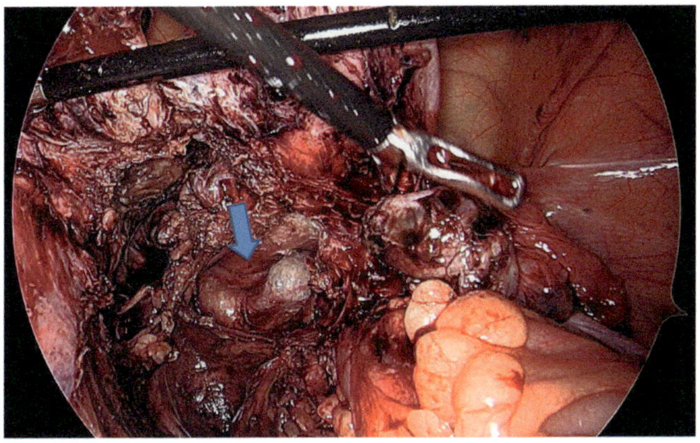

Fig. 10.12 Rectovaginal space started appearing

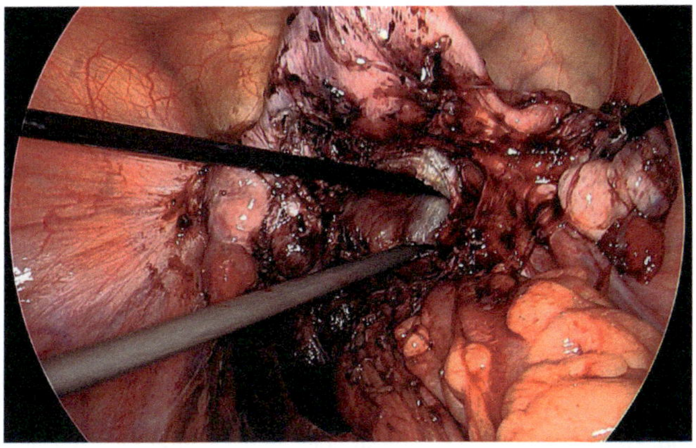

Fig. 10.13 Dissection further proceeds to clear up the rectovaginal space by following the cotton candy plane

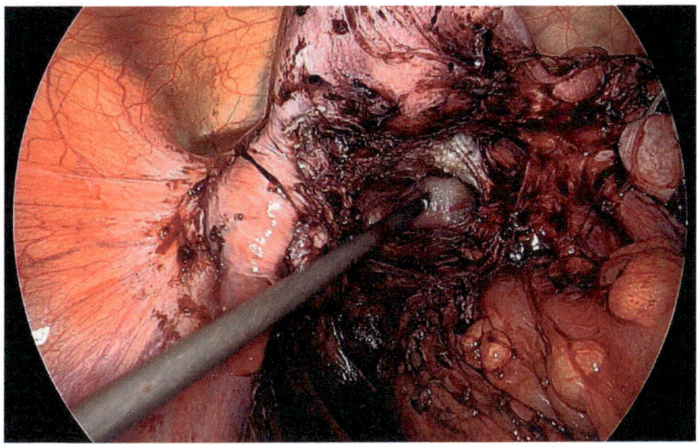

Fig. 10.14 Rectovaginal space fully exposed from the left side

rectovaginal space by dissecting the adhesions of rectum and retro cervical region. The rectum is fully brought down opening up the cotton candy recto vaginal space. The rectal nodule management is done according to the pre-operative assessment with shaving, disc or end to end resection anastomosis.

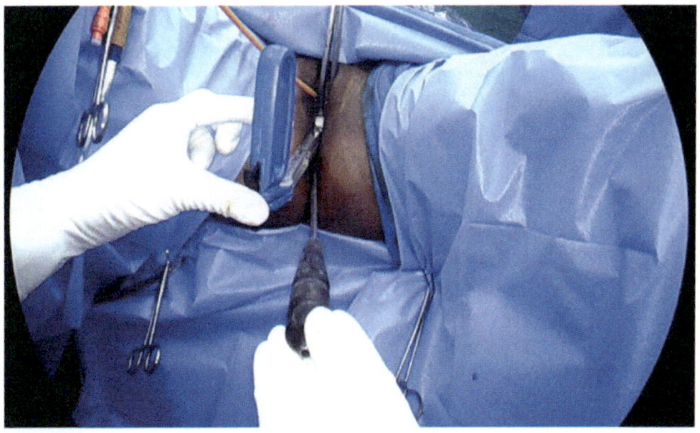

Fig. 10.15 RUMI uterine manipulator and rectal probe

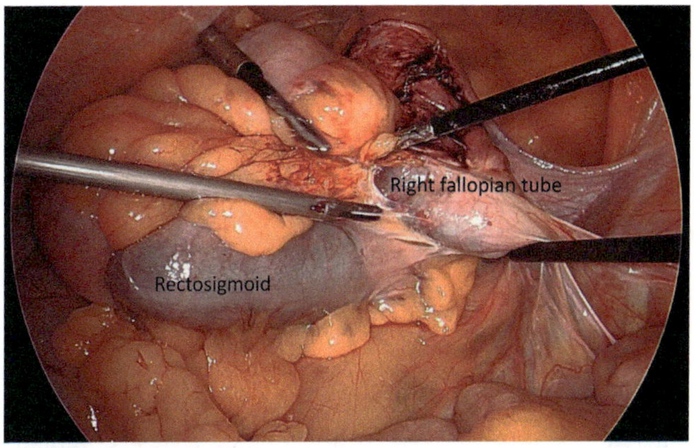

Fig. 10.16 Adhesiolysis on right side

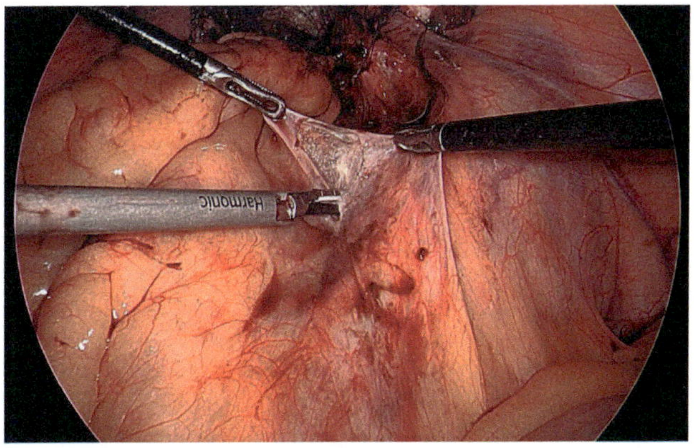

Fig. 10.17 Opening presacral space

After the pouch of douglas is fully cleared and the parametrial and ovarian endometriosis has been taken care of, we proceed to the steps of TLH (Figs. 10.29, 10.30, 10.31, 10.32, 10.33, 10.34, 10.35, 10.36, 10.37, 10.38, 10.39, 10.40, 10.41, 10.42, 10.43, 10.44, 10.45 and 10.46).

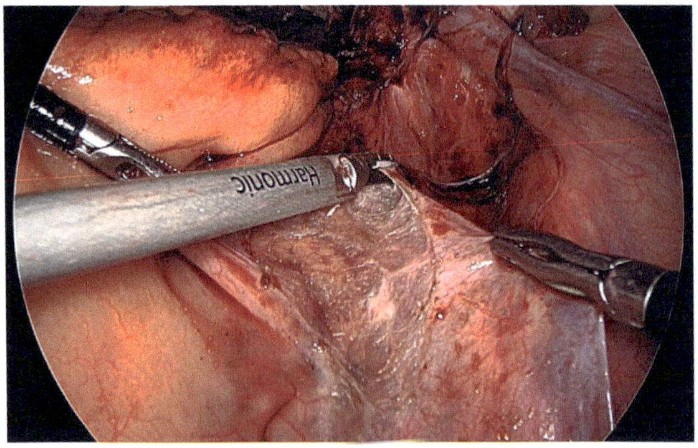

Fig. 10.18 Cutting the presacral fascia

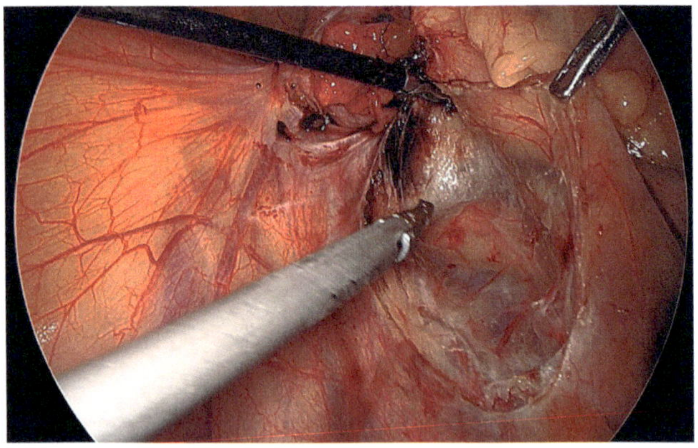

Fig. 10.19 Sacral promontory exposed and entry in to presacral space

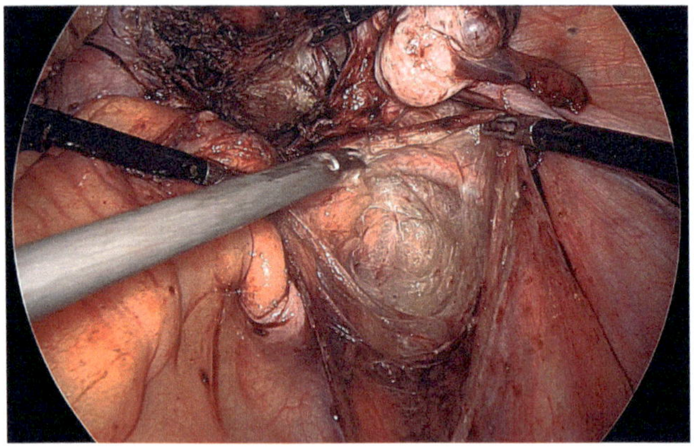

Fig. 10.20 Right ureterolysis done and pararectal space cleared

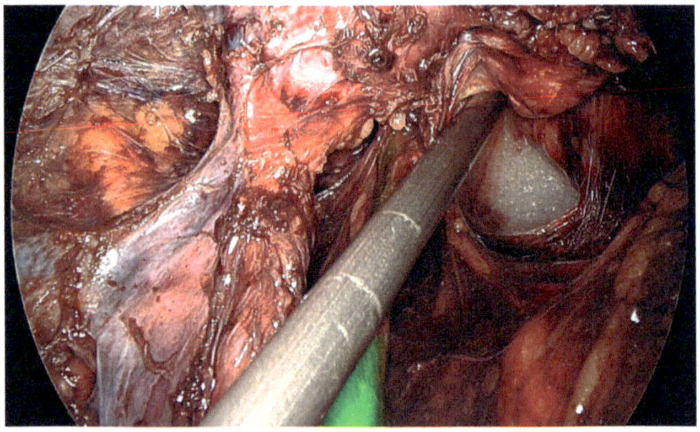

Fig. 10.21 Cotton candy rectovaginal space visualized

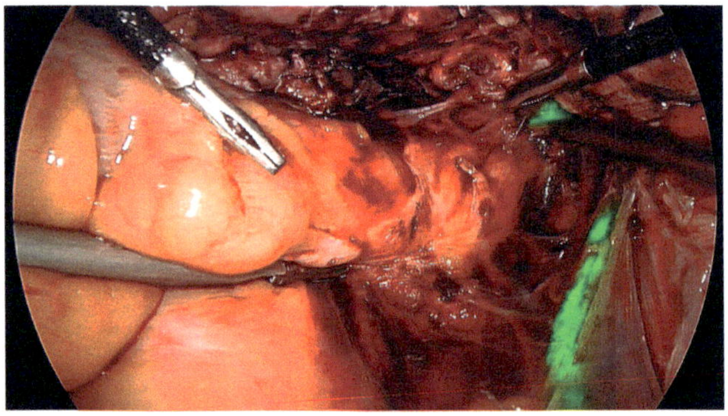

Fig. 10.22 Right side ureterolysis done till the uterosacral ligament

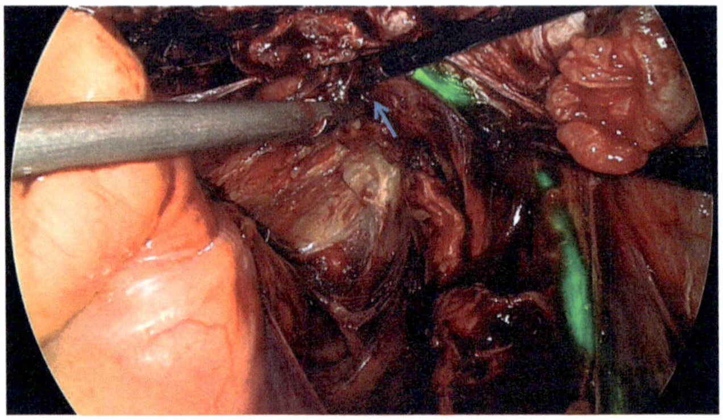

Fig. 10.23 Atraumatic grasper deflecting the ureter laterally and making way for further dissection to reach the rectovaginal space

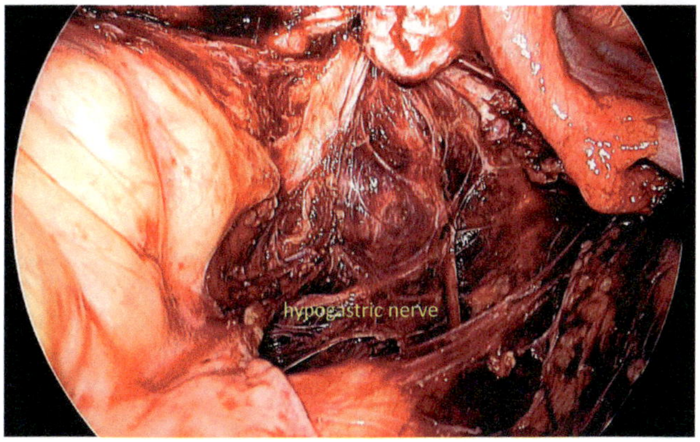

Fig. 10.24 Right side hypogastric plexus exposed to ensure a nerve sparing procedure

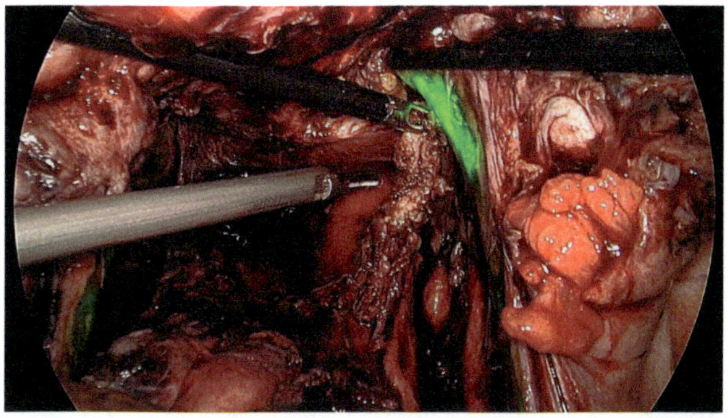

Fig. 10.25 Excision of rectovaginal nodule

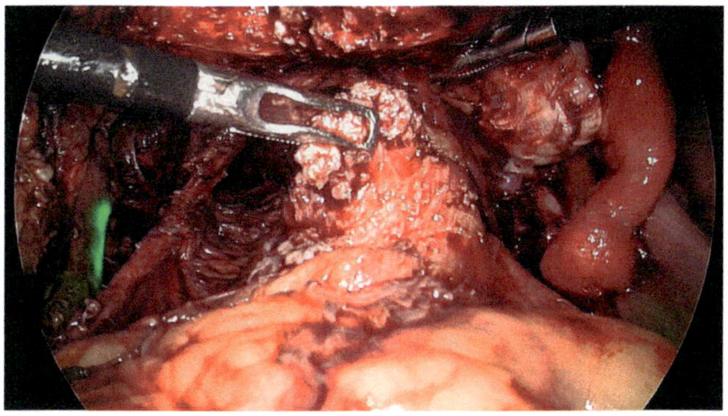

Fig. 10.26 Shaving of rectovaginal endometriotic nodule from the rectum

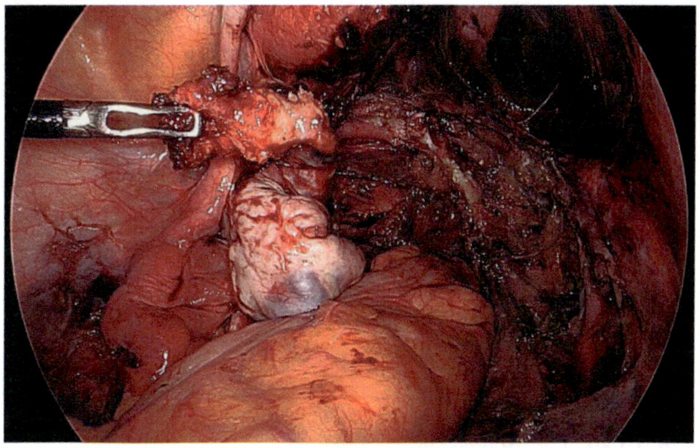

Fig. 10.27 POD cleared of all rectovaginal endometriotic nodules and now patient is set for TLH

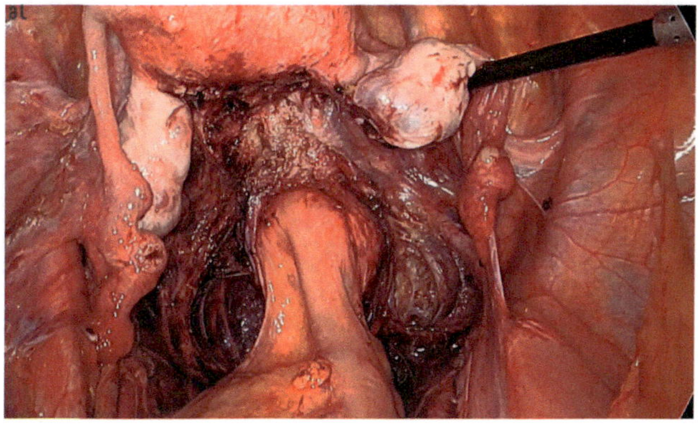

Fig. 10.28 Hour glass appearance after dissection done on right and left side

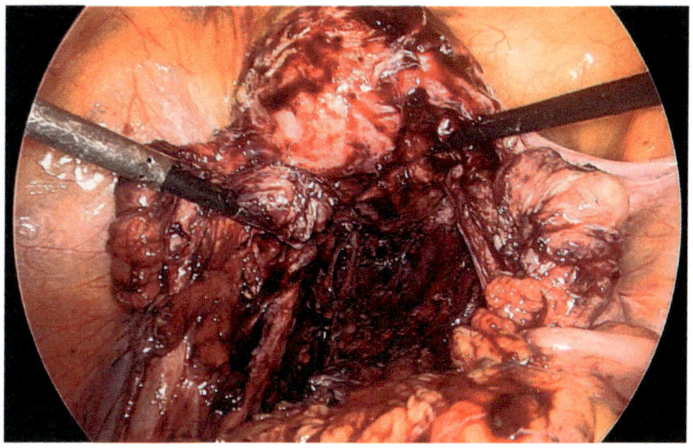

Fig. 10.29 Ante grade dissection of ovaries is carried out

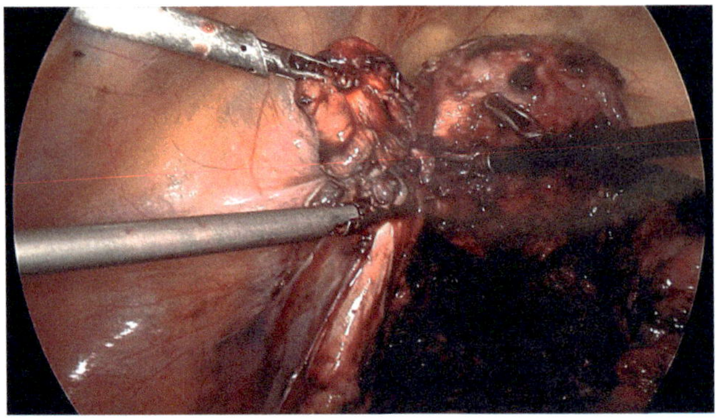

Fig. 10.30 Left IP ligament coagulated

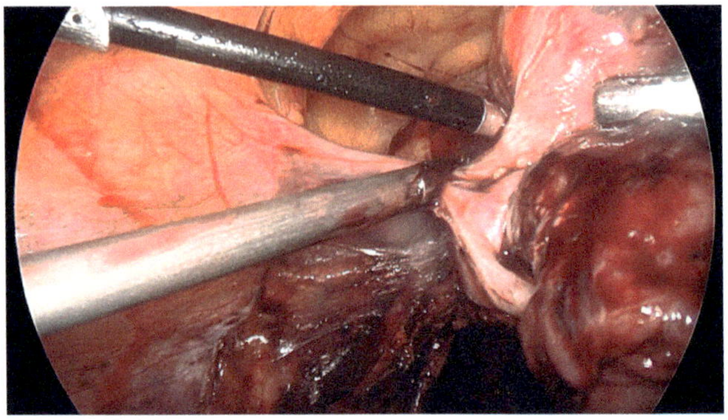

Fig. 10.31 Left round ligament coagulated

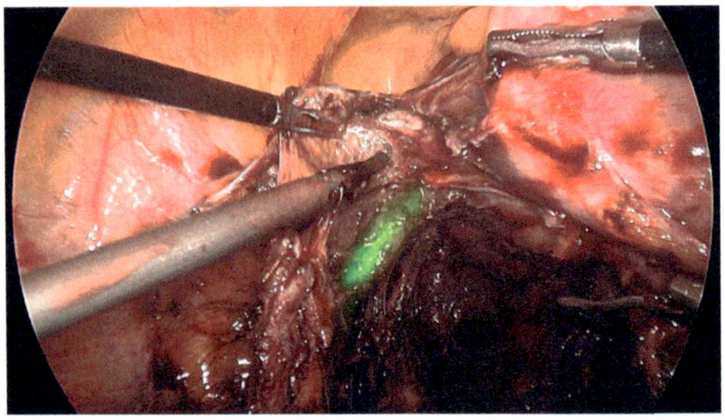

Fig. 10.32 Left uterine artery crossing over the ureter, depicting water under the bridge sign. Bladder adherent to the anterior surface of uterus

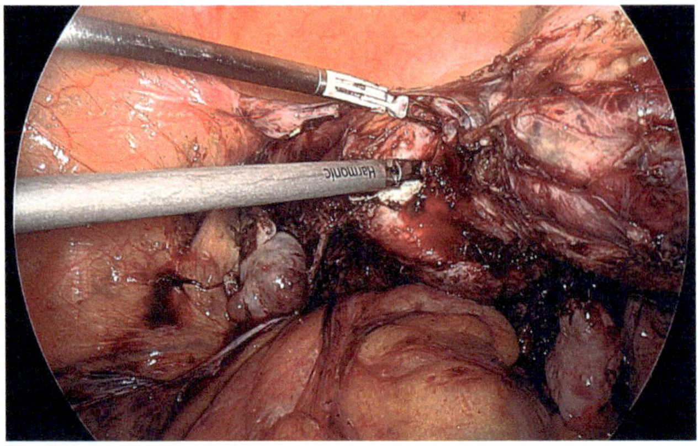

Fig. 10.33 Coagulating and cutting the left uterine artery first, before the bladder dissection

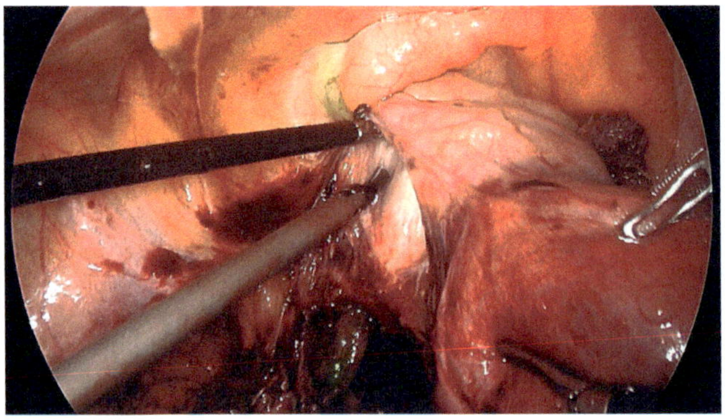

Fig. 10.34 After transecting the uterine artery, dissection of 1 cm area just adjacent to uterine artery done to develop the bladder canopy

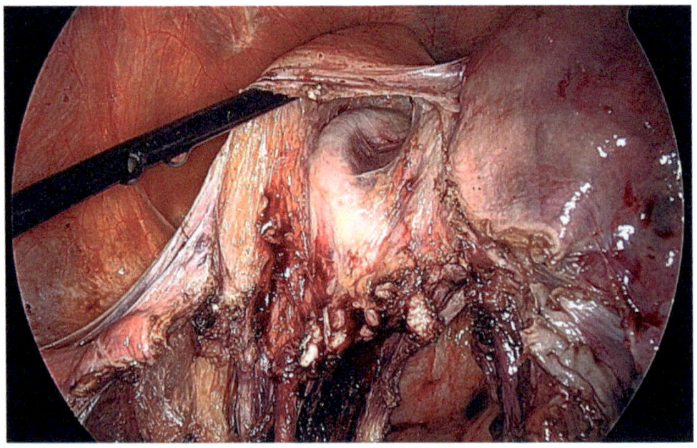

Fig. 10.35 Canopy concept of bladder dissection

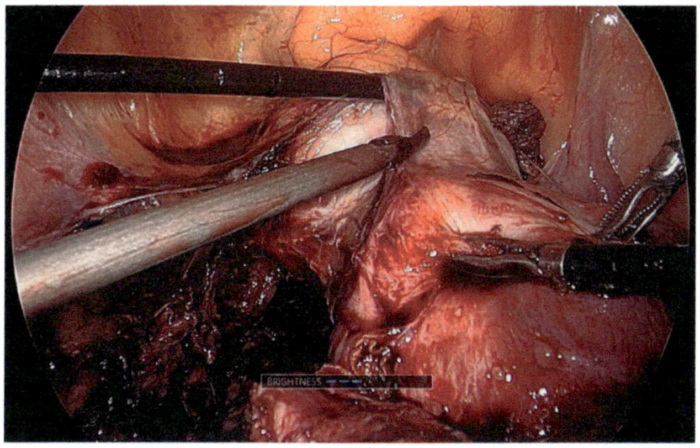

Fig. 10.36 Cutting the UV fold, after the UV space dissection is completed

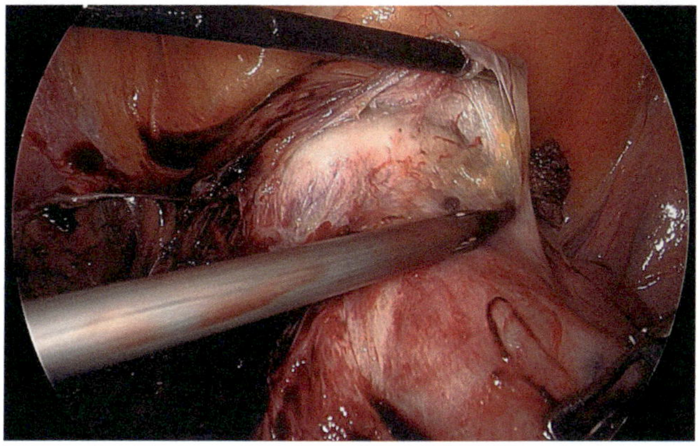

Fig. 10.37 Dissection continues widely till the contralateral round ligament to expose the contralateral uterine artery from the anterior approach

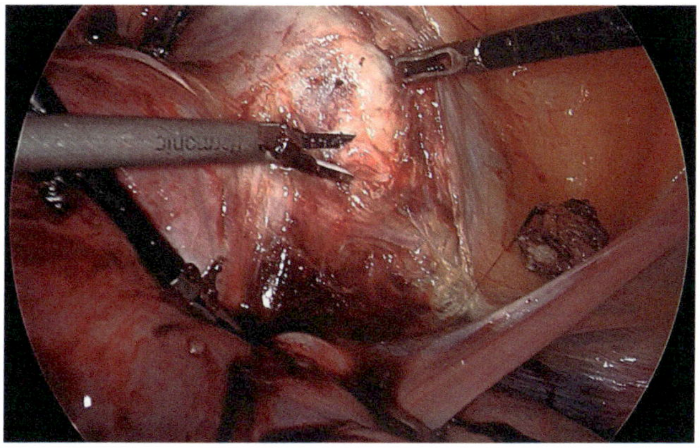

Fig. 10.38 Uterine artery widely exposed by the anterior approach

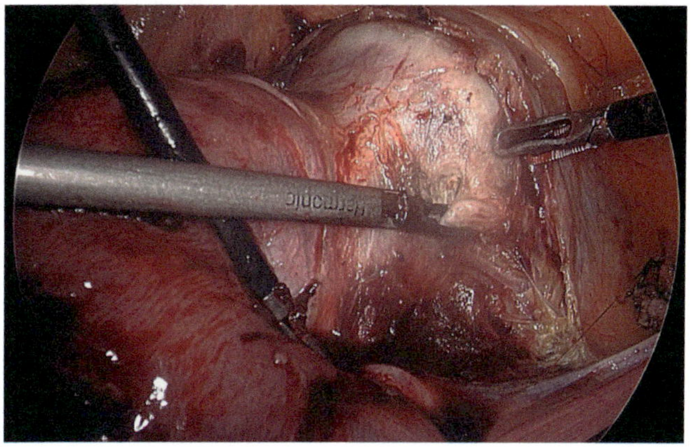

Fig. 10.39 Right uterine artery coagulated and cut

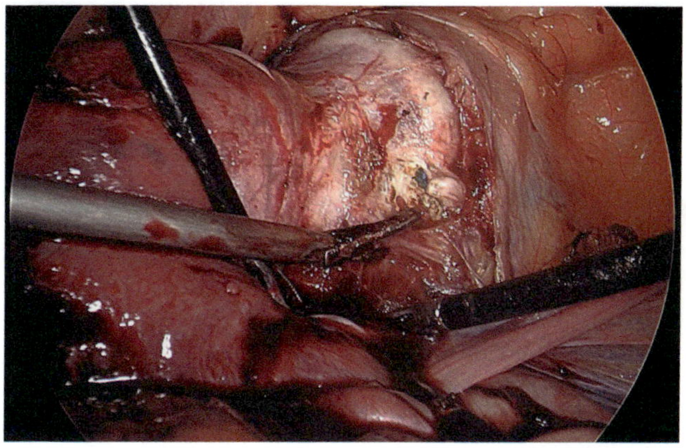

Fig. 10.40 Uterine artery shaved off the manipulator cup

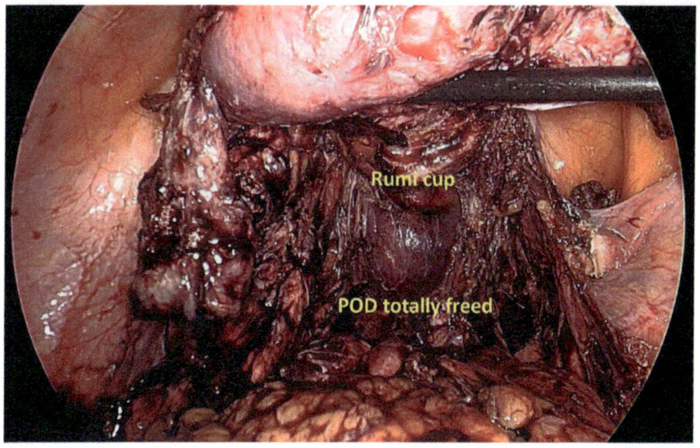

Fig. 10.41 POD totally free and patient ready for culdotomy

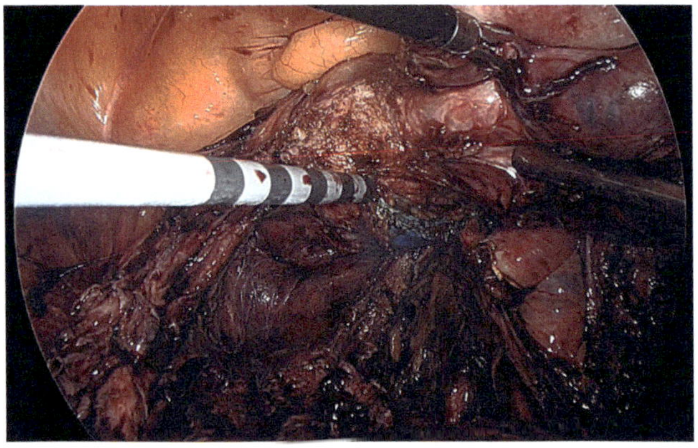

Fig. 10.42 Circumferential culdotomy done by monopolar hook

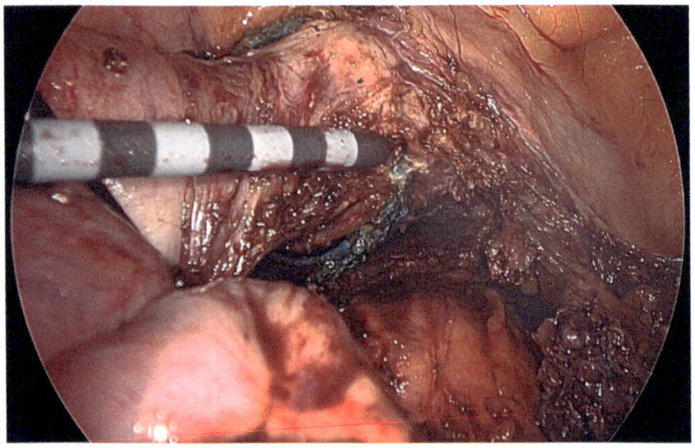

Fig. 10.43 Culdotomy carried anteriorly

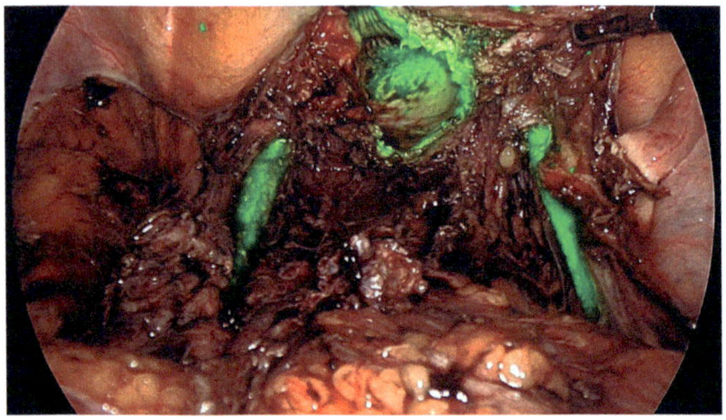

Fig. 10.44 Uterus delivered out with both edges of vault and ureters seen clearly with ICG staining

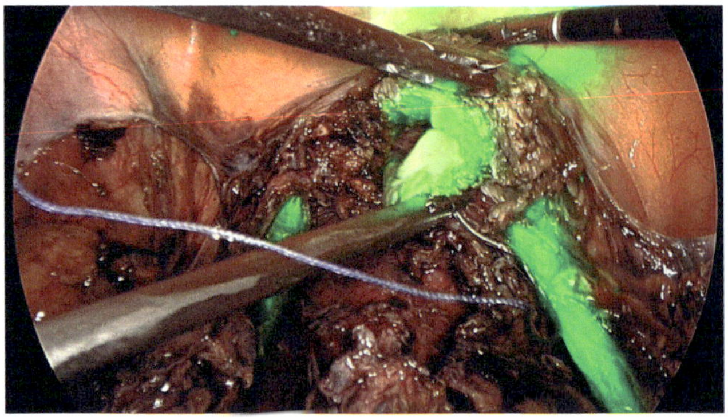

Fig. 10.45 Vault closure done with polygalactin sutures

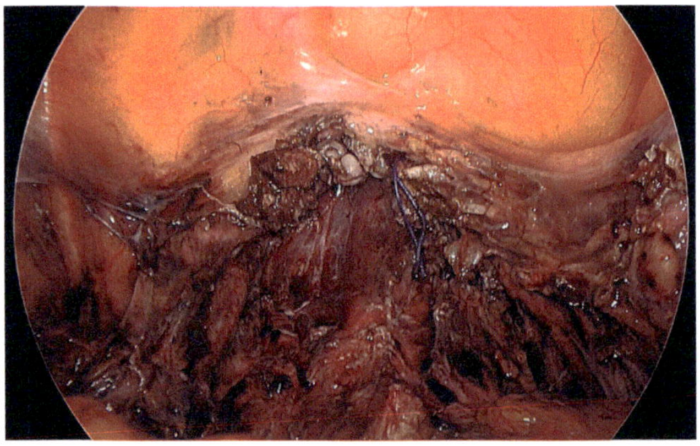

Fig. 10.46 Vault suspension and closure done in two layers

10.5 TLH in Endometriosis

- We start dealing with the adenexa. If the tubes and the ovaries are stuck to the utero sacral ligaments and the back of the retro cervical region, ante-grade dissection of the tube and ovary is carried out till they are made absolutely free for their management during the course of TLH.
- The energy source used for TLH is usually the LigaSure™ (COVIDIEN, USA) or the Enseal PTC (Ethicon Johnson & Johnson Surgical, USA) and even at times, it can be done by HARMONIC ACE™ 1000 HD (Ethicon Johnson & Johnson Surgical, USA). The use of energy device is largely dependent upon the surgeon's choice, the institu-

tional norms and dictate of that particular case. Our comprehensive canopy approach to bladder dissection in TLH unfolds in three steps using Comprehensive Canopy Concept, 'The 3 Step Technique':

1. **Step 1: Posterior approach of uterine artery ligation**—We do not usually prefer to do the uterine artery ligation at origin [30]. As a very wide posterior dissection has already been done and all retroperitoneal structures are laid open, the uterine artery is easily skeletonized by posterior approach as its location is close to the cervix. Due to injecting of the ureter with ICG, uterine artery is very nicely seen as water under the bridge sign [31]. We ligate and coagulate the uterine artery first and then we find the plane of cleavage to enter for the bladder dissection, as the plane of uterine artery is the same as bladder dissection. We do not touch the adherent bladder and work in the cotton candy uterovesical space below to create the bladder canopy.
2. **Step 2: Comprehensive canopy concept of bladder dissection**—We do the bladder dissection by canopy approach, meaning that even if the patient has had previous caesarean sections, ventrifixed uterus [32], adhesions or obliteration in the anterior pouch; we start from the posterior approach, section the uterine artery and then find the plane of cleavage of the bladder flap. Finding the correct plane is the key to forming a successful canopy, thereby ensuring avascular dissection of the bladder flap. This is accomplished by dissecting the area immediately 1–2 cm anterior to the coagulated uterine artery. Dissection proceeds further in this avascular plane over the manipulator cup, under the stretched out bladder canopy of adhesions.
3. **Step 3: Anterior approach of contralateral uterine artery ligation**—We keep working from one end to other in the cotton candy space till we reach the contralateral uterine artery by the side of the manipulator cup. We skeletonize and coagulate the right uterine artery and the bladder remains stretched above like a canopy. We do not carry out adhesiolysis of the bladder. We simply go in a retrograde manner to dissect the cotton candy space, opened up beneath the bladder canopy.

- In case of severely ventrifixed uterus, sometimes we go for the adnexal removal on the right side first, by opening the posterior leaf of broad ligament. Due to extensive adhesiolysis and dissection, the uterine artery and ureter are seen very clearly. The uterine artery is easily coagulated and cut; if not already done by the anterior approach.
- We then carry out circumferential culdotomy by using a monopolar hook, starting from one end to the other, trying to conserve the uterosacral ligaments.

These steps highlight the efficiency of the technique as with a single maneuver, we do uterine artery dissection and section, followed by bladder dissection under the stretched out canopy and the sequential progression from the posterior approach to the canopy-based uterine artery ligation, anteriorly on the other side.

- **Vault closure and suspension**: After the culdotomy, the uterus is delivered vaginally and we do the vault closure along with a stout vault suspension [33]. The vault suspension means that we take bites through the uterosacral ligaments and close the angle sutures on both the sides separately and then we take a running continuous suture from one end to the other end in double layers using polyglactin sutures. Since the day we began doing TLH, we have always closed the vault in this way. Our long-term post-operative results show no incidence of vault prolapse in any of our cases.
- **Check cystoscopy**—After the vault closure, the suction irrigation and lavage is carried out and we do a check cystoscopy. It is not needed when the ureteric catheters are already in place. In many cases of ureteric endometriosis [34], we have to almost strip off the ureter from the rectum or from the surrounding and encircling parametrial endometriosis. In these cases, we assess the potential of thermal damage to the ureter and then bilateral or unilateral ureteric stenting [35] is done under the guidance of C-Arm.

Postoperative Care The patient in the post-operative phase is kept on clear liquid diet on day one of the surgery and once she passes flatus, she is allowed on a semisolid diet gradually progressing to solid diet and the patient is discharged in 48 h. If the stents are in place, they are removed after 3–6 [36] weeks depending upon the amount of risk of thermal injury to the ureter. We follow individualized, patient-centred approach for optimal surgical outcomes using the enhanced recovery after surgery (ERAS) protocol [37].

Learning Points

- Comprehensive preoperative assessment is essential for a tailored surgical planning in extensive endometriosis cases.
- Strategic counselling regarding ovarian conservation and removal offers informed patient choices.
- Diluted ICG injection enhances ureter visualization, minimizing the risk of injury during laparoscopic procedures.
- Vasopressin use aids in controlled vasoconstriction, reducing blood loss, and facilitating hydrodissection for avascular plane creation.

- Ultrasonic energy is effective in dissecting pelvic structures amidst challenging adhesions, ensuring safer surgeries.
- TLH procedure involves a posterior approach to uterine artery ligation, optimizing surgical outcomes.
- Canopy-based bladder dissection proves beneficial in cases of anterior adhesions, allowing precise and safe manoeuvres.
- Anterior approach helps in simplifying the TLH, as with a single sweep, the contralateral uterine artery ligation is accomplished, even in challenging extensive endometriosis.
- Consistent vault closure technique contributes to favourable long-term postoperative results.
- Individualized, patient-centred approaches following ERAS protocol are emphasized for optimal surgical outcomes in complex cases.

Competing Interest The author declares no conflict of interest that is relevant to content of this chapter.

Ethical Approval Informed consent was obtained from individual participants and patients regarding publication and documentation without disclosing their identity.

References

1. Garcia Garcia JM, Vannuzzi V, Donati C, Bernacchioni C, Bruni P, Petraglia F. Endometriosis: cellular and molecular mechanisms leading to fibrosis. Reprod Sci. 2023;30(5):1453–61. https://doi.org/10.1007/s43032-022-01083-x. Epub 2022 Oct 26. PMID: 36289173; PMCID: PMC10160154.
2. Abd El-Kader AI, Gonied AS, Lotfy Mohamed M, Lotfy Mohamed S. Impact of endometriosis-related adhesions on quality of life among infertile women. Int J Fertil Steril. 2019;13(1):72–6. https://doi.org/10.22074/ijfs.2019.5572. Epub 2019 Jan 6. PMID: 30644248; PMCID: PMC6334013.
3. Sinha R, Sundaram M, Lakhotia S, Hedge A, Kadam P. Total laparoscopic hysterectomy in women with previous cesarean sections. J Minim Invasive Gynecol. 2010;17(4):513–7. https://doi.org/10.1016/j.jmig.2010.03.018.
4. Douglass L, Tu F, Senapati S. Anterior cul-de-sac obliteration resulting in acute pain during pregnancy. J Minim Invasive Gynecol. 2012;19(6):S119. https://doi.org/10.1016/j.jmig.2012.08.745.
5. Lee SY, Koo YJ, Lee DH. Classification of endometriosis. Yeungnam Univ J Med. 2021;38(1):10–8. https://doi.org/10.12701/yujm.2020.00444. Epub 2020 Aug 7. PMID: 32764213; PMCID: PMC7787892.
6. Lorusso F, Scioscia M, Rubini D, et al. Magnetic resonance imaging for deep infiltrating endometriosis: current concepts, imaging technique and key findings. Insights Imaging. 2021;12:105. https://doi.org/10.1186/s13244-021-01054-x.
7. Yin S, Lin Q, Xu F, Xu J, Zhang Y. Diagnosis of deep infiltrating endometriosis using transvaginal ultrasonography. Front Med (Lausanne). 2020;7:567929. https://doi.org/10.3389/fmed.2020.567929. PMID: 33330527; PMCID: PMC7719798.
8. Nezhat C, Li A, Falik R, Copeland D, Razavi GM, Shakib A, Mihailide C, Bamford H, DiFrancesco L, Tazuke S, Ghanouni P, Rivas H, Nezhat A, Nezhat C, Nezhat F. Bowel endometriosis: diagnosis and management. Am J Obstet Gynecol. 2017;218:549. https://doi.org/10.1016/j.ajog.2017.09.023.
9. Donnez O. Conservative management of rectovaginal deep endometriosis: shaving should be considered as the primary surgical approach in a high majority of cases. J Clin Med. 2021;10(21):5183. https://doi.org/10.3390/jcm10215183. PMID: 34768704; PMCID: PMC8584847.
10. Roman H. Disc excision using transanal circular stapler for deep endometriosis of the rectum in 10 steps. J Minim Invasive Gynecol. 2021;28(1):14–5. https://doi.org/10.1016/j.jmig.2020.04.017. Epub 2020 Apr 23. PMID: 32335183.
11. Malzoni M, Rasile M, Coppola M, Iuzzolino D, Casarella L, Di Giovanni A, Falcone F. Totally laparoscopic resection with transanal natural orifice specimen extraction for deep endometriosis infiltrating the rectum. J Minim Invasive Gynecol. 2022;29(1):19. https://doi.org/10.1016/j.jmig.2021.07.015. Epub 2021 Jul 30. PMID: 34333148.
12. Erekson EA, Martin DK, Ratner ES. Oophorectomy: the debate between ovarian conservation and elective oophorectomy. Menopause. 2013;20(1):110–4. https://doi.org/10.1097/gme.0b013e31825a27ab. PMID: 22929033; PMCID: PMC3514564.
13. Guo S-W. Recurrence of endometriosis and its control. Hum Reprod Update. 2009;15(4):441–61. https://doi.org/10.1093/humupd/dmp007.
14. Kobayashi H, Oda A, Matsuzaki Y, Kondo Y, Hamada Y, Nagashima M, Kobayashi M, Takaki Y, Adachi H. Ureter injury in total laparoscopic hysterectomy. Case Rep Obstet Gynecol. 2023, 2023, 10 pages.:5071080. https://doi.org/10.1155/2023/5071080.
15. Boni L, David G, Mangano A, Dionigi G, Rausei S, Spampatti S, Cassinotti E, Fingerhut A. Clinical applications of indocyanine green (ICG) enhanced fluorescence in laparoscopic surgery. Surg Endosc. 2015;29(7):2046–55. https://doi.org/10.1007/s00464-014-3895-x. Epub 2014 Oct 11. PMID: 25303914; PMCID: PMC4471386.
16. Alander JT, Kaartinen I, Laakso A, Pätilä T, Spillmann T, Tuchin VV, Venermo M, Välisuo P. A review of indocyanine green fluorescent imaging in surgery. Int J Biomed Imaging. 2012;2012:940585. https://doi.org/10.1155/2012/940585. Epub 2012 Apr 22. PMID: 22577366; PMCID: PMC3346977.
17. Pg P, Shabnam K, Bhosale SA, et al. Laparoscopic hysterectomy in frozen pelvis—an alternative technique of retrograde adhesiolysis. Gynecol Surg. 2013;10:285–90. https://doi.org/10.1007/s10397-013-0810-8.
18. Benoit L, Dabi Y, Bazot M, Thomassin-Naggara I, Ferrier C, Puchar A, Owen C, Touboul C, Darai E, Bendifallah S. Parametrial endometriosis: A predictive and prognostic factor for voiding dysfunction and complications. Eur J Obstet Gynecol Reprod Biol. 2022;276:236–43. https://doi.org/10.1016/j.ejogrb.2022.07.035. Epub 2022 Aug 4. PMID: 35961258.
19. Treschan TA, Peters J, Warltier DC. The vasopressin system: physiology and clinical strategies. Anesthesiology. 2006;105:599–612. https://doi.org/10.1097/00000542-200609000-00026.
20. Modi R. Laparoscopic myomectomy with aquadissection and barbed sutures. J Gynecol Endosc Surg. 2011;2(1):47–52. https://doi.org/10.4103/0974-1216.85283. PMID: 22442536; PMCID: PMC3304286.
21. Broughton D, Welling AL, Monroe EH, Pirozzi K, Schulte JB, Clymer JW. Tissue effects in vessel sealing and transection from an ultrasonic device with more intelligent control of energy delivery. Med Devices (Auckl). 2013;6:151–4. https://doi.org/10.2147/MDER.S51663. PMID: 24072978; PMCID: PMC3783500.
22. Kostov S, Slavchev S, Dzhenkov D, Mitev D, Yordanov A. Avascular spaces of the female pelvis-clinical applications in obstetrics and gynecology. J Clin Med. 2020;9(5):1460. https://doi.org/10.3390/jcm9051460. PMID: 32414119; PMCID: PMC7291144.

23. Jacob GP, Vilos GA, Al Turki F, Bhangav G, Abu-Rafea B, Vilos AG, Ternamian A. Ureteric injury during gynaecological surgery—lessons from 20 cases in Canada. Facts Views Vis Obgyn. 2020;12(1):31–42. PMID: 32696022; PMCID: PMC7363243.
24. Li L, Bi Y, Wang L, et al. Identification and injury to the inferior hypogastric plexus in nerve-sparing radical hysterectomy. Sci Rep. 2019;9:13260. https://doi.org/10.1038/s41598-019-49856-w.
25. Uccella S, Gisone B, Serati M, Biasoli S, Marconi N, Angeretti G, Gallotta V, Cardinale S, Rausei S, Dionigi G, Scambia G, Ghezzi F. Functional outcomes of nerve-sparing laparoscopic eradication of deep infiltrating endometriosis: a prospective analysis using validated questionnaires. Arch Gynecol Obstet. 2018;298(3):639–47. https://doi.org/10.1007/s00404-018-4852-z. Epub 2018 Jul 30. PMID: 30062386.
26. Darwish B, Roman H. Nerve sparing and surgery for deep infiltrating endometriosis: pessimism of the intellect or optimism of the will. Semin Reprod Med. 2017;35(1):72–80. https://doi.org/10.1055/s--0036-1597305. Epub 2016 Dec 12. PMID: 27951614.
27. Puntambekar S, Manchanda R. Surgical pelvic anatomy in gynecologic oncology. Int J Gynaecol Obstet. 2018;143(Suppl 2):86–92. https://doi.org/10.1002/ijgo.12616. PMID: 30306582.
28. Koh CH. A new technique and system for simplifying total laparoscopic hysterectomy. J Am Assoc Gynecol Laparosc. 1998;5:187–92.
29. Donnez J, Jadoul P, Colette S, et al. Deep rectovaginal endometriotic nodules: perioperative complications from a series of 3,298 patients operated on by the shaving technique. Gynecol Surg. 2013;10:31–40. https://doi.org/10.1007/s10397-012-0759-z.
30. Choi HJ, Kim MS, Kim TJ. Uterine artery ligation at its origin following retroperitoneal space development decreases blood loss during single-port total laparoscopic hysterectomy. Taiwan J Obstet Gynecol. 2020;59(2):262–8. https://doi.org/10.1016/j.tjog.2020.01.015. PMID: 32127148.
31. Chaudhry R, Chaudhry K. Anatomy, abdomen and pelvis: uterine arteries. 2023 Sep 4. In: StatPearls [Internet]. Treasure Island: StatPearls Publishing; 2023 Jan–. PMID: 29489202.
32. El-Shawarby S, Salim R, Lavery S, et al. Uterine adherence to anterior abdominal wall after caesarean section. BJOG. 2011;118:1133.
33. Crigler B, Zakaria M, Hart S. Total laparoscopic hysterectomy with laparoscopic uterosacral ligament suspension for the treatment of apical pelvic organ prolapse. Surg Technol Int. 2012;22:195–202. PMID: 23225594.
34. Palla VV, Karaolanis G, KataFig. 10.Iotis I, Anastasiou I. Ureteral endometriosis: a systematic literature review. Indian J Urol 2017;33(4):276–282. doi: https://doi.org/10.4103/iju.IJU_84_17. PMID: 29021650; PMCID: PMC5635667.
35. Weingertner AS, Rodriguez B, Ziane A, Gibon E, Thoma V, Osario F, Haddad C, Wattiez A. The use of JJ stent in the management of deep endometriosis lesion, affecting or potentially affecting the ureter: a review of our practice. BJOG. 2008;115(9):1159–64. https://doi.org/10.1111/j.1471-0528.2008.01795.x. Epub 2008 May 30. PMID: 18518868.
36. Rozsnyai F, Roman H, Resch B, Dugardin F, Berrocal J, Descargues G, Schmied R, Boukerrou M, Marpeau L, CIRENDO Study Group. Outcomes of surgical management of deep infiltrating endometriosis of the ureter and urinary bladder. JSLS. 2011;15(4):439–47. https://doi.org/10.4293/108680811X13176785203798. PMID: 22643496; PMCID: PMC3340950.
37. Melnyk M, Casey RG, Black P, Koupparis AJ. Enhanced recovery after surgery (ERAS) protocols: time to change practice? Can Urol Assoc J. 2011;5(5):342–8. https://doi.org/10.5489/cuaj.11002. PMID: 22031616; PMCID: PMC3202008.

11 Total Laparoscopic Hysterectomy (TLH) with Large Uterus by Comprehensive Canopy Concept, 'The 3 Step Technique'

Nutan Jain, Vandana Jain, and Sakshi Srivastava

11.1 Introduction

TLH for a large uterus is a daunting task and requires skilful management in a preoperative phase as well as on the table and after the surgery [1].

Initially designed for moderate-sized uteri, the increasing incidence of patients with larger uteri and their growing acceptance of laparoscopic procedures have paved the way for TLH in patients with large uterus. The one kilo club which was supposed unimaginable in the early years of evolution of TLH, over the years has become a reality. Surgeons, once constrained to smaller uteri, are now venturing into TLH for larger uteri, breaking the one-kilo club barrier and still larger [2, 3].

Before undertaking TLH for a large uterus, a thorough preoperative workup is essential. This involves recording the patient's surgical history, noting the number and types of previous surgeries, evaluating the scar length and type, and assessing the height of the uterus. A comprehensive physical examination is crucial to determine if the uterine pathology extends into the cervical region, lower uterine segment (Fig. 11.1), or fornices, as this can impact the relationship of ureters and uterine arteries during surgical dissection in TLH. In patients with ultrasound report suggestive of large fibroids, it's very important to see whether they are subserosal or deeply stuck in the lower pelvis causing distortion of the course of the ureters and causing difficulty in tackling the uterine artery [4] and increasing risk ureter injury.

The patient's surgical history, including number of previous caesarean sections, myomectomies, laparotomies for ectopic or septic abortions, or other surgeries, should be thoroughly studied, as these may contribute to adhesions, increasing the complexity of the procedure.

During physical examination, we take a note of the position of the cervix, whether it is normally placed or pulled up behind the pubic symphysis as can happen in previous caesarean section cases, whether the fornices are free or there is fullness due to cervical myoma is also observed. The fundal height is the next important thing to see till where the masses are reaching or whether they are deviated to one side or the other. After this, we subject the patient to complete imaging

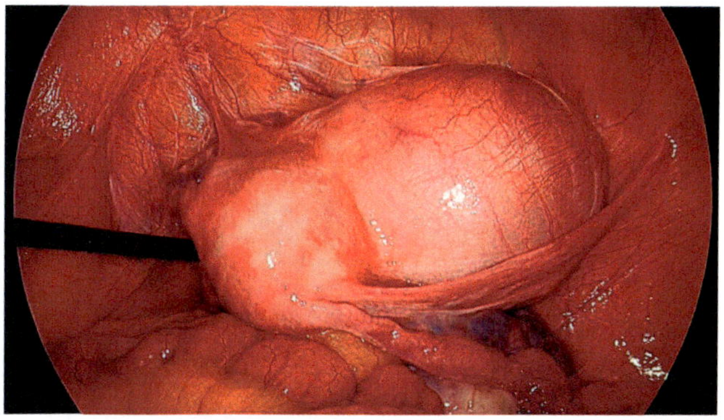

Fig. 11.1 Huge cervical myoma with adherent bladder

Supplementary Information The online version contains supplementary material available at https://doi.org/10.1007/978-981-97-3226-5_11. The videos can be accessed individually by clicking the DOI link in the accompanying figure caption or by scanning this link with the SN More Media App.

N. Jain (✉)
Obstetrics and Gynaecology, GSVM Medical College, Affiliated by Kanpur University, Kanpur, Uttar Pradesh, India

Department of Obstetrics and Gynecology, Vardhman Trauma and Laparoscopy Centre Pvt. Ltd., Muzaffarnagar, Uttar Pradesh, India

V. Jain
Department of Obstetrics and Gynecology, Vardhman Trauma and Laparoscopy Centre Pvt. Ltd., Muzaffarnagar, Uttar Pradesh, India

Obstetrics and Gynaecology, Kasturba Hospital, Affiliated by Delhi University, Delhi, India

S. Srivastava
Obstetrics and Gynecology, Rohilkhand Medical College and Hospital, Affiliated by Bareilly International University, Bareilly, Uttar Pradesh, India

Gynae Endoscopy, Vardhman Trauma and Laparoscopy Centre Pvt. Ltd., Muzaffarnagar, Uttar Pradesh, India

N. Jain (ed.), *Complex Total Laparoscopic Hysterectomy (TLH) with Newer Approaches in Bladder Dissection*,
https://doi.org/10.1007/978-981-97-3226-5_11

studies which include a full bladder ultrasound per abdomen and transvaginal ultrasound. In cases of multiple fibroids or the suspicion of endometriosis, along with sonography we carry out an MRI also to know the exact location of the myomas and the obliteration of the pouch of Douglas. MRI significantly adds to the findings already achieved by physical examination and ultrasound. Sonographic appearances which look neither like well circumscribed myoma, nor the appearance of adenomyoma & adenomyosis, just diffusely merging masses in to one another and the myometrium, should, raise the suspicion of sarcomatous changes. So be careful in taking up these cases for surgery and first carry out necessary lab investigation and tumour markers relevant to large uteri, which are CA125, LDH [5–7].

Now, next important thing is to get proper lab investigations, anesthesiologist and physician clearance as the surgery could last longer. Her BMI is very important and also the location of the fat, whether it is central or truncal around the hip area. So, all this evaluation really adds up to a good planning, to make the TLH in large uterus safe.

In the preoperative phase, on the night before the surgery, it is a good plan, in larger uterus to do a good bowel preparation, and the patient is put on a low residual diet as this helps to keep the bowels flat as ribbon and not obscuring the surgical field at all.

During the induction of anesthesia, a nasogastric tube is always put by the anesthesiologist and the anesthesia team is expected not to use nitrous oxide which could bloat up the bowel. In the face of a large uterus, this step is extremely important. The next crucial step is to how to make the primary first blind entry port. As we said earlier, the examination of the abdomen and the per-vaginal examination is carried out again under anesthesia and according to the size of the uterus. All the ports are put above and outside the mass. But the first port is extremely important so that we enter safely and we do not bang upon the fibroid and excite bleeding even before the telescope has gone in [8, 9]. In our setup, we use the far lateral, paraumbilical port, the Jain point [10], and it is usually inserted from the left side, it is at the level of the umbilicus but in cases of large uteri, we can use a higher Jain point [11] which can be anywhere between the umbilicus and one finger beneath the subcostal margin, on the same line above as the surface marking of Jain Point (Fig. 11.2).

After the first blind port, we optimize the 10 mm port which is usually entered with a 30 degree scope for better visualization of the entire surgical field and the anterior and the posterior pouches during the course of the surgery. We go to the point highest in the epigastrium. To avoid the falciparum ligament we remain about a centimeter towards the right side of the midline for 10 mm port. This is done under the vision of 5 mm Jain Point port (Fig. 11.3a, b). Other ports from the surgeon side, which is the left side, are ipsilateral. The second lower port on the left side is also made according to the position of the myomas. Usually we try to keep the distance between the two ports on the left side that is the upper Jain point port and the lower port to be around 10–12 cm for good ergonomic working (Fig. 11.4). On the assistant side that is from the right side, first lower port is standard that is

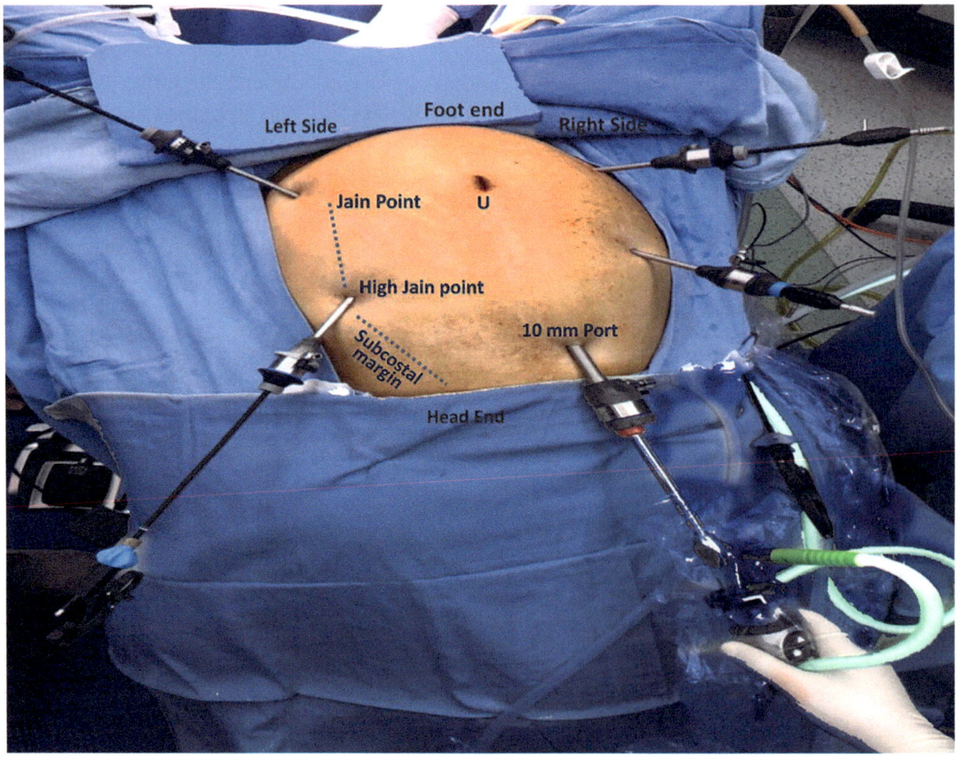

Fig. 11.2 High Jain point port

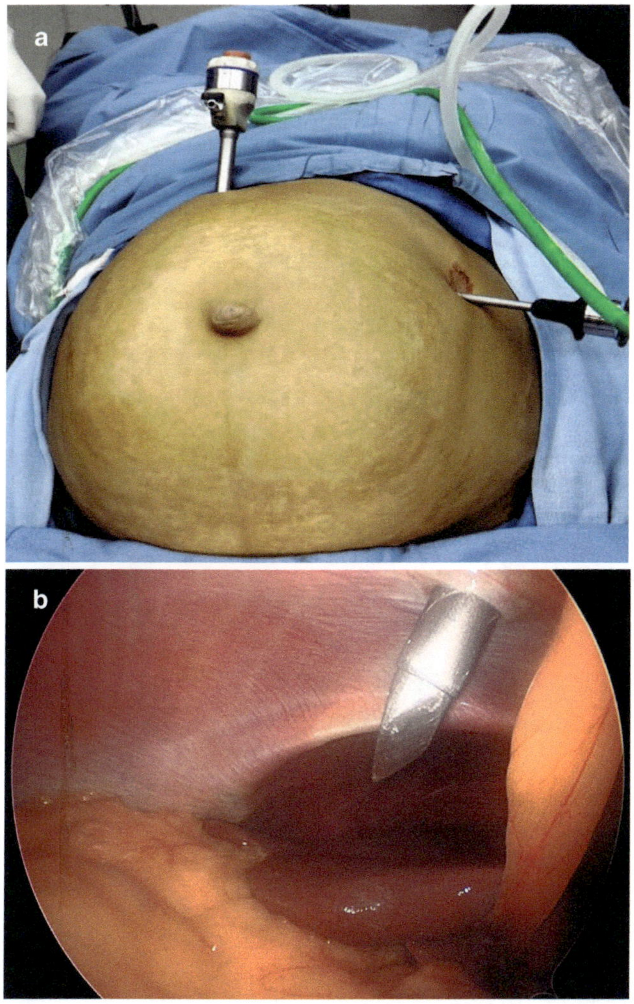

Fig. 11.3 **a** 10 mm trocar inserted high up, under vision of 5mm Jain point port. **b** 10 mm trocar inserted under vision of 5 mm Jain point port

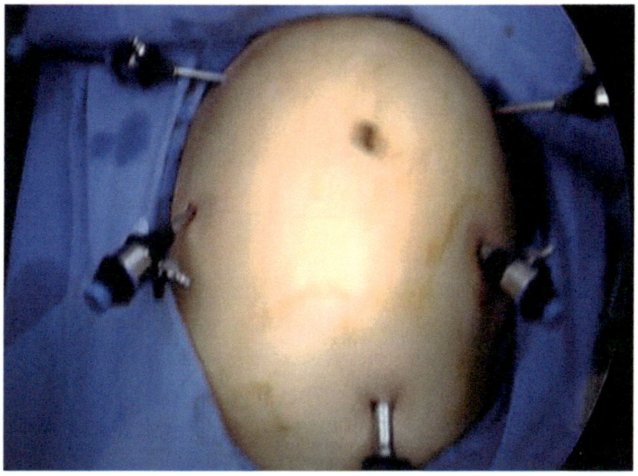

Fig. 11.4 Port placement for large uterus

closer to the left ASIS and the upper port is placed as needed for extra hand for manipulation because in larger uterus, the uterine manipulators applied from below may not work efficiently. So an extra port is applied to give traction and counter traction during the various manoeuvre and movements for coagulating and sectioning of the adenexa and the uterine arteries. The upper port for the assistant can be placed anywhere between the subcostal margin and the umbilicus. Usually at the level of the umbilicus it works fine.

In instances of heightened complexity, such as when dealing with a large uterus with multiple previous Caesarean sections leading to increased adhesions, the surgical approach necessitates the incorporation of an additional port. This supplementary port is strategically placed at the umbilical level and serves the purpose of facilitating manipulation and the application of a myoma screw.

After establishing the necessary ports, the selection and application of a proficient uterine manipulator become pivotal in ensuring a successful surgical procedure [12]. Most of the manipulators available by various manufacturers in the endoscopy arena offer one benefit or the other and the surgical team chooses the one that aligns best with their specific requirements. Manipulators typically come with varying sizes of tips; however, even the largest tip may prove insufficient when dealing with a uterus at 24 weeks or larger, particularly in the presence of large multiple myomas. In such cases, the largest available tip is employed, supplemented by an additional laparoscopic instrument for manipulation, which could be a tenaculum or a myoma screw. With the gadgets available, any size of myoma can be tackled by the laparoscopic route.

For the hysterectomy, we adhere to our standard technique of Comprehensive Canopy Concept, 'The 3 Step Technique', extensively described in several chapters of the book. This approach is characterized by its adaptability, and is feasible even in the face of adhesions in the anterior cul-de-sac, ventrifixed uterus or scarred bladder flap. Despite these complexities, we follow the comprehensive canopy concept and start the TLH with the posterior approach of uterine artery ligation. Avoiding big vessels on the surface of the myoma, we inject large quantity diluted vasopressin (Figs. 11.5 and 11.6).

Step 1 We start on the left side, and we systematically tackle the adnexa, according to mandate of the case and the patient's preferences for ovarian conservation. In instances where ovarian conservation is a priority, we commence with the coagulation and transection of the ovarian ligament (Fig. 11.7), followed by the fallopian tube, and then the round ligament.

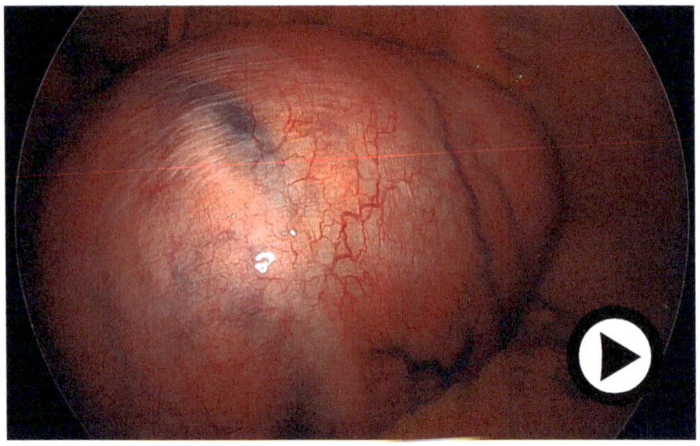

Fig. 11.5 26 weeks size large uterus (Video.11.5 TLH with Large uterus) (▶ https://doi.org/10.1007/000-c97)

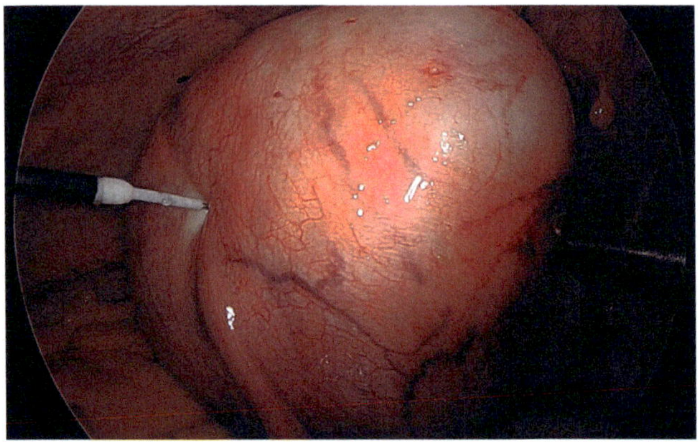

Fig. 11.6 Injecting dilute vasopressin

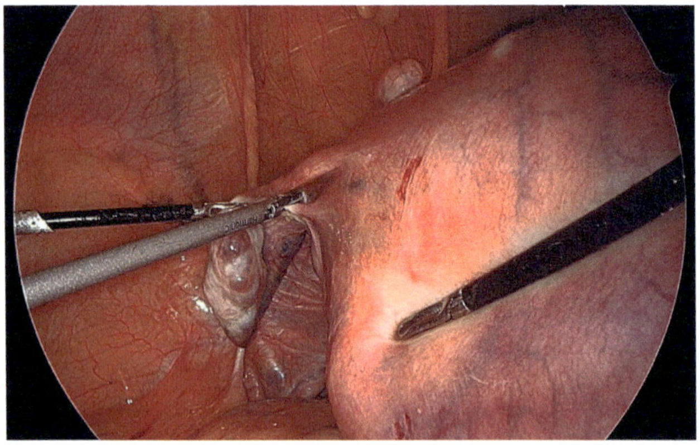

Fig. 11.7 Tackling left adnexa

After the round ligament is transected, the pelvic end assistant gives a smart cephalad push over the manipulator cup and retracts the uterus to the other side. By performing these actions simultaneously, the posterior leaf of broad ligament (Fig. 11.8) opens up and we focus our attention to widely opening up the posterior leaf of broad ligament till the *Arcus Taurinus*. The uterosacral ligament and that the adjoining retroperitonium is freely mobilized and that brings the uterine

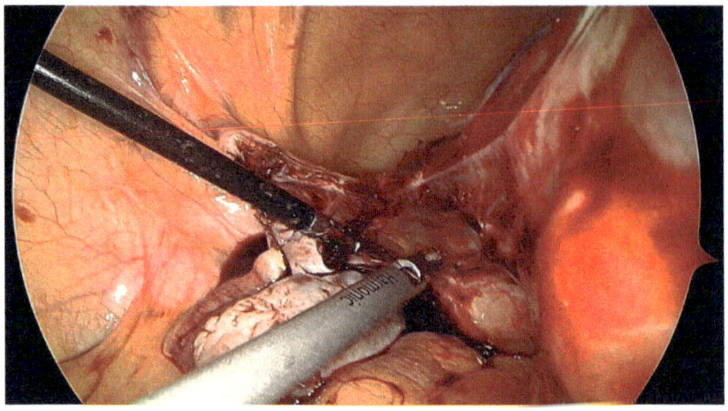

Fig. 11.8 Opening up the posterior leaf of broad ligament

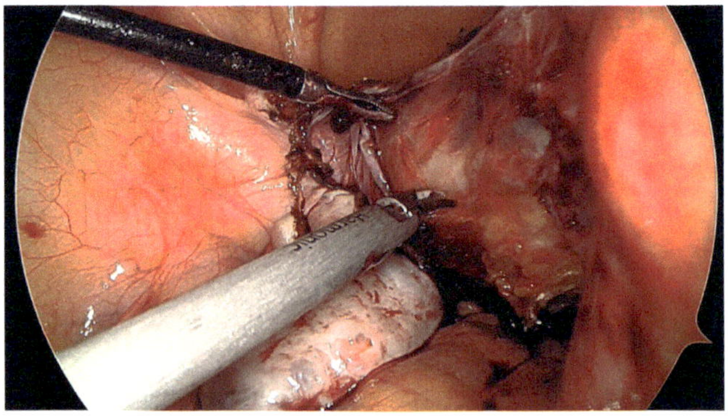

Fig. 11.9 Exposing left uterine artery

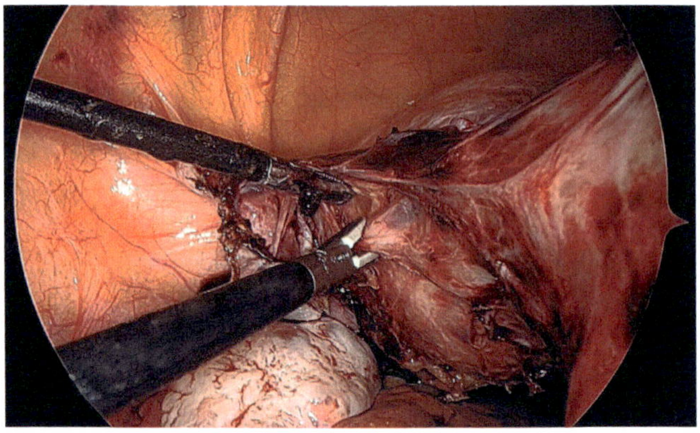

Fig. 11.10 Coagulating left uterine artery

pedicle into the surgical field. First the uterine vein, which is easily recognized by the bluish color, appears and then the spiral winding uterine artery becomes visible (Fig. 11.9). If one does not do too many maneuvers at this point and just remain in the retroperitonium, an excellent view of uterine pedicle comes up and there is no risk of bleeding. The energy source we usually employ at this point to dissect and skeletonize the uterine artery is ultrasonic energy or the ligasure (COVIDIEN Inc., Mansfield, MA, USA), 5 mm. Irrespective of the energy source used, our primary focus is complete skelotonization and coagulation (Fig. 11.10) of the uterine artery.

Step 2 We do not make any endeavour to touch the bladder flap at this point. Our philosophy being that when we cut the uterine artery first, along with it the anterior cervical ligament is also transected. This causes the ureter to move downwards and laterally, and subsequently we gain access into the pubo-vesico cervical space. The 1.5 cm area immediately medial and anterior to the cut uterine artery pedicle is most important for dissecting and reaching the pubovesical fascia (Fig. 11.11). Once we expose the pubo-vesico-cervical fascia and the plane of the bladder dissection, the vaginal assistant continues to give a smart cephalad push over the manipulator cup (Fig. 11.12). The assistant at the laparoscopic end gives traction over the uterine fundus and we keep moving in the pubo-vesico-cervical fascia plane and the cotton candy uterovesical space is opened up. As the anatomic principle, that bladder is densely adherent at the top and loosely adherent at the level of the cervical isthmus. This anatomical principle comes into play and very avascularly and without much effort, the champagne bubbles or the cotton candy plane appears (Fig. 11.13).

Step 3 We keep working with the grasper further and further till we reach the contralateral round ligament. At times it may be needed to cut the bladder flap (Fig. 11.14) by the time we reach the other side of the manipulator cup rim; and after that we can open up the peritoneal fold till the round ligament (Figs. 11.15 and 11.16). As we keep pushing the manipulator cup and we open up bladder flap up to the round ligament, this brings forth in all its glory, the contralateral uterine artery and the uterine vein. It is such a wonderful sight to see the uterine artery and vein by the side of the manipulator cup in the champagne bubbles and the cotton candy space which was exposed from the left side. We further skeletonize, coagulate and cut the right sided uterine artery by vessel sealer or ultrasonic device (Figs. 11.17, 11.18, and 11.19). We call this the anterior approach of uterine artery ligation. So if we see that the whole of the TLH can be finished just by starting in the correct retroperitoneal plane and dissection, by posterior approach of uterine artery ligation itself.

By these manoeuvres the bladder has already walked down. We don't need to do any special maneuver to push the bladder down. It simply walks down. Now the stage is set for a circumferential culdotomy (Figs. 11.20 and 11.21) and in our setup we carry out the culdotomy by a monopolar hook. The vault closure and vault suspension are done by number 1–0 VICRYL™ (polyglactin 910) suture and we always do it in two layers. The first layer takes the deeper layer of the vaginal cuff, both the mucosa on the anterior and the posterior rim should be taken, and it is an absolute must to take the mucosa. In the second layer which we come in a continuous non -locking fashion we take the recto vaginal fascia posteriorly and the pubo-vesico-cervical fascia anteriorly and we tie the knot at the starting point. We always incorporate the uterosacral ligaments in closure thus we call it the vault suspension [13] (Fig. 11.22).

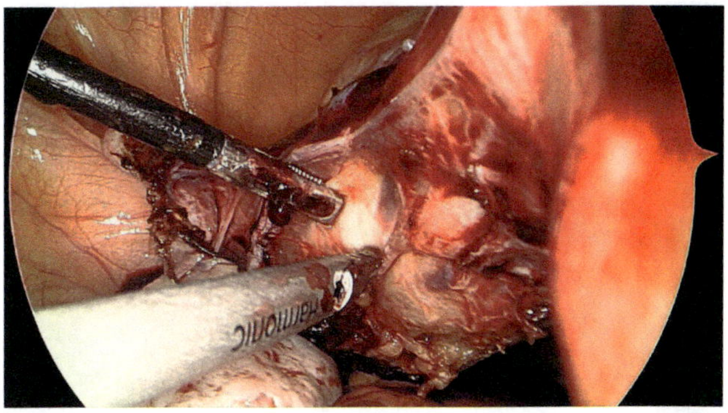

Fig. 11.11 1 cm area immediately medial and anterior to the cut uterine artery pedicle is most important for dissecting and reaching the pubovesical fascia

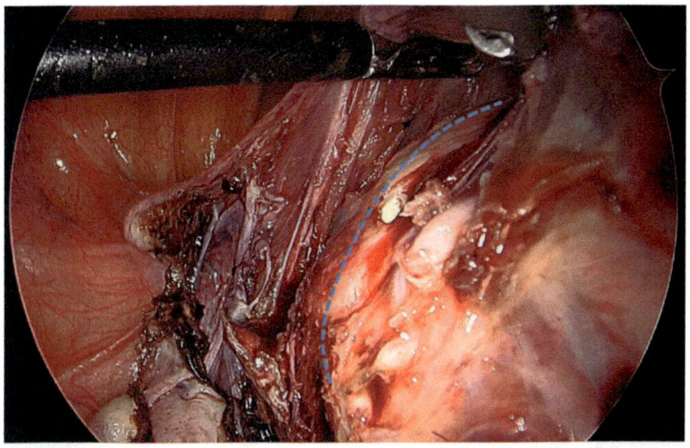

Fig. 11.12 Raising the bladder canopy by cephalad push of manipulator cup

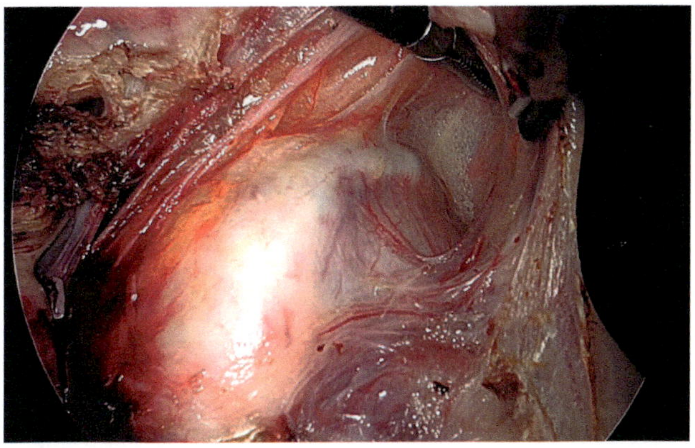

Fig. 11.13 Uterovesical cotton candy space

In larger uteri, for uterus retrieval we always try to do it from the vaginal end and the technique used are the coring [14] or making the serial ribboning out of the uterus by

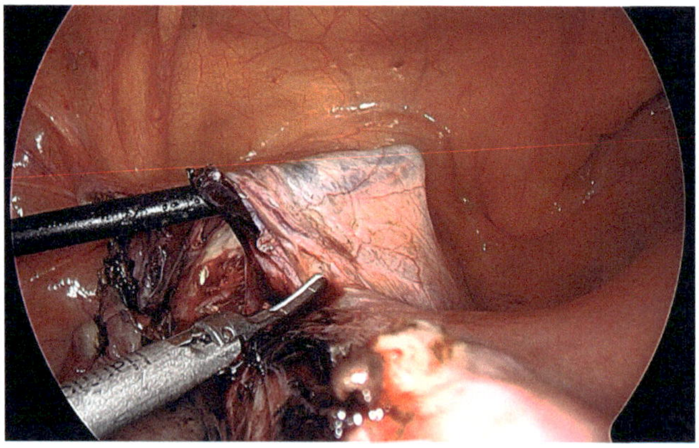

Fig. 11.14 Bladder canopy lifted up and uterovesical cotton candy space dissected beneath it

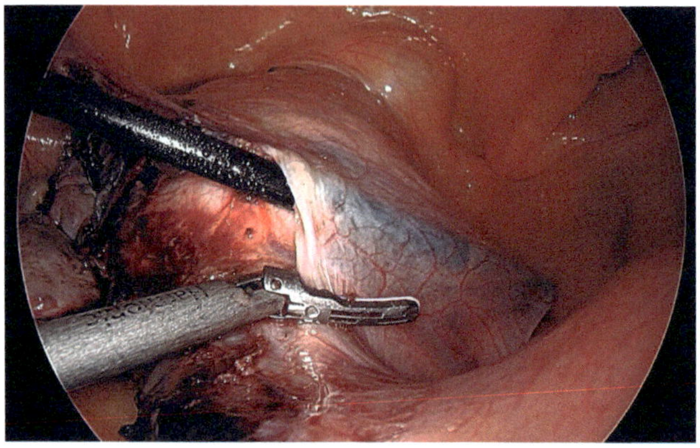

Fig. 11.15 Cotton candy space developed below till the round ligament

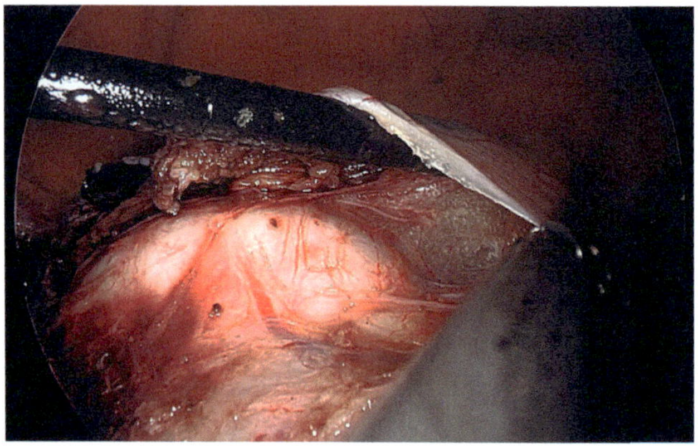

Fig. 11.16 Exposing the cotton candy space to expose the uterine artery from anterior approach

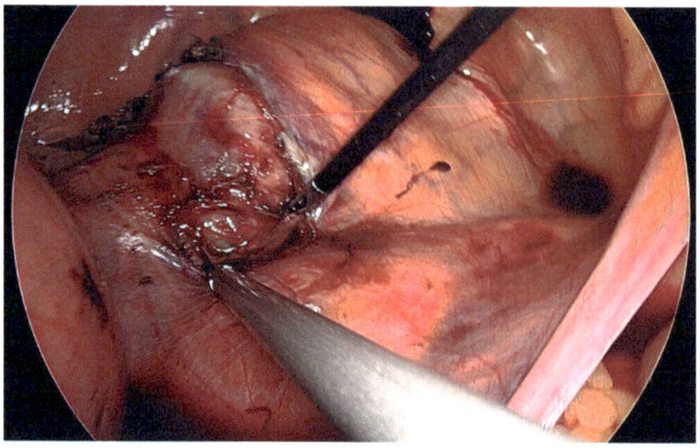

Fig. 11.17 Starting exposure of the uterine artery from anterior approach

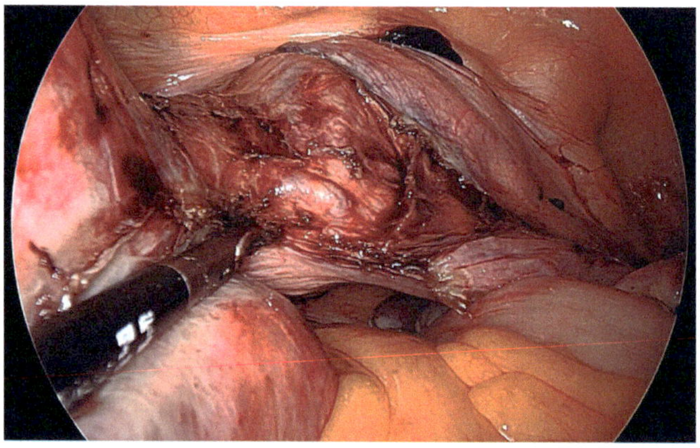

Fig. 11.18 Exposing uterine artery from anterior approach before tackling the adnexa of right side

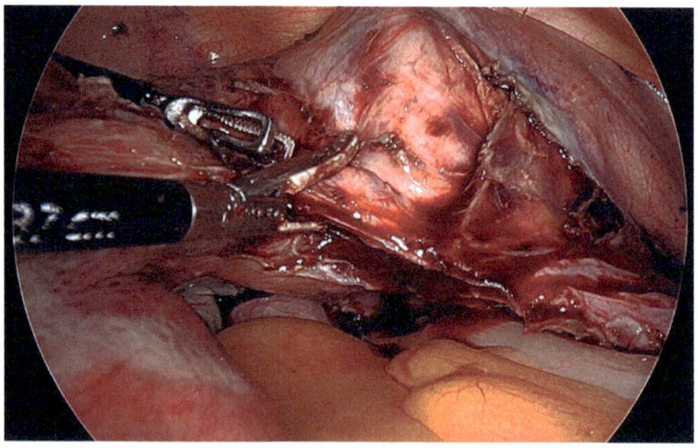

Fig. 11.19 Coagulating right side uterine artery

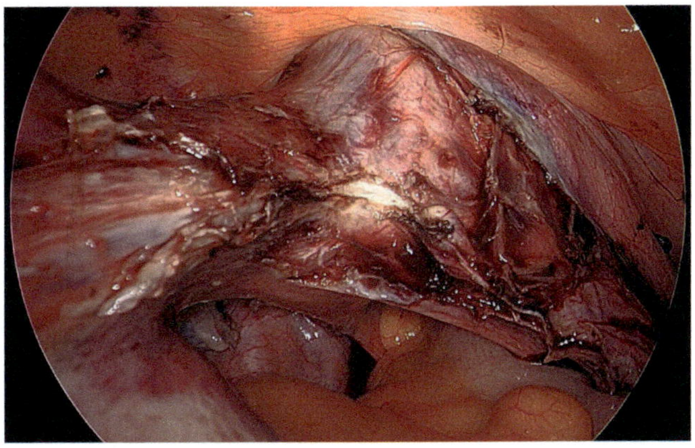

Fig. 11.20 Right sided uterine artery cut from anterior approach and uterus is set to be removed

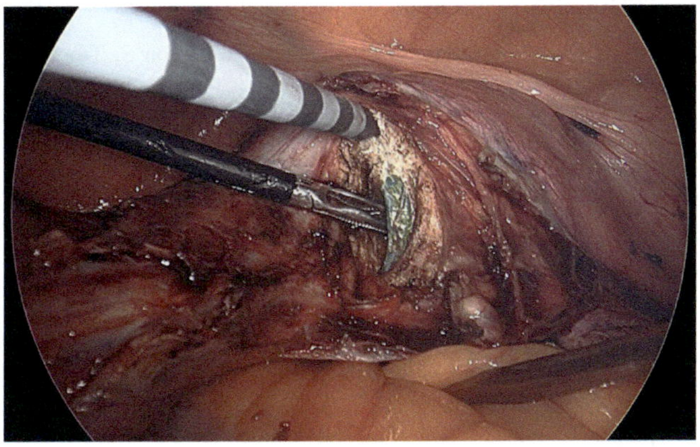

Fig. 11.21 Culdotomy performed by monopolar hook

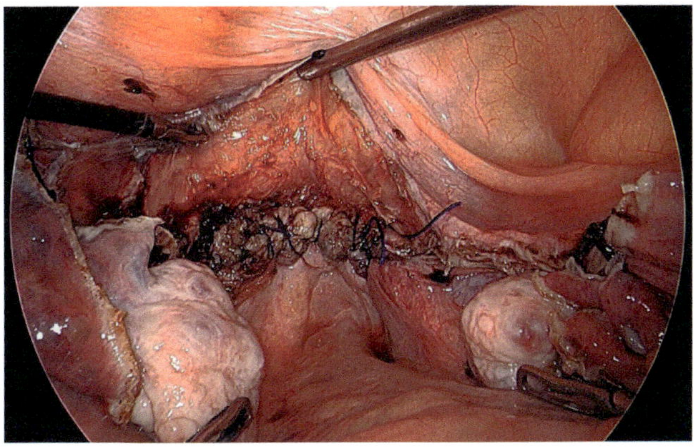

Fig. 11.22 Vault closure and suspension completed

sequentially moving the uterus clockwise and anti-clockwise and coring it out with a scalpel blade. We always try to avoid using a laparoscopic morcellation but if it becomes necessary then we try to do it in bag morcellation. In cases where there are large myomas which are bulging out especially at the lower body of uterus or cervix myomectomy can be done leaving the myomas somewhat attached to the uterus. This brings the larger myomas out easily from vaginal end.

A check cystoscopy is always done and we give the patient pyridium, two tablets in the night before the surgery so that the urine becomes orange and it becomes very easy to document the ureter jet as soon as we put in the cystoscope. The entire check of the bladder is done to see for any interstitial cystitis, any stone or any other pathology of the bladder. So this way we conclude our TLH with closure of all the ports and only the port which are larger than the 10 mm we do the facial closure otherwise a routine mattress suture is given for all the ports.

The patient is returned to the ward and we retain the foley's catheter in for the next 24 hours as the patient might be obese, patients may have other comorbidities and increased surgical time. All these patients receive broad spectrum antibiotics, DVT prophylaxis is always given and we enforce early ambulation, breathing exercises following the ERAS protocol and the patient is discharged 24 hours after the surgery.

Learning Points

- Comprehensive preoperative workup is crucial for planning TLH in large uteri, involving patient history, scar assessment, and advanced imaging.
- Careful consideration of previous surgeries and potential adhesions is essential to asses complexities during TLH.
- Primary port placement, particularly the strategic use of the Jain point, plays a pivotal role in ensuring safe and effective entry into the abdominal cavity.
- The posterior approach to uterine artery ligation is emphasized, providing a clear view and minimizing the risk of bleeding.
- The Comprehensive Canopy Concept, 'The 3 Step Technique', adaptable to varying complexities, is a key surgical technique for TLH in large uteri.
- Vault closure and suspension, conducted meticulously, contribute to successful outcomes, and careful uterus retrieval techniques are discussed.
- Check cystoscopy plays an important role at the end of procedure.
- Postoperative care, including early ambulation and adherence to ERAS protocols, is essential for optimized recovery in patients with large uteri undergoing TLH

Competing Interest The author declares no conflict of interest that is relevant to content of this chapter.

Ethical Approval Informed consent was obtained from individual participants and patients regarding publication and documentation without disclosing their identity.

References

1. Macciò A, Kotsonis P, Lavra F, et al. Laparoscopic removal of a very large uterus weighting 5320 g is feasible and safe: a case report. BMC Surg. 2017;17:50. https://doi.org/10.1186/s12893-017-0248-4.
2. Cesta M, Kennedy B, Pasic R. Total laparoscopic hysterectomy of a 7400 g uterus. J Minim Invasive Gynecol. 2021;28(4):748–9. https://doi.org/10.1016/j.jmig.2020.06.019. PMID: 32610076.
3. Walid MS, Heaton RL. Total laparoscopic hysterectomy for uteri over one kilogram. JSLS. 2010;14:178–82.
4. Nakayama K, Tsukao M, Ishikawa M, et al. Total laparoscopic hysterectomy for large uterine cervical myoma. Mol Clin Oncol. 2017;6(5):655–60. https://doi.org/10.3892/mco.2017.1217. PMID: 28515917; PMCID: PMC5431257.
5. Kil K, Chung JE, Pak HJ, Jeung IC, Kim JH, Jo HH, Kim MR. Usefulness of CA125 in the differential diagnosis of uterine adenomyosis and myoma. Eur J Obstet Gynecol Reprod Biol. 2015;185:131–5. https://doi.org/10.1016/j.ejogrb.2014.12.008. ISSN 0301-2115.
6. Kim A, Boyd L, Ringel N, Meyer J, Bennett G, Lerner V. Preoperative MRI and LDH in women undergoing intra-abdominal surgery for fibroids: effect on surgical route. PLoS One. 2021;16(2):e0246807. https://doi.org/10.1371/journal.pone.0246807. PMID: 33561167; PMCID: PMC7872248.
7. Hatta K, Terai Y, Okuda K, et al. Preoperative assessment by magnetic resonance imaging is useful for planning the treatment of an enlarged uterus by total laparoscopic hysterectomy. J Obstet Gynaecol Res. 2013;39(4):814–9. https://doi.org/10.1111/j.1447--0756.2012.02065.x. PMID: 23379476.
8. Jansen FW, Kapiteyn K, Trimbos-Kemper T, Hermans J, Trimbos JB. Complications of laparoscopy: a prospective multicentre observational study. Br J Obstet Gynaecol. 1997;104(5):595–600. https://doi.org/10.1111/j.1471-0528.1997.tb11539.x. PMID: 9166204.
9. Jansen FW, Kolkman W, Bakkum EA, de Kroon CD, Trimbos-Kemper TC, Trimbos JB. Complications of laparoscopy: an inquiry about closed- versus open-entry technique. Am J Obstet Gynecol. 2004;190(3):634–8. https://doi.org/10.1016/j.ajog.2003.09.035. PMID: 15041992.
10. Jain N, Sareen S, Kanawa S, Jain V, Gupta S, Mann S. Jain point: a new safe portal for laparoscopic entry in previous surgery cases. J Hum Reprod Sci. 2016;9(1):9–17. https://doi.org/10.4103/0974-120.
11. Jain N, Jain V, Gupta S. 10225 high Jain point in large masses. J Minim Invasive Gynecol. 2023;30(6):343. https://doi.org/10.1016/j.jmig.2023.08.343.
12. Abdel Khalek Y, Bitar R, Christoforou C, Garzon S, Tropea A, Biondi A, Sleiman Z. Uterine manipulator in total laparoscopic hysterectomy: safety and usefulness. Updat Surg. 2020;72(4):1247–54. https://doi.org/10.1007/s13304-019-00681-w. Epub 2019 Oct 12. PMID: 31606857.
13. Peters A, Ali R, Miles S, Foley CE, Buffie A, Ruppert K, Mansuria SM. Two-layer compared with one-layer vaginal cuff closure at the time of total laparoscopic hysterectomy to reduce complications. Obstet Gynecol. 2021;138(1):59–65. https://doi.org/10.1097/AOG.0000000000004428.
14. Hendessi P, Rindos N, Schiff L, Shainker S. Fundal coring: a technique to facilitate delivery of uterine specimens. J Minim Invasive Gynecol. 2013;20(6 Suppl):S189. https://doi.org/10.1016/j.jmig.2013.08.662.

12 Total Laproscopic Hysterectomy (TLH) in Frozen Pelvis by the Comprehensive Canopy Technique, '3 Step Technique'

Nutan Jain, Vandana Jain, and Sakshi Srivastava

12.1 Introduction

Frozen pelvis refers to a surgical condition where reproductive organs and other adjacent pelvis structures are distorted by extensive adhesive disease and fibrosis, which obscure the normal anatomical landmarks and surgical planes, making dissection extremely difficult and increasing the risk of injury to vital organs [1] (Fig. 12.1a, b). A frozen pelvis typically stems from specific conditions such as endometriosis [2], malignancies [3, 4] or infections affecting the parietal and urogenital regions, including Pelvic Inflammatory Disease, (PID) [5]. Notably, genital tuberculosis in the Indian subcontinent significantly contributes to the manifestation of a frozen pelvis [6]. This may manifest as bowel and omental adhesion to the uterus, tubes, and adnexa, or present as caseous materials, resembling cheesy, creamy, thick yellowish pus (Fig. 12.2). Clinical manifestations are menorrhagia and pelvic pain. Many a times, these indications predispose the patients to undergo TLH [7].

In this chapter, we will delve into the techniques employed to address the challenges presented by the frozen pelvis, focusing particularly on Total Laparoscopic Hysterectomy (TLH) by the Comprehensive Canopy Technique, '3 Step Technique' [8]. The section on endometriosis has been thoroughly covered in a separate chapter; therefore, readers are encouraged to refer to the dedicated content on endometriosis. Here, our focus will be on infectious pathologies.

Supplementary Information The online version contains supplementary material available at https://doi.org/10.1007/978-981-97-3226-5_12. The videos can be accessed individually by clicking the DOI link in the accompanying figure caption or by scanning this link with the SN More Media App.

N. Jain (✉)
Obstetrics and Gynaecology, GSVM Medical College, Affiliated by Kanpur University, Kanpur, Uttar Pradesh, India

Department of Obstetrics and Gynecology, Vardhman Trauma and Laparoscopy Centre Pvt. Ltd., Muzaffarnagar, Uttar Pradesh, India

V. Jain
Department of Obstetrics and Gynecology, Vardhman Trauma and Laparoscopy Centre Pvt. Ltd., Muzaffarnagar, Uttar Pradesh, India

Obstetrics and Gynaecology, Kasturba Hospital, Affiliated by Delhi University, Delhi, India

S. Srivastava
Obstetrics and Gynecology, Rohilkhand Medical College and Hospital, Affiliated by Bareilly International University, Bareilly, Uttar Pradesh, India

Gynae Endoscopy, Vardhman Trauma and Laparoscopy Centre Pvt. Ltd., Muzaffarnagar, Uttar Pradesh, India

N. Jain (ed.), *Complex Total Laparoscopic Hysterectomy (TLH) with Newer Approaches in Bladder Dissection*,
https://doi.org/10.1007/978-981-97-3226-5_12

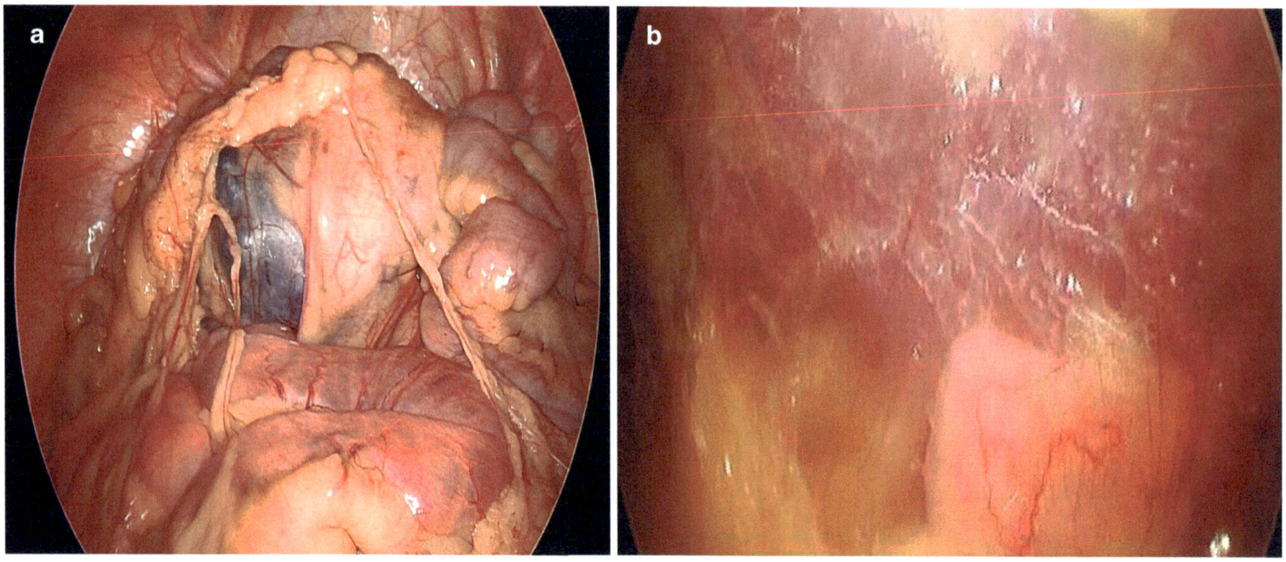

Fig. 12.1 Frozen pelvis. **a** Bilateral tubo-ovarian mass. **b** Bowel and omental adhesions totally warding off the uterus and adnexa

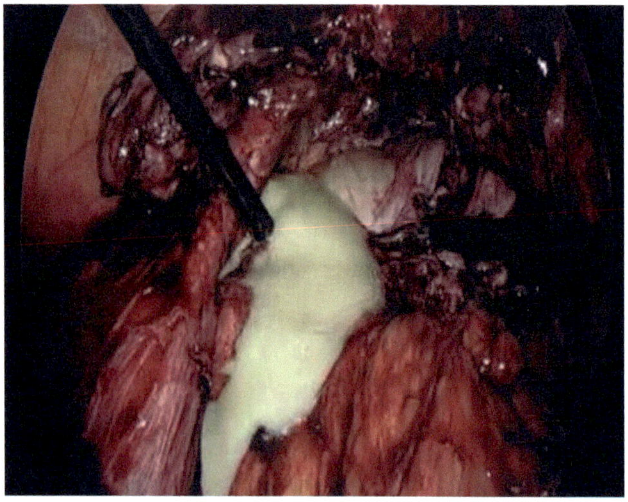

Fig. 12.2 Caseous pus like cheesy material drained during adhesiolysis

12.2 Clinical Presentation

History of menstrual disorders, characterizes these patients along with lower abdomen pain, with or without radiation to the legs and back which is a common complaint. Additionally, patients may present with undiagnosed tub-ovarian masses [9], experiencing abdominal pain and discomfort. Past medical history may include abdomino-genital infections, like Koch's, PID, septicaemia, previous surgeries, a history of carcinoma, and a background of undergoing radiations or chemotherapy for the same.

12.3 Investigation

Pelvic examination (P/V), Per speculum (P/S), and trans vaginal ultrasound (TVS) may provide essential clues suggestive of a frozen pelvis. Findings may include the presence of vaginal discharge, infections in the vagina and cervix, and tender, palpable masses in the pelvis, potentially causing probe tenderness. While sonographic evaluation is typically adequate, the addition of an MRI can enhance clinical findings when combined with ultrasound.

12.3.1 USG Findings

Ultrasound is typically the initial imaging choice for patients presenting with lower abdominal pain. In Pelvic Inflammatory Disease (PID), early ultrasound findings often reveal [10]:

1. Indistinct uterine margins
2. Echogenic pelvic fat
3. Thickening of the fallopian tubes.

Some less specific findings include fluid in the cul-de-sac, fluid in the endometrial cavity, increased ovarian volumes, and heightened thickness and vascularity of the endometrium.

In severe cases, ultrasound may detect adnexal masses with a heterogeneous echo-pattern. Tubal inflammation is associated with specific sonographic signs, such as thickened or dilated fallopian tubes, incomplete septa in the tube, fluid collection (hydrosalpinx), increased vascularity around the tube on color Doppler, echogenic fat around the tube, and occasionally, a small amount of reactive free fluid in the pelvis. In some instances, there might be echogenic fluid within the tube, indicating pyosalpinx [10].

12.3.2 Lab Investigation

In addition to routine tests, specific investigations such as those for Koch's, and Chlamydia may be necessary. Consideration of the patient's history, including previous surgeries and any instances of septicaemia, is crucial. The per-operative evaluation is comprehensive, encompassing clinical, radiological, and laboratory investigations to formulate the surgical approach effectively.

Before proceeding with surgery, a comprehensive consultation is conducted with the patient and her husband to discuss the management of the adnexa during the procedure. Adnexal management is typically straightforward as these patients are scheduled for hysterectomy and have concluded their childbearing. The condition of the fallopian tubes, whether normal or affected by hydrosalpinx, is considered for removal. During the preoperative consultation, the patient's wishes and findings are crucial in determining the management of the ovaries. The patient is informed that efforts will be made to conserve the ovaries whenever possible. However, the dilemma arises when leaving the ovaries may lead to the persistence of infectious pathology postoperatively. It is emphasized that, in consultation with the patient, there is a possibility of on-table decisions to remove the adnexa if deemed necessary. Provisional consent is obtained from the patient and her husband, particularly when dealing with dense tubo-ovarian masses that may recur in the postoperative phase. This meticulous workup, involving a thorough history, radiological findings, investigations, and counselling, forms the basis for the surgical approach.

12.3.3 Surgical Technique

Entry In such complex cases, Jain Point is the most preferred method of entry as infectious pathologies cause the Fitz-Hugh syndrome, causing extensive adhesions in the liver bed and upper quadrant of abdomen. In extensive Koch's many occasions we found Palmer's point not free of adhesions. Jain Point being lower and lateral at level of umbilicus is spared of these adhesions [11] (Fig. 12.3a–d). This entry point typically involves a 5 mm trocar after $CO2$ insufflation with veress needle from Jain Point. Once entry is established, a thorough examination is conducted to identify additional adhesions and assess the feasibility of placing a 10 mm telescope.

The surgical technique for Total Laparoscopic Hysterectomy (TLH) in a frozen section involves the following steps:

12.3.4 Bowel Adhesiolysis

When considering potential complications associated with frozen pelvis cases, it becomes imperative to perform adhesiolysis to free the bowel and omentum, allowing for a clearer view of the uterus and adnexa. In severe instances, the uterus, adnexa, or the entire pelvic region may be extensively adhered to omental and bowel structures, not only within the pelvis but also spanning the entire abdominal cavity. This adherence can extend from the hepatic and splenic areas to both flanks, including the central, umbilical area, and the pelvis itself.

Bowel adhesiolysis is the initial step in addressing a frozen pelvis (Fig. 12.4a–f). The primary objective is to create accessibility for the surgeon to address the pelvis structures, including the uterus and adnexa, and facilitate the execution of Total Laparoscopic Hysterectomy (TLH).

Bowel adhesiolysis is a nuanced skill, laden with specific challenges. The presence of bowel adhesions poses a substantial risk of bowel injury, ranging from minor serosal damage to through-and-through injuries, especially when encountered with the initial blind trocar insertion. Conditions such as tuberculosis, pelvic inflammatory disease (PID), Chlamydia, and the aftermath of septic abortions may result in densely adherent bowel loops, situated just beneath the peritoneal layer making second layer of abdominal wall.

In cases of such intricate adhesions, achieving complete adhesiolysis is nearly impossible. Consequently, our focus shifts to targeted adhesiolysis, concentrating only on the necessary areas. This approach becomes particularly crucial when addressing adhesions involving the bowel loops adhered to the pelvis, uterus, bladder, and the pouch of Douglas. The surgical priority lies in meticulous attention to these specific adhesion, ensuring a comprehensive and effective procedure.

Extreme caution is exercised when dealing with bowel loops, emphasizing the use of solely atraumatic graspers. The objective is to meticulously create a plane of cleavage between the anterior abdominal wall and the adhered bowel, specifically navigating through the intricacies of the bowel adhesiolysis.

Our approach consistently employs the method of traction and counter-traction. We refrain from intervening unless a distinct white plane of cleavage emerges between the bowel and its adhered structure. In such instances, the use of any means to separate the bowel from its adherence is strictly prohibited until the cleavage plane is identified. It is crucial to utilize only cold scissors, steering clear of energy sources such as, ultrasonic energy, monopolar or bipolar cautery

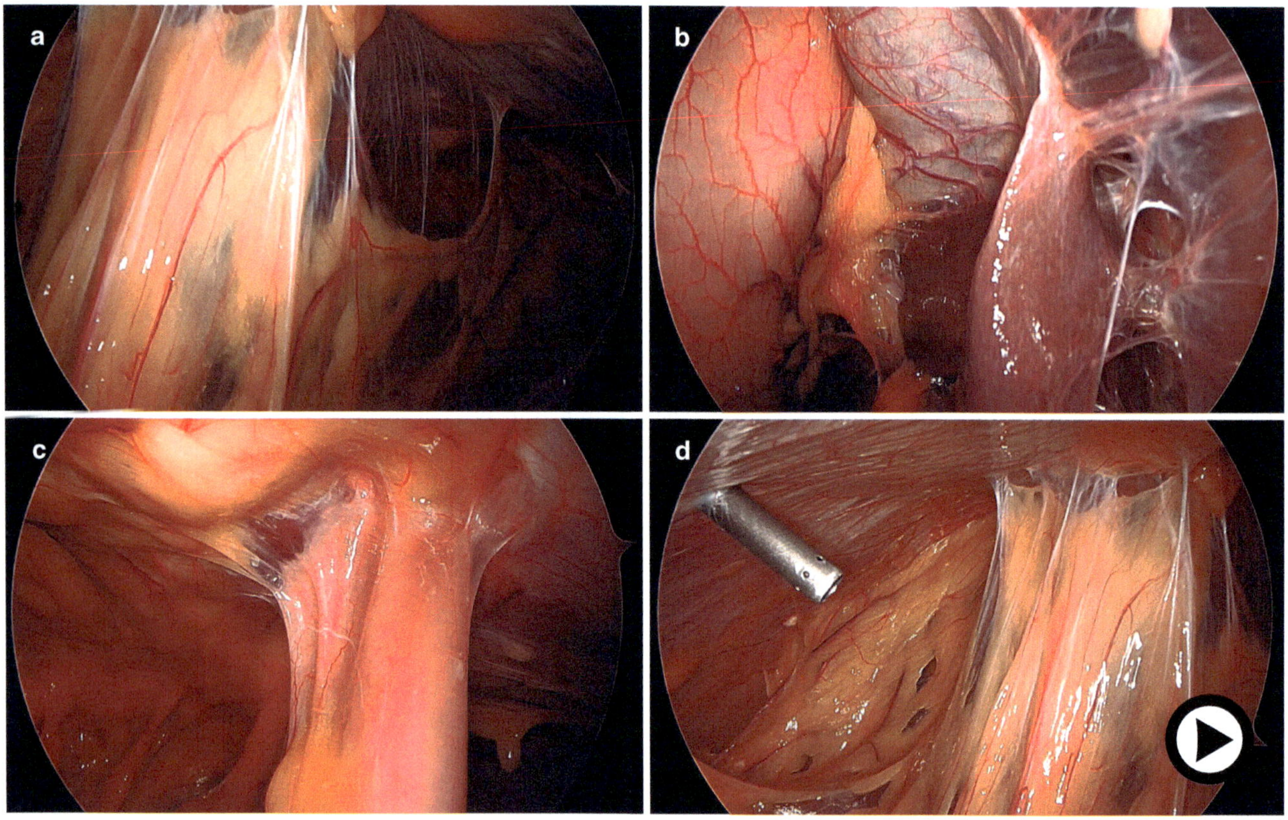

Fig. 12.3 **a** Dense omental adhesions noted all over abdomen. **b** Adhesions noted in upper quadrant over the gall bladder & liver. **c** Bowel loops stuck to anterior abdominal wall. **d** Dense omental adhesions noted with Jain point totally free (Video.12.3d TLH with Frozen pelvis) (▶ https://doi.org/10.1007/000-c98)

instruments, or the shearer in any form. The preference is to rely on cold scissors. The initial emphasis is on attempting to create a cleavage plane through meticulous traction and counter-traction.

A specific precautionary measure is exercised when addressing adhesions involving the omentum. It is imperative to recognize that there might be a hidden bowel loop behind the omental adhesion. Using 30° scope and turning the light cable and telescope to thoroughly assess the region ensures the absence of any concealed bowel loops. This precautionary step significantly contributes to preventing bowel complications. Noteworthy is the fact that over the past 40 years, we proudly report no incidents of bowel injury, whether thermal or mechanical, during the adhesiolysis process in our set up.

Upon successfully separating the bowel loop from the abdominal wall or adjacent visceral adherence, a thorough inspection is conducted to assess any damage to the bowel wall beyond the serosa. If the damage is found to extend slightly beyond the serosa, it is advisable to secure the area with a stitch or two, preventing the potential consequences of postoperative complications associated with bowel injury.

Bowel adhesions commonly occur in the pouch of Douglas, attaching to the fundus of the uterus, especially in cases of previous cesarean sections. With the escalating frequency of cesarean sections leading to an increase in multiple surgery patients, bowel adherence is also observed in the anterior utero-vesical fold. Regardless of the specific location of bowel adhesions, the guiding principles for bowel adhesiolysis remain consistent:

1. Utilization of atraumatic graspers,
2. meticulous creation of a cleavage plane through traction and counter-traction,
3. strict avoidance of thermal or any energy sources,
4. thorough inspection of the bowel loop after its descent to identify and address any potential issues of bleeding or breach in bowel integrity.

We describe the case of a 42 years old patient, with one cesarean section. Patient also had three previous laparoscopies for pain abdomen due to abdomino-genital koch's and she received anti tubercular treatment. Inspite of this she continued to have pain abdomen & severe menorrhagia for which she was posted for TLH at another centre and the pro-

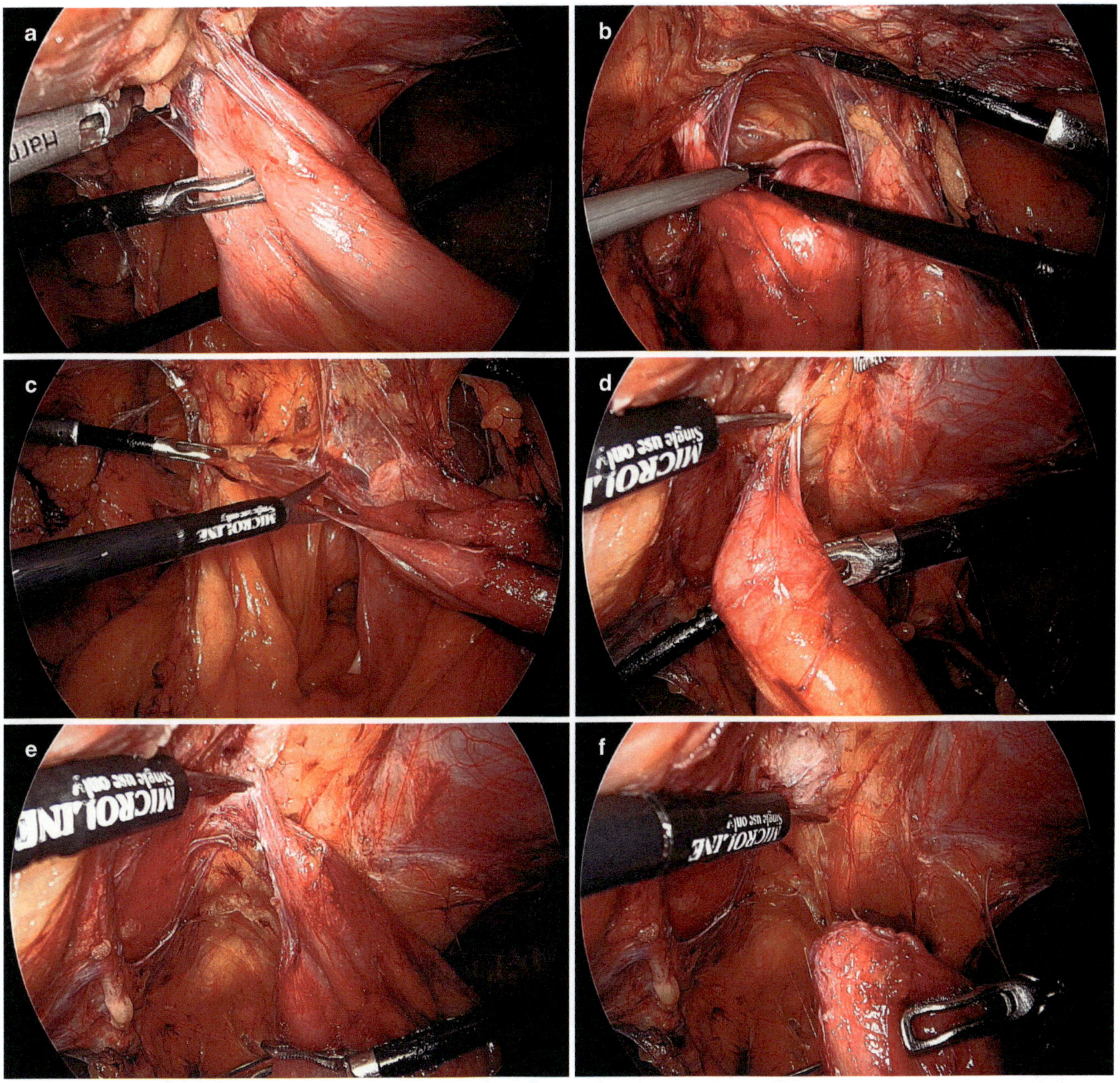

Fig. 12.4 **a** Adhesiolysis for bowel loops. Traction and counter traction is the key. **b** Bowel loops and uterus stuck to anterior abdominal wall. **c** Bowel adhesiolysis done carefully with scissors. **d** Bowel adhesiolysis being done. **e** Adhesiolysis in progress. **f** The serosal surface of the bowel which has been brought down is inspected

cedure was abandoned because of severe adhesions. Making it a total of 5 previous surgeries leading to severely adherent uterus, bladder and bowel loops. Patient now presented to us with complaints of severe pain abdomen, dysmenorrhea, dyspareunia and menorrhagia. She was posted for hysterectomy (TLH) after through clinical and radiological work up. Jain Point entry was safe even though intense bowel adhesions criss crossed the whole abdomen. Being a complete case of frozen pelvis, the uterus and adnexa was not visible even after an hour of adhesiolysis. ICG (indocyanine green) helped to keep the ureters safe in such surgeries with severe adhesions. Even though it was an extraordinary case of 'frozen pelvis' due to Koch's, the hysterectomy was done successfully, and the patient recovered well. In this case after careful lysis of bowel adhesions as mentioned before we found uterus still covered by dense omental and bowel adhesions on all sides, anterior and posterior, cul-de-sac totally obliterated (Fig. 12.5). Uterus stuck to anterior abdominal wall, a band of adhesions was divided (Fig. 12.6) and uterus brought down (Fig. 12.7). Both adenexa totally covered with omental and bowel adhesions (Fig. 12.8). Very careful bowel adhesiolysis is done from the left adenxa (Fig. 12.9).

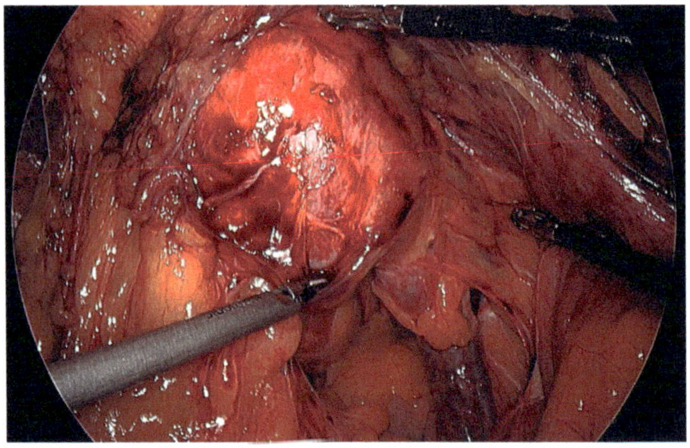

Fig. 12.5 Uterus covered by omental and bowel adhesions on all sides, started showing up after adhesiolysis

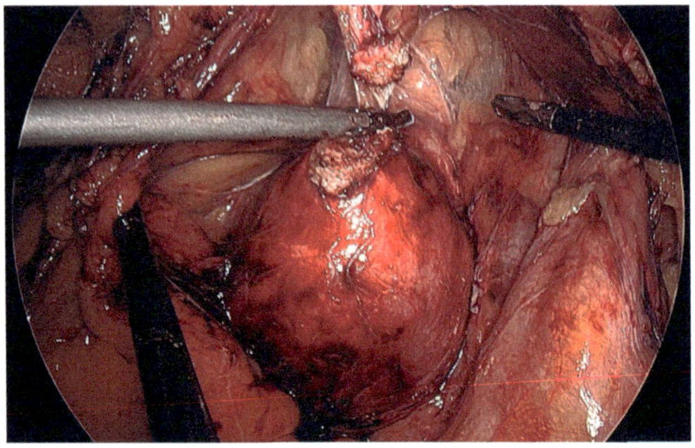

Fig. 12.6 Band of adhesion divided

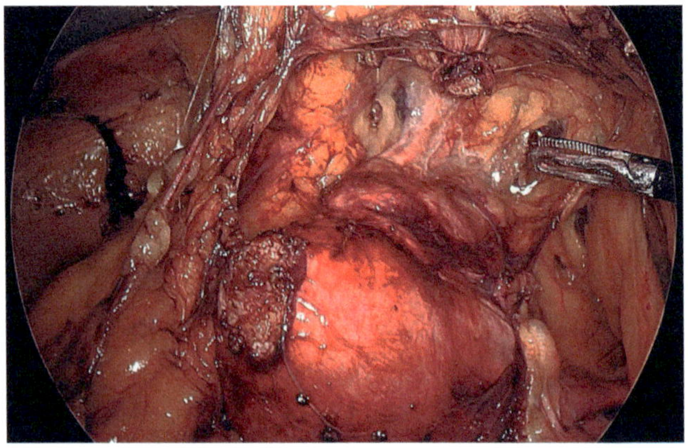

Fig. 12.7 Uterus brought down

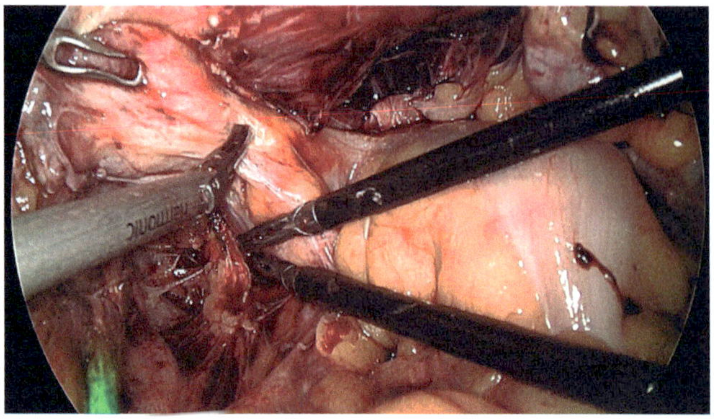

Fig. 12.8 Bowel stuck to left adnexa

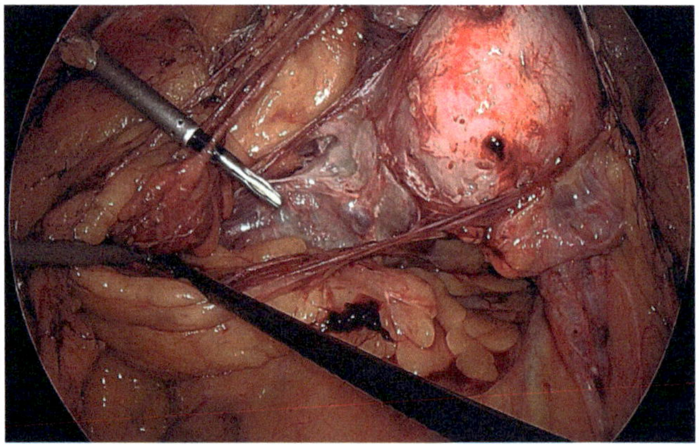

Fig. 12.9 Adhesiolysis on left adnexa

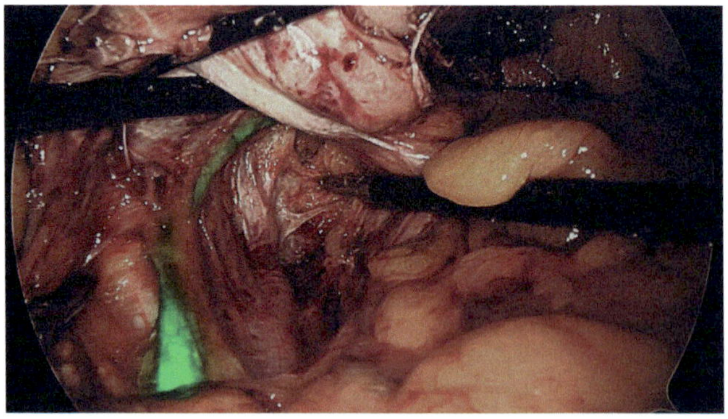

Fig. 12.10 Left ureter tagged by ICG, dissection being done

Preparation of the ureters is done, either through indocyanine green (ICG) injection or exposure.

After ensuring careful management of the bowels, the next critical system susceptible to complications in severe adhesion is the urinary tract. For effective visualization of the ureters, a surgeon must possess the expertise to identify them at the pelvic brim. The ureters are most easily identified as they traverse over the common iliac vessels and assume their pelvic sidewall position. In advanced cases and with the aid of modern technological advancements, the injection of indocyanine green (ICG) (Fig. 12.10) into the ureters can be performed using a cystoscope and ureteric catheters in a precise manner. Further details on this procedure can be found in Chap. 21.

During the operative workup, the cases that stand to benefit the most from indocyanine green (ICG) injection are identified. Typically, these include patients with a history of multiple previous surgeries, a severe history of tuberculosis, or sequelae of pelvic inflammatory disease (PID) manifesting as collections such as straw-colour collections of Koch's, tubo-ovarian abscesses, or the presence of smooth cheesy pus or caseous materials. These conditions exhibit distinctive sonographic appearances, easily distinguishable from normal cases. In such instances, equipped with the appropriate camera systems and expertise in ureteric catheterization, we opt for ICG injections to enhance visualization and precision during the procedure.

In less severe cases, our reliance is primarily on visual inspection during ureteric dissection, observing peristalsis. Occasionally, we may collaborate with the anesthesiologist to administer furosemide, enhancing ureteric peristalsis and facilitating smoother adhesiolysis.

TLH: (Figs. 12.11, 12.12, 12.13, 12.14, 12.15, 12.16, 12.17, 12.18, 12.19, 12.20, 12.21 and 12.22) Once the pelvis is accessible for TLH, we initiate the procedure at the left pelvic brim. Initially addressing sigmoid and other bowel adhesion, along with omental adhesions, on the left pelvic sidewall. Subsequently, the peritoneum adjacent to the ureter is opened, followed by an incision extending towards the sacral promontory. This allows us to approach the rectum, opening the medial and lateral para-rectal spaces proximate to the rectum. Importantly, this maneuver is performed with due consideration to maintaining a safe distance from the ureters and inferior hypogastric nerves. This technique is not only applicable to endometriosis but also proves beneficial for various types of frozen pelvis conditions.

The subsequent step involves comprehensive ureterolysis from the pelvic brim to the point where the classical sign of 'water under the bridge' emerges, indicating the crossing of the uterine artery over the ureter. The dissection proceeds in the medial and para-rectal spaces, opening them adequately. Although the initial appearance of the case may seem challenging, adopting a centrifugal approach, starting from the lateral pelvic sidewall and progressing to the medial pararectal space, allows for the systematic encounter of adhesions. A profound understanding of anatomy aids in predicting the sequence of retroperitoneal structures encountered during the procedure. Adhering to this surgical principle, we progress with adhesiolysis, gradually opening up the space from the pelvic brim to the region where the ureter descends beneath the uterine artery and the rectovaginal space medial to the uterosacral ligaments.

Confidence in surgical techniques, along with the assistance provided by a reliable uterine manipulator, such as the RUMI® uterine manipulator (Cooper Surgical, Trumbull, CT, USA), is crucial. This device not only facilitates anteversion and retroversion of the uterus but also allows a complete 360-degree maneuverability for optimal traction and countertraction among adherent bowels, omentum, adnexa, and the uterus. The RUMI® uterine manipulator (Cooper Surgical, Trumbull, CT, USA), proves invaluable in navigating through adhesions obscuring the pouch posteriorly, anteriorly, and laterally. This tool is particularly useful when unveiling the uterus hidden beneath layers of adhesions. Gentle movements of the manipulator from the pelvic end create avenues for adhesiolysis, employing a combination of traction and counter-traction.

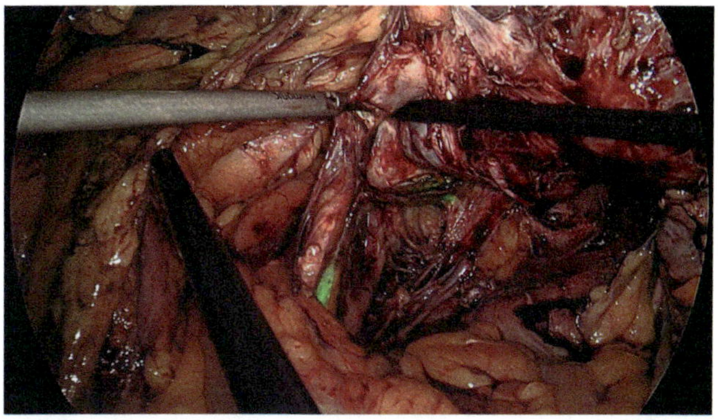

Fig. 12.11 Left IP ligament transected

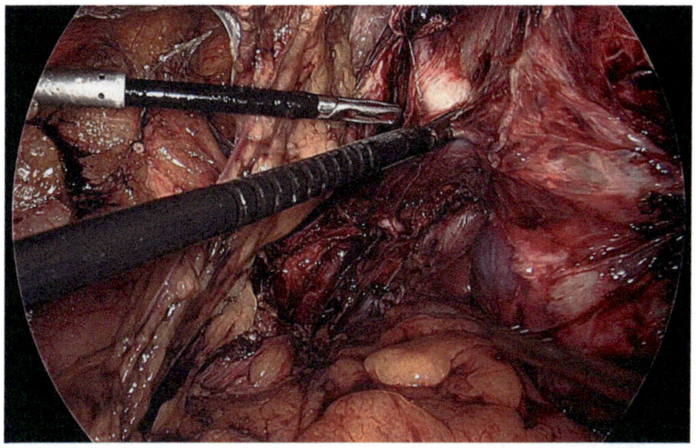

Fig. 12.12 Left uterine artery coagulated

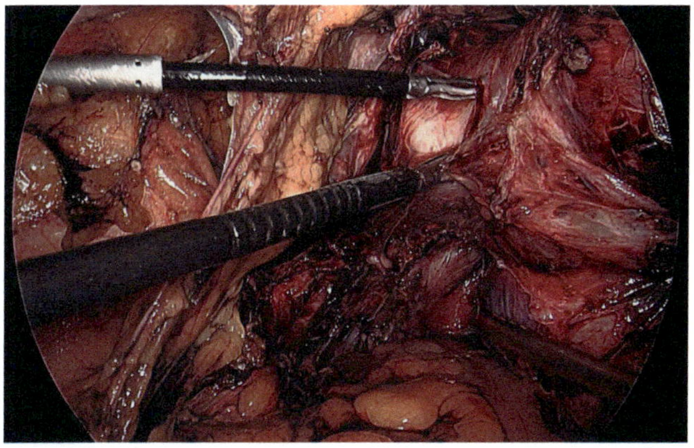

Fig. 12.13 1 cm area immediately anteromedial to the cut uterine artery pedicle most important for dissecting and reaching pubocervical fascia. Left uterine artery coagulated

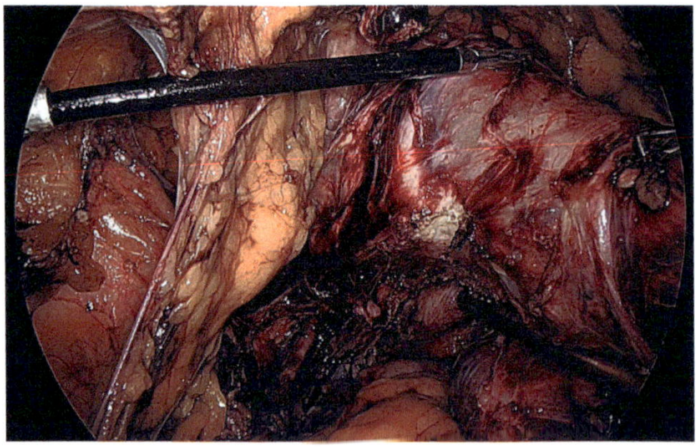

Fig. 12.14 Left uterine artery transected

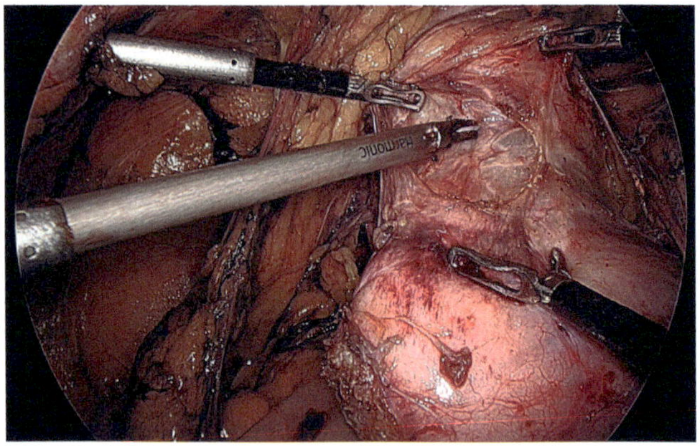

Fig. 12.15 Dissecting the bladder down

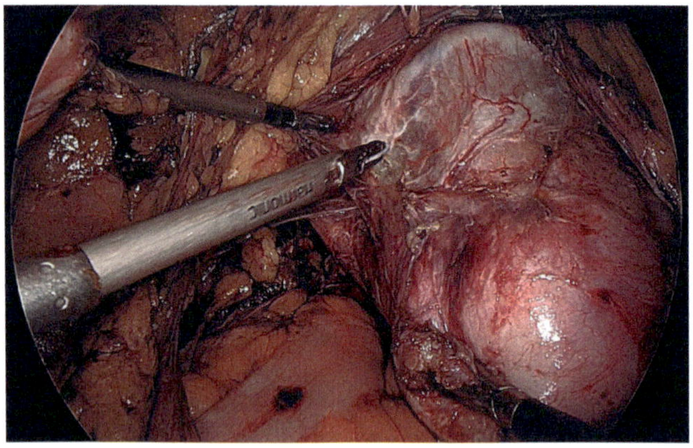

Fig. 12.16 Bladder totally brought down

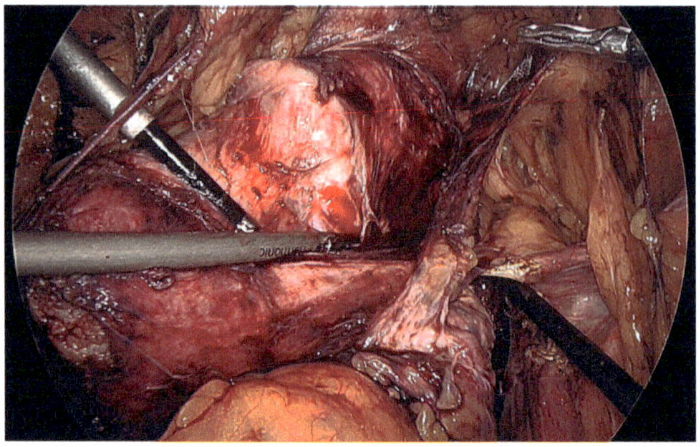

Fig. 12.17 Right uterine artery exposed from anterior approach

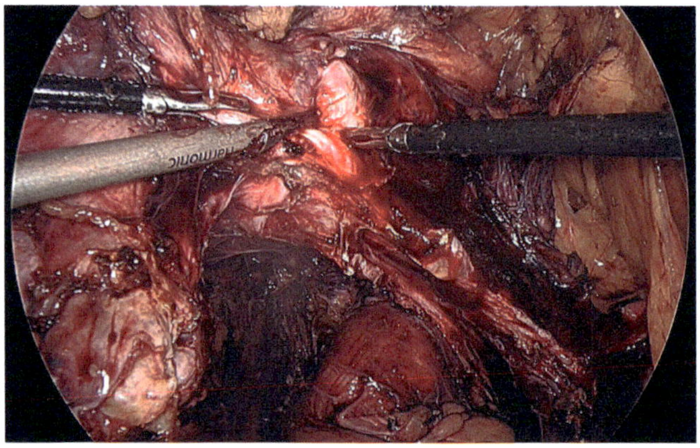

Fig. 12.18 Right uterine artery coagulated

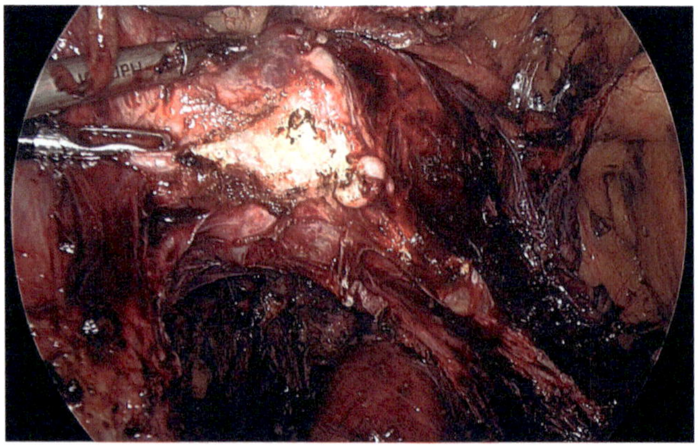

Fig. 12.19 Right uterine artery coagulated & transected

After successfully clearing the left pelvic side wall, our focus shifts to the pouch of Douglas. Unlike in endometriosis cases, adhesion in the pouch of Douglas is generally not as extensive. While Koch's may contribute to adhesion, they typically exhibit a less dense nature and seldom extend beyond the boundary to the rectovaginal septum. Consequently, addressing adhesions in conditions other than endometriosis tends to be more manageable and can be brought down in a comparatively easier fashion, but remember that risk of bowel injury is more in infectious pathologies.

Similarly, our attention turns to the right side, which is notably more straightforward compared to the left side. Beginning the dissection at the pelvic brim, precisely adjacent to the sacral promontory, where the ureter crosses over the common iliac vessels and establishes its root in the retro-

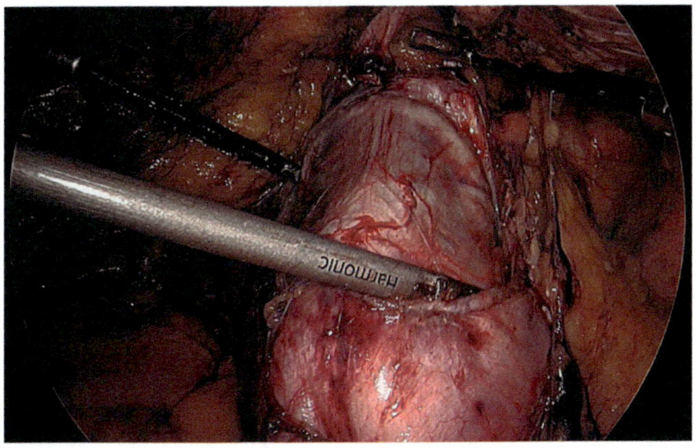

Fig. 12.20 Vault ready for culdotomy

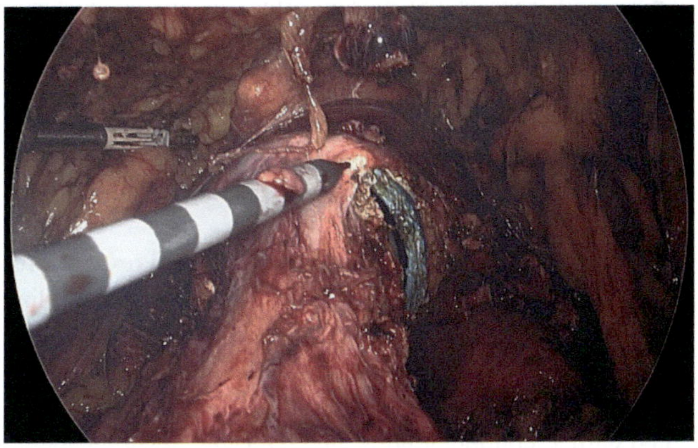

Fig. 12.21 Colpotomy

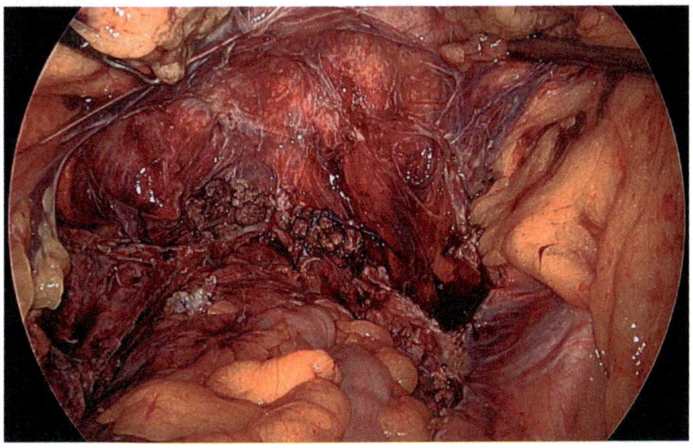

Fig. 12.22 Vault closure & suspension done

peritoneal space within the pelvis. Employing the same technique as on the left side, we utilize a pinch-up, lift-up fold of the peritoneum over the sacral promontory, widening the opening closer to the rectum. As a substantial portion is lifted, outward traction is applied by the assistant opposite me. In cases of frozen pelvis, we commonly use two ports for the surgeon or the assistant standing opposite the main surgeon. Additionally, a separate camera person is employed to manipulate the camera, 30-degree scope, and most crucial moving the light cable in such scenarios.

As the ureter becomes visible and we approach the rectum, we proceed to open up the presacral space, followed by the medial para-rectal space. Maintaining a safe distance from the hypogastric nerve and the ureters, we continue the descent until we reach just medial to the uterosacral ligaments. If the ureters have been traced with ICG, even in challenging adhesions, we can confidently rely on the assistance provided by the green glowing fluorescent ureters throughout their entire course. Modern camera systems, equipped with the onlay mode, allow for a natural laparoscopic view along with the green fluorescent ICG mode, facilitating the dissection in the posterior pouch.

The second step involves addressing the adnexa. In the context of Total Laparoscopic Hysterectomy (TLH), the fallopian tubes are sacrificed. Various conditions, such as blockage, hydrosalpingis filled with straw-colour fluid, or containing caseous materials or purulent materials, may necessitate cautious dissection for removal of the fallopian tubes. Additionally, considerations are made for scenarios where the tubes may be the site of tubo-ovarian abscess. The decision regarding the conservation or removal of the ovary takes into account these factors, ensuring a comprehensive and tailored approach based on the specific conditions observed during the procedure.

The decision regarding ovarian removal is judiciously discussed with the patient and her attendant during the preoperative phase. In younger patients with bilateral tubo-ovarian masses, we make efforts to preserve at least one ovary, extracting any viable tissue from the densely adherent and complex adhesions. In cases where only tubal involvement is present, the ovary can be easily dissected out, simplifying the procedure.

In cases of Koch's and pelvic inflammatory disease (PID), especially in peri-menopausal patients, it might be prudent to discuss the possibility of deciding, on the operating table, whether to conserve or remove the ovary. This suggestion is presented to the patient during pre-operative counselling, involving both the patient and her husband in the decision-making process. A provisional consent is obtained, acknowledging that if deemed necessary to avoid persistent infections in the pelvis, ovarian removal may be considered and carried out during the procedure.

Step 1 After completing adhesiolysis in the pouch of Douglas and deciding on the conservation or removal of the adnexa, we proceed to address the round ligament. At this juncture, the pelvic assistant provides a well-coordinated cephalad push. Upon transecting the round ligament and performing an additional pedicle sectioning, the leafs of the broad ligament are opened. A strategic cephalad push from the manipulator, coupled with the pneumoperitoneum, aids in smoothly unfurling the two leaves of the broad ligament. As they open up, our dissection progresses toward the posterior rim of the manipulator cup, allowing for a wide exposure of the retroperitoneum. This reveals the uterine vein, followed by the uterine artery.

The dissection progresses from behind to the front, exposing and refining further with strokes of the ultrasonic device, an effective dissector with a curved tip. In case of a small bleed, the ultrasonic device, serving as an energy source during adhesiolysis, can be employed. At this stage, we avoid going anteriorly, even if the bladder is densely adherent, it is allowed to remain untouched. Our focus remains on dissecting the uterine artery pedicle, coagulating it, and subsequently cutting it. While cutting, we are mindful that the anterior cervical ligament is also transected alongside the uterine artery pedicle. As we push the transected uterine pedicle below the rim of the manipulator cup, the anterior cervical ligament moves downward, concurrently displacing the ureter downwards. This strategic approach minimizes the risk of ureteric injury.

Step 2 Now, we direct our attention to the 1 or 1.5 cm area immediately adjacent to the cut pedicle of the uterine artery. In this region, we persist with slow and deliberate movements using the ultrasonic energy source. The dissection continues in a manner that ensures the correct plane of cleavage is achieved, considering that the plane of cleavage for the uterine artery aligns with that of the bladder dissection. This negotiation of the plane unfolds through a series of four or five movements, requiring persistence in this specific area to expose the shiny, glistening, pubo-vesical fascia. Once this fascia is unveiled, applying further cephalic pressure and traction on the manipulator cup allows us to insinuate the grasper deeper into the uterovesical space. Swiftly, we are able to expose the avascular uterovesical space resembling cotton candy, setting the foundation for the development of the bladder canopy. As mentioned earlier, there is no attempt to separate the bladder flap from its attachments either to the body of the uterus or the abdominal wall. Instead, we work beneath the stretched-out bladder canopy within the easily accessible cotton candy space at the level of the cervical isthmus mimicking an underpass. This area is readily delineated in Total Laparoscopic Hysterectomy (TLH) by the manipulator cup.

Step 3 Taking a step forward, we endeavour to expose the uterine artery from the anterior approach. Working beneath the canopy, we extend our efforts laterally from the left side to the right, directing the grasper towards the round ligament. Opening the retroperitoneal space is facilitated by the pneumoperitoneum, allowing us to precisely identify the plane of the cotton candy or the champagne bubbles of the uterovesical folds. This makes the task of continuous opening quite straightforward. We persist in working within the canopy until further progress becomes impossible.

Subsequently, we proceed to transect the uterovesical fold of peritoneum while remaining in close proximity to the uterus, precisely at the level of adherence of the uterovesical fold. The cutting initiates from the left side and continues up to the contralateral side of the round ligament. This step completes the dissection and exposure of the uterine artery on the right side, which was pending during the initial phase. The uterine artery of the right side is thoroughly exposed, skeletonized, transected.

In the Comprehensive Canopy Concept, 'The 3 Step Technique', three key maneuvers are undertaken to streamline Total Laparoscopic Hysterectomy (TLH). Initially, we expose and transect the uterine artery using the posterior approach. Subsequently, we create a bladder canopy, facilitating easy dissection of the uterovesical space. The third aspect involves exposing the uterine artery from the anterior approach. These three steps collectively constitute the Comprehensive Canopy Concept, promising to simplify and streamline TLH significantly.

Following the completion of these manoeuvres, we proceed with the removal of pedicles on the right side, including the ovary and the tube, based on the preoperative decisions or the need for on-table decisions to remove the ovaries. Subsequently, the patient is prepared for colpotomy, executed with a monopolar hook, and the vault closure is meticulously carried out in two layers.

Cystoscopy is routinely performed in these cases for thorough examination. In instances where there is uncertainty, particularly in severe frozen pelvis cases where there is concern about potential thermal injury to the ureter, prophylactic stenting is considered. The decision on stenting is based on the site of greater adherence, and these stents are typically scheduled for removal after 3–4 weeks.

Learning Points

- Frozen pelvis, characterized by extensive adhesive disease and fibrosis, poses surgical challenges, often associated with endometriosis, cancers, or infectious pathologies.
- Total Laparoscopic Hysterectomy (TLH) is a complex technique for managing frozen pelvis, especially in cases of infectious pathology.
- Clinical presentation includes menstrual disorders, abdominal pain, and diagnosed tub-ovarian masses.
- Diagnostic approaches encompass pelvic examination, ultrasound, and MRI, with ICG injection enhancing visualization in complex cases.
- Surgical techniques involve meticulous bowel adhesiolysis, emphasizing targeted adhesiolysis in severe cases, and careful adnexal management.

- Innovative methods like Comprehensive Canopy Concept, 'The 3 Step Technique' and contribute to systematic dissection in TLH.
- Individualized decision-making, on-table considerations, and patient consultations are crucial in managing adnexal removal.
- A case study highlights the successful application of TLH in a challenging frozen pelvis scenario.
- Urological care involves routine cystoscopy, prophylactic stenting in uncertain cases, and follow-up examinations for optimal outcomes.

Competing Interest The author declares no conflict of interest that are relevant to content of this chapter.

Ethical Approval Informed consent was obtained from individual participants and patients regarding publication and documentation without disclosing their identity.

References

1. Donald PG, Michael JC. Surgical strategies to untangle a frozen pelvis. OBG Manag. 2007;19(3):62
2. Kataoka ML, Togashi K, Yamaoka T, Koyama T, Ueda H, Kobayashi H, Rahman M, Higuchi T, Fujii S. Posterior cul-de-sac obliteration associated with endometriosis: MR imaging evaluation. Radiology. 2005;234(3):815–23.
3. Hudson CN. Victor Bonney lecture, 1980. Ovarian cancer—a gynaecological disorder? Ann R Coll Surg Engl. 1981;63:118–25.
4. Volpi E, Bernardini L, Ferrero AM. The retrograde and retroperitoneal totally laparoscopic hysterectomy for endometrial cancer. Int J Surg Oncol. 2012;2012:263850.
5. Jennings LK, Krywko DM. Pelvic inflammatory disease. StatPearls. 2023 Mar 13.
6. Sharma JB, Sharma SK, Dharmendra S, Singh UB, Kumar S, Roy KK. Laparoscopic evaluation of female genital tuberculosis in infertility: an observational study. Indian J Med Res. 2023;157(2&3):183–91. https://doi.org/10.4103/ijmr.ijmr_2498_21. PMID: 37202937; PMCID: PMC10319378.
7. Stovall TG. Hysterectomy. In: Berek JS, editor. Berek & Novak's gynecology. 14th ed. Philadelphia: Lippincott Williams & Wilkins; 2007. p. 805–46.
8. Paul PG, Shabnam K, Bhosale SA, Kaur H, Talwar P, Thomas T. Laparoscopic hysterectomy in frozen pelvis—an alternative technique of retrograde adhesiolysis. Gynecol Surg. 2013;10(4):285–90. https://doi.org/10.1007/s10397-013-0810-8.
9. Walid SM, Heaton RL. Total laparoscopic extirpation of a fixed uterus from benign gynecological disease. Gynecol Surg. 2011;8:157–9.
10. Radswiki T, Campos A, Knipe H, et al. Pelvic inflammatory disease. Reference article, Radiopaedia.org. https://radiopaedia.org/articles/14987. Accessed 26 Jan 2024.
11. Jain N, Sareen S, Kanawa S, Jain V, Gupta S, Mann S. Jain point: a new safe portal for laparoscopic entry in previous surgery cases. J Hum Reprod Sci. 2016;9(1):9–17. https://doi.org/10.4103/0974-1208.178637. PMID: 27110072; PMCID: PMC4817291.

Total Laparoscopic Hysterectomy (TLH) in Obese Patients by the Comprehensive Canopy Technique, '3 Step Technique'

13

Nutan Jain, Sakshi Srivastava, and Divyanee Gulati

13.1 Introduction

Obesity is an epidemic in both affluent and developing countries with more than 500 million clinically obese individuals worldwide [1]. This prevalence is increasing by roughly 20% each year and if this explosion continues, majority of surgical patients will be obese too [2]. In 1910, Dr. Kelly described obesity, "*to be a storehouse for useless adipose tissue and to carry this handicap around, openly displayed wherever one goes, is one of the most distressing of life's minor ailments* [3]." As per the World Health Organization (WHO), obesity is defined as having a body mass index (BMI) equal to or exceeding 30, and its classification is as per BMI range, spanning from class 1 (30–34.9), class 2 (35–39.9), to class 3 (BMI > 40) [4]. In obese patients, minimally invasive surgical approach is preferred over open surgery [5], [6] as open surgery in the face of obesity leads to significant wound complications [7]. However, gaining primary access to the abdomen remains challenging due to the substantial presence of adipose tissue in the abdominal wall and a higher prevalence of prior surgical scars. This challenge persists, as there exists a clear correlation between obesity and various gynaecological conditions. Conditions such as type 2 diabetes mellitus, hypertension, obstructive sleep apnea, atherosclerosis, and angina, pose significant challenges in the perioperative period [8–14].

Supplementary Information The online version contains supplementary material available at https://doi.org/10.1007/978-981-97-3226-5_13. The videos can be accessed individually by clicking the DOI link in the accompanying figure caption or by scanning this link with the SN More Media App.

N. Jain (✉)
Obstetrics and Gynaecology, GSVM Medical College, Affiliated by Kanpur University, Kanpur, Uttar Pradesh, India

Department of Obstetrics and Gynecology, Vardhman Trauma and Laparoscopy Centre Pvt. Ltd., Muzaffarnagar, Uttar Pradesh, India

S. Srivastava
Obstetrics and Gynaecology, Rohilkhand Medical College and Hospital, Affiliated by Bareilly International University, Bareilly, Uttar Pradesh, India

Gynaecology Endoscopy, Vardhman Trauma and Laparoscopy Centre Pvt. Ltd., Muzaffarnagar, Uttar Pradesh, India

D. Gulati
Obstetrics and Gynecology, GMC Patiala, Affiliated by Baba Farid University of Health Sciences, Patiala, Punjab, India

Gynaecology Endoscopy, Vardhman Trauma and Laparoscopy Centre Pvt. Ltd., Muzaffarnagar, Uttar Pradesh, India

13.2 Preoperative Considerations

Proper assessment of the patient's panniculus and body morphology is conducted, with particular emphasis placed on the distribution of weight and the waist-to-hip ratio (i.e., a higher waist circumference relative to hip circumference). Patients exhibiting a concentration of adipose tissue around the waist pose greater technical challenges compared to those with adiposity predominantly around the hips. In the preoperative assessment phase, the panniculus is elevated to locate the ischial spines and to ascertain the positioning of the aortic bifurcation concerning the patient's umbilicus, both while standing and in the supine position. Preoperatively, various measurements are taken, including height, weight, neck circumference, width of mouth opening, sternomental distance, and thyromental distance. It is important to note that while BMI itself is not indicative of a challenging airway, studies have revealed that a high Mallampati score (3 or higher) and a larger neck circumference elevate the likelihood of encountering difficulties during laryngoscopy and intubation. Specifically, a neck circumference of 40 cm poses a 5% risk, whereas 60 cm carries a 35% risk of encountering challenges during intubation [15].

Obesity is often associated with comorbidities like coronary artery disease (CAD), hypertension, diabetes mellitus, obstructed airway and obstructive sleep apnea. Obstructive sleep apnea can be associated with postoperative respiratory

N. Jain (ed.), *Complex Total Laparoscopic Hysterectomy (TLH) with Newer Approaches in Bladder Dissection*,
https://doi.org/10.1007/978-981-97-3226-5_13

complications like pneumonia, postoperative hypoxemia, and unplanned re-intubation. So pre-operative optimization of these underlying medical co-morbidities is crucial as they could affect intra-operative and postoperative care. A multidisciplinary team, comprising clinicians, physicians, anesthetists, intensivists, and surgeons, assesses these cases collectively. Subsequently, a surgical and post-operative plan is developed based on their combined expertise and insights.

Mechanical bowel preparation is performed on the night preceding the surgery. Pre-operative administration of prophylactic antibiotics is tailored to the patient's weight, and thromboprophylaxis is administered based on Caprini scoring [16] to mitigate the risk of venous thromboembolism [17].

13.3 Intraoperative Considerations

Special considerations have to be given to anaesthesia, patient positioning, creation of pneumoperitoneum and trocar entry. For gynaecological laparoscopy, obese patients are placed in trendelenberg position. So proper patient positioning is crucial to prevent undue injuries. To prevent slippage, a surgical mattress and chest strapping are employed, while the legs are adequately supported to minimize trauma. Proper padding of the knees and calves is ensured, and leg stirrups are used to decrease the chances of nerve injuries. Additionally, measures such as shoulder blade and arm extenders, along with padding of pressure points like elbows and wrists, are implemented for patient safety. To mitigate the risk of deep venous thrombosis, leg stockings or sequential compression devices are utilized (Fig. 13.1).

Very active and thorough management by the anaesthetist is crucial for safe laparoscopy in obesity. The role of anaesthetist is essential as it may pose challenges as follows:

- Difficult airway
- Pulmonary vital capacity is low in obese patients especially expired volume
- Performing procedures in the pelvic region often requires the Trendelenburg position, which may complicate ventilation of the patient
- For better visualization, we need higher pneumoperitoneal pressure which can potentially impede the ability to ensure sufficient ventilation.
- Longer operating time in obese patients.

Before induction, preoxygenation with 100% oxygen is administered while maintaining a 25-degree head-up position for 3–5 min to mitigate hypoxemia. The application of positive pressure ventilation during pre-oxygenation is cru-

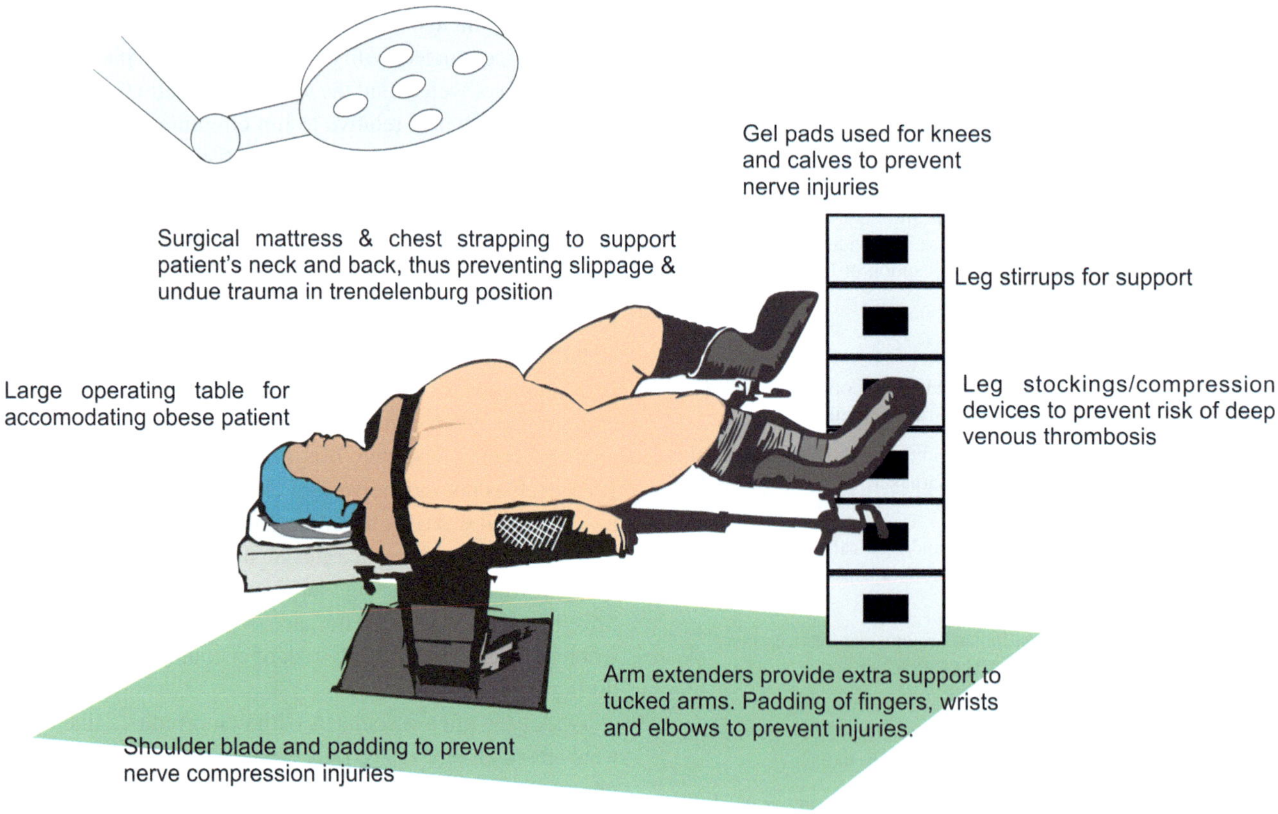

Fig. 13.1 Obese patient positioning on operation table

cial. PEEP (positive end-expiratory pressure) is the only ventilatory parameter that consistently has been shown to enhance respiratory function in obese subjects. Following induction, maintaining an intraoperative PEEP of 10–12 cm H_2O is reasonable, although vigilance is necessary to address any hypotension that may arise.

Laparoscopic Access In any laparoscopic surgery, the initial stage involves primary access through the abdominal wall, a process not devoid of risks. Literature indicates that 25% of injuries occurring in laparoscopic procedures arise during the initial blind port placement [18], with bowel injuries reported in 1.8 per 1000 and vascular injury in 0.9 per 1000 cases [19]. In obese patients, entry is more challenging.

In obese patients, the most frequent laparoscopic entry point is through the umbilicus. This necessitates entering the abdomen in a vertical direction, contrary to the typical 45° inclination towards the pelvis in individuals of normal weight. This vertical entry raises the risk of encountering major retroperitoneal vessels (MRV) [20], as the umbilicus is situated merely 4–5 cm from these vessels. Additionally, raising the abdominal wall for umbilical entry becomes challenging in obese patients. If both the surgeon and assistant are involved in this process, there's a risk of applying unequal forces, which can lead to incorrect placement [21] or, worse, major retroperitoneal vessel injury. In laparoscopic entry after previous surgery there is risk of adhesions under the umbilicus [22]. Consequently, umbilical entry can make primary blind port insertion hazardous [23], prompting consideration for a lateral port alternative [24]. This lateral approach mitigates the risk of MRV injury and avoids peri-umbilical adhesions common in cases with previous surgeries. To address this concern, the Jain point, situated 10–13 cm from the umbilicus, has become a routine choice, particularly in cases with a history of previous surgeries [25].

When making entry in obese patients, a crucial aspect involves evaluating patient's weight distribution and mobility of panniculus. A high waist circumference, i.e. central obesity, can result in more technical challenges compared with patients whose weight is more concentrated along hips, i.e. truncal obesity (Fig. 13.2a). The Jain Point proves particularly advantageous in cases of central obesity, where there tends to be less adipose tissue in the region situated 10–13 cm lateral to the umbilicus. It is identified by a fixed and prominent bony landmark, the ASIS, which remains palpable even in obese patients (Fig. 13.2b). This characteristic, along with it's short learning curve, alleviates the fear associated with the initial blind entry and major retroperitoneal vessel injury, particularly for beginners.

The Hassan's open technique, an established alternative entry port, presents limitations in obese patients due to the necessity of penetrating through 8–10 cm of adipose tissue before reaching the fascia which is impractical due to excess abdominal fat and risk of port site hernia [26]. In our study, conducted over an extended follow-up period, we did not encounter any instances of port site hernia or infection at the Jain Point port. This can be attributed to its smaller size, measuring 5 mm, in contrast to the 2 cm incision required for the Hasson technique. Moreover, Hasson's open entry technique is hazardous in type 2 bowel adhesions [27], where bowel is adherent right under the umbilicus, making the second layer of abdomen.

Another commonly utilized entry point is the Palmer's point [28], which, as noted in the literature, carries certain limitations. These include occasional liver lacerations attributed to peri-visceral fat deposition and the presence of distorted anatomy, particularly in obese patients [29, 30] Jain point, free of vessel, viscera, adhesion and bowel, is relatively found to be safe [31, 32] (Fig. 13.3). To overcome increased abdominal fat, we use longer Veress needle of 150 mm length and longer trocars (Fig 13.4a, b) There is no need to lift the abdominal wall or change in angle of Veress insertion with change in BMI (Figs. 13.5, 13.6a, b, 13.7a, b).

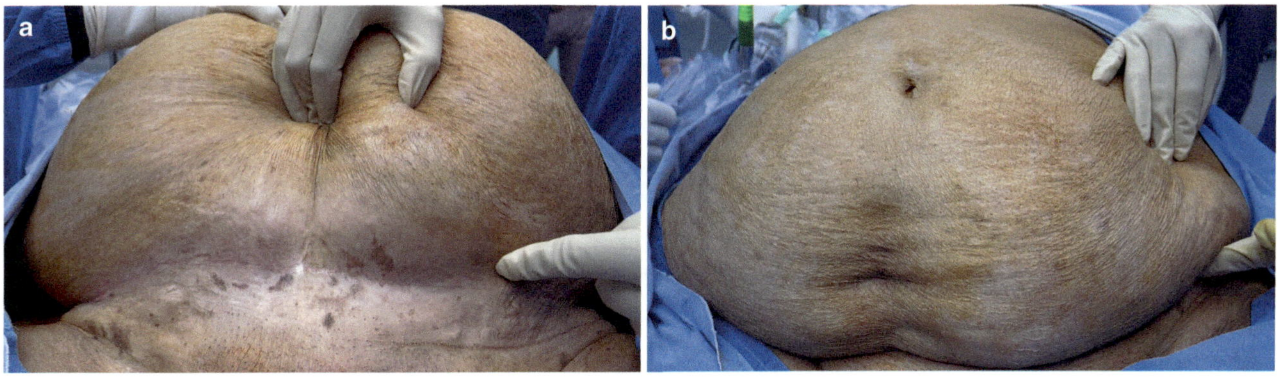

Fig. 13.2 **a** Frontal view of an obese patient(weight 120 kg; BMI 48.4 kg/m^2) with a large pannus lifted up to demonstrate persistent skin rash in the suprapubic area. **b** Jain point is located by a single prominent bony landmark, the ASIS, which remains fixed even in obese patients where umbilicus droops down

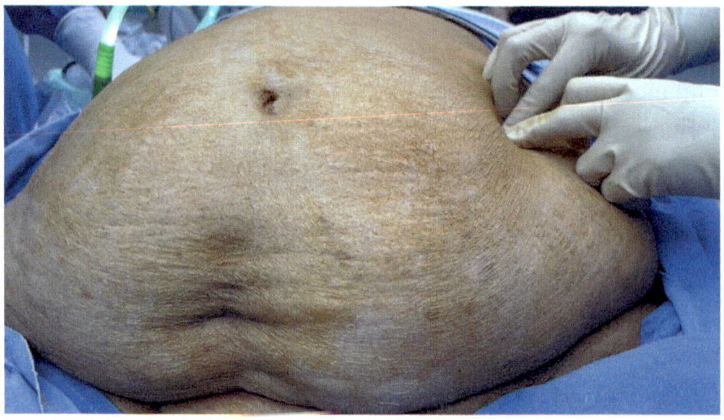

Fig. 13.3 Finger pointing at Jain point which lies at paraumbilical level, 2.5 cm medial to ASIS

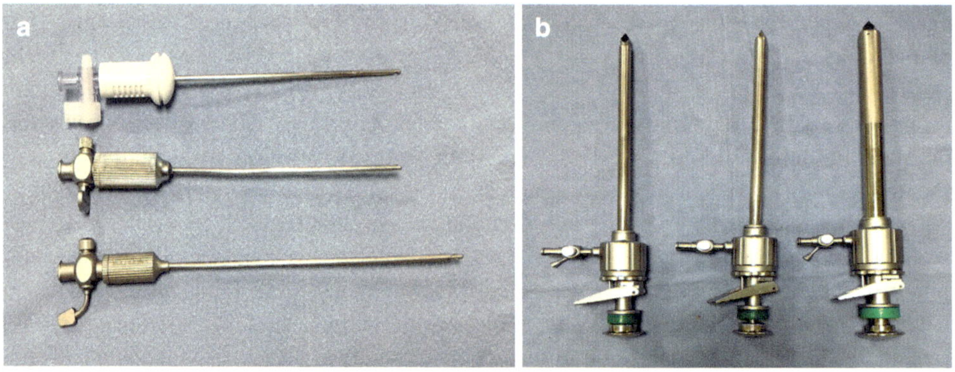

Fig. 13.4 **a** Long Veress needle of 150 mm length is used to traverse increased abdominal fat. **b** Longer ancillary trocars of 15 cm length used

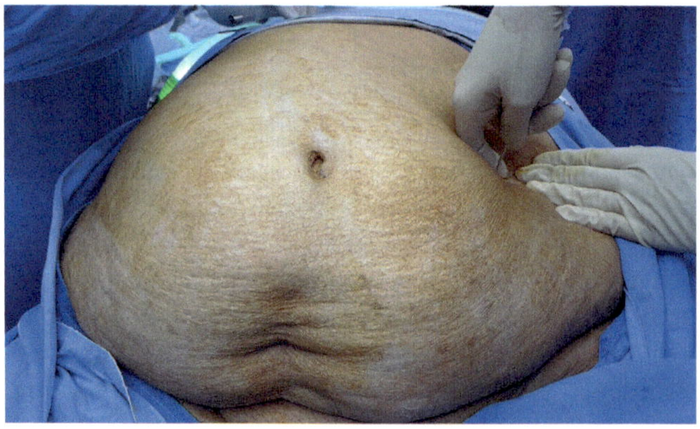

Fig. 13.5 Veress needle entry in vertical direction at Jain point, no need of lifting the abdomen or changing the angle

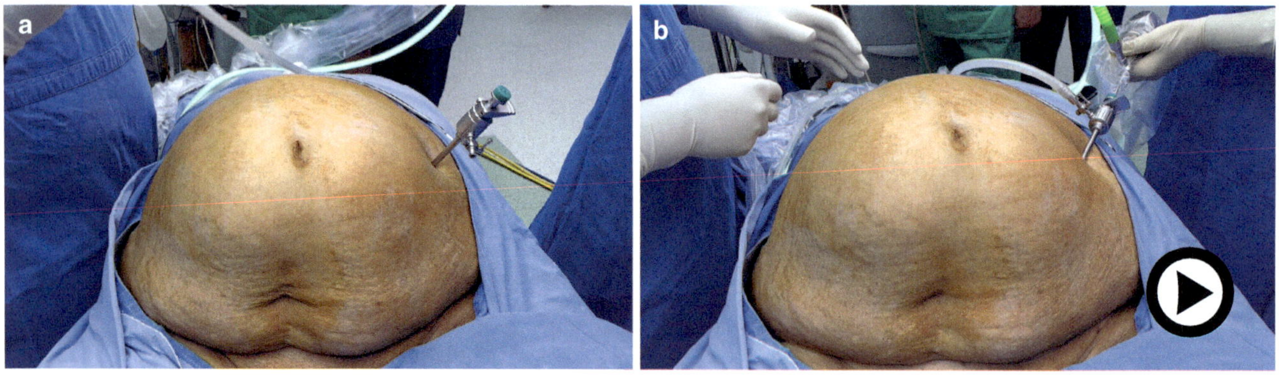

Fig. 13.6 **a** Primary long trocar insertion in vertical direction at Jain point (Video 13.6a TLH in Obese Patient) (▶ https://doi.org/10.1007/000-c99). **b** 5 mm telescope inserted through primary port to make a 360 degree check of abdomen

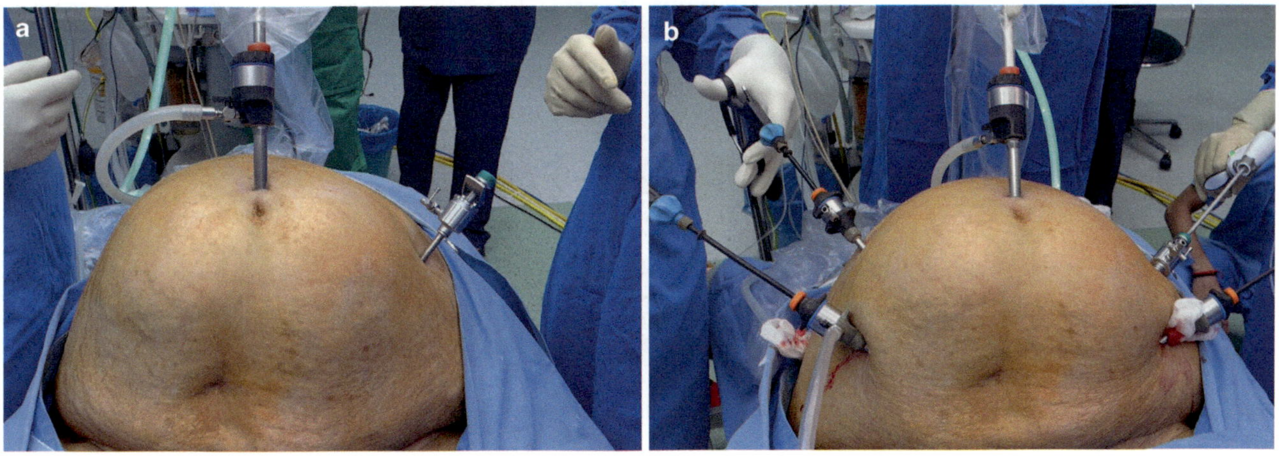

Fig. 13.7 **a** 10 mm supraumbilical optical port optimized through 5 mm telescope. **b** Final port placement

13.4 Surgical Steps in Total Laparoscopic Hysterectomy

- Several studies have highlighted visceral adiposity as having a stronger correlation with increased morbidity and mortality. Hence, both BMI and visceral adiposity should be regarded as influential factors impacting a patient's health status both during surgery and throughout the recovery period [33].
- The propensity of visceral and peritoneal fat in obese patients pose a significant challenge to the operating surgeon, hampering the visualization and manipulation (Fig. 13.8a). The usage of uterine manipulator, rectal probe and enhanced visualization in cases of dense adhesions with Indocyanine Green (ICG) and special camera system aids us in the technique (Fig. 13.8b).
- For the bothersome peritoneal and bowel fat, we often use an extra port either suprapubic or right upper paraumbilical for better retraction.
- In patients with previous caesarean sections, we usually find uterus densely adherent to anterior abdominal wall (Fig. 13.9). Due to marked perivascular fat in obese patients, the visualization of uterine pedicle is also challenging. Our Comprehensive Canopy Concept, 'The 3 Step Technique' comes as a saviour in such cases as it helps in easy skeletonization of uterine artery and vein.
- Articulating vessel sealer instruments and other longer instruments are very useful for reaching the deepest part of the pelvis with ease (Fig. 13.10).

Our standardized steps of Comprehensive Canopy Concept to TLH unfolds in three distinct steps:

Injection of Diluted Vasopressin Prior to commencing TLH, we inject diluted vasopressin (20 units in 400 ml normal saline) into the uterus. This vasoconstrictor aids in minimizing bleeding during the procedure, and helps open up surgical planes.

Coagulation and Cutting of Left Adnexal Pedicle We initiate the TLH with the coagulation and sequential cutting of the left adnexal pedicle, encompassing the ovarian ligament, fallopian tube, and round ligament (Fig. 13.11a, b).

1. **FIRST STEP—Posterior approach of uterine artery dissection:** We transect the posterior leaf of the broad ligament, widely from utero sacral ligaments to arcus torinus over the cephalad pushed manipulator cup. This posterior approach exposes the uterine artery pedicle easily, which is skeletonized, coagulated and cut with the help of ultrasonic energy, before developing the bladder flap. Early uterine artery sectioning cuts the transverse cervical ligament too, thereby facilitating lateral and inferior movement of the ureter, minimizing the risk of ureteric injury (Fig. 13.12a–f).
2. **SECOND STEP—Canopy concept of bladder dissection:** Utilizing the plane of the uterine artery as a guide, we dissect 1–1.5 cm anterior to the coagulated uterine artery and we navigate an atraumatic grasper anterior to the coagulated uterine artery. The dissection continues until we reach the shiny glistening pubocervical fascia. We usually notice that even in case of excessive visceral fat over bladder and dense bladder adhesions, the adherence is more at the body of uterus; while the cervical isthmus is found to be free, which is delineated by the manipulator cup. Negotiating under the canopy of bladder adhesions, we access the avascular uterovesical space. Once the uterovesical space is opened completely, then the stuck bladder flap at the top is dissected down, allowing for avascular effortless downward movement of the densely adherent bladder flap (Fig. 13.13a–f).

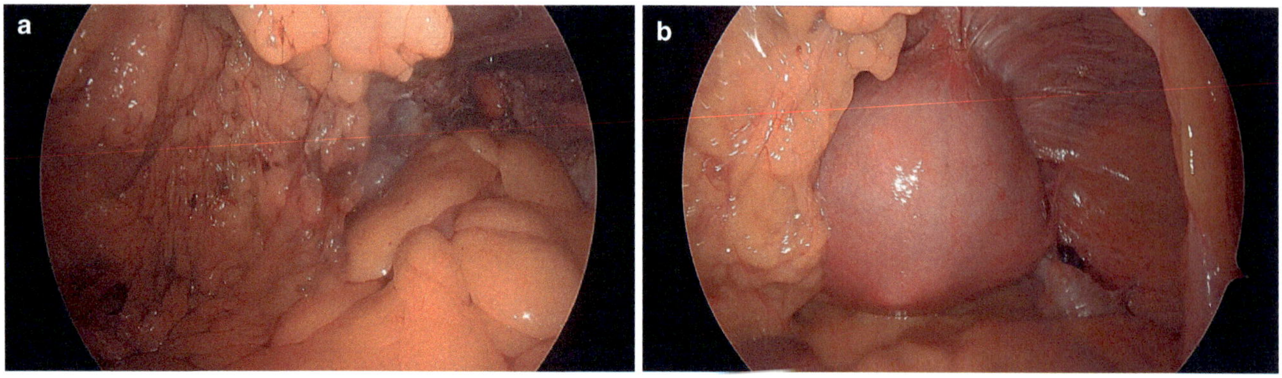

Fig. 13.8 **a** Abdominal cavity full of visceral and peritoneal fat and adhesions. **b** Patient's initial picture of pelvis after retracting the abdominal fat

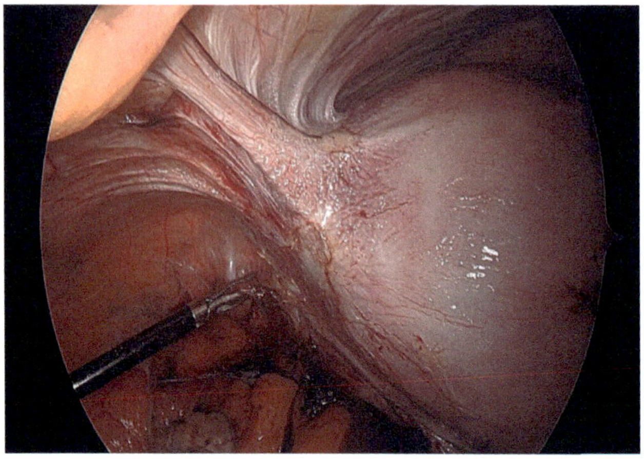

Fig. 13.9 Uterus densely adherent with bladder and anterior abdominal wall

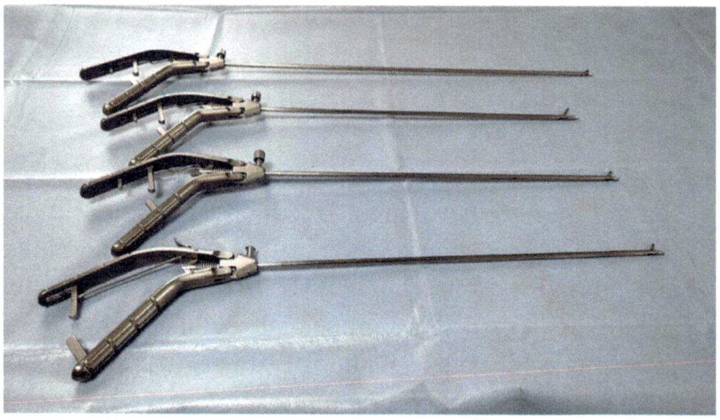

Fig. 13.10 Long needle holders used to reach the depth of pelvis with ease

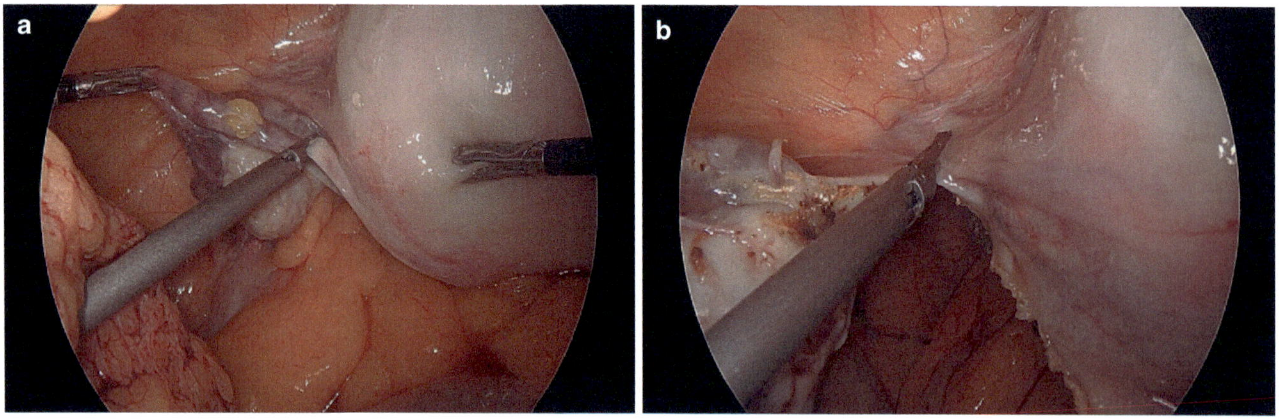

Fig. 13.11 **a** Left fallopian tube and ovarian ligament coagulated and cut. **b** Left round ligament coagulated and cut

3. **THIRD STEP—Anterior approach of contralateral uterine artery dissection:** Working within the avascular plane till the round ligament, we reach the right uterine artery and vein alongside the manipulator cup rim, which is coagulated and cut (Fig. 13.14a, b). Coagulation and cutting are then executed in a similar manner for the right-sided adnexa. In severely ventrifixed uterus, sometimes it might not be possible to go straight to the third step of anterior approach of uterine artery dissection. In such instances, we coagulate and cut the right cornual pedicle first and then proceed to right uterine artery coagulation (Fig. 13.15a–f).

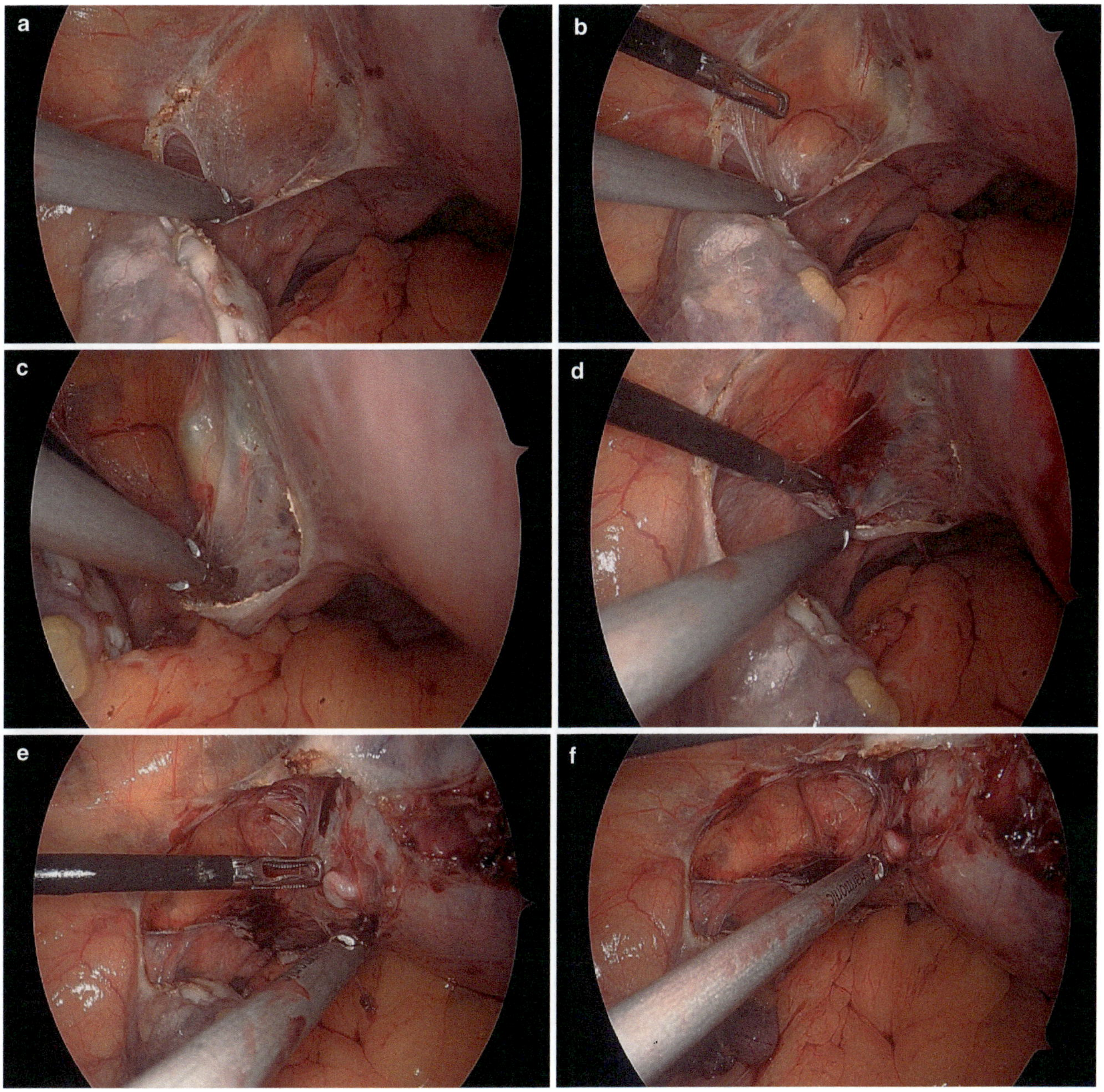

Fig. 13.12 First step of comprehensive canopy concept- 'The 3 Step Technique': Posterior approach of uterine artery dissection. **a** Opening of posterior leaf of broad ligament. **b** Posterior leaf of broad ligament dissected widely from uterosacrals to arcus torinus. **c** Posterior approach easily skeletonizes the uterine artery pedicle. **d** Left uterine vein skeletonized by posterior approach. **e** Left uterine artery skeletonized by posterior approach. **f** Left uterine pedicle coagulated and cut

Colpotomy and Uterus Extraction Ensuring the manipulator cup is free of bowel and bladder adhesions, we proceed to circumferential colpotomy using a monopolar hook (Fig. 13.16). The uterus is delivered, and prophylactic salpingectomy is performed. The decision regarding ovarian removal depends on the disease and is subject to discussion with the patient.

Vault Closure and Suspension Closure of the vault is conducted in double layers using polyglactin sutures. Vault suspension is accomplished by taking bites separately through the utero sacral ligaments. This step is implemented to prevent vault prolapse, which is extremely important in obese individuals (Fig. 13.17a).

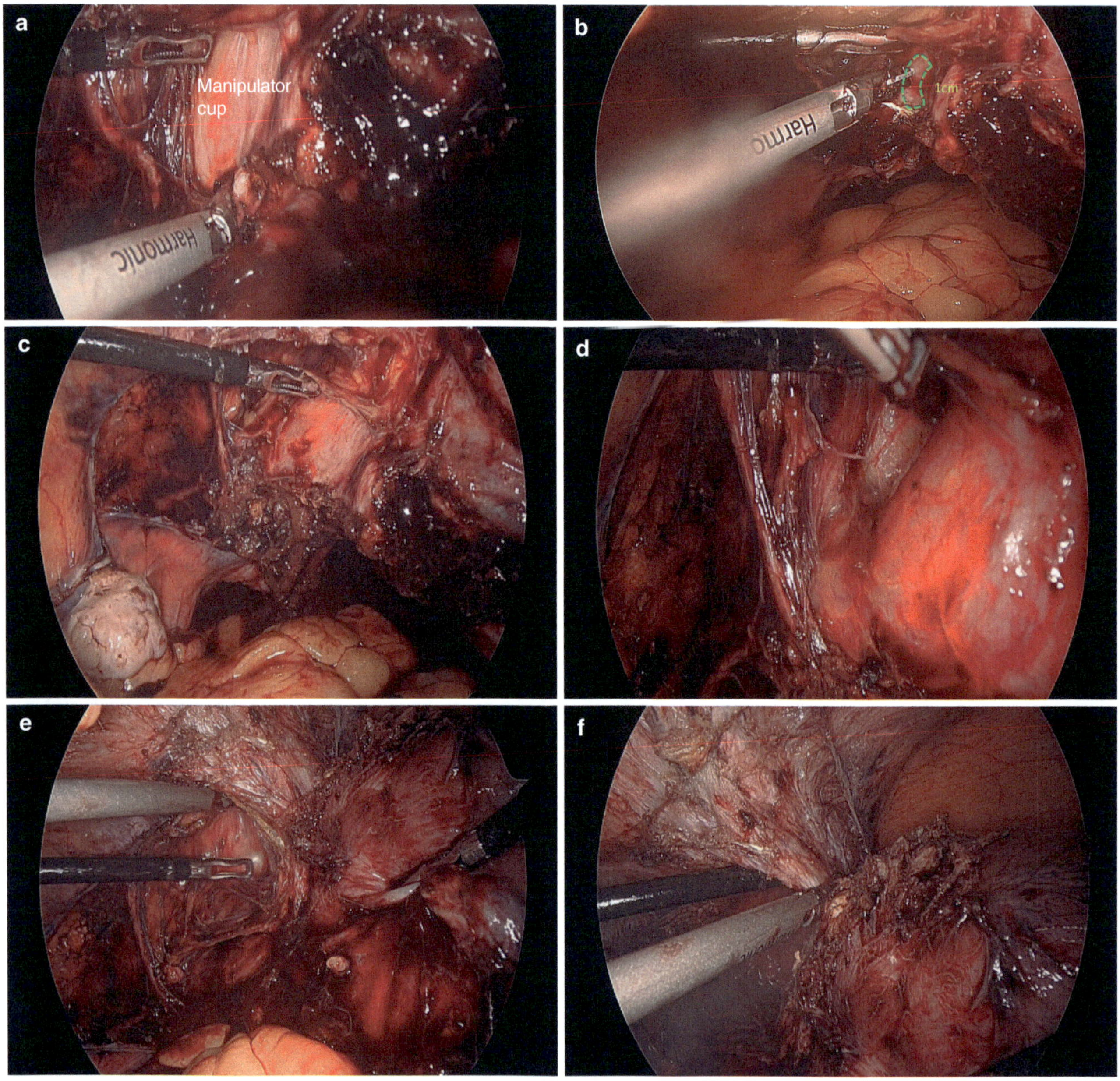

Fig. 13.13 **a** Coagulated left uterine artery shaved off the manipulator cup rim. **b** Bladder dissection begins just 1 cm anteromedial to the coagulated uterine artery. **c** Dissection continues over the cranially pushed manipulator cup till we reach the shiny glistening pubocervical fascia. **d** Further dissection beneath the stretched out canopy opens up the cotton candy uterovesical space. **e** Bladder still densely adherent to the body of uterus, and curve harmonic ace helps in finding the plane of cleavage. **f** Grasper inserted in the loose uterovesical space and then bladder flap dissected off the uterus

Finally, a meticulous process of suction, irrigation, and drainage is carried out to ensure a clean and clear surgical field (Fig. 13.17b). Ports more than 10 mm are closed using port closure device. A routine check cystoscopy is carried out to confirm bilateral ureteric jet and peristalsis.

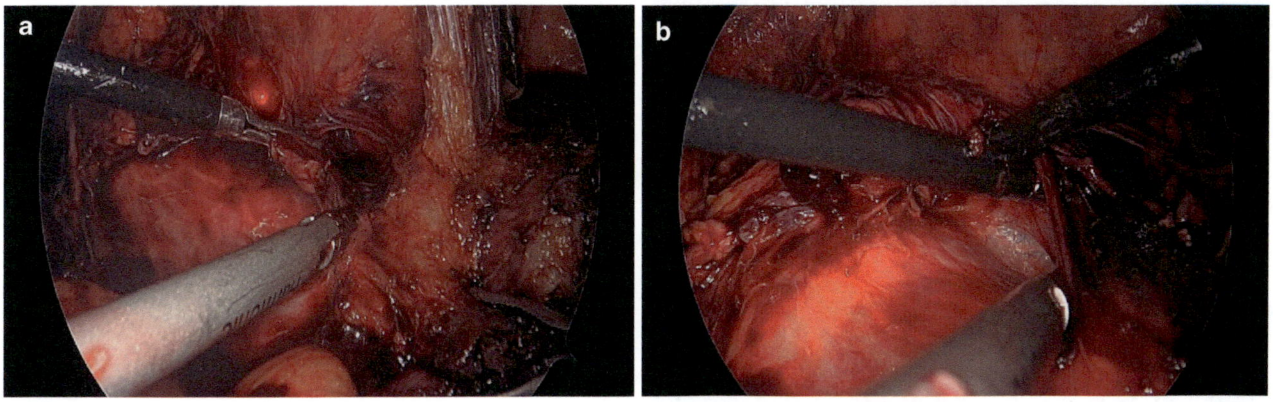

Fig. 13.14 **a** Dissection continues upto contralateral right round ligament. **b** Dissection extended from the cotton candy uterovesical space towards the right broad ligament to expose the contralateral uterine artery and vein

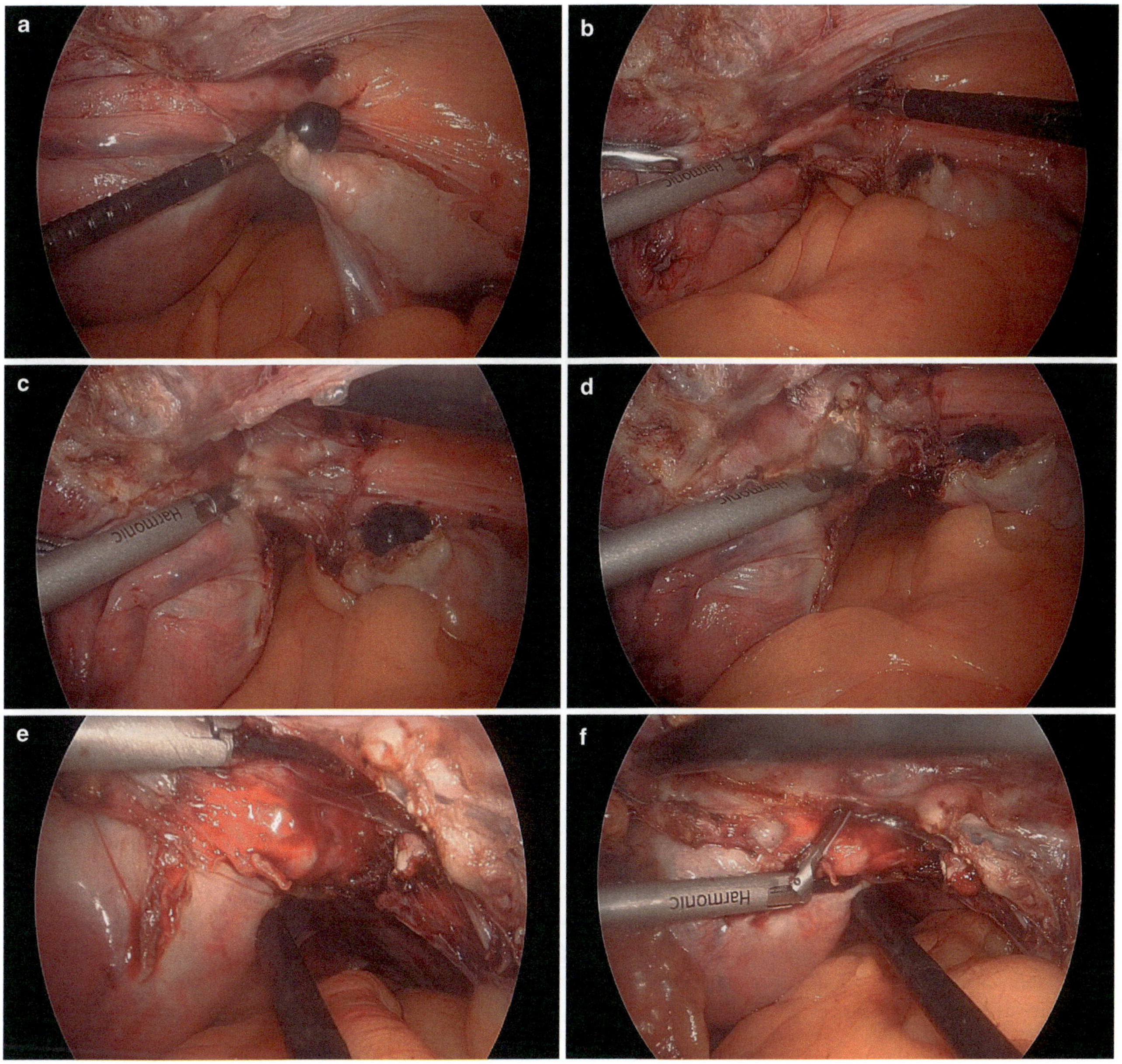

Fig. 13.15 **a** Right ovarian ligament coagulated and cut. **b** Right fallopian tube coagulated and cut. (**c**) Right round ligament coagulated and cut. **d** Incision over posterior leaf of right broad ligament. **e** Right uterine artery skeletonized. **f** Right uterine artery coagulated and cut

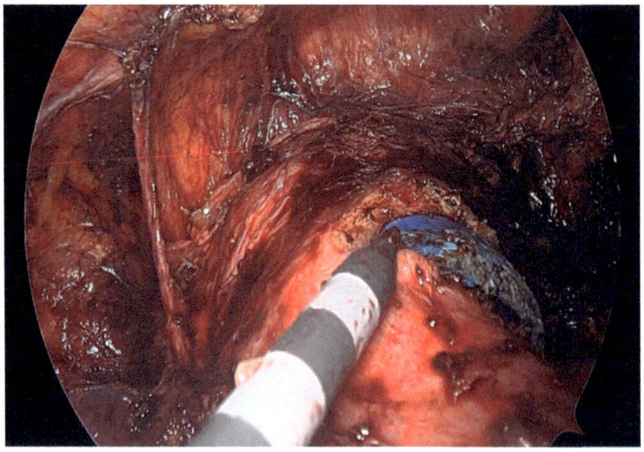

Fig. 13.16 Circumferential culdotomy done with monopolar hook

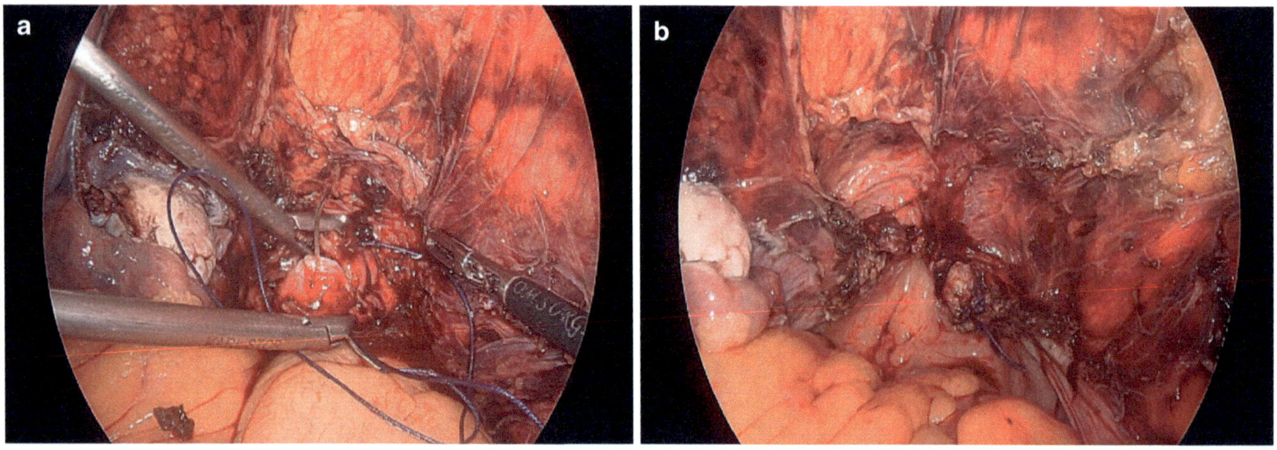

Fig. 13.17 **a** Vault closure and suspension done in double layers using polygalactin suture. **b** Final picture of pelvis showing sutured vault and retained ovaries

13.5 Postoperative Considerations

Obese patients may face a higher risk of postoperative complications, owing to risk of thrombosis and reduced oxygenation.

1. Postoperatively, expert care is diligently administered in strict adherence to Enhanced Recovery After Surgery (ERAS) protocols [34], which prioritize early ambulation. This is further facilitated by actively encouraging breathing exercises and leg movements, all aimed at enhancing positive outcomes for the patient.
2. Pain management is done with non-opioid, NSAIDS and regional anaesthesia to avoid breathing difficulty. Intensive care is offered in morbidly obese patients.
3. O_2 supplementation is done to combat hypoxemia. Aggressive pulmonary care is given in semi recumbent position.
4. Thromboprophylaxis, comprising the use of compression stockings and subcutaneous heparin, is maintained until the patient resumes spending the majority of their time out of bed.
5. Postoperative fluid is administered judiciously to prevent overload at the rate of 10–12 ml/kg/h.

Learning Points

- Interdisciplinary collaboration between gynecologists, anesthesiologists, intensivists and other specialists is crucial to optimize preoperative assessment, perioperative care, and postoperative management for obese patients undergoing laparoscopic surgery.
- Longer Veress and longer trocar is recommended to traverse the thick adipose layer.
- For primary entry port, surface marking of other non-umbilical ports is difficult, so the Jain Point is advocated for routine use due to its identification by a single prominent

bony landmark, the ASIS, which remains discernible even in cases of morbid obesity. Furthermore, it serves as the primary ergonomic working port throughout the surgery.

- Establishing standardized steps like Comprehensive Canopy Concept, 'The 3 Step Technique' for laparoscopic surgery in obese patients can improve consistency, reduce complications, and enhance outcomes.
- Post-operative early ambulation and optimal care should be provided to reduce the incidence of embolism and hypoxia.
- Weight loss should be emphasized, to further reduce their morbidity and mortality.

Competing Interest The author declares no conflict of interest that are relevant to content of this chapter.

Ethical Approval Informed consent was obtained from individual participants and patients regarding publication and documentation without disclosing their identity.

References

1. Frühbeck G, Yumuk V. Obesity: a gateway disease with a rising prevalence. Obes Facts. 2014;7(Suppl 2):33–6. https://doi.org/10.1159/000361004. PMID: 24853349; PMCID: PMC5646210.
2. McTigue KM, Garrett JM, Popkin BM. The natural history of the development of obesity in a cohort of young U.S. adults between 1981 and 1998. Ann Intern Med. 2002;136(12):857–64. https://doi.org/10.7326/0003-4819-136-12-200206180-00006. PMID: 12069559.
3. Kelly HA. Excision of the fat of the abdominal wall lipectomy. Surg Gynecol Obstet. 1910;10:229.
4. Obesity: preventing and managing the global epidemic. Report of a WHO consultation. World Health Organ Tech Rep Ser 2000;894:i–xii, 1–253. PMID: 11234459.
5. Chan JK, Gardner AB, Taylor K, Thompson CA, Blansit K, Yu X, Kapp DS. Robotic versus laparoscopic versus open surgery in morbidly obese endometrial cancer patients—a comparative analysis of total charges and complication rates. Gynecol Oncol. 2015;139(2):300–5. https://doi.org/10.1016/j.ygyno.2015.09.006. PMID: 26363212.
6. Shabanzadeh DM, Sørensen LT. Laparoscopic surgery compared with open surgery decreases surgical site infection in obese patients: a systematic review and meta-analysis. Ann Surg. 2012;256(6):934–45. https://doi.org/10.1097/SLA.0b013e318269a46b. PMID: 23108128.
7. Matory WE Jr, O'Sullivan J, Fudem G, Dunn R. Abdominal surgery in patients with severe morbid obesity. Plast Reconstr Surg. 1994;94(7):976–87.
8. Barber TM, Hanson P, Weickert MO, Franks S. Obesity and polycystic ovary syndrome: implications for pathogenesis and novel management strategies. Clin Med Insights Reprod Health 2019;13. doi: https://doi.org/10.1177/1179558119874042.
9. Barber TM, McCarthy MI, Wass JA, Franks S. Obesity and polycystic ovary syndrome. Clin Endocrinol (Oxf). 2006;65:137–45.
10. Onstad MA, Schmandt RE, Lu KH. Addressing the role of obesity in endometrial cancer risk, prevention, and treatment. J Clin Oncol. 2016;34(35):4225–30. https://doi.org/10.1200/JCO.2016.69.4638. PMID: 27903150; PMCID: PMC5455320.
11. Schmandt RE, Iglesias DA, Co NN, Lu KH. Understanding obesity and endometrial cancer risk: opportunities for prevention. Am J Obstet Gynecol 2011;205(6):518–525. doi: 10.1016/j.ajog.2011.05.042. PMID: 21802066; PMCID: PMC4264838.
12. Park CY, Kim JC, Kim DY, Kim SK. Inguinal hernia repair in overweight and obese patients. J Korean Surg Soc. 2011;81(3):205–10. https://doi.org/10.4174/jkss.2011.81.3.205. PMID: 22066122; PMCID: PMC3204546.
13. Novitsky YW, Cobb WS, Kercher KW, Matthews BD, Sing RF, Heniford BT. Laparoscopic ventral hernia repair in obese patients: a new standard of care. Arch Surg. 2006;141(1):57–61. https://doi.org/10.1001/archsurg.141.1.57.
14. Liu T, Wang W, Ji Y, Wang Y, Liu X, Cao L, Liu S. Association between different combination of measures for obesity and new-onset gallstone disease. PLoS One. 2018;13(5):e0196457. https://doi.org/10.1371/journal.pone.0196457. PMID: 29772027; PMCID: PMC5957348.
15. Brodsky JB, Lemmens HJ, Brock-Utne JG, Vierra M, Saidman LJ. Morbid obesity and tracheal intubation. Anesth Analg. 2002;94(3):732–6; table of contents. https://doi.org/10.1097/00000539-200203000-00047. PMID: 11867407.
16. Tadesse TA, Kedir HM, Fentie AM, Abiye AA. Venous thromboembolism risk and thromboprophylaxis assessment in surgical patients based on caprini risk assessment model. Risk Manag Healthc Policy. 2020;13:2545–52. https://doi.org/10.2147/RMHP.S272852. PMID: 33204195; PMCID: PMC7667181.
17. Laryea J, Champagne B. Venous thromboembolism prophylaxis. Clin Colon Rectal Surg. 2013;26(3):153–9. https://doi.org/10.1055/s-0033-1351130. PMID: 24436666; PMCID: PMC3747284.
18. Chapron CM, Pierre F, Lacroix S, Querleu D, Lansac J, Dubuisson JB. Major vascular injuries during gynecologic laparoscopy. J Am Coll Surg. 1997;185(5):461–5. PMID: 9358090.
19. Ahmad G, O'Flynn H, Duffy JM, Phillips K, Watson A. Laparoscopic entry techniques. Cochrane Database Syst Rev. 2012;(2):CD006583. https://doi.org/10.1002/14651858.CD006583.pub3. Update in: Cochrane Database Syst Rev. 2015;8:CD006583. PMID: 22336819.
20. Giannios NM, Gulani V, Rohlck K, Flyckt RL, Weil SJ, Hurd WW. Left upper quadrant laparoscopic placement: effects of insertion angle and body mass index on distance to posterior peritoneum by magnetic resonance imaging. Am J Obstet Gynecol. 2009;201(5):522.e1–5. https://doi.org/10.1016/j.ajog.2009.07.017. Epub 2009 Sep 17. PMID: 19761999; PMCID: PMC3966431.
21. Ahmad G, Baker J, Finnerty J, Phillips K, Watson A. Laparoscopic entry techniques. Cochrane Database Syst Rev. 2019; Issue 1. Art. No.: CD006583. https://doi.org/10.1002/14651858.CD006583.pub5.
22. Audebert AJ, Gomel V. Role of microlaparoscopy in the diagnosis of peritoneal and visceral adhesions and in the prevention of bowel injury associated with blind trocar insertion. Fertil Steril. 2000;73(3):631–5. https://doi.org/10.1016/s0015-0282(99)00555-5.
23. Royal College of Obstetricians and Gynaecologists. Green-top guideline No. 49. Preventing entry-related gynaecological laparoscopic injuries. London: RCOG; 2008.
24. Sharp HT. Overview of gynecologic laparoscopic surgery and non-umbilical entry sites. In: Falcone T, editor, UpToDate. 2019. p. 10.
25. Jain N, Sareen S, Kanawa S, Jain V, Gupta S, Mann S. Jain point: a new safe portal for laparoscopic entry in previous surgery cases. J Hum Reprod Sci. 2016;9(1):9–17. https://doi.org/10.4103/0974-1208.178637.
26. Hasson HM. Open laparoscopy as a method of access in laparoscopic surgery. Gynecol Endosc. 1999;8:353–62. https://doi.org/10.1046/j.1365-2508.1999.00316.x.

27. Magos A, Frappell J. Laparoscopic entry after previous surgery. Obstet Gynecol. 2013;15:68–9. https://doi.org/10.1111/j.1744-4667.2012.00146_1.x.
28. Palmer R. Safety in laparoscopy. J Reprod Med. 1974;13(1):1–5. PMID: 4276707
29. Womack AS, Mourad J. Liver laceration with Palmer's point entry in the super obese patient. J Minim Invasive Gynecol. 2020;27(7, Supplement):S58. https://doi.org/10.1016/j.jmig.2020.08.413.
30. McIntosh PG, Andrew CG, Needle insufflation into the liver as a cause of massive gas embolus and CVA, J Surg Case Rep, 2021, Issue 10, 2021, rjab448, https://doi.org/10.1093/jscr/rjab448.
31. Jain N, Jain V, Chandi A, Srivastava S, Singh S, Vasundhara N. Jain point: an alternate laparoscopic non-umbilical first blind entry port to avoid vessel, viscera, adhesions and bowel (VVAB). Updates Surg. 2021;73(6):2321–9. https://doi.org/10.1007/s13304-021-01099-z. Epub 2021 Jun 13. PMID: 34121164; PMCID: PMC8606393.
32. Jain N, Srivastava S, Bayya SLP, Jain V. Jain point laparoscopic entry in contraindications of Palmer's point. Front Surg. 2022;9:928081. https://doi.org/10.3389/fsurg.2022.928081.
33. Reis JP, MacEra CA, Araneta MR, Lindsay SP, Marshall SJ, Wingard DL. Comparison of overall obesity and body fat distribution in predicting risk of mortality. Obesity. 2009;17(6):1232–9.
34. Melnyk M, Casey RG, Black P, Koupparis AJ. Enhanced recovery after surgery (ERAS) protocols: time to change practice? Can Urol Assoc J. 2011;5(5):342–8. https://doi.org/10.5489/cuaj.11002. PMID: 22031616; PMCID: PMC3202008.

14 Total Laparoscopic Hysterectomy (TLH) with Hernia Repair

Siddharth Gupta, Sunil Gupta, and Nutan Jain

14.1 Introduction

Combining TLH with Laparoscopic ventral hernia mesh repair has gained wide acceptance due to its benefits of shorter hospital stay, simultaneous recovery, from both procedures, and improved patient outcome, and. Combining procedures at different quadrants of the abdomen provides an additional advantage. In this chapter, we will discuss the safety aspects of integrating laparoscopic intraperitoneal onlay mesh (IPOM) repair with laparoscopic hysterectomy, which is a clean contaminated surgery.

Surgical wounds are characterized into clean, clean contaminated, contaminated and infected. Clean-contaminated surgeries involve procedures in which there is an incision made into the respiratory, alimentary, or genitourinary tract. These surgeries occur under controlled conditions but are subject to potential contamination during the operation.

In clinical practice, the decision to undertake hernia repair along with TLH depends on various factors, including the size of the hernia, the patient's overall health status, and the inherent risks and benefits of the combined procedure.

Additionally, we have to take several steps from preoperative period to stave off infection in combining TLH with mesh repair, a procedure already known for complications of mesh infection.

14.2 Hernia

A hernia is bulging of part of the contents of abdominal cavity through a weakness in abdominal wall. Hernia of the anterior abdominal wall (ventral hernia) represents noninguinal nonhiatal defect in the parietal abdominal wall fascia and muscle through which intraabdominal or preperitoneal contents can protude [1]. These defects can be spontaneous or acquired (Fig. 14.1).

Ventral hernia is on rising trend with increase in obesity, with approximately 30% of patients having a BMI greater than 35 [2]. In the majority of cases, acquired hernias typically occur after surgical incisions and are therefore termed incisional hernias. In the postoperative setting, patients face approximately a 10% risk of developing a hernia following a midline laparotomy, a 5% risk after a transverse muscle splitting incision, and less than 1% risk following a laparoscopic procedure [3, 4].

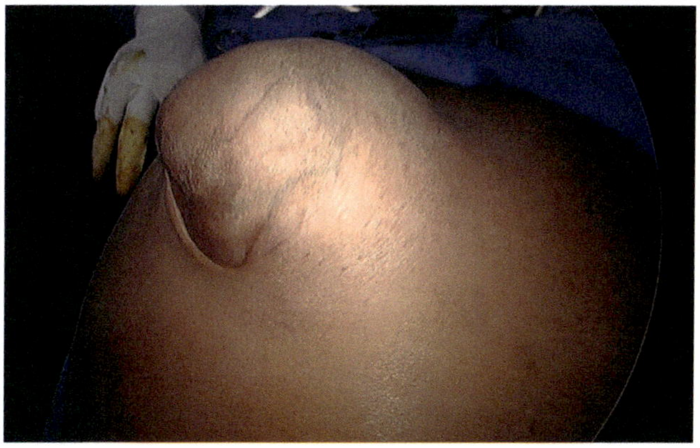

Fig. 14.1 Large Hernia seen after creating Pneumoperitoneum

S. Gupta (✉)
Advanced Laparoscopy and Robotics, GEM Hospital Coimbatore, Coimbatore, Tamil Nadu, India

S. Gupta
Jyoti Nursing Home, Muzaffarnagar, Uttar Pradesh, India

N. Jain
Obstetrics and Gynaecology, GSVM Medical College, Affiliated by Kanpur University, Kanpur, Uttar Pradesh, India

Department of Obstetrics and Gynecology, Vardhman Trauma and Laparoscopy Centre Pvt. Ltd., Muzaffarnagar, Uttar Pradesh, India

N. Jain (ed.), *Complex Total Laparoscopic Hysterectomy (TLH) with Newer Approaches in Bladder Dissection*,
https://doi.org/10.1007/978-981-97-3226-5_14

14.3 Anatomy of Anterior Abdominal Wall

Lateral musculature consists of three layers, with the fascicles of each layer directed obliquely at different angles, collectively forming a strong envelope for the abdominal contents. Each of these muscles gives rise to an aponeurosis that inserts into the linea alba, a midline structure that connects both sides of the abdominal wall. External oblique, the most superficial muscle of lateral abdominal wall, features fibers coursing in an inferomedial direction. The deepest layer is comprised of the transversus abdominis muscle, which courses horizontally. These three lateral muscles contribute aponeurotic layers lateral to the rectus muscle, forming both the anterior and posterior rectus sheath.

External oblique and internal oblique aponeurosis medially forms anterior layer of rectus sheath. At midline two anterior rectus sheath forms linea alba. On both sides of linea alba lie rectus abdominis muscle directed longitudinally along the length of anterior abdominal wall.

Interior oblique and transversus abdominis aponeurosis passes posterior to rectus muscle to form posterior rectus sheath, which also contributes to the linea alba.

Arcuate line an important landmark in anterior abdominal wall, located 3–6 cm below the umbilicus. It is the point below which posterior rectus sheath is absent and rectus abdominis muscles are fused with transversalis fascia.

Nerves (intercostal 7–12 and L1, L2) traverse through lateral abdominal wall between tansversus abdominis and internal oblique to innervate lateral abdominal muscles, rectus muscle and overlying skin (Fig. 14.2).

Lower three or four intercostal arteries, deep circumflex iliac artery and lumbar arteries supply lateral muscles. Rectus abdominis receives its blood from Superior, inferior epigastric artery and lower intercostal arteries.

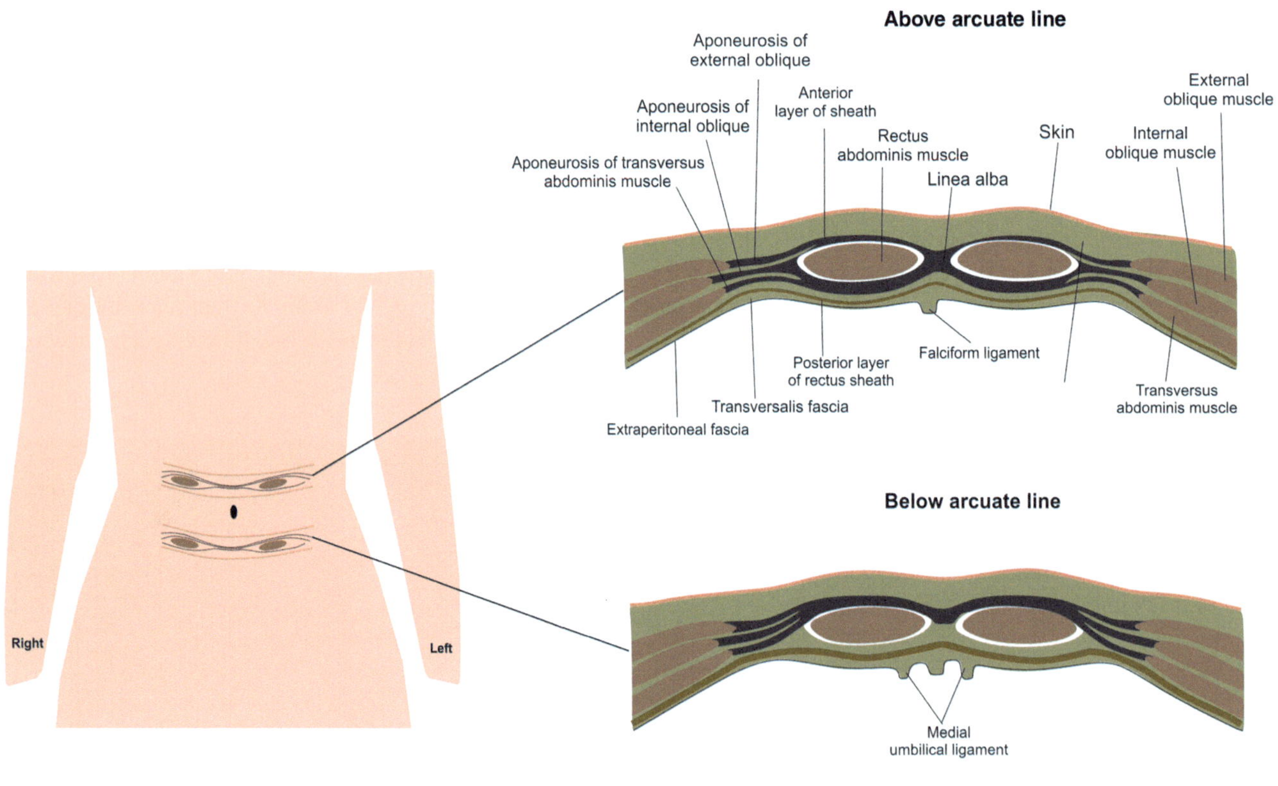

Fig. 14.2 Anatomy of anterior abdominal wall

14.4 Causes of Ventral Hernia

Despite of complex design of the abdominal wall, the primary cause is weakness of abdominal wall which leads to ventral hernia. Common causes are

- Weaknesses can develop in the abdominal wall due to structures entering and exiting the abdomen, potentially resulting in umbilical or epigastric hernias.
- Developmental failure to close the umbilicus.
- Sharp trauma e.g. surgical scar, stabbing lead to incisional hernia
- Weakness due to ageing and pregnancy
- Excessive intrabdominal pressure e.g. Obesity, pregnancy, ascites, constipation Childbirth chronic coughing etc. lead to microscopic tears of tissue which gradually diminishing its strength over time and ultimately resulting in the formation of a hernia.
- Various contributory factors can increase the risk of hernia formation, including obesity, wound infection, defects in primary wound healing, multiple prior procedures, previous incisional hernias, technical errors during repair, the nutritional status of the patient, anemia, hypoproteinemia, diabetes, immunosuppression, and smoking [5].

14.5 Classification

Umbilical hernia: occurs at umbilical ring present either at birth or develop gradually during lifetime. Congenital one usually closes spontaneously by 2 years of age. Acquired one is common in ladies.

Epigastric hernia: occurs from xyphoid process to the umbilicus. Causes pain out of proportion due to incarceration of peritoneal fat.

Hypogastric hernia: that occurs below the umbilicus in the midline.

Incisional hernia: 80% of ventral hernia. 10–20% incidence after laparotomy.

14.6 Concomitant TLH with Hernia Repair

A recent study conducted by Raj PP et al. has proposed the safety of combining clean-contaminated surgeries with mesh repair, encouraging surgeons to undertake such procedures without causing additional morbidity. Combining hernia repair with other laparoscopic surgeries not only eliminates the risk of subjecting the patient to anesthesia twice but also reduces hospital stays and associated costs. Furthermore, it diminishes the likelihood of hernia-related complications arising during the interval period [6].

It has been observed that mean operating time for combined laparoscopic IPOM with hysterectomy was 224 min (range, 196–285 min) which can be reduced with use of modern gadgets like vessels sealer and HARMONIC ACE™ (Ethicon Johnson & Johnson Surgical, USA), better imaging system and better experience of surgeons carrying out these extensive surgeries.

When two procedures are taken together it is not that time spent will be twice as for one individual procedure, in the pre-operative planning the surgeons and the gynecologist sit together, examine the patient and see all the pelvic findings and the size and site of hernia, according to both the pathologies, the team agrees to common surgical plan to cut short the time spent in port placement and planning the sequence of surgery.

At the end, clearing up of the pelvis, and suction irrigation is done as a common step for both procedures hence we can justify that the time taken for one TLH and fixing up the mesh (which is done by absorbable tacker) rather than getting doubled remains the same.

Simultaneous laparoscopic intraperitoneal onlay mesh (IPOM) procedures can be conducted alongside clean-contaminated surgeries with acceptable morbidity rates. The infectious complications associated with combined procedures do not significantly differ from those observed with IPOM performed alone. Moreover, combining certain selected clean-contaminated surgeries does not adversely affect the outcome of the procedure. However, it is advisable to undertake such combined procedures only after acquiring adequate experience in the treatment of laparoscopic ventral hernia repairs.

14.7 Advantages of Combined Procedure [6, 7]

The decision to combine TLH and hernia repair is based on several factors like patient's BMI and associated medical comorbidities, and size and location of hernia.

Combined procedure leads to early recovery, and it becomes cost effective for both healthcare system and patient thus reducing the overall medical cost for separate surgery.

Patients are exposed to anesthesia only once, which can be beneficial. The risks associated with undergoing multiple surgeries, such as infection and complications from anesthesia, are further reduced when procedures are combined. Usage of same laparoscopic ports also gives an added benefit to patient. Patient's mental and physical stress also gets centered around one single setting of surgery and recovery.

14.8 Pre-operative Care

It is also important to select patient properly before planning a combined procedure,

Preoperative care for patients undergoing combined laparoscopic hysterectomy and hernia repair is crucial for ensuring patient safety and optimizing surgical outcomes. It includes:

(a) Pelvic pathology -all necessary blood test for associated co morbidities and imaging using ultrasonography and MRI are done to asses targeted pelvic pathology, vaginal swab and PAP smear testing is done
(b) Hernia—CT scan to asses size and content of hernia is done
(c) General -BMI is evaluated and all necessary preoperative tests are done for medical and anesthesia fitness including cardiovascular evaluation.

Preparation of vagina—vagina is prepared 1–2 weeks prior to surgery. Any cervical or vaginal infections should be noted and treated before the patient is taken for surgery. A normal pap smear is also checked for any pathology.

Preoperative examination of patient is done to see any signs of infections, and in case of any positive signs we defer the surgery for a week, and give her targeted antibiotic according to culture and sensitivity and patient is taken up for surgery when there is no vaginal infection.

On admission—preoperative broad spectrum antibiotic protocol is started for gram negative anaerobic coverage in form of third generation cephalosporin, amikacin and metronidazole are given and bowel Preparation is done using polyethylene glycol.

Preoperatively vaginal douching and packing of vagina is done and betadine pessaries are given.

In operation theatre—Betadine douching is done again to prevent the chances of any infection. Since TLH is a clean contaminated surgery, we take all efforts so that the mesh should not get in contact with any of the instruments used in surgery, In our set up we use a separate trolley over which, on sterile surface the mesh is opened up with pre tied sutures and the mesh is rolled over and directly delivered into peritoneal cavity via grasper from the 10 mm optical port by withdrawing the 10 mm telescope so that the mesh doesn't come in contact with any of used instruments.

All these efforts have borne fruit and we have been routinely combining these two procedures at our set up without any postoperative complications.

14.9 Repair Methods

Primary repair/closure can be done when defect size is small i.e. <2 cm and viable surrounding tissue is there. High Recurrence rate of 43% is seen after 3 years of primary closure. Recurrence rate after open tissue repair is 18–20% while with open mesh repair is 13–15% [8].

The component separation technique involves the creation of large subcutaneous flaps lateral to the fascial defect, followed by incisions of the external oblique muscle and, if necessary, the posterior rectus sheath bilaterally to facilitate primary closure under reduced tension. However, studies report a high wound infection risk of 20% and a recurrence rate of 18% at 1 year following this repair. Despite these challenges, this technique is frequently employed in settings with contaminated or potentially contaminated surgical fields [9].

For hernia defect >2 cm tension free mesh repair is the gold standard management. Recurrence rate reduces by 50% with the use of prosthetic mesh.

Mesh can be placed as an-

- Underlay deep to fascial defect (intraperitoneal or preperitoneal).
- Interlay between defect edges or within abdominal wall musculoaponeurotic layers(intraparietal)
- Onlay superficial to the fascial defect
- Open mesh hernia repair has recurrence rate of over 20% using underlay technique and 8% using onlay technique [10, 11].

In hernia repair we use absorbable tack to fix the mesh using AbsorbaTack™ which is a 5 mm fixation device containing 30 violet absorbable tacks. The tack used here is made of an absorbable synthetic polyester copolymer derived from lactic and glycolic acid. Its absorption profile in first 2 weeks is minimal; significant absorption rate is seen in the period from 3 to 5 months, following this significant breakdown the polymer absorption is essentially completed prior to 1 year. Due to this, absorbable tackers result in a significant decrease in post-operative pain, compared to titanium non absorbable tackers which cause chronic pain and hence decreased patient compliance.

Laparoscopic hernia repair was first described by LeBlanc and Booth in 1993 [12]. The utilization of laparoscopic techniques is statistically linked to fewer wound complications and a lower recurrence rate, reported at 3.4% [13]. with a quicker return to normal activities with less pain, short hospital stay, etc. as with any other laparoscopy procedure. In addition to above, laparoscopic repair offers the advantage of visualizing the entire undersurface of the abdominal wall, often uncovering multiple secondary defects that might not be otherwise detected.

14.10 Types of Meshes Used in Incisional Hernia

Table 14.1

Table 14.1 Meshes used intraperitoneally for the repair of Ventral and Incisional hernias

Group/mesh	Material	Company
ePTFE		
Dulex Dual mesh	ePTFE ePTFE	Bard Davol, Inc., Warwick, RI W. L. Gore
Composite mesh with absorbable coated barrier		
Proceed Parietene Parietex Composite Symbotex Physiomesh	PP with ORC layer PP with collagen coated Polyester with collagen coated Polyester with collagen film PP with polyglecaprone 25	Ethicon, Somerville, NJ Covidien, Mansfield, MA Covidien Covidien Ethicon
Composite mesh with permanent coated barrier		
Composix Ventrio	PP/ePTFE PP/ePTFE	Bard Davol, Inc. Bard Davol, Inc.

ePTFE expanded polytetrafluoroethylene, *PP* polypropylene, *ORC* oxidized regenerated cellulose

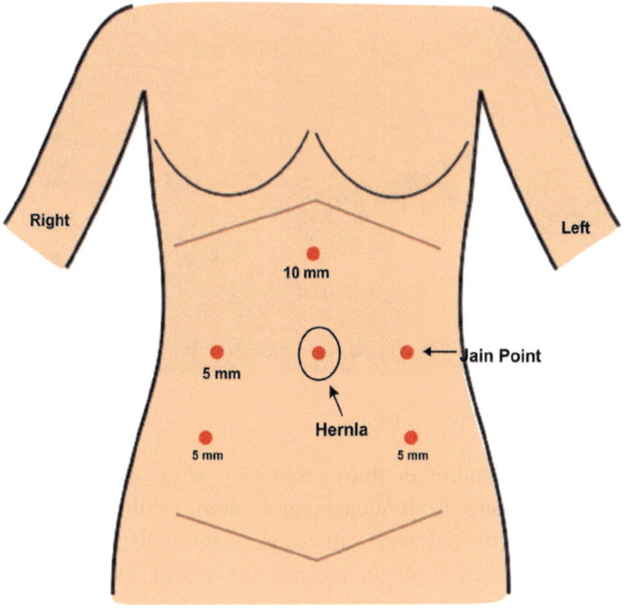

Fig. 14.3 Port position in combined procedure

14.11 Intraperitoneal Mesh Repair with Primary Closure of the Defect (IPOM Plus)

This repair is performed to mitigate postoperative bulging and seroma formation. According to Laplace's law, a central nonfunctional portion of the abdominal wall behaves like a sail in the wind, rendering it susceptible to bulging. Advantage of primary closure of defect under physiologic tension restores abdominal wall function [14, 15]. This can only be done for defects upto 5 cm, which can be approximated without any tension.

The combined procedure of TLH with mesh hernia repair involves these steps

- We have an obese patient, weight—100 kg, BMI- 40 kg/m^2 and previous three caesarian section with history of premature rupture uterus with bladder injury, now presented with very large cervical fibroid of about 12 cm and the uterus sitting on top like a lantern top and concomitant incisional hernia. The case was a nightmare due to obesity, large incisional hernia, 3 caesarean, previous bladder injury, a large cervical myoma.
- *Position:* The patient is positioned on the operating table in a dorsal lithotomy position, which allows access to the pelvic and abdominal areas.
- *Anesthesia*: patient is placed under general anesthesia
- *Pneumoperitoneum:* created using long Veress needle introduced through Jain point [16],so that it is able to stay away from midline adhesions and also much lateral to make a feasible working port to apply mesh comfortably
- *Optical entry and working ports:* The patient is reviewed by both surgeon and gynecologist and they decide about entry points as per findings of the patient.
- Since we have been working together as team, we find paraumbilical far lateral port the jain point, works well as 5 mm blind entry port in combined procedure as well as in cases with history of previous surgery
- First the entry point is made by Veress needle and 5 mm telescope is placed through Jain point and then a 10 mm port with 30 degree scope is introduced and both surgeons and gynecologist take a stock of situation about the adhesions and pelvic findings and the hernia defect. Rest of the optical and working ports are placed accordingly as shown in Fig. 14.3. In laparoscopic repair of ventral hernia ports needs to be placed at least 10 cm lateral to the midline defect [17]. For lateral defects contralateral ports should be placed.
- *Delineation of defect:* contents of the hernia sac are reduced using traction and counter traction along with ultrasonic energy to facilitate the visualization of abdomen and pelvis and to proceed for hysterectomy (Fig. 14.4).
- Before proceeding for TLH we close the hernial defect by robust suturing with V- loc™ sutures in two layers, the suturing begins 1 cm distal to the edge of hernial defect, to ensures no contamination from hernial defect. This becomes the first step of IPOM plus
- Laparoscopic Hysterectomy is done first by the Gynecological team.
- Our *steps of TLH* are same as described in comprehensive canopy concept- 'The 3 Step Technique' chapter. Extreme adhesions are noted all around due to previous antenatal

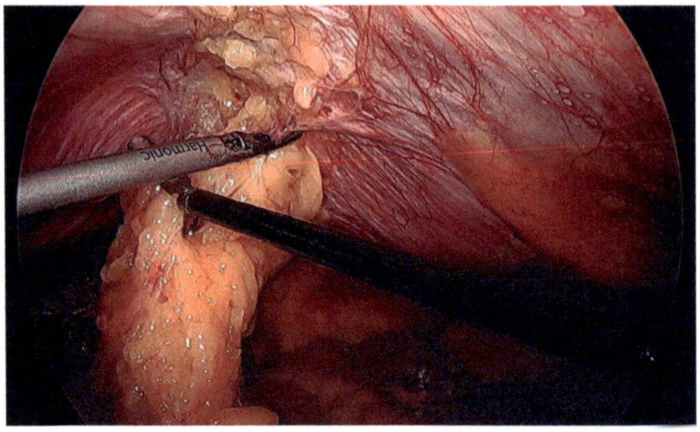

Fig. 14.4 Reducing the hernia

uterine rupture in third pregnancy with bladder injury repair done. Both adenexa and anterior cul-de-sac were totally covered with adhesions. After performing adequate adhesiolysis in the anterior cul-de-sac and both adenexa, we started the TLH from right side which was relatively free. We started with the adenexa, right round ligament is coagulated and divided.

1. **Step 1: Posterior approach of uterine artery ligation**—The posterior leaf of broad ligament was opened up widely upto the arcus taurinus. This helps in easy skelotonization of the uterine artery pedicle which is coagulated and cut. We do this step entirely before any dissection of the bladder.
2. **Step 2: Canopy concept of bladder dissection**—We proceed with dissection from the side of cut uterine artery pedicle to expose the shiny glistening pubocervical fascia, by persisting in dissection of immediate 1–2 cm area anterior to uterine artery cut stump. With a combined movement of cephalad push of the uterine manipulator cup and correct plane of cleavage, the cotton candy utero vesical space opens up. We may need to put a surgical bougie to identify the limits of bladder in tough cases like this. Since the bladder adherence on the uterine corpus is not tampered so it creates a bladder canopy stretched up over the cotton candy space. We navigate beneath the canopy using the underpass of the cotton candy uterovesical space.
3. **Step 3: Anterior approach of uterine artery ligation**—Dissection continues till we reach the contralateral round ligament. This helps in exposure of the contralateral uterine artery by the anterior approach. In cases with dense adhesions, once the dissection of pubo-vesico-cervical fascia is completed and bladder fully pushed down, we move over to the left side, where more adhesiolysis had to be performed before starting the adnexal removal (Fig. 14.5a–r).

- The *uterine artery* is ligated in a manner that the stump remains below the manipulator cup. A circumferential culdotomy is performed with monopolar hook. The uterus and cervical myoma removed by vaginal morcellation. Vault suspension and meticulous double layer vault closure is done using vicryl 1–0 incorporating the utero sacral ligaments and involving endo pelvic fascia namely recto-vaginal fascia posteriorly and pubo-vesical fascia anteriorly.
- A *check cystoscopy* is done at the end to re-confirm ureteric peristalsis by visualizing ureteric spurt, which are made more conspicuous by giving pyridium tablets to the patient a night before. This simple endeavor of staining the urine orange by Pyridium becomes handy in difficult and prolonged cases.
- *After vaginal closure* and thorough suction irrigation and lavage, the case is handed over to surgical colleague for placing the mesh and suturing the hernial defect.
- Once the area encompassing all fascial defects is defined, the defect is closed intracorporeally using VLoc™ 1 number or ETHIBOND EXCEL™ Suture number 1 in a way that there is no tension using ipsilateral ports of left side.
- *Mesh size* to be used is determined by the size of defect plus 5 cm overlap all around the defect edge of the defect circumferentially.
- Composite mesh is introduced via 10 mm epigastric port and is fashioned to allow atleast 5 cm overlap under the healthy abdominal wall.
- Mesh is anchored to the abdominal wall via 4 transfacial sutures preplaced on mesh before inserting into abdominal cavity
- Mesh is secured with absorbable spiral tacks placed circumferentially at 1 cm margin of mesh to prevent bowel from incarceration between mesh and abdominal wall (Fig. 14.6a–j)
- The patient received pre-operative and post-operative antibiotics, DVT prophylaxis and very active ambulatory and breathing exercise protocol in the post-operative phase.

Limitations of IPOM

- Loss of domain: large hernia sac > 30% abdominal contents, reduction will cause abdominal hypertension
- Incarcerated hernia
- Active enterocutaneous fistula
- Large abdominal defects

TIPS

- Use principles of Traction and Counter traction while reducing the contents.
- Ask Assistant to press the content not skin over defect
- Minimal use of energy source for adhesiolysis (scissors > harmonic > bipolar > monopolar)
- Avoid extra adhesiolysis. Do not remove adhesions where mesh is not going to stick the abdominal wall.
- Beware of bowel behind every omentum and adhesion near the defect.

- In case of bleeding fix it then and there
- Remain close to the anterior abdominal wall
- Take small bites to avoid inadvertent injury to bowel.
- Structures such as the falciform ligament and ligamentum teres hepatis are dissected, and the prevesical space is opened to facilitate sufficient fixation and integration of the mesh.
- Preoperative CT scan is valuable to diagnose occult hernias, multiple defects, hematoma, incarcerated hernia, abdominal wall neoplasm.

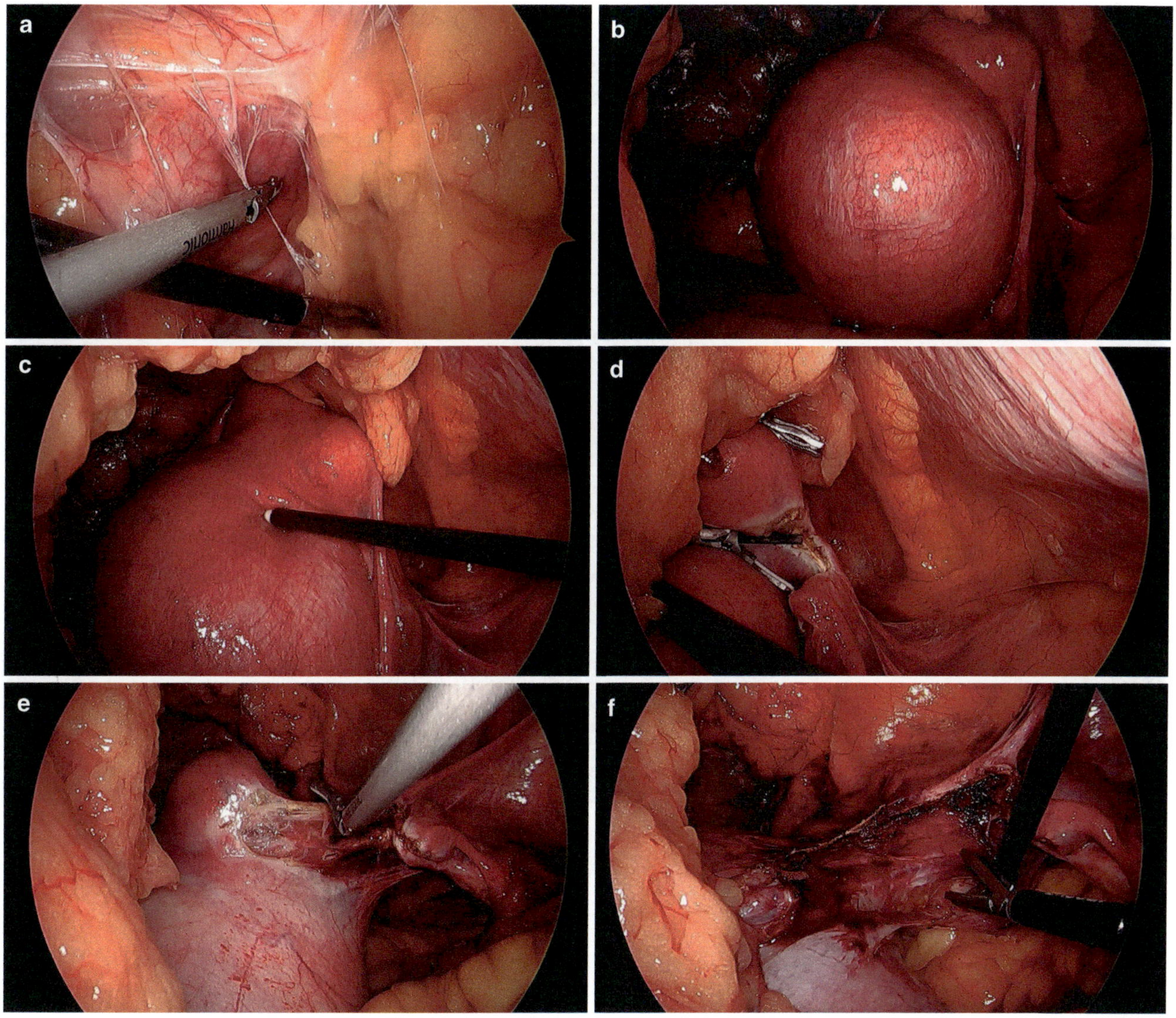

Fig. 14.5 **a** Extensive adhesions in anterior cul de sac in a case of previous 3 caesarean section. **b** Huge cervical myoma with lantern top uterus. **c** Dilute vasopressin injection. **d** Right side adnexa being coagulated and cut. **e** Round ligament transected. **f** Opening posterior leaf of broad ligament. **g** Exposed posterior leaf of broad ligament. **h** Coagulating right uterine artery. **i** Boogie placed in bladder to delineate after right uterine artery coagulated and cut. **j** Dissection in 1 cm area immediately anterior and medial to uterine artery stump exposes the pubo-vesical cervical fascia. **k** Bladder dissected down after sectioning uterine artery. **l** Bladder completely pushed down over the manipulator cup. **m** Tackling the left adnexa. **n** Left uterine artery cut pedicle is visualized. **o** Colpotomy in progress. **p** Vault suspension, right angle suture initiated. **q** Securing the right angle. **r** Completed vault closure

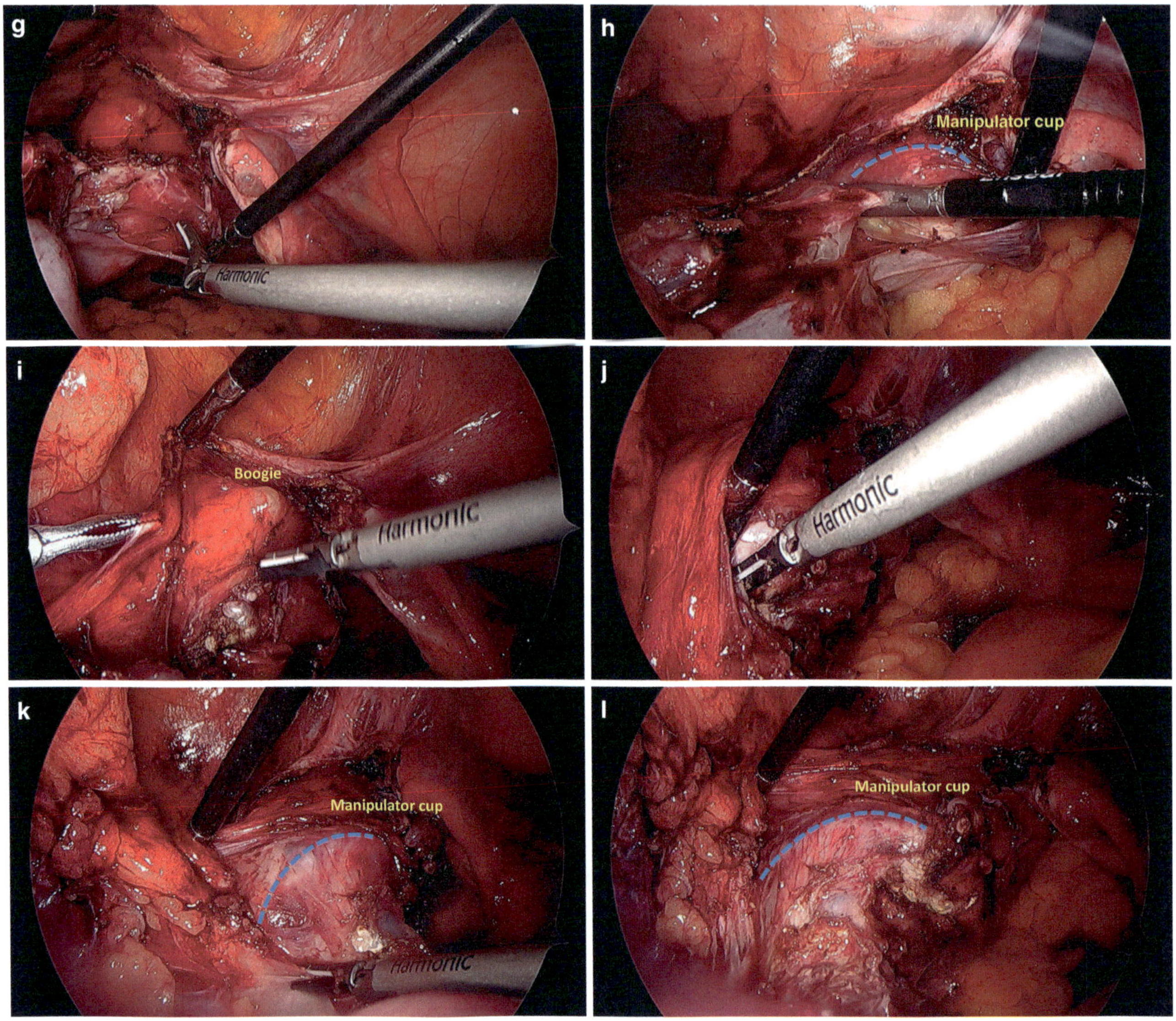

Fig. 14.5 (continued)

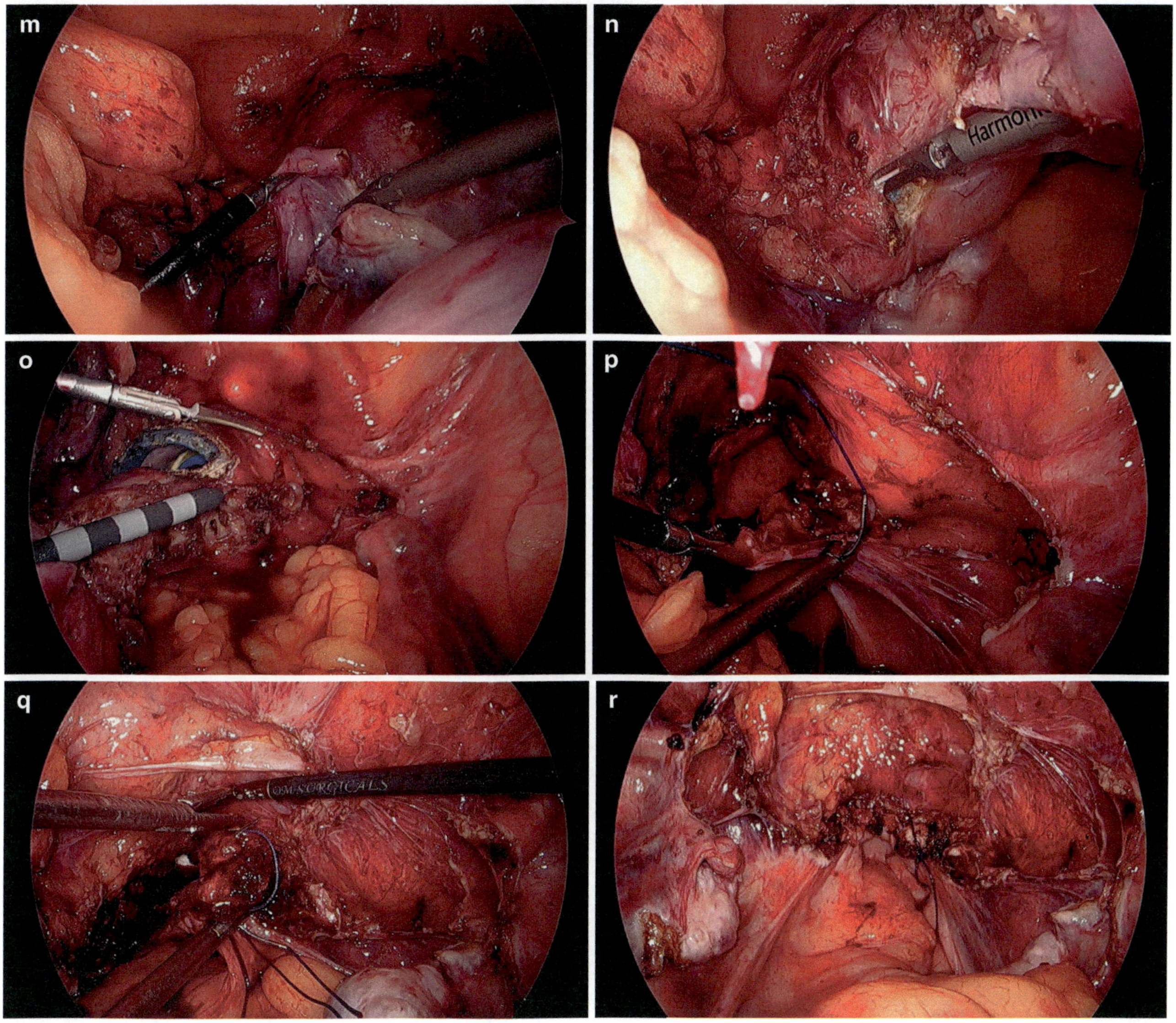

Fig. 14.5 (continued)

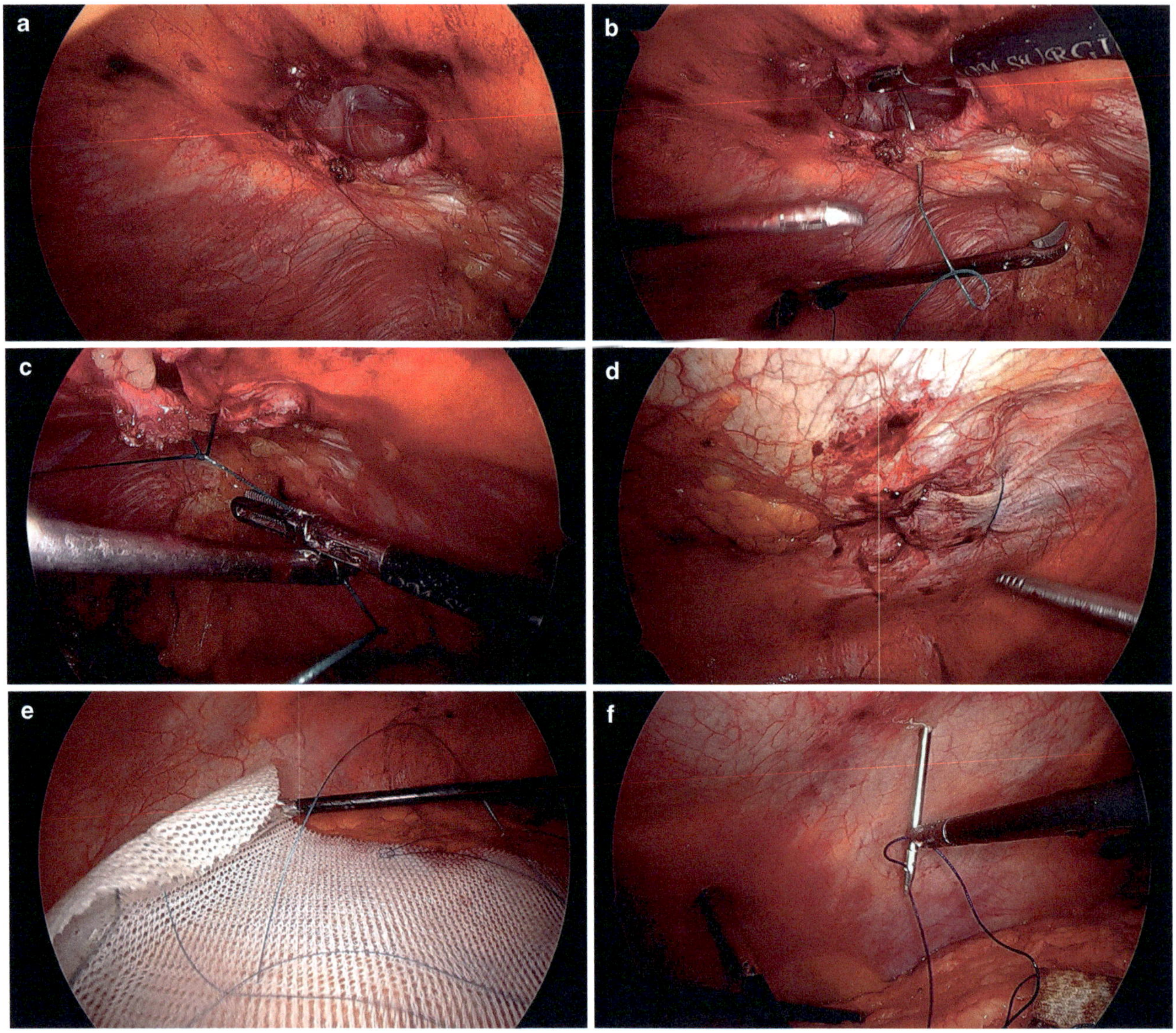

Fig. 14.6 **a** Big hernia defect seen. **b** Hernia defect being closed with ETHIBOND EXCEL™ Suture number. **c** Tying the first knot. **d** Closed hernial Defect. **e** Spreading rolled out mesh. **f** Prefixed suture being held. **g** Mesh anchored with transfascial suture. **h** Spiral tacks being tacked. **i** Mesh anchored with spiral tacks. **j** Final view with mesh placement

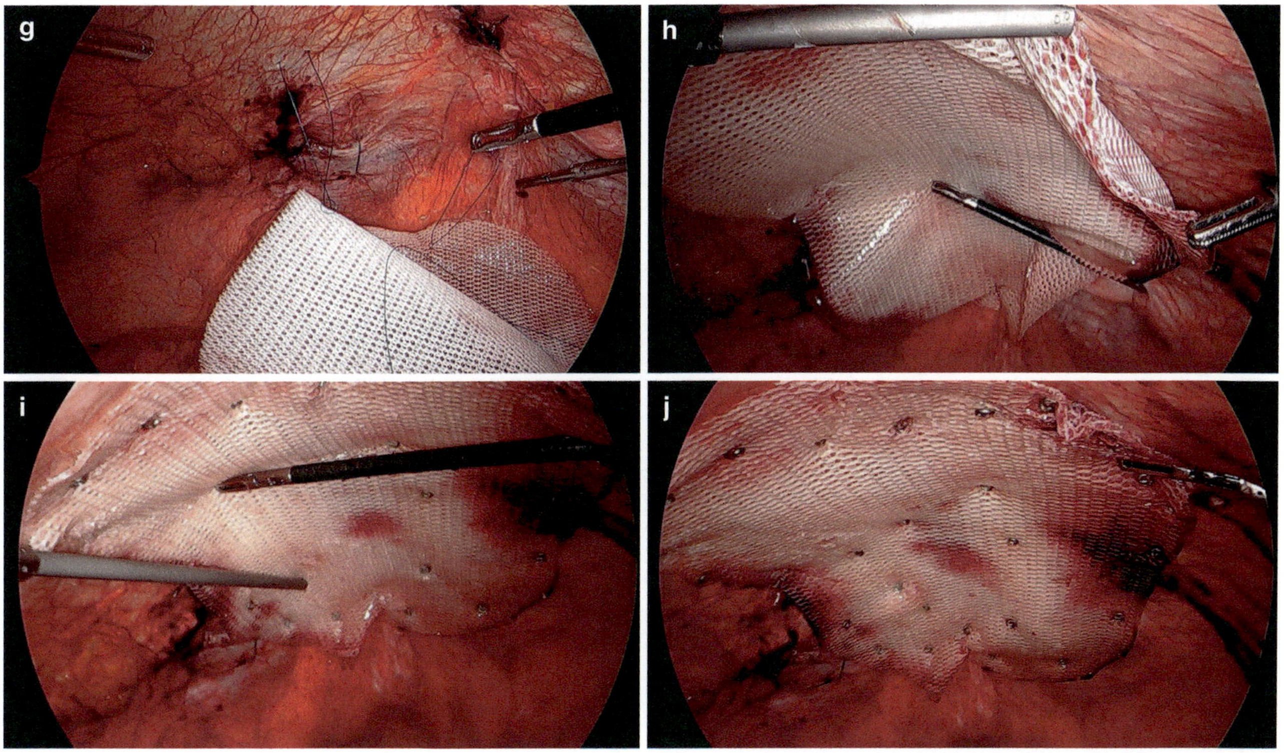

Fig. 14.6 (continued)

14.12 Conclusion

In conclusion, it can be affirmed that laparoscopic intraperitoneal onlay mesh (IPOM) repair can be safely conducted concurrently with clean-contaminated surgery, yielding acceptable morbidity rates. Combining these procedures does not adversely affect the outcomes, provided that they are performed with sufficient expertise and experience.

Patient can undergo recovery for two procedures concurrently, requiring only one period of absence from work. It effectively minimizes both physical and mental stress. For a successful concomitant surgery proper preoperative planning, precautions taken during the procedures and the collaborative efforts of both teams are important.

Learning Points

- Combined TLH and hernia repair is a modern approach in minimally invasive surgery (MIS).
- Ventral hernia is classified as umbilical, epigastric, hypogastric and incisional hernia
- Time in combined procedure is not doubled rather it gets balanced with few steps being same in both procedures like—common entry ports, initial adhesiolysis for reducing contents, suction irrigation and port closure
- Decision of combined IPOM is based on patient's BMI, associated comorbidities, size and location of hernia
- Proper preoperative assessment for pelvic pathology, site and location of hernia with proper preparation of vagina to decrease contamination is important
- The use of prosthetic mesh in tension-free repair significantly reduces recurrence rates, making it a gold standard in hernia management..
- Instead of titanium tackers, absorbable tackers are used nowadays for hernia repair as it causes less postoperative pain and better patient compliance.
- Close cooperation between the gynecologist and surgical team along with anesthesiologist is required for successful outcomes of combined surgery.

Competing Interest The author declares no conflicts of interest that are relevant to content of this chapter.

Ethical Approval Informed consent was obtained from individual participants and patients regarding publication and documentation without disclosing their identity.

References

1. Korenkov M, Paul A, Sauerland S, Neugebauer E, Arndt M, Chevrel JP, et al. Classification and surgical treatment of incisional hernia. Results of an experts' meeting. Langenbeck's Arch Surg. 2001;386:65–73.

2. Dietz UA, Kudsi OY, Gokcal F, Bou-Ayash N, Pfefferkorn U, Rudofsky G, Baur J, Wiegering A. Excess body weight and abdominal hernia. Visc Med. 2021;37(4):246–53. https://doi.org/10.1159/000516047. Epub 2021 Apr 28. PMID: 34540939; PMCID: PMC8406351.
3. Cherla DV, Poulose B, Prabhu AS. Epidemiology and disparities in care: the impact of socioeconomic status, gender, and race on the presentation, management, and outcomes of patients undergoing ventral hernia repair. Surg Clin North Am. 2018;98(3):431–40. https://doi.org/10.1016/j.suc.2018.02.003. Epub 2018 Mar 21. PMID: 29754613.
4. Zavlin D, Jubbal KT, Van Eps JL, Bass BL, Ellsworth WA 4th, Echo A, Friedman JD, Dunkin BJ. Safety of open ventral hernia repair in high-risk patients with metabolic syndrome: a multi-institutional analysis of 39,118 cases. Surg Obes Relat Dis. 2018;14(2):206–13. https://doi.org/10.1016/j.soard.2017.09.521. Epub 2017 Sep 22. PMID: 29122528.
5. Sorensen LT, Hemmingsen U, Kallehave F, Wille-Jorgensen P, Kjaergaard J, Moller LN, et al. Risk factors for tissue and wound complications in gastrointestinal surgery. Ann Surg. 2005;241:654–8.
6. Raj PP, Ganesh MK, Senthilnathan P, Parthasarathi R, Rajapandian S, Palanivelu C. Concomitant laparoscopic intraperitoneal onlay mesh repair with other clean contaminated procedures—study of feasibility and safety. J Laparoendosc Adv Surg Tech. 2015;25(1):33–6. https://doi.org/10.1089/lap.2014.0001.
7. Wadhwa A, Chowbey PK, Sharma A, Khullar R, Soni V, Baijal M. Combined procedures in laparoscopic surgery. Surg Laparosc Endosc Percutan Tech. 2003;13(6):382–6. https://doi.org/10.1097/00129689-200312000-00007.
8. Smith J, Parmely JD. Ventral Hernia. [Updated 2023 Aug 8]. In: StatPearls [Internet]. Treasure Island (FL): StatPearls Publishing; 2024 Jan-. Available from: https://www.ncbi.nlm.nih.gov/books/NBK499927/
9. Sailes FC, Walls J, Guelig D, Mirzabeigi M, Long WD, Crawford A, Moore JH Jr, Copit SE, Tuma GA, Fox J. Synthetic and biological mesh in component separation: a 10-year single institution review. Ann Plast Surg. 2010;64(5):696–8. https://doi.org/10.1097/SAP.0b013e3181dc8409. PMID: 20395790.
10. Köckerling F. Onlay technique in incisional hernia repair-a systematic review. Front Surg. 2018;5:71. https://doi.org/10.3389/fsurg.2018.00071. PMID: 30538992; PMCID: PMC6277585.
11. Timmermans L, de Goede B, van Dijk SM, Kleinrensink GJ, Jeekel J, Lange JF. Meta-analysis of sublay versus onlay mesh repair in incisional hernia surgery. Am J Surg. 2014;207(6):980–8. https://doi.org/10.1016/j.amjsurg.2013.08.030. Epub 2013 Oct 26. PMID: 24315379.
12. Leblanc KA, Booth WV. Laparoscopic repair of incisional abdominal hernias using polytetrafluoroethylene: preliminary findings. Surg Laparosc Endosc. 1993;3:39–41.
13. Sánchez LJ, Piccoli M, Ferrari CG, Cocozza E, Cesari M, Maida P, Iuppa A, Pavone G, Bencini L. Laparoscopic ventral hernia repair: results of a two thousand patients prospective multicentric database. Int J Surg. 2018;51:31–8. https://doi.org/10.1016/j.ijsu.2018.01.022. Epub 2018 Feb 3. PMID: 29367031.
14. Kurmann A, Visth E, Candinas D, et al. Long term follow-up of open and laparoscopic repair of large incisional hernias. World J Surg. 2011;35:297–301.
15. Nguyen DH, Ngugen MT, Askenasy EP, Kao LS, Liang MK. Primary fascial closure with laparoscopic ventral hernia repair: systematic review. World J Surg. 2014;38:3097–104.
16. Jain N, Srivastava S, Bayya SLP, Jain V. Jain point laparoscopic entry in contraindications of Palmers point. Front Surg. 2022;9:928081. https://doi.org/10.3389/fsurg.2022.928081. PMID: 36439525; PMCID: PMC9696343.
17. Earle D, Roth JS, Saber A, Haggerty S, Bradley JF 3rd, Fanelli R, Price R, Richardson WS, Stefanidis D, SAGES Guidelines Committee. SAGES guidelines for laparoscopic ventral hernia repair. Surg Endosc. 2016;30(8):3163–83. https://doi.org/10.1007/s00464-016-5072-x. Epub 2016 Jul 12. PMID: 27405477.

Total Laparoscopic Hysterectomy (TLH) with Cholecystectomy

15

Siddharth Gupta, Sunil Gupta, and Nutan Jain

15.1 Introduction

Laparoscopic surgery, with its minimally invasive nature and advancements in anaesthesia, has revolutionized surgical interventions. This progress has paved the way for performing multiple surgeries in a single session, marking a significant shift in contemporary medical practices. Coupled with the expanding expertise in surgical techniques and a multidisciplinary approach to patient care, the integration of laparoscopic cholecystectomy with other procedures like Total Laparoscopic Hysterectomy (TLH) has become not only feasible but also highly beneficial.

The combined approach brings forth a myriad of advantages, streamlining the patient's healthcare journey.

Patients with symptomatic gall stones and even asymptomatic cases with gall stones with underlying indications for hysterectomy can be operated at same time with single admission, single surgery, single anesthesia, not to say it will ensure a one-time abstinence from work and patient's mental and physical stress of two surgeries get combined in a single simultaneous surgical endeavor. It also reduces financial burden, consistent post-operative medication, and comparable safety and efficacy when compared to individual surgeries [1]. This combination of procedures also underscores a patient-centric approach to healthcare.

Gallbladder stone disease is one of the most prevalent disorders affecting the digestive tract [2], and women, in particular, exhibit a higher susceptibility to gallstones compared to men. The incidence of gallstones is multifactorial, influenced by age, gender, diet, obesity, and pregnancy [3]. A fatty fertile flatulent female of Fifty (5 F's of gall stone disease) is more prone to develop gallstone disease. Mostly, this is the age when there are maximum indications of hysterectomy; hence getting patients of gall stones with hysterectomy indication are very common and rightfully taken up for combined surgery.

Ultrasonography is the diagnostic test of choice, being 90–95% sensitive [3].Interestingly, a significant number of patients with gallstones remain asymptomatic, often discovered incidentally during abdominal imaging for during work up for hysterectomy.

Symptomatic gallstones typically manifest when they obstruct the biliary system, especially the cystic duct. This obstruction leads to gallbladder distension after meals, resulting in biliary colic (epigastric and right upper quadrant pain associated with nausea or vomiting occurring 30–60 min after meals) [3]. Symptomatic gall stones disease may progress to complications related to the gall stones [4]. These include acute cholecystitis, choledocholithiasis with or without cholangitis, gall stone pancreatitis, cholecystocholedochal fistula, cholecystoduodenal fistula, cholecystoenteric fistula leading to gallstone ileus and gall bladder carcinoma. Once gallstones become symptomatic, patients may experience recurrent attacks of biliary pain. Approximately 30% of patients with asymptomatic gallstone disease progress to symptomatic gallstones within 20 years [5].

Certain risk factors elevate the likelihood of complications associated with gallstones. Patients with a porcelain gallbladder (characterized by a calcified wall), large stones (>2.5 cm), long bile and pancreatic ducts, and long-standing gallstones (>20 years) face an increased risk of developing gallbladder cancer [6–8]. In such cases, asymptomatic patients are recommended to undergo surgery upon diagnosis.

Cholecystectomy, stands as the definitive treatment for gallstone disease. Previously, open approaches were the pre-

S. Gupta (✉)
Advanced Laparoscopy and Robotics, GEM Hospital Coimbatore, Coimbatore, Tamil Nadu, India

S. Gupta
Jyoti Nursing Home, Muzaffarnagar, Uttar Pradesh, India

N. Jain
Obstetrics and Gynecology, GSVM Medical College, Affiliated by Kanpur University, Kanpur, Uttar Pradesh, India

Department of Obstetrics and Gynecology, Vardhman Trauma and Laparoscopy Centre Pvt. Ltd., Muzaffarnagar, Uttar Pradesh, India

N. Jain (ed.), *Complex Total Laparoscopic Hysterectomy (TLH) with Newer Approaches in Bladder Dissection*,
https://doi.org/10.1007/978-981-97-3226-5_15

ferred method, but the scenario changed with the advent of laparoscopic cholecystectomy. Dr. Erich Muhe performed the pioneering laparoscopic cholecystectomy in 1985 in Germany, marking a transformative moment in surgical history. In India, Dr. TE Udwadia replicated this achievement with the first laparoscopic cholecystectomy in 1990.

Since then, the evolution of laparoscopic techniques has been remarkable, with a multitude of procedures being performed laparoscopically. The benefits extend beyond the efficiency of the surgery itself. Shorter hospital stays, reduced postoperative pain, early ambulation, and a quicker return to work contribute to the appeal of laparoscopic surgery. Importantly, studies and clinical experience have established that laparoscopic procedures are not only safe but also equally efficacious when compared to traditional open methods.

15.2 Concomitant TLH and Cholecystectomy

Combining TLH with Laparoscopic cholecystectomy in a single sitting is not only beneficial to the patient, but also appears to be cost-effective both for the patient as well as to the MIS facility. Additionally it gives benefits of single hospital admission, single pre-operative evaluation, single time anesthesia for surgical intervention for multiple pathologies and only one-time post-operative medication. Thus, the patient has the dual benefit of receiving surgical therapy for two coexisting pathologies concurrently while experiencing substantially less perioperative pain and morbidity than would have been expected with two discrete procedures [9].

15.3 Advantages of Combined Procedure

Study done by Resutra et al. [9] evaluated the safety and efficacy of such surgeries when paired in a single sitting with laparoscopic cholecystectomy and concluded that all the combined surgical procedure were done successfully and the mean operative time of the combined surgical procedures was shorter than the total time taken if both the procedures were done separately. The mean operating time for combined procedure was 70 min (50–180 min) and the longest time was for the patient who had undergone laparoscopic cholecystectomy with laparoscopic vaginal hysterectomy (180 min).

Intraoperatively the time taken for both the procedures is not like summing up the two, for a TLH and cholecystectomy, rather the time spent in port placement and creation of pneumoperitoneum is same for both the surgeries, With a regular team of gynecologist and surgeon performing the procedure, the port for such cases becomes standardized over time. These are comfortable and ergonomic for both teams. Likewise, the time aspect at the end of both procedures of suction irrigation and port closure is also summed up. Gall bladder removal and extraction does not add significantly to the time taken for an average TLH.

Apart from the surgeon and gynecologist working as an efficient team it is of great importance to work together with the anesthesiologist and post-operative recovery team also. Good level of competence of both gynecologist and surgeon and their compatibility with the laparoscopy assistant is paramount to smooth outcomes.

In our setup we are routinely combining laparoscopic cholecystectomy, not only TLH, but with many other gynecological surgeries like ovarian and adenexal masses and patients of infertility who concomitantly present with sonography showing gall stones and are desirous of getting both procedures done simultaneously.

As long as the basic surgical principles and indications for combined procedures are adhered to, more patients with concomitant pathologies in the abdomen can enjoy the benefits of minimal access surgery and also one time anesthesia without significant addition in post-operative morbidity and hospital stay [9].

So this way by performing both procedures concurrently eliminates the need for multiple surgeries, reducing overall risk, anesthesia exposure, and recovery time.

15.3.1 Pre-operative Preparation

Preoperative care for patients undergoing combined laparoscopic hysterectomy and cholecystectomy is crucial for ensuring patient safety and optimizing surgical outcomes.

It is important to assess the patient's medical history, surgical risks, and perform a detailed physical examination to assess the patient's general health, cardiovascular and respiratory status, and abdominal/pelvic findings.

Focus on gynecological examination for hysterectomy and abdominal examination for cholecystectomy.

All thorough pre-operative lab investigations for laparoscopic cholecystectomy and laparoscopic Hysterectomy are done.

Evaluation by Ultrasonography to assess Gall bladder stones and pelvic organs to see the extent of gynecological disease is done.

Gynecological Evaluation (for Hysterectomy): including per speculum, per-vaginal examination and imaging to evaluate pelvic pathology is done. Pap Smear testing is done, and important to treat any cervical or vaginal infection.

Obtain informed consent from the patient after counseling the nuances of combined surgical procedure, potential risks, and alternatives. Usually, as there are none, most patients are willing for the opportunity of getting both procedures done with the benefits of one-time admission, single surgery and anesthesia.

Concomitant gall bladder removal does not alter the post-operative course in any way, and patient enjoys the abstinence from work one time only.

15.4 Technique of combined surgery

Anesthesia Patient is placed under general anesthesia. Additionally 2.5 mg Indocyanine green (ICG) dye is given intravenously diluted in 10 ml normal saline after induction of anesthesia [10, 11].

Position The patient is positioned on the operating table in a dorsal lithotomy position, which allows access to the pelvic and abdominal areas.

Pneumoperitoneum Creation of pneumoperitoneum is done using Veress needle introduced through Jain point. (2.5 cm medial to anterior superior iliac spine in horizontal plane and from this point vertical line drawn upward upto the level of umbilicus) [12]. Jain point is safe and ergonomic point in naive abdomen as well as in patient with previous abdominal scars.

Visualisation & Working Ports It is reviewed by both surgeon and gynecologist and they formulate a combined plan for port placement or make changes deemed necessary as per the case. After creating pneumoperitoneum by Veress needle, 5 mm incision is made at Jain point and 5 mm trocar is placed through which 5 mm telescope is placed to see the abdomen. Other working ports are made in accordance, as shown in figure below (Fig. 15.1). Then we introduce the 10 mm port and 5 mm port which is 2.5 cm medial to ASIS, and both teams together take the stock of the situation about the adhesions at gall bladder site and about the pelvic findings. TLH is done first, for which Jain point becomes the main operating port. 10 mm epigastric port works as optical port for doing hysterectomy and working port for Cholecystectomy and for gall bladder Jain point becomes the optical port. Thereby using the same port in different applications during the surgery. In our technique of doing laparoscopic Cholecystectomy using same ports as for hysterectomy, Jain point offers an extra advantage of using it as entry as well as working port.

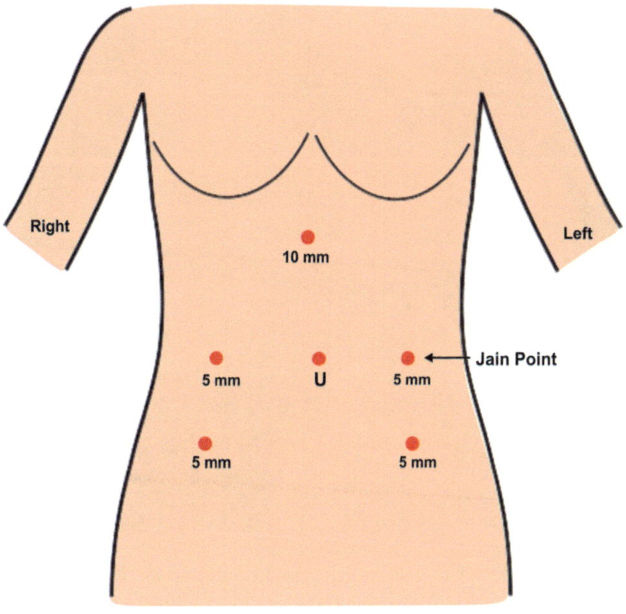

Fig. 15.1 Port position for combined TLH and Cholecystectomy surgery

Which Surgery First? We start with the laparoscopic part of TLH which is done by the Gynecological team following the *Comprehensive Canopy Concept, 'The 3 Step Technique' to bladder dissection in TLH* (Fig. 15.2a–l):

1. **Step 1: Posterior approach of uterine artery dissection and ligation-** We start with injecting dilute pitressin. The left adnexal pedicle is then coagulated and cut. The posterior leaf of broad ligament is transected widely from uterosacral ligament to arcus torinus. This helps in skelotonization of uterine artery and vein, which is coagulated and cut, without dissecting the bladder flap. Transecting the uterine artery also cuts the transverse cervical ligament thereby causing downward movement of the ureter, preventing ureteric injury. At this moment, we do not touch the adherent bladder and work in the cotton candy uterovesical space below to create the bladder canopy which is described in step 2.
2. **Step 2: Canopy concept of bladder dissection-** Dissection continues just 1 cm anterior to the coagulated uterine artery till the shiny glistening pubocervical fascia is exposed. Further dissection is continued over the manipulator cup in this cotton candy space, below the stretched out bladder canopy. Once the uterovesical space is opened completely, the uterovesical fold of peritoneum is cut. This helps in avascular effortless downward movement of the bladder flap.
3. **Step 3: Anterior approach of contralateral uterine artery dissection-** Dissection continues further till we reach the contralateral round ligament. This helps in skelotonization of the contralateral uterine artery anteriorly by the side of the manipulator rim. The skeletonized uterine artery is coagulated and dissected off the manipulator cup rim. The right sided adnexa is then coagulated and cut. After retrieval of the uterus and vault closure, the case is handed for cholecystectomy which is done by surgical team.

Identification of Calots Triangle We use Jain point as optical port using 5 mm telescope. Gallbladder body is retracted using port at mirror image of Jain Point, from the right side.

A 2.5 mm Alligator micro-forceps is introduced through right hypochondrium to hold the Gallbladder neck. After retracting the gallbladder using microforceps the hepatocystic triangle is dissected out.

Critical View of Safety After careful adhesiolysis and dissection of Calot's triangle is done Critical view of safety is achieved and confirmed with the help of Infrared imaging camera system (Stryker® 1688 4 K in our setting).ICG is a tricarbocyanine dye which binds to albumin and is selectively taken up by hepatocytes and excreted into bile [13]. after binding to albumin, it emits light in the infrared region of the electromagnetic spectrum at approximately 835 nm [14]. An infrared camera detects infrared light identified as strong fluorescence in response to ICG [15]. this is very useful in verification of biliary anatomy without risk of bile duct and cystic artery injury.

After confirming in ICG mode, cystic duct is doubly clipped using LT 300 or LT 400 depending on width of cystic duct. Cystic artery is fulgurated using HARMONIC ACE™ (Ethicon Johnson & Johnson Surgical, USA) before dividing the cystic duct. After securing haemostasis cystic duct is divided.

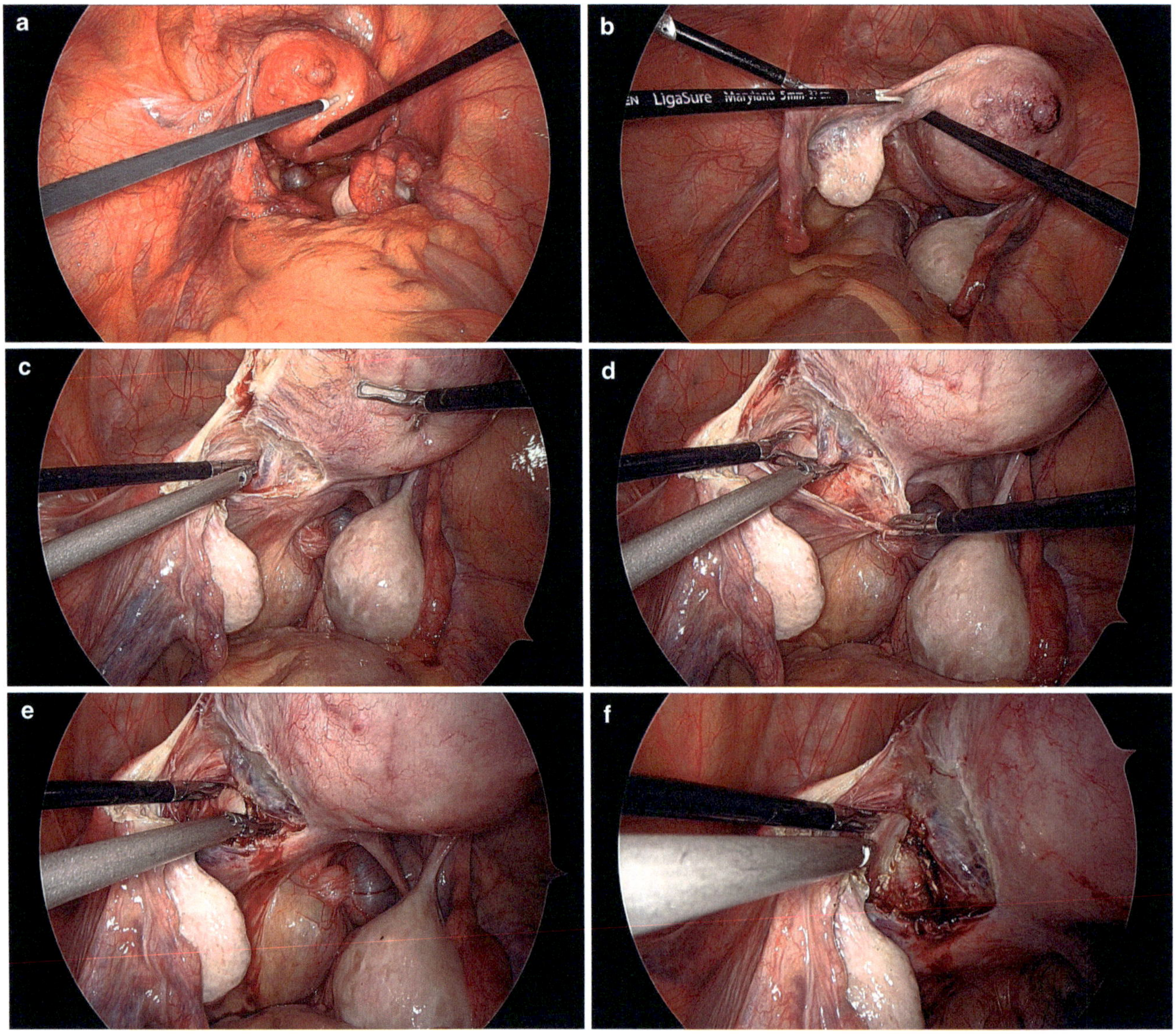

Fig. 15.2 **a** Dilute vasopressin injected. **b** Coagulating and cutting the left adnexa. **c** Left sided uterine artery and vein skeletonized by posterior approach. **d** Coagulating the left uterine artery. **e** Dissection begun in the 1 cm area immediately next to cut uterine artery pedicle. **f** Opening the plane adjacent to cut pedicle of uterine artery. **g** Developing the bladder canopy and visualizing cotton candy space. **h** Bladder canopy created. **i** Right sided uterine artery dissected using anterior approach. **j** Right sided uterine artery coagulated. **k** Coagulating and cutting the right adnexa. **l** Colpotomy proceeded with monopolar hook. **m** Vault closure and suspension done

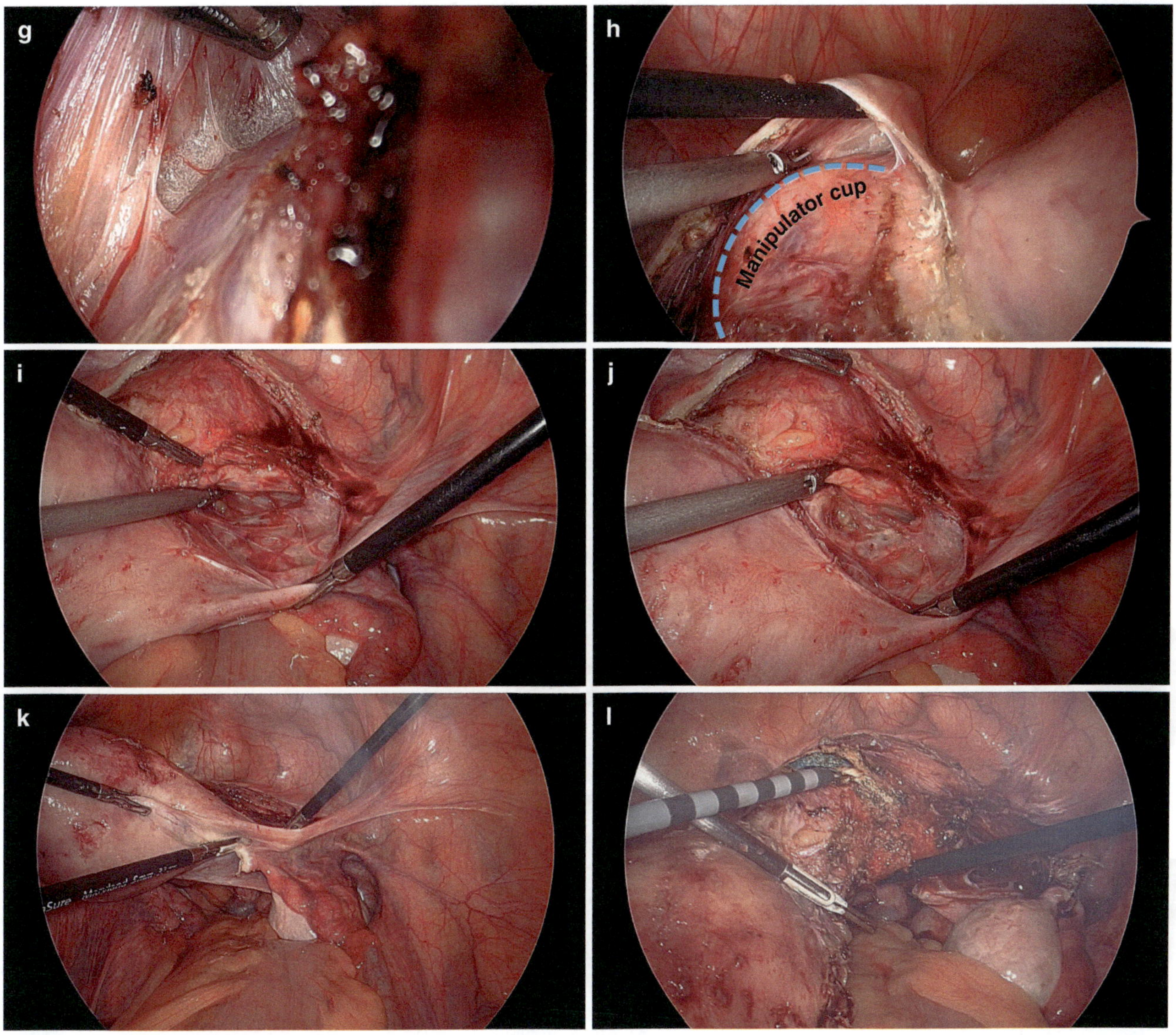

Fig. 15.2 (continued)

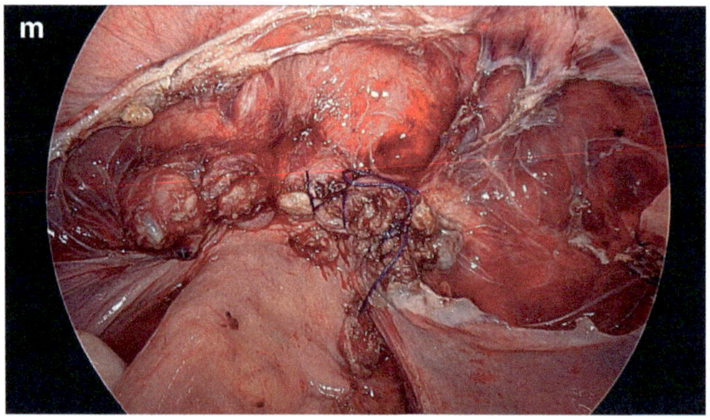

Fig. 15.2 (continued)

Gall bladder is dissected from the liver bed separating it from surrounding tissues using HARMONIC ACE™ (Ethicon Johnson & Johnson Surgical, USA) gallbladder is then kept in endobag and is removed via 10 mm epigastric port. (Which was optical port for gynecological team).

After removing gallbladder haemostasis check is done, suction irrigation done. 14 fr drain is placed in right sub hepatic space and pneumoperitoneum is deflated under vision.

Drain fixation is done and ports are closed in subcuticular fashion (Fig. 15.3a–l).

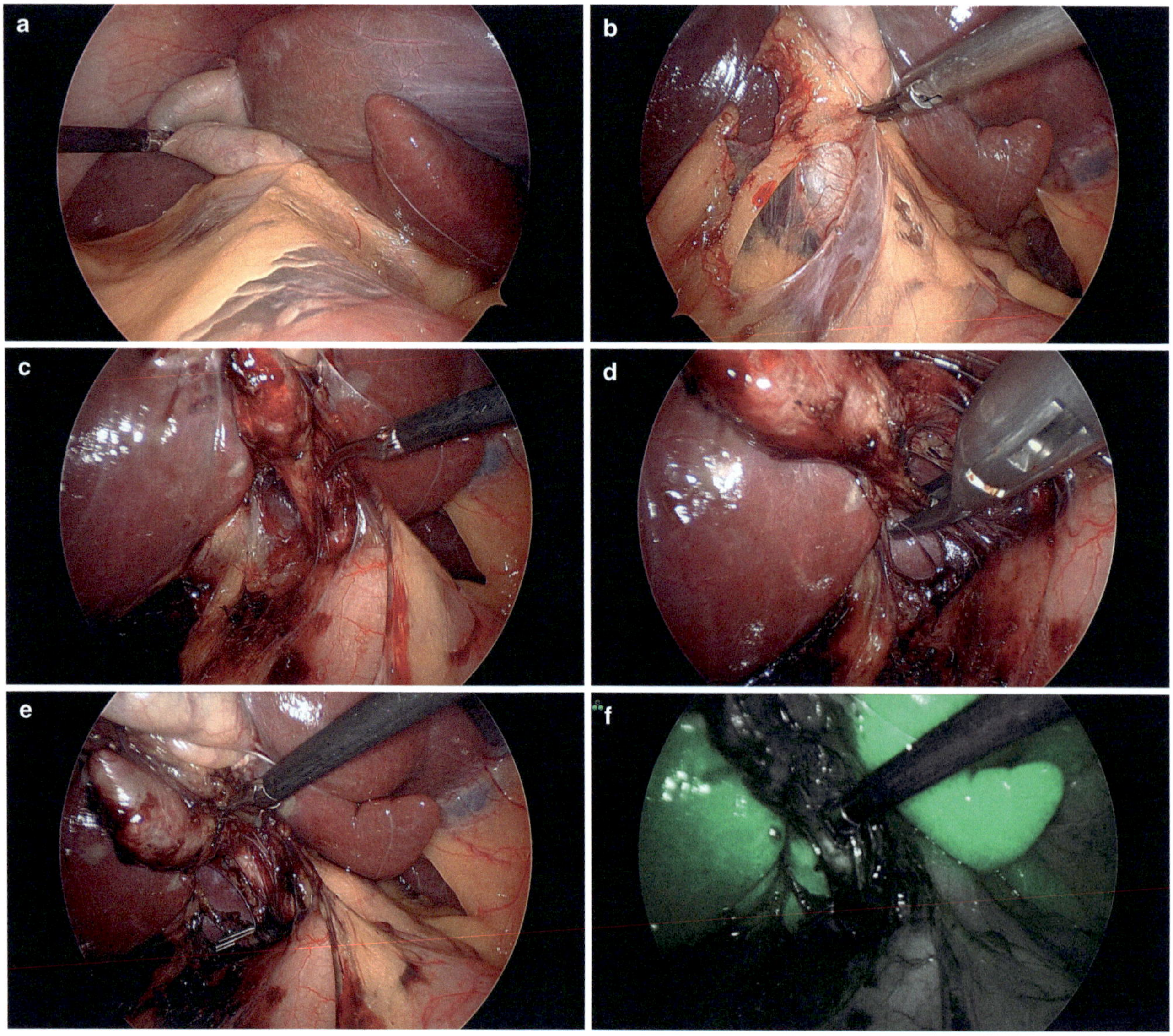

Fig. 15.3 **a** Gall bladder visualised. **b** Adhesiolysis done using harmonic ACE. **c** Calots being dissected. **d** Posterior cystic artery with fibrinous band being clipped. **e** Calots dissection continued. **f** Triangle of safety visualized using ICG. **g** Cystic duct being clipped. **h** Cystic clipped. **i** Cystic artery dissected. **j** Cystic artery being fulgurated with Harmonic Ace. **k** Gall Bladder removed from Gb bed. **l** Gall Bladder removed through 10 mm port

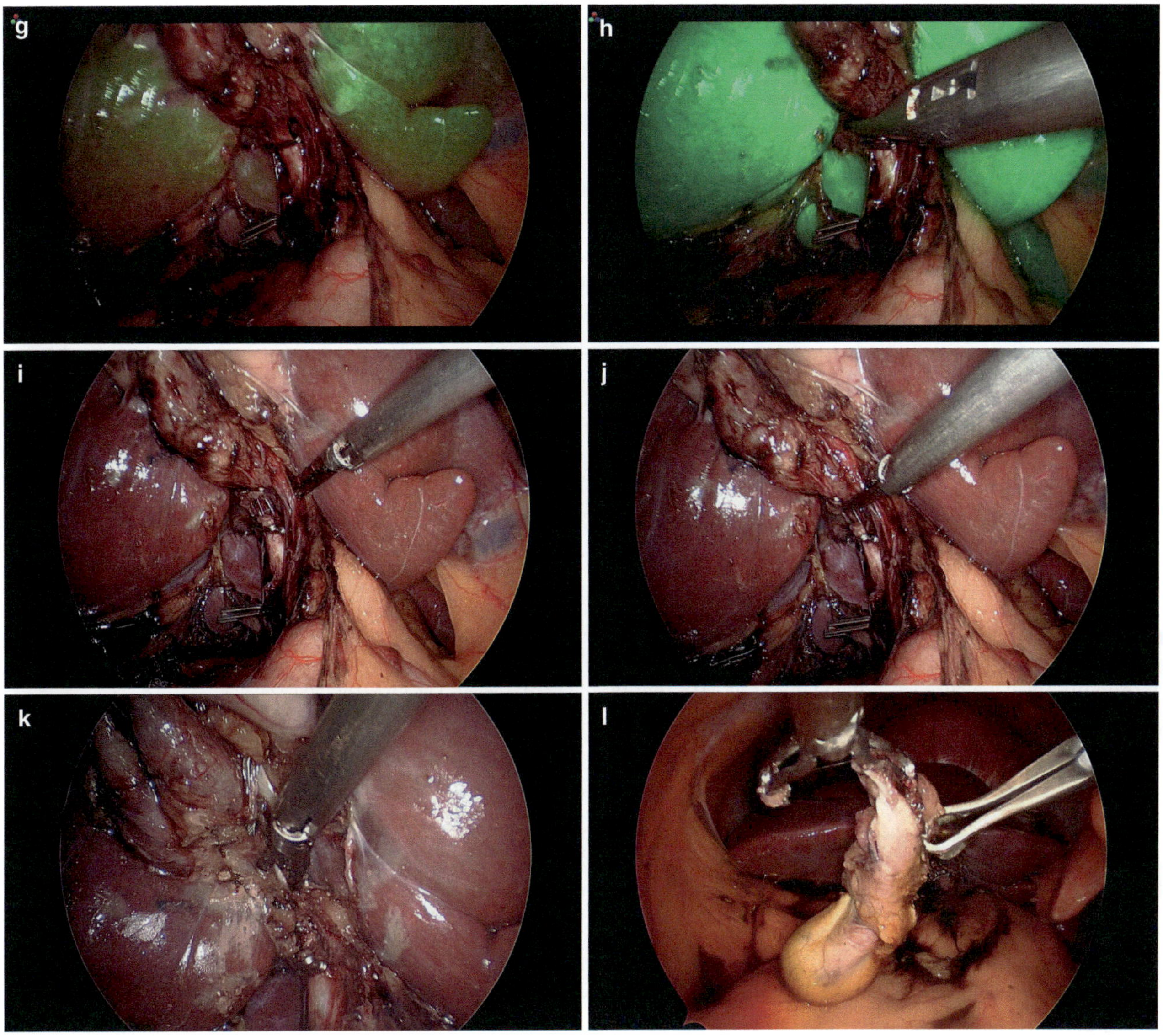

Fig. 15.3 (continued)

15.4.1 Tips to Improve Safety Profile of Cholecystectomy

These are few useful tips for laparoscopic gall bladder removal:

- Always take proper informed written consent (including chance of conversion, need for subtotal cholecystectomy, risk if bile duct injury etc.)
- Good quality imaging system with Infrared imaging capability and good thermal energy source like HARMONIC ACE™ (Ethicon Johnson & Johnson Surgical, USA), THUNDERBEAT®.
- Better to use 30 degree angled telescope
- Introduce, use and remove instruments under vision.
- If required do aspirate the over distended gallbladder
- Gallbladder fundus to be retracted by assistant up towards the right shoulder of patient
- Gallbladder neck should be retracted down and out towards the right elbow of patient
- Use an extra 5 mm port whenever needed
- Work above the Rouviere sulcus
- Remain right to the cystic lymphnode
- Remain and work close to the galllbaldder
- Define hepatocystic triangle by dissecting posterior one third of gallbladder off from bed
- In case of doubt calots anatomy should be defined using ICG
- Do not try to find the cystic duct- CBD junction.
- Take care of cystic artery before dividing the cystic duct
- Never clip the cystic duct flush with CBD

- Gallbladder bed should be washed and examined for any bile or blood leak
- Pressure with mobilized gallbladder, or gauze will help in controlling bleeding
- Always extract the gallbladder under vision

Postoperative Care Patient is put on clear liquid diet on day of surgery and from next morning she is allowed semi-solid diet progressing to solid diet and patient is discharged on next day of surgery.

In the current times when everybody is up for cosmesis, short hospital stay, quick return to work, less financial and mental burden this combined approach of involving surgical and gynecological disciplines in a single setting and setup is safe and costeffective [16] procedure with optimal outcomes.

15.5 Conclusion

The integration of laparoscopic cholecystectomy with other surgeries shows the progress and adaptability of minimally invasive surgery, advancement of MIS that two procedures, in different quadrant of abdomen can be easily done which could not have been imagined with open surgery.

Learning Points

- Combined surgery can safely be done with competent surgical and gynaecological team along with modern technology with proper intraoperative and post-operative care
- Advantages include a single hospital stay, single anesthesia administration, single mental and physical exertion and reduced financial burden, and comparable safety and efficacy.
- incidence of gallstones is multifactorial, a fatty fertile flatulent female of Fifty (5 F's of gall stone disease) is more prone to develop gallstone disease
- Thorough pre-operative assessments, including imaging and lab tests, are crucial for the combined procedure's success.
- Operating time in combined surgery is not summed up, rather it gets balanced with few steps being same in both procedures like - common entry ports, suction irrigation and port closure
- Good quality imaging system with Infrared imaging capability and good thermal energy source like HARMONIC ACE™ (Ethicon Johnson & Johnson Surgical, USA), THUNDERBEAT® and using 30 degree angled telescope improves surgical outcomes
- Jain point is safe and ergonomic point in naive abdomen as well as in patient with previous abdominal scars.
- Infrared imaging and Indocyanine green usage enhance safety by verifying biliary anatomy during cholecystectomy.

Competing interest The author declares no conflict of interest that are relevant to content of this chapter.

Ethical Approval Informed consent was obtained from individual participants and patients regarding publication and documentation without disclosing their identity.

References

1. Savita K, Khedkar I, Bhartia VK. Combined procedures with laparoscopic cholecystectomy. Indian J Surg. 2010;72(5):377–80.
2. Jones MW, Weir CB, Ghassemzadeh S. Gallstones (Cholelithiasis). 2023. In: StatPearls [Internet].
3. Schirmer BD, Winters KL, Edlich RF. Cholelithiasis and cholecystitis. J Long-Term Eff Med Implants. 2005;15(3):329–38.
4. Brasca A, Berli D, Pezzotto SM, et al. Morphological and demographic associations of biliary symptoms in subjects with gallstones: Findings from a population-based survey in Rosario, Argentina. Dig Liver Dis. 2002;34:577.
5. Attili AF, De Santis A, Capri R, et al. The natural history of gallstones: the GREPCO experience. The GREPCO Group. Hepatology. 1995;21:655–60.
6. Stephen AE, Berger DL. Carcinoma in the porcelain gallbladder: a relationship revisited. Surgery. 2001;129:699–703.
7. Lowenfels AB, Walker AM, Althaus DP, et al. Gallstone growth, size, and risk of gallbladder cancer: An interracial study. Int J Epidemiol. 1998;18:50–4.
8. Serra I, Calvo A, Baez S, et al. Risk factors for gallbladder cancer. An international collaborative case-control study. Cancer. 1996;78:1515–7.
9. Resutra R, Mahajan N, Gupta R. Pairing surgery with Laparoscopic Cholecystectomy in single sitting. Int Surg J. 2019;6:3991–5.
10. Ishizawa T, Bandai Y, Ijichi M, et al. Fluorescent cholangiography illuminating the biliary tree during laparoscopic cholecystectomy. Br J Surg. 2010;97:1369–77.
11. Gotoh K, Yamada T, Ishikawa O, et al. A novel image-guided surgery of hepatocellular carcinoma by indocyanine green fluorescence imaging navigation. J Surg Oncol. 2009;100:75–9.
12. Jain N, Srivastava S, Bayya SLP, Jain V. Jain point laparoscopic entry in contraindications of Palmer's point. Front Surg. 2022;9:928081. https://doi.org/10.3389/fsurg.2022.928081. PMID: 36439525; PMCID: PMC9696343.
13. Cherrick GR, Stein SW, Leevy CM, et al. Indocyanine green: observations on its physical properties, plasma decay, and hepatic extraction. J Clin Invest. 1960;39:592–600.
14. Landsman ML, Kwant G, Mook GA, et al. Light-absorbing properties, stability, and spectral stabilization of indocyanine green. J Appl Physiol. 1976;40:575–83.
15. Mitsuhashi N, Kimura F, Shimizu H, et al. Usefulness of intraoperative fluorescence imaging to evaluate local anatomy in hepatobiliary surgery. J Hepato-Biliary-Pancreat Surg. 2008;15:508–14.
16. Wadhwa A, Chowbey PK, Sharma A, Khullar R, Soni V, Baijal M. Combined procedures in Laparoscopic Surgery. Surg Laparosc Endosc Percutan Tech. 2003;13:382–6.

Complex Robotic Hysterectomy: Tackling the Bladder with Previous Cesarean Section

16

Rooma Sinha and Rupa Bana

16.1 Introduction

Laparoscopic Hysterectomy was first described in 1989 by Harry Reich [1]. However, despite this milestone; the abdominal approach remains the primary method in many centers [2]. It's worth noting that in 2005, the FDA approved the use of the daVinci robotic system in gynaecology and since then it has been used world-wide to perform minimal access hysterectomy. A new technology can often perplex surgeons and delay universal adoption in their surgical practice. According to World Health Organization statistics, the global cesarean section (CS) rate has significantly increased since 1980. In India, the overall prevalence of CS was recorded at 21.50% (49,634 out of 230,870 births), reflecting an increase from 16.72% (2312 out of 13,829 births) in 1998–99 [3]. This fact translates to an increased rate of bladder complications when these women need hysterectomy in the later years. There is a 2.5% chance of bladder complications in patients with 1 or 2 previous cesarean sections, which increases to 21.1% in patients with 3 or more previous cesarean sections. The rate of inadvertent cystotomy in patients with 3 or more cesarean sections is 18 times higher than in patients with no history of cesarean section [4].

This chapter aims to discuss

1. A simple reproducible Sinha Apollo technique- A "Two arm Three instruments "method to do Robotic Hysterectomy.
2. Strategies to tackle bladder adhesion while doing hysterectomy using the robotic platform

16.2 Sinha Apollo Technique-"Two Arms Three Instrument"

We developed a surgical technique to optimize operating time and cost. It is a reproducible two arms three instrument "Sinha Apollo Technique" [5]. Using only 3 daVinci's EndoWrist® instruments (Fenestrated bipolar, Hot Shears and Needle driver) which limits the instrument exchanges during the procedure and using a 15 cm barbed suture to avoid intracorporeal knot-tying during vault suturing reduces the overall time. We employ the Rumi® uterine manipulator system in along with the Advincula Arch® (Cooper Surgical, Trumbull, CT, USA), utilizing an appropriately sized Rumi tip and KOH cup. This efficient uterine manipulation technique obviates the necessity for a third robotic arm. The bevelled edge of the KOH cup identifies the trajectory of colpotomy at the cervico-vaginal junction.

16.2.1 Port Placement & Positioning

The primary optic port (8 mm) is typically positioned using a modified Hassan's technique, usually at the umbilicus. In our practice, a supra-umbilical position is rarely utilized.

Supplementary Information The online version contains supplementary material available at https://doi.org/10.1007/978-981-97-3226-5_16. The videos can be accessed individually by clicking the DOI link in the accompanying figure caption or by scanning this link with the SN More Media App.

R. Sinha (✉)
Gynecology, AHERF, Hyderabad, Telangana, India

Macquarie University, Sydney, NSW, Australia

Gynecological Robotic Surgery, Apollo GROUP of Hospitals, Hyderabad, Telangana, India

Apollo Health City, Hyderabad, Telangana, India

AGRS (Association of Gynecological Robotic Surgeons of India), Hyderabad, Telangana, India

ASGRS (Asian Society of Gynecological Robotic Surgeons), Singapore, Singapore

SERGS (Society of European Robotic Gynecological Surgeons), Waregem, Belgium

R. Bana
Apollo Health City, Hyderabad, Telangana, India

N. Jain (ed.), *Complex Total Laparoscopic Hysterectomy (TLH) with Newer Approaches in Bladder Dissection*,
https://doi.org/10.1007/978-981-97-3226-5_16

The left and right robotic trocars (8 mm, Intuitive Surgical, Inc., Sunnyvale, CA, USA) are then placed 8–10 cm lateral to the midline and 3–4 cm inferior to the optic trocar. A line is drawn from the left 8 mm trocar to the optic trocar, and at the midpoint of this line, a perpendicular line is drawn in the cranial direction. A 5 mm assistant port is then placed 4–5 cm from this line (Fig. 16.1a) The Trendelenburg position of 15–20 degrees is done. Attention to the position is important as this cannot be changed once the patient's cart is docked. The patient cart is positioned on the left side, allowing ample space between the patient's legs for the utilization of the uterine manipulator. Following the completion of targeting, the robotic arms are docked on either side.

16.3 Surgical Steps

For Robotic Hysterectomy, we employ a 30-degree telescope and advocate a sequential approach. We first complete all left-sided ligaments and the uterine complex up to the colpotomy ring before proceeding to the right side. The ureters are identified at the pelvic brim, and their path is traced either transperitoneally or dissected retroperitoneally, especially in cases involving endometriosis. In Arm 3, we utilize fenestrated bipolar with a power setting of 40 watts, while in Arm 1, we select hot shear monopolar scissors with a power setting of 30 watts (Fig. 16.1b). The arm 2 has the telescope.

Steps (Figs. 16.2a–d, 16.3a–d, 16.4a–c, 16.5a, b)

1. We begin by coagulating and transecting the left round ligament and ovarian pedicle. Salpingectomy and/or oophorectomy are performed towards the conclusion of the procedure.
2. The dissection progresses by opening the anterior leaf of the broad ligament using hot shears. We then proceed anteriorly to incise the vesico-uterine peritoneal reflection, followed by dissecting the bladder inferiorly.
3. Next, we coagulate and transect the posterior left leaf of the broad ligament along with the left utero-sacral ligament.
4. Skeletonization of the uterine vessels is performed, followed by applying the bipolar forceps with a tension-free technique, ensuring a slightly loose grip. This approach guarantees adequate tissue effect and robust sealing of the vessels before transection, while minimizing lateral thermal spread.
5. The uterine artery and vein is then coagulated and transected by a synchronised movement of fenestrated bipolar and hot shears. We describe this as the "Salsa manoeuvre"

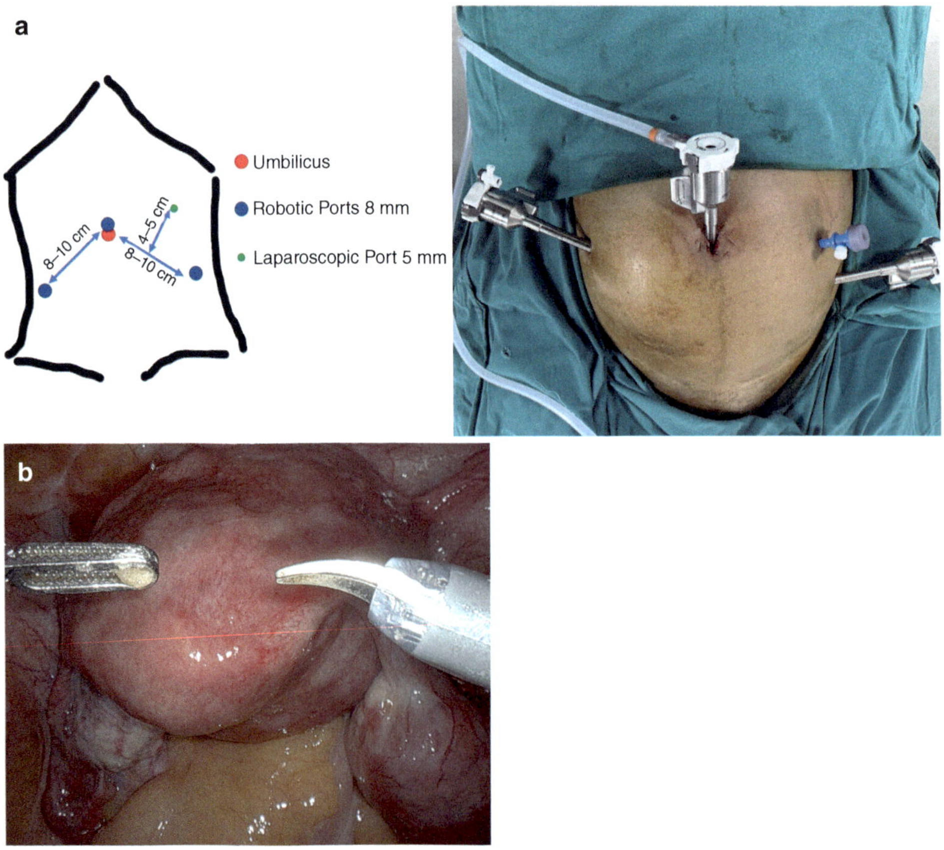

Fig. 16.1 **a** Port Placement—Sinha Apollo Technique. **b** Fenestrated Bipolar forceps in arm 2(left) and Hot shears inarm 4(right); 30 degree telescope in arm 3 in the center

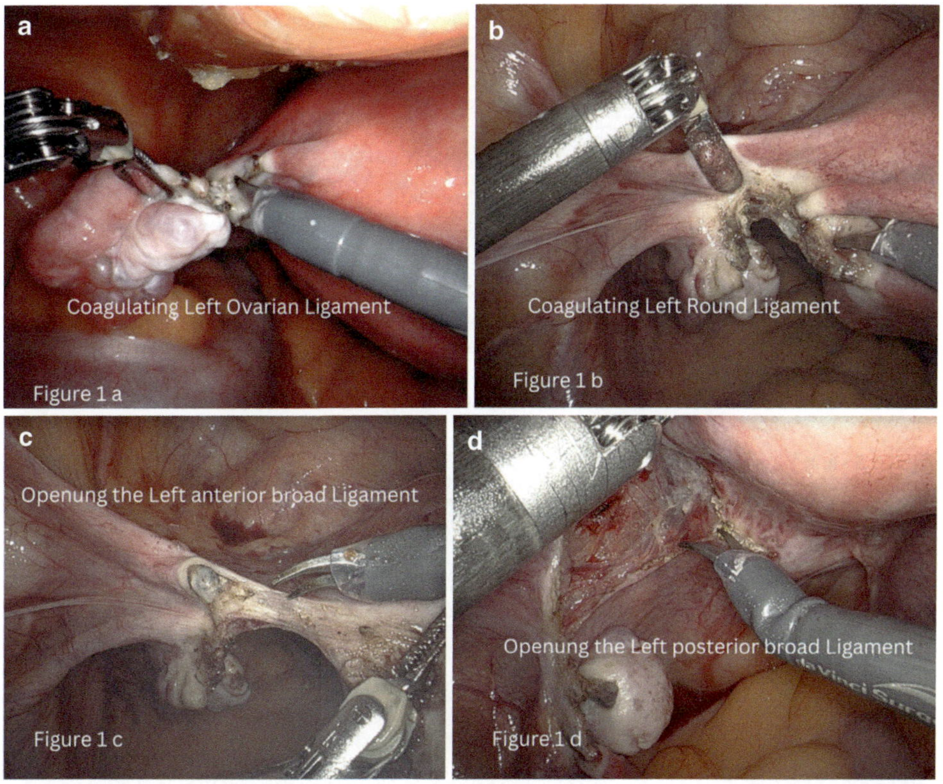

Fig. 16.2 **a–d** Surgical steps of Sinha Apollo Technique Robotic Hysterectomy

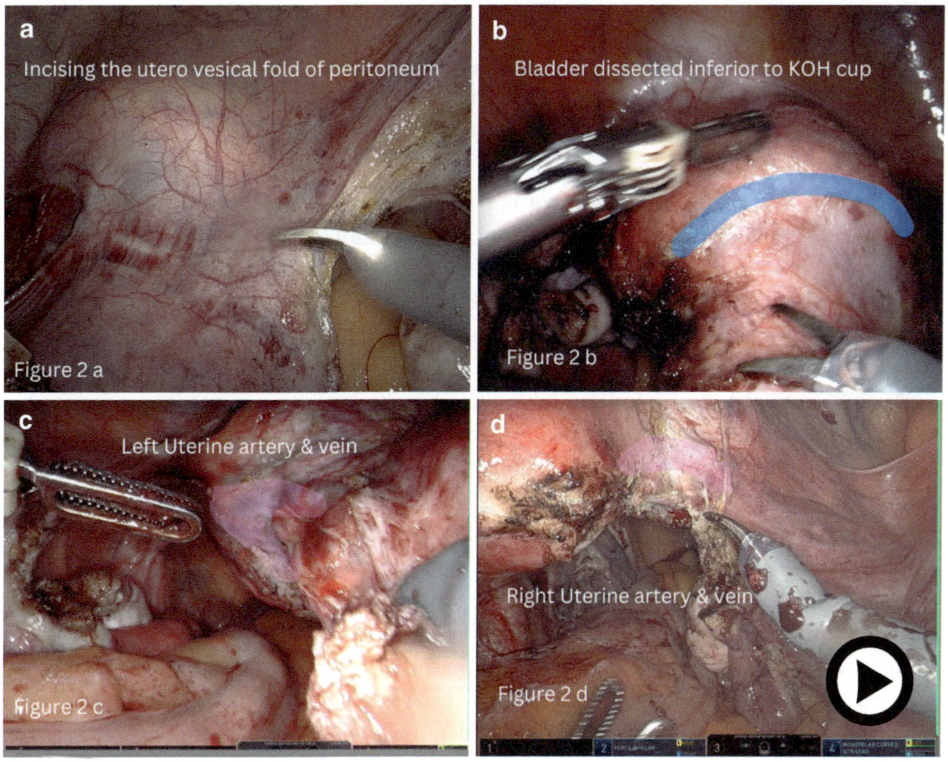

Fig. 16.3 **a–d** Surgical steps of Sinha Apollo Technique Robotic Hysterectomy (Video 16.3b Robotic Complex Hysterectomy) (▶ https://doi.org/10.1007/000-c9a)

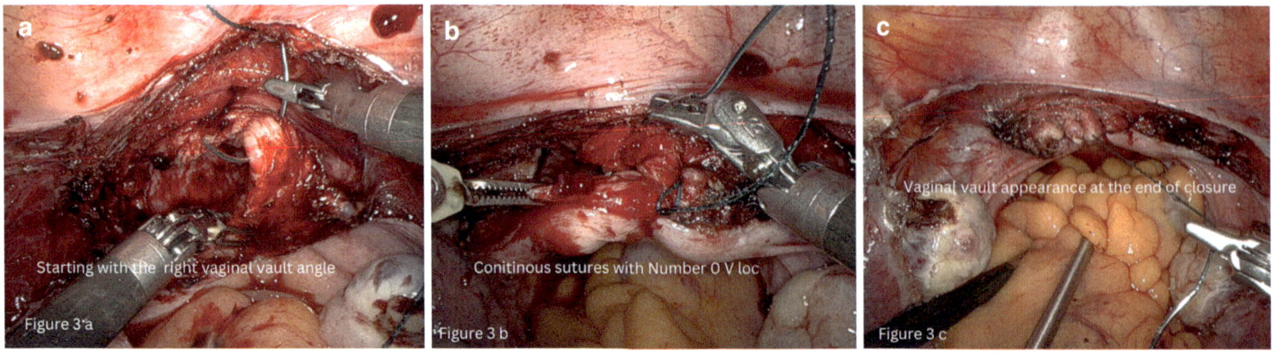

Fig. 16.4 a–c Surgical steps of Sinha Apollo Technique Robotic Hysterectomy

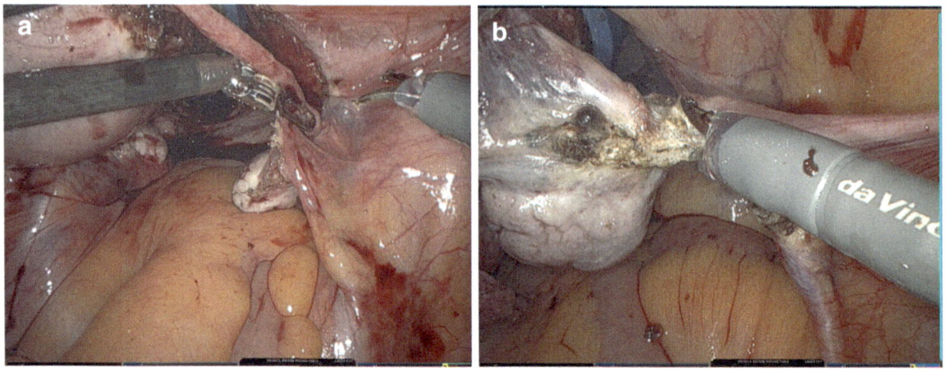

Fig. 16.5 a, b Right Salpingectomy & Right Salpingoophorectomy

6. Colpotomy is then begun from the anterior vaginal vault. The cardinal ligament complexes of the left side are then divided using monopolar hot shears, followed by the right side, consistent with an intra-fascial hysterectomy approach. Subsequently, the camera is rotated upwards by 300 degrees, and the posterior aspect of the colpotomy is completed. At this point, pneumoperitoneum is upheld by inflating the pneumo-occluder balloon and positioning it in the vagina. This represents a sequential approach to accessing the vaginal
7. At this stage, the removal of the tubes and/or ovaries is conducted. Following the identification of the infundibulopelvic ligaments and the ureters, bipolar coagulation is performed using fenestrated bipolar forceps, and the pedicle is transected with hot shears. The adnexa are then placed in the vaginal canal for retrieval.
8. The closure of the vaginal cuff is achieved using fenestrated forceps in arm 3 to grasp and evert the edges of the vaginal cuff, while a mega needle driver in arm 1 is utilized for suturing. Following the 5x5 rule, each vaginal bite is taken at a distance of 5 mm and to a depth of 5 mm on the cut edge, encompassing both the vaginal fascia and vaginal epithelium in each bite. A 15 cm 1–0 V-Loc™ barbed suture (Medtronic, Minneapolis, MN, USA) on a GS2 needle is employed for closure. This is executed in a single layer, incorporating the uterosacral ligament to prevent future vault prolapse. Finally, the end of the barbed suture is trimmed flush with the vault, and the needle is retrieved.

Before closure, all operative sites are irrigated, and a low insufflation pressure check is conducted to ensure hemostasis. Subsequently, the patient cart is undocked after removing all instruments, and ports are removed under direct vision. The pneumoperitoneum is released using the smoke evacuation system. The rectus sheath of the primary port at the umbilicus is identified and closed with a number 1/0 polypropylene suture. However, the rectus sheath of the 8 mm ports is not routinely closed. All port skin is closed with number 3/0 polyglecparone absorbable suture.

16.3.1 Why Robotics for Complex Hysterectomy- Advantages to the Surgeon

1. Magnified (10X) stereoscopic binocular vision
2. Wristed movements at the end of the operative instruments
3. Intuitive motion of the instruments in the pelvis
4. Near control of the surgical field
5. Tremor filtration

16.3.2 Tackling the Bladder Adhesions

Intraoperative adhesions, particularly between the uterus and bladder and between the uterus and the anterior abdominal wall, are commonly observed in patients with a history of cesarean sections. These adhesions significantly increase the risk of serious intraoperative complications, such as bowel or bladder injury during hysterectomy. However, it's important to note a word of caution—adhesiolysis is a highly skilled and demanding procedure associated with a high risk of complications. To mitigate these risks, adhesiolysis should only be undertaken by experienced surgeons, and intraoperative strategies should be employed to ensure safe surgery, even if it necessitates calling in a colleague for assistance. One must also remember that not every possible adhesiolysis should be conducted just because a surgeon can perform it. In general adhesions do not cause pain, infertility, or future bowel obstruction. Hence the lysis of asymptomatic adhesions should be done only if it blocks the access to the pelvis thus hampering the intended operation as in our case hysterectomy.

Adhesions develop due to post-surgical imbalance between fibrin deposition and fibrinolysis. As a normal response to trauma, fibrin is deposited at the surgical site. These should normally get lysed in a few days and prevent development of permanent adhesions. However, tissue hypoxia or excessive inflammatory reaction can disrupt the fibrinolytic system. This subsequently invaded by fibroblasts leading to development of connective tissue that may contain vessels and nerves. It is reported that there is a 20% incidence of adhesion development. A surgeon may encounter the presence of adhesions in approximately one-fifth of patients undergoing hysterectomy with a previous history of cesarean section. Therefore, it's crucial for every surgeon to be acquainted with strategies aimed at averting complications during surgery in patients with existing adhesions.

Following a cesarean section, the anatomical relationships of the post-gravid uterus are altered. This alteration leads to a direct apposition of the uterus with the anterior abdominal wall, without an interposition of the intestines or omentum. Such adhesions can hinder the descent of the uterus into the pelvic cavity during its involution. Consequently, the uterus remains positioned as an abdominal organ, resulting in elongation of the uterus and cervix, while the bladder is typically left unaffected by this ascension. Over time, superior adhesions may form a musculo-connective cordon, suspending the uterus. Consequently, the uterus remains adherent to the anterior abdominal wall, with the bladder becoming completely hidden. Clinically symptoms like dyspareunia, voiding problems or chronic pelvic pain may suggest such adhesions in cases with previous caesarean section. On pelvic examination the cervix is not visible as it is usually fixed behind the symphysis pubis.

Intra-abdominal adhesiolysis in such situations is associated with a high risk of intraoperative complications, however, before one can perform intra-abdominal adhesiolysis, the first critical step is to access to the abdominal cavity especially in cases with previous longitudinal incision. Entry is the most specialised step in such patients. We generally prefer a modified Hasson technique at the upper border of umbilicus [6]. Other points of entry can be Palmar's point [7] or Jain Point [8]. Advantage being Jain point entry can be used in contraindications of Palmar's Point. Using an optic port can also help to enter a scarred abdomen under vision [9].

Once entry has been established one can encounter two situations

1. OBLITERATED ANTERIOR COMPARTMENT (Captive Uterine Syndrome)/Ventro-suspended uterus
2. DENSE BLADDER ADHESIONS AT THE PREVIOUS UTERINE SCAR

1. OBLITERATED ANTERIOR COMPARTMENT (Captive Uterine Syndrome)/Ventro-suspended uterus

These adhesions between the uterus and abdominal wall along with the obliterated vesico-uterine space has been describe as three levels. (Fig. 16.6)

1. Superior adhesions, particularly those located at the uterine fundus, can fix the uterus high on the anterior abdominal wall.
2. Velamentous adhesions at the middle third of the uterus
3. Severe adhesions that affect the anterior surface of the uterus and completely obliterating the vesico uterine space. Upper border of bladder is masked and hidden in the adhesions.

Similar description has been also mentioned by Hardy et al. in their paper published in 2018. [10]

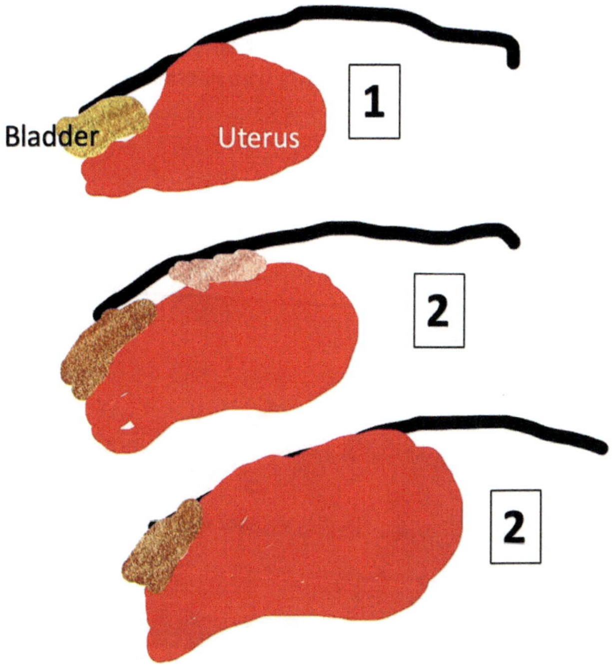

Fig. 16.6 Captive Uterine Syndrome—3 types of Adhesions

Begin with careful lysis of abdominal wall adhesions first for better visibility of the lesser pelvis. It can be difficult to maintain the orientation in dense obliterative adhesions. The uterus is first freed from the anterior abdominal wall. In instances of adhesions in the omentum, particular attention must be paid to ensuring adequate hemostasis. Identifying bleeders in the adipose tissue can become challenging once retraction occurs.

16.3.3 5 Steps Structured Approach to Obliterated Anterior Compartment During Robotic Hysterectomy (Figs. 16.7, 16.8, 16.9, 16.10, 16.11, 16.12, 16.13, 16.14, 16.15 and 16.16)

Step 1—Release the central fibro-muscular band down to up to the previous caesarean scar.

Step 2—Identify and transect left round ligament and open the anterior fold of the peritoneum to identify the lateral space. The sidewall of the lesser pelvis, identifying the left adnexa or beginning with left ureterolysis at the pelvic brim if associated endometriosis and then proceed in to the pelvis can be alternate paths to reach for the lateral space.

Step 3—Identify the left lateral space between the bladder and the vesico-uterine ligament. This space then identifies the dense adhesion between the bladder and scar.

Step 4—Identify the left uterine artery, coagulate and transect. Helps to prevent clean surgical field.

Step 5—Hold the bladder up, away from the vesico-uterine ligament, separate the adhesion between the bladder and the caesarean scar sharply with hot shears either with monopolar current (180 watts Level3) or without electro surgery. From this point proceed slowly with inferior and caudal dis-

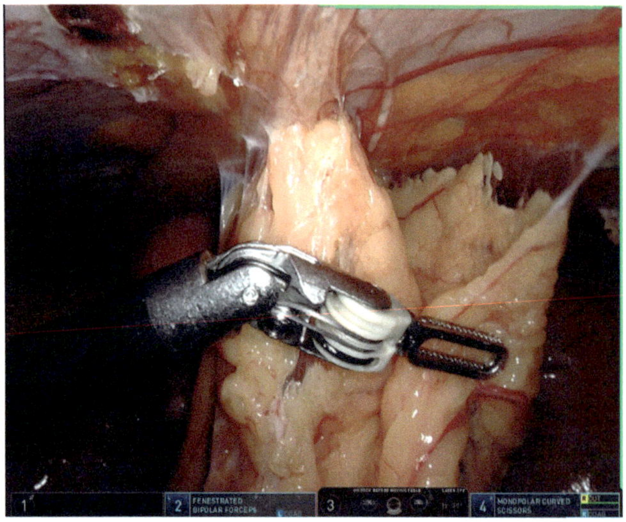

Fig. 16.7 Captive Uterine Syndrome Initial picture; omental adhesions to anterior abdominal wall

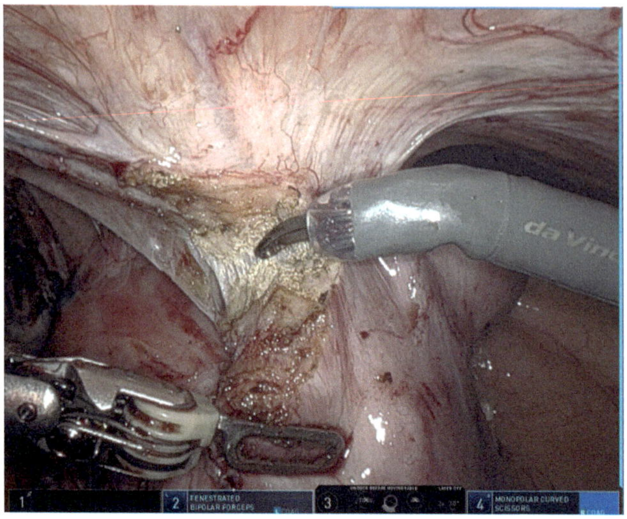

Fig. 16.8 Releasing the central fibro muscular band

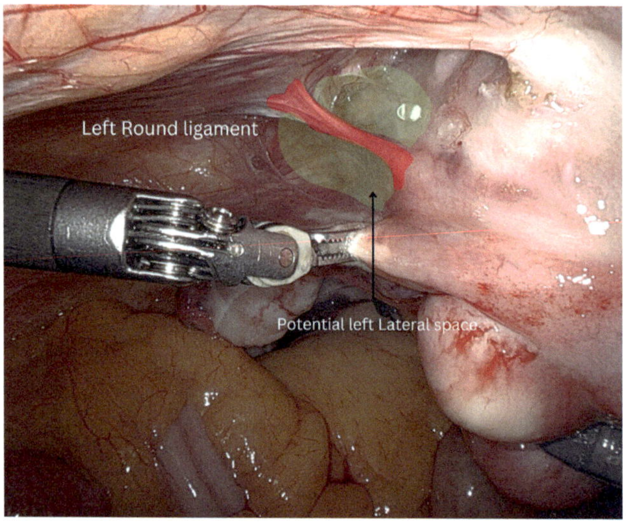

Fig. 16.9 Identifying the Left Round ligament and the potential lateral space

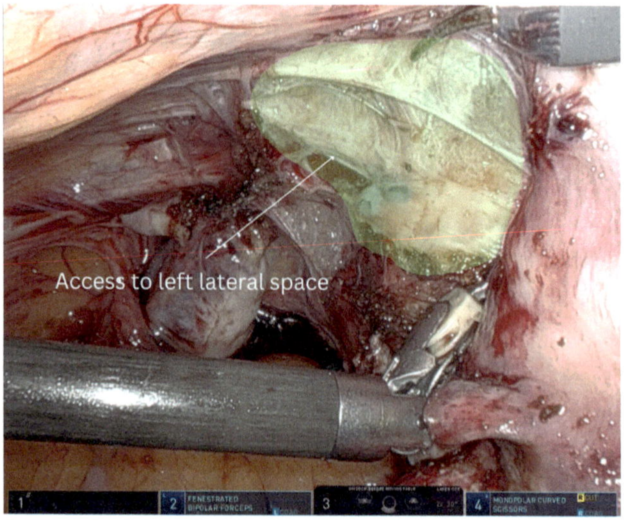

Fig. 16.10 Access to left lateral space

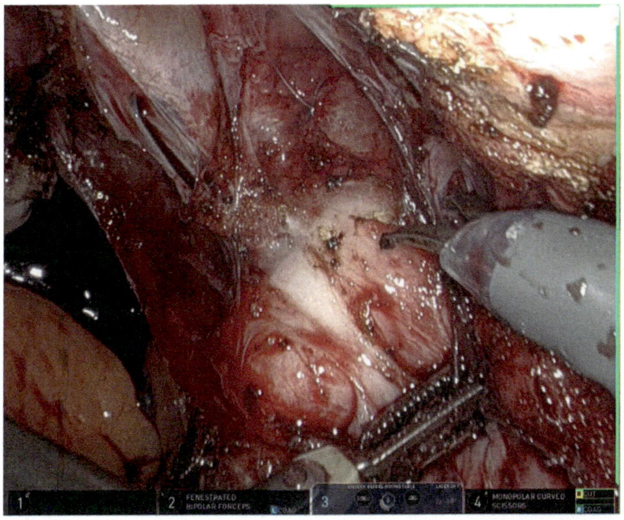

Fig. 16.11 Identification of glistening cervico vaginal ligament under the adherent bladder

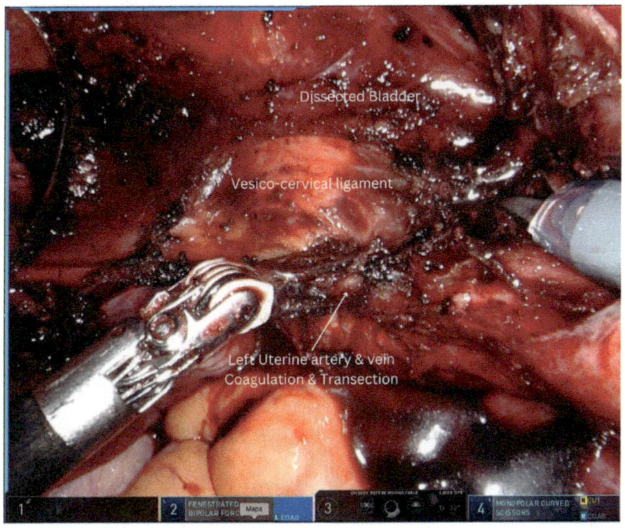

Fig. 16.12 Left Uterine artery & vein Coagulation & Transection

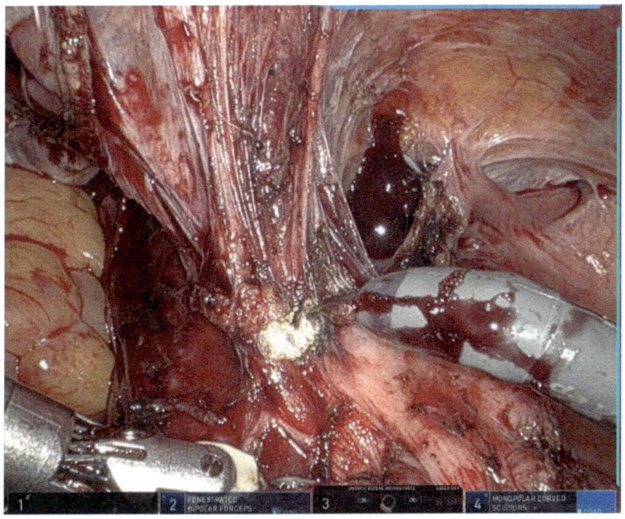

Fig. 16.13 Dissection of bladder adherent fibers by head on approach

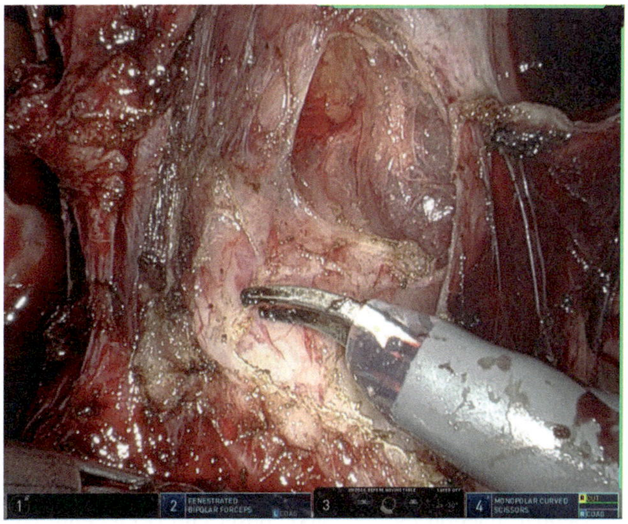

Fig. 16.14 Glistening cervico vaginal fascis on right side

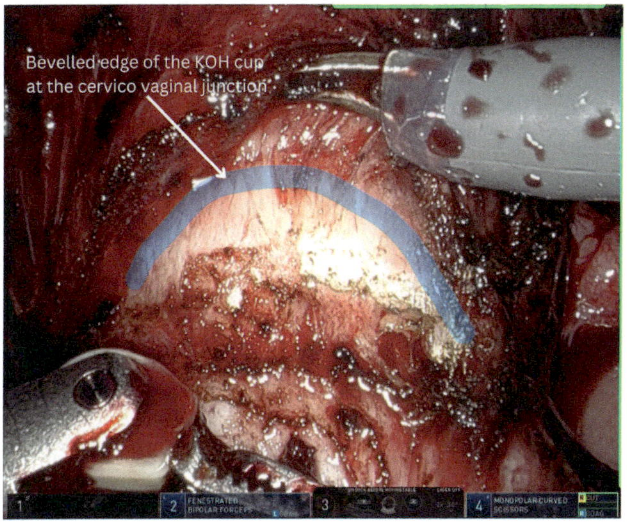

Fig. 16.15 Dissection of bladder beyond the bevelled edge of the KOH cup at the cervico vaginal junction

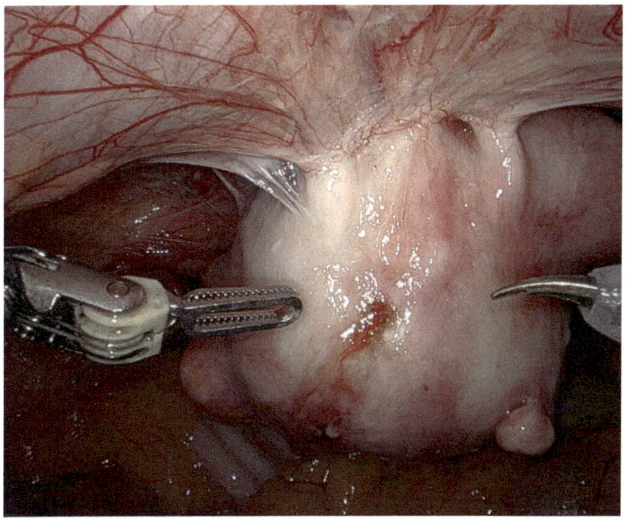

Fig. 16.16 Ventro suspended uterus

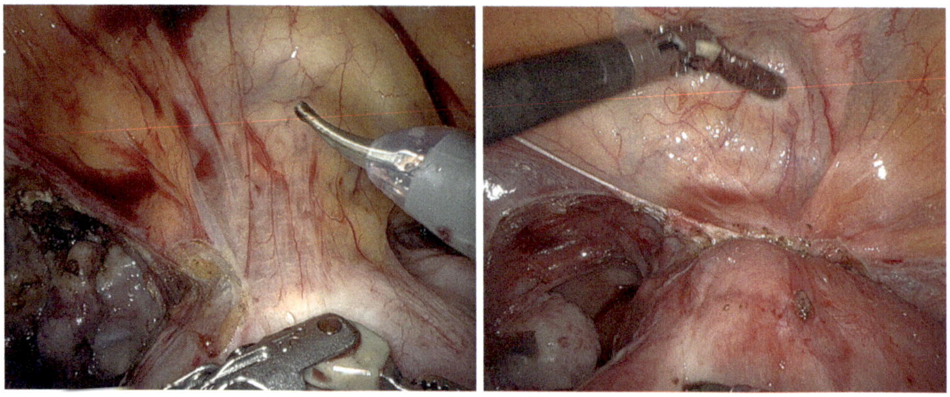

Fig. 16.17 Bladder adherent to previous cesarean scar, ideal for head on approach

section of the bladder in the vesico-cervical and subsequently vesico vaginal space. The delineation of the cervico vaginal junction by the colpomotiser cup (KOH cup with Rumi Uterine manipulator) can guide the level of caudal dissection. Dissect the bladder caudally beyond the cup as this can help in opening the vaginal vault safely as well as provide a 5-10 mm vaginal wall pave for vault suturing.

2. DENSE BLADDER ADHESIONS AT THE PREVIOUS UTERINE SCAR.

We describe three methods for bladder adhesiolysis during robotic hysterectomy.

(a) Head on Approach
(b) Lateral Window approach
(c) Reverse Bladder dissection

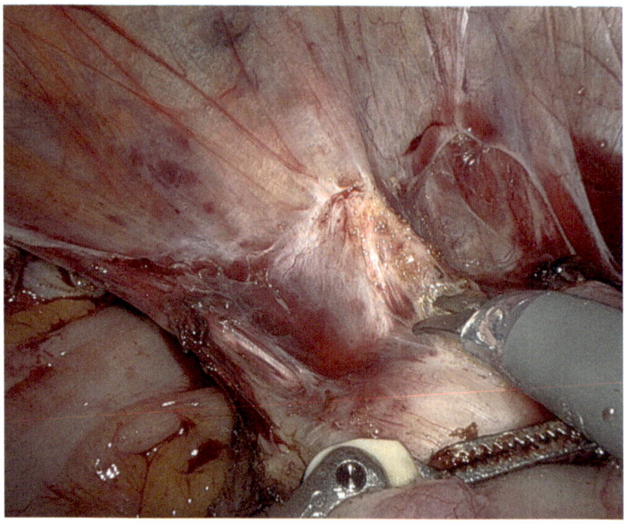

Fig. 16.18 Dissection begins from the central adhesions

16.3.4 Head on Approach

This approach is for bladder dissection when the classically described lateral window is not visible. This approach is possible only with robotic platform and involve superior to inferior dissection (Figs. 16.17, 16.18, 16.19, 16.20, 16.21 and 16.22).

It is based on five concepts with the use of Robotic System.

1. There is an HEAD ON view while doing surgery using the robotic platform. This means that the camera that if fixed at the midline optic port gives a view to the surgeon as if she/he is sitting at the head end of the operating table and viewing the pelvis. This view is impossible in laparoscopy leave alone open surgery as in both the surgeon stands on the side of the patient.

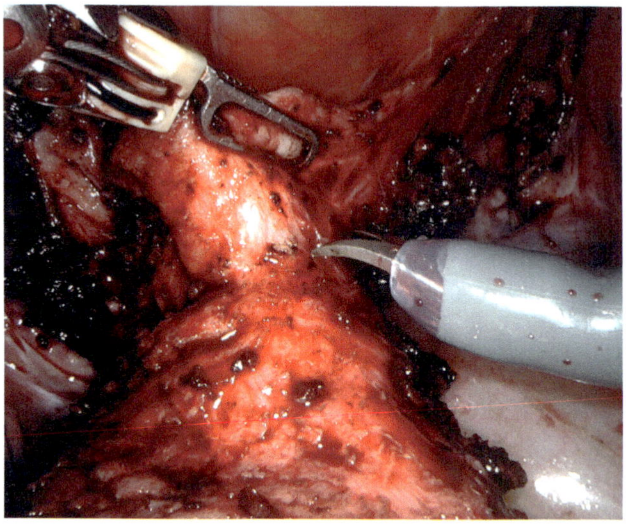

Fig. 16.19 Hold the central band and dissect

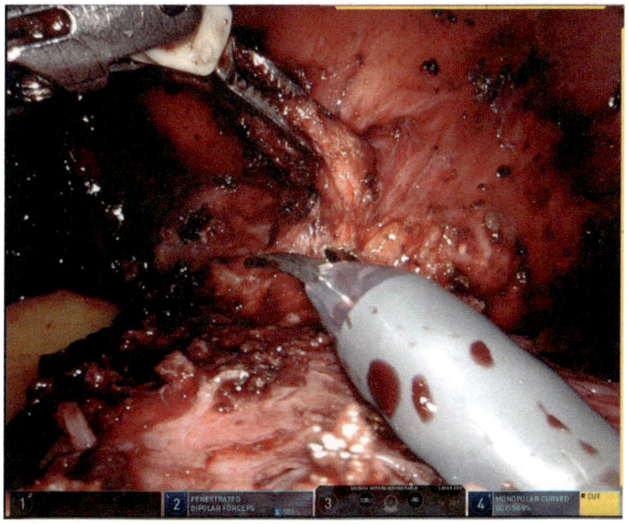

Fig. 16.20 Dissect the bladder adhesion off the vesico cervical ligament

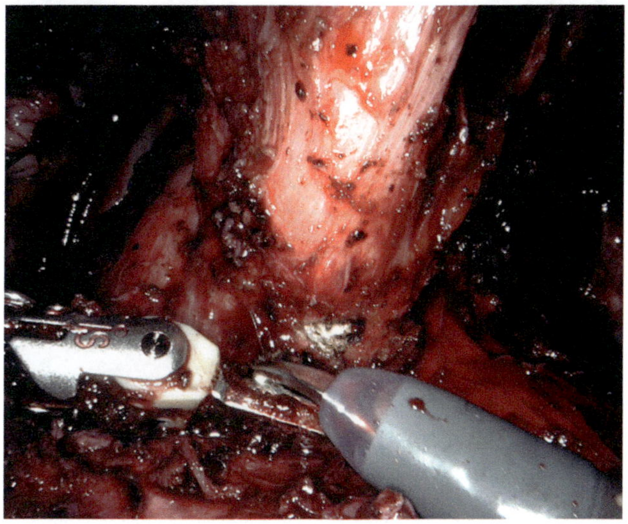

Fig. 16.21 central band of adhesion opening up with use of short burts of monopolar current.

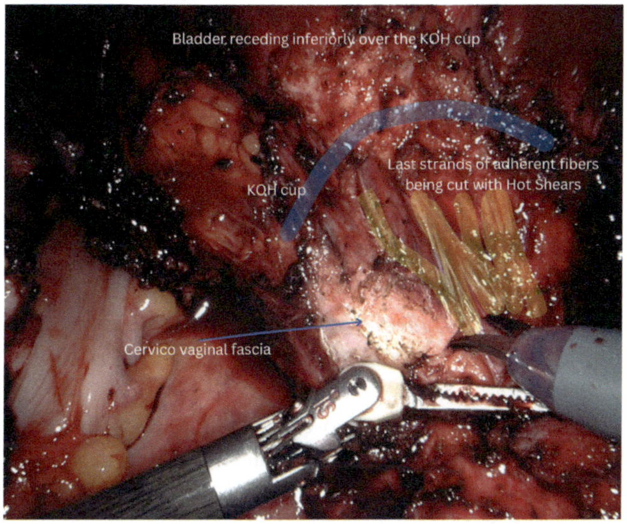

Fig. 16.22 Bladder receding inferiorly over the KOH cup

2. The wrist like movements of the hot shears can help lyse the bladder adhesions PERPENDICULAR to the line of adhesiolysis.
3. The use of short bursts of mono-polar current with a rock steady scissors due to the TREMOR FILTRATION PROPERTY of the robotic platform can help in doing fibre by fibre dissection with confidence. The monopolar currents give excellent assistance in the dissection of fibrous bands with the bladder on one side and utero vesical ligament in the other side.
4. The use of the fenestrated bipolar forceps as a HUMAN HAND which is from the left robotic port to hold the uterus and stretch the vesico uterine fold of peritoneum upwards. These stretched fibres with the glistening vesico-uterine peritoneum and subsequently the ligament under the peritoneum below confirms the correct dissection plane.
5. The judicious use of a colpomotiser at the cervico-vaginal junction helps to dissect the bladder caudally once the cervico vaginal ligament can be visualised at any point during dissection.

16.3.5 Lateral Window Approach (Figs. 16.23, 16.24, 16.25, 16.26, 16.27 and 16.28)

The lateral window is a potential space that is accessed by transecting the round ligament is first on the left side. This dissection is then extended posteriorly to utero ovarian ligament and the posterior leaf of the broad ligament thus deflecting the ureters laterally. Idea is to transect both utero-sacral ligaments at this point. This helps in up-ward mobilisation of the uterus. The anterior leaf of the broad ligament is extended inferiorly and medially to access the space lateral and parallel to the bladder pillar down to the cervical region.

This dissection is done to identify the vesicocervical and subsequently vesicovaginal ligaments. Having identi-

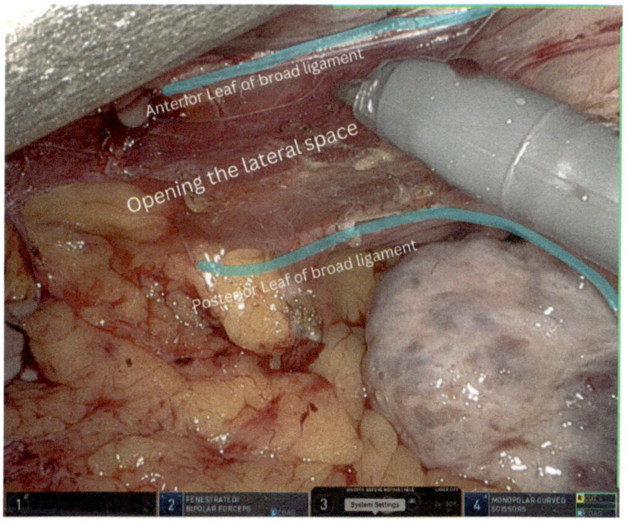

Fig. 16.23 Opening the lateral space between the anterior and posteror leaf of broad ligament

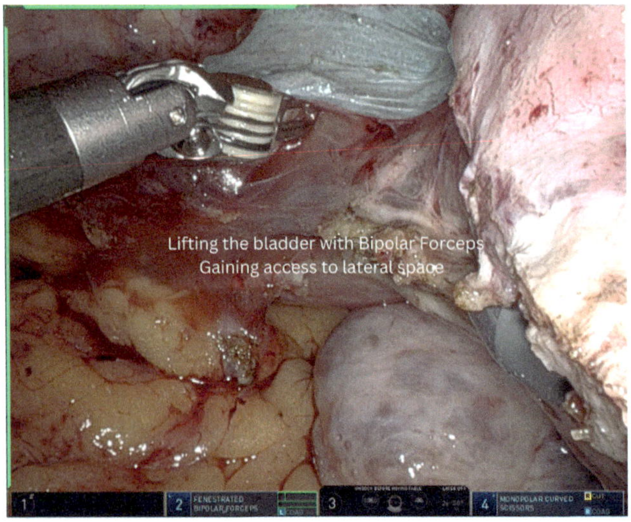

Fig. 16.24 Lifting the bladder with Bipolar Forceps Gaining access to lateral space

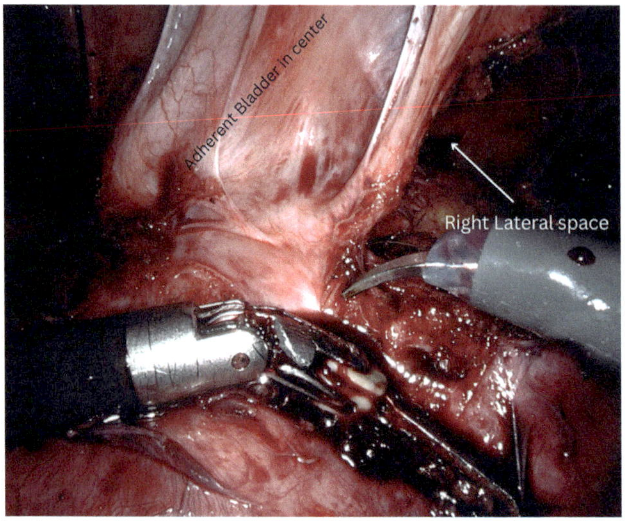

Fig. 16.27 Right Lateral space

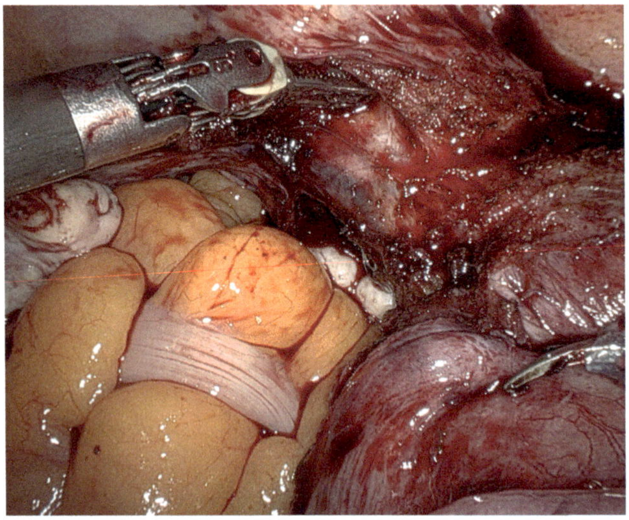

Fig. 16.25 Lateral approach lifting the bladder off the vesico cervical ligament

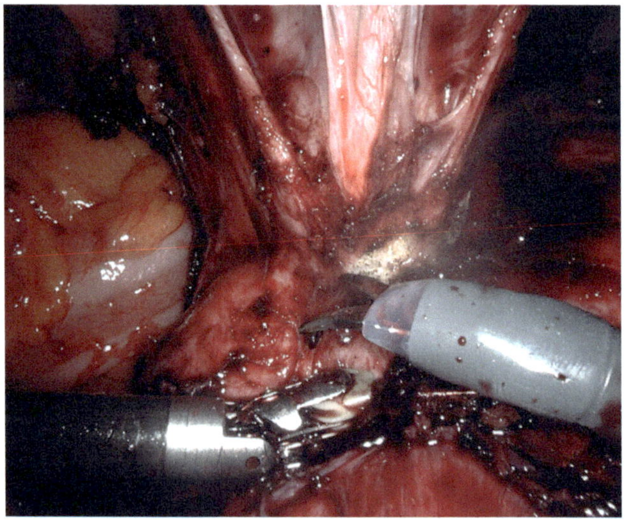

Fig. 16.28 Head on approach of bladder dissection after creating both the lateral spaces

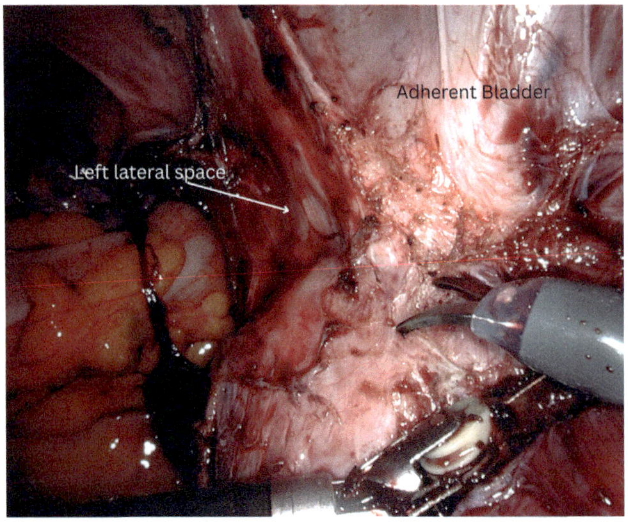

Fig. 16.26 Left lateral space

fied these ligaments, one is sure about the correct plane of dissection. This lateral space in the vesicovaginal plane has the vesicocervical–vaginal ligament (bladder pillar) and the bladder medially, some part of anterior leaf of the broad ligament on the anterior aspect and posteriorly by the parametrium. This dissection can define the margin of the midline adhesions secondary to the cesarean delivery scar. The potential space between the anterior and posterior leaves of the broad ligament is opened up. This manoeuvre exposes the uterine vessels, which are then skeletonized, coagulated, and transected at this juncture. Subsequently, these steps are replicated on the contralateral side.

The white shining vesico-cervical ligament is the guide regarding the right plane. The fenestrated bipolar is used to lift and deflect the bladder medially and the hot shears is used to transect the fibrous band between the bladder and previous scar. Usually, this dissection is done from left to right, unless the fibers found to be very dense on the left side, and in such situations, one might need to go on the right side to find the right plane. Keeping an eye on the upper border of the bladder helps to prevent any inadvertent cystotomy. Hot shears can be used either cold or with short burst of monopolar cutting current. (daVinci 180 watts @ level 3). This dissection can then be combined with a head on approach as described above. The short burst of monopolar current identifies the plane between the fibrous tissue and the nascent adipose tissue at the base of the bladder. Dissection is easier once we identify the KOH cup.

16.3.6 Reverse Bladder Dissection (Figs. 16.29, 16.30, 16.31, 16.32, 16.33, 16.34, 16.35 and 16.36)

The lateral space is developed in the same manner as described above. Once this lateral space is identified and you find that the adhesion of bladder to the previous scar does not budge, one can try to get in a clean and nascent space beyond and inferior the adhesions. The lateral vesicovaginal space can be furthered dissected and a space can be entered inferiorly by sharp and blunt dissection using fenestrated bipolar for blunt and hot hears for sharp dissection. Once the inferior space is identified, the dissection in the vesicovaginal space is proceeded from inferior to superior (caudal to cranial) by using a reverse dissection concept. This helps in completely mobilizing the bladder safely from the dense adhesions. This technique was also described by Nezhat et al. for laparoscopic hysterectomy in previous caesarean section cases which we have modified for our robotic hysterectomy cases [11].

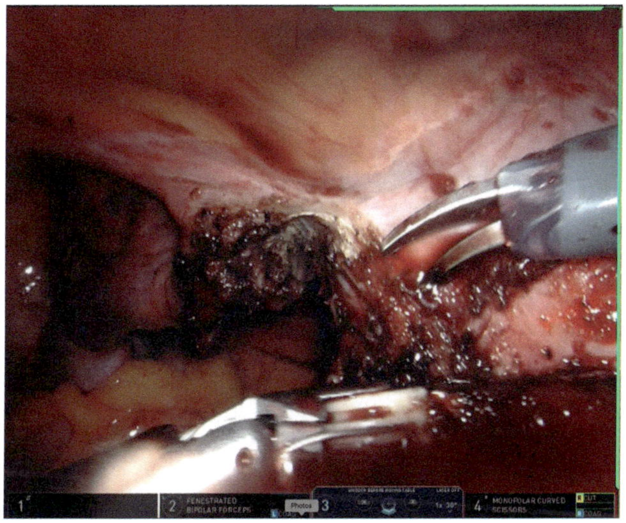

Fig. 16.29 Round Ligament is cut Adherent bladder seen

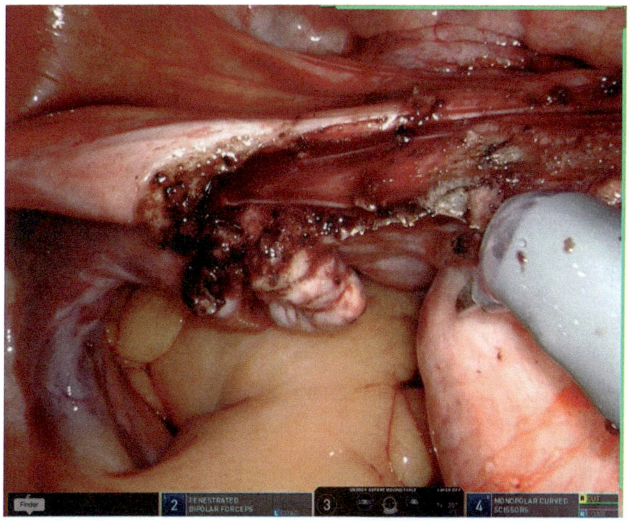

Fig. 16.30 potential space between ant and post leaf peritoneum

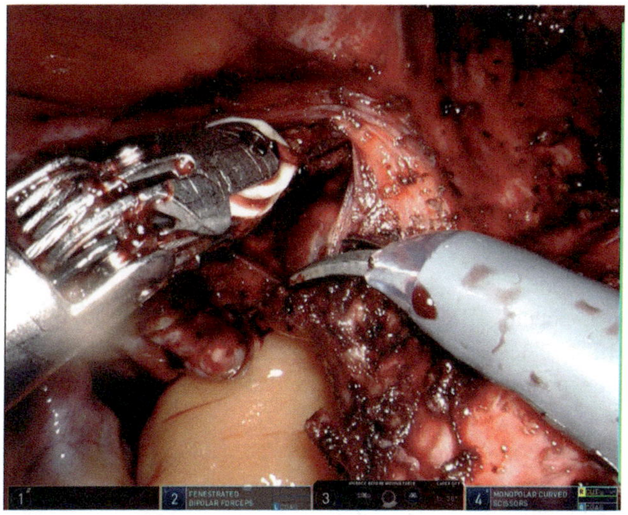

Fig. 16.31 bipolar forceps is beyond the bladder adhesions -in the nascent plane below the adherent bladder

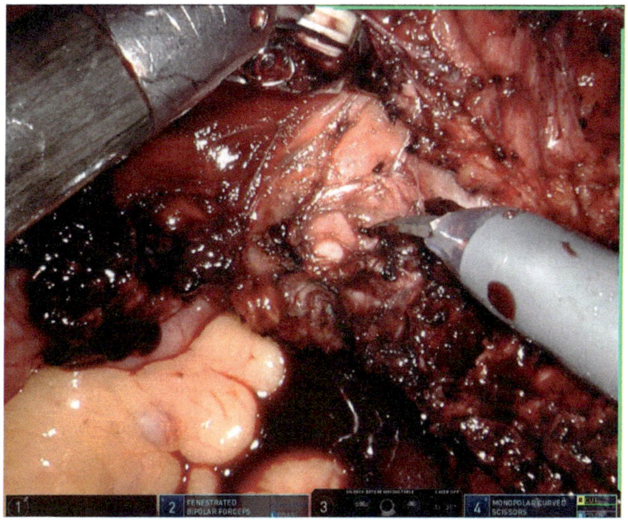

Fig. 16.32 bipolar in the area below the adherent bladder in the scar and monopolar releasing the dense adherent fibers

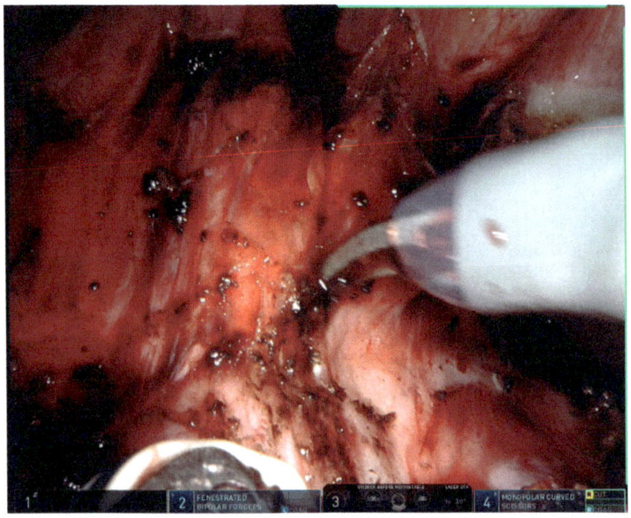

Fig. 16.33 Righ potential lateral space

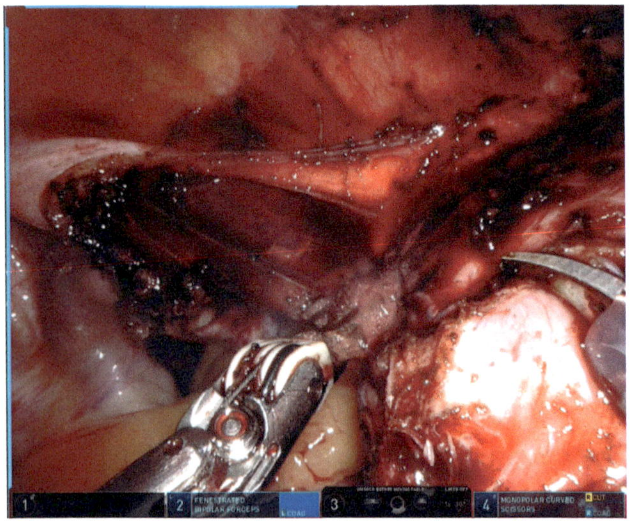

Fig. 16.34 Potential left lateral space coagulation of left uterine vessels before reverse dissection

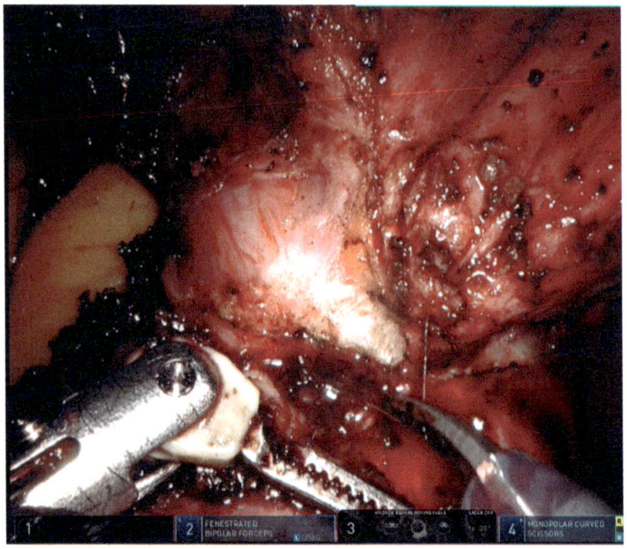

Fig. 16.35 Bladder receding over the KOH cup

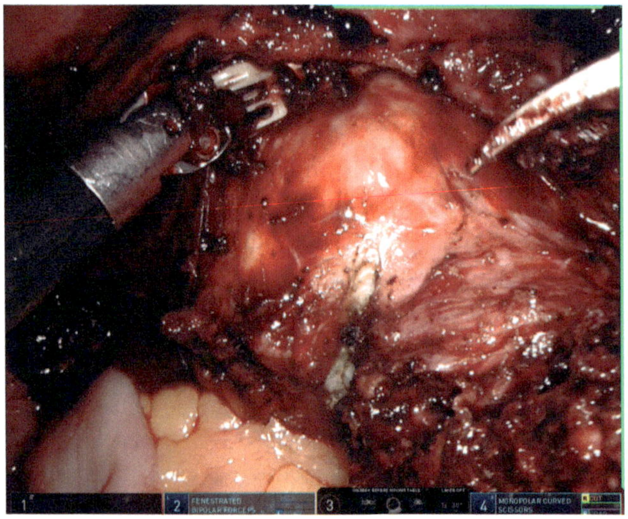

Fig. 16.36 Naked KOH cup

16.4 Conclusions

With increase in incidence of caesarean sections, surgeons will often encounter dense bladder adhesions at hysterectomies. Minimal access is the recommended technique for hysterectomy however, genital tract injuries remains a potential problem. Robotic surgeries with its advantages of wrist like intuitive movements helps in bladder dissection in narrow pelvis with dense bladder adhesions or in situations with completely obliterated anterior compartment can be the way forward in difficult hysterectomies. The knowledge of anatomy and the identification of correct dissection planes will help prevent such complication. The techniques described in the chapter have developed by authors with large experience in doing robotic hysterectomies.

Learning Points

- Minimal Access is the preferred method of doing hysterectomy
- Robotic technology is an advanced form of endoscopic surgery
- Magnified (10X) stereoscopic binocular vision with tremor filtered wristed intuitive movements are the advantages with robotic surgery
- Dense bladder adhesion requires anatomical knowledge and special surgical techniques to prevent potential injuries
- Uterine manipulator with a colpotomizer can aid in bladder dissection in cases with altered anatomy.

Competing Interest The author declares no conflict of interest that is relevant to content of this chapter.

Ethical Approval Informed consent was obtained from individual participants and patients regarding publication and documentation without disclosing their identity.

References

1. Reich H, DeCaprio J, McGlynn F. Laparoscopic hysterectomy. J Gynecol Surg. 1989;5(2):213–6.
2. Cohen SL, Vitonis AF, Einarsson JI. Updated hysterectomy surveillance and factors associated with minimally invasive hysterectomy. J Soc Laparoendosc Surg. 2014;18(3):e2014.00096.
3. Pandey AK, Raushan MR, Gautam D, Neogi SB. Alarming trends of cesarean section-time to rethink: evidence from a large-scale cross-sectional sample survey in india. J Med Internet Res. 2023;(25):e41892. https://doi.org/10.2196/41892. PMID: 36780228; PMCID: PMC9972201.
4. Wang L, Mranzcog H, Merkur F, Hardas G, Franzcog S, Franzcog S, Lujic S, MBiostat. Laparoscopic hysterectomy in the presence of previous caesarean section: a review of one hundred forty-one cases in the Sydney West Advanced Pelvic Surgery Unit. J Minim Invasive Gynecol. 2010;17:186–91.
5. Sinha R, Bana Rupa, Girija Shankar Mohanty, Two arms-three instruments robot-assisted laparoscopic hysterectomy: a reproducible technique, Laparosc Endosc Robot Surg, Volume 4, Issue 2, 2021, Pages 44–47, ISSN 2468-9009.
6. Sinha R, Rupa B. Non umbilical midline entry- a modified Hassan technique. Non umbilical laparoscopic entry points. Jaypee Brothers Medical Publishers; 2020. ISBN-13-978-9389776454.
7. Palmer R. Safety in laparoscopy. J Reprod Med. 1974;13:1–5.
8. Jain N, Jain V, Chandi A, Srivastava S, Singh S, Vasundhara N. Jain point: an alternate laparoscopic non-umbilical first blind entry port to avoid vessel, viscera, adhesions and bowel (VVAB). Updates Surg. 2021;73(6):2321–9. https://doi.org/10.1007/s13304-021-01099-z. Epub 2021 Jun 13. PMID: 34121164; PMCID: PMC8606393.
9. String A, Berber E, Foroutani A, Macho JR, Pearl JM, Siperstein AE. Use of the optical access trocar for safe and rapid entry in various laparoscopic procedures. Surg Endosc. 2001;15(6):570–3.
10. Hardy I, Rousseau S. Captive uterus syndrome: an unrecognized complication of cesarean sections? Med Hypotheses. 2019;122:98–102. https://doi.org/10.1016/j.mehy.2018.10.010. Epub 2018 Oct 24. PMID: 30593433.
11. Nezhat C, Grace LA, Razavi GM, Mihailide C, Bamford H. Reverse vesicouterine fold dissection for laparoscopic hysterectomy after prior cesarean deliveries. Obstet Gynecol. 2016;128(3):629–33. https://doi.org/10.1097/AOG.0000000000001593.

Minimally Invasive Sentinel Lymph Node Mapping for Cancer of Endometrium

17

Nutan Jain, Shivam Vatsal, and Sakshi Srivastava

17.1 Introduction

Cancer stands as the leading cause of mortality and morbidity worldwide [1]. Endometrial cancer poses a global challenge, with approximately 417,000 new cases reported annually and the incidence and mortality rates are increasing every year [2]. In the United States, endometrial cancer is the fourth most frequently diagnosed cancer among females and the sixth leading cause of mortality [3]. In the Asian countries, the incidence is also increasing probably due to increased body weight and physical inactivity [4]. Data suggests that 67% of cases with cancer endometrium at diagnosis are confined to the uterus [5]. Regional and distant disease comprises about 21% and 8% of cases respectively. The most important prognostic factor in the disease being the depth of myometrial invasion and lymph node metastasis; other being the grade of invasion, lymphovascular space invasion, and lower uterine segment invasion. Metrorrhagia and postmenopausal bleeding are generally the presenting symptoms, usually first screened by ultrasonography. If found suspicious, then office endometrial biopsy is done. Fractional dilatation and curettage is done if office endoscopy is negative in suspicious patients. Hysteroscopy guided biopsy is needed in case of endometrial polyps. MRI, USG and FDG-PET CT scans are required for disease assessment and staging as per the indication, symptoms and need. TAH/BSO (Total laparoscopic hysterectomy with/without bilateral salpingo-oophorectomy) either open/laparoscopic/robotic with pelvic and para-aortic lymphadenectomy was the standard surgical management of carcinoma endometrium for long. But to reduce the long and short-term morbidity associated with lymphadenectomy and with better understanding of the disease behavior, and depth of myometrial invasion; currently a more selective and tailored approach is followed. Based on preoperative imaging denoting the grade and depth of myometrium invasion; nodal evaluation with SLN mapping of early-stage disease or low risk patients, and a complete lymphadenectomy for locally advanced disease and high-risk patients is proposed. Adjuvant treatment modality is primarily radiation therapy or systemic chemotherapy. Minimally invasive hysterectomy is the preferred method, which offers less hospital stay, less morbidity and less blood loss and has better recovery rate as compared to open hysterectomy. Laparoscopic hysterectomy has been now the standard of care in cancer endometrium. Due to the drawbacks associated with systematic lymphadenectomy, the National Comprehensive Cancer Network (NCCN) [6] and European Society of Medical Oncology (ESMO) [7] have advocated the concept of sentinel lymph node (SLN) mapping and biopsy in patients with early-stage endometrial cancer.

17.2 Sentinel Lymphatic Mapping in endometrial cancer

The word "sentinel" in oxford dictionary refers to a guardian, and the SLN represents the initial lymph node or group of lymph nodes in a lymphatic chain where cancer is likely

Supplementary Information The online version contains supplementary material available at https://doi.org/10.1007/978-981-97-3226-5_17. The videos can be accessed individually by clicking the DOI link in the accompanying figure caption or by scanning this link with the SN More Media App.

N. Jain (✉)
GSVM Medical College, Kanpur Affiliated by Kanpur University, Kanpur, India

Department of Obstetrics and Gynecology, Vardhman Trauma and Laparoscopy Centre Pvt. Ltd., Muzaffarnagar, Uttar Pradesh, India

S. Vatsal
HOD Surgical Oncology, Metro Hospital, Faridabad, India

S. Srivastava
Rohilkhand Medical College and Hospital, Affiliated by Bareilly International University, Bareilly, India

Gynaecological Endoscopic, Vardhman Trauma and Laparoscopy Centre Pvt. Ltd., Muzaffarnagar, Uttar Pradesh, India

N. Jain (ed.), *Complex Total Laparoscopic Hysterectomy (TLH) with Newer Approaches in Bladder Dissection*,
https://doi.org/10.1007/978-981-97-3226-5_17

to spread from its organ of origin. Identifying the SLN is crucial, as it has the highest risk of metastasis. If cancer is present in the first lymph node, it suggests the potential for metastasis in the rest of the lymphatic chain [8]. The SLN mapping strategy holds promise in reducing the morbidity associated with systematic lymphadenectomy, as it exposes fewer patients to these potential complications of performing a routine pelvic lymphadenectomy in all cases. This chapter aims to give an overview of how to perform laparoscopic SLN mapping and dissection; and hysterectomy for cancer endometrium. The lymphatic drainage of the endometrium is intricate. The lymph nodes of lower uterine segment and cervix drain through the parametrium to the iliac and obturator nodes at the pelvic sidewall, common iliac lymph nodes, para-aortic lymph nodes and beyond. For the uterine fundus, an alternative drainage route develops along the gonadal vessels directly to the para-aortic nodes. The uterine body lymphatics usually cross over the obliterated umbilical artery and SLN is most commonly seen medial to the external iliac, superior part of the obturator region and ventral to the hypogastric nerve. Less common location of SLN is along common iliacs in the presacral region [9]. If the sentinel lymph node (SLN) is located in the para-aortic region, it may be missed by standard SLNB techniques that primarily target pelvic nodes. A prospective study involving 742 patients reported that only 3% of patients had isolated positive para-aortic nodes when pelvic nodes were negative [10]. This suggests that the risk of isolated positive para-aortic nodes is relatively low when pelvic nodes are negative.

17.3 Importance of lymph node assessment

The majority of these women typically present with early-stage disease (around 67%), showing no signs of metastasis [11]. Since most of these tumours are confined to the uterus (International Federation of Gynaecology and Obstetrics [FIGO] stage I), the 5-year overall survival rate for this patient population ranges from 80% to 90% [12]. It's noteworthy that about 10% to 15% of these patients may have metastatic nodal disease, and almost 15% initially classified with grade 1 tumours through office biopsy or dilatation and curettage may, in fact, exhibit higher-grade disease upon final pathologic review after hysterectomy [11]. Therefore, accurately staging and treating these patients is crucial to prevent overlooking undetected metastatic disease that could lead to upstaging the patient [9].

Decisions regarding whether to perform lymphadenectomy and the extent of the procedure, such as dissection of pelvic nodes only or both pelvic and para-aortic nodes, can be guided by a combination of preoperative and intraoperative findings. Criteria have been proposed to indicate low risk for nodal metastases [13], including:

1. less than 50% myometrial invasion;
2. tumour size less than 2 cm; and
3. well or moderately differentiated histology.

The above are the inclusion criteria for SLN in cancer endometrium. Recently SLN mapping is also considered in high risk histology cases (Grade 3, serous, clear cell, carcinosarcoma pathology and depth of invasion >50%). However, accurately determining these criteria before final pathology results are available, can be challenging.

Nodal evaluation plays a crucial role in identifying patients with nodal metastasis, guiding the appropriate adjuvant treatment, that has demonstrated improvements in survival and reduced loco regional recurrence. The debate surrounding whether to include para-aortic lymphadenectomy in pelvic node dissection has been ongoing. Previous studies have presented conflicting information regarding the risk of para-aortic nodal metastases in patients without pelvic node involvement [14]. For selective patients, including those with pelvic lymphadenectomy or high-risk histologic features, consideration may be given to extending para-aortic lymphadenectomy up to the renal vessels. Lymph node dissection serves to identify patients who may benefit from adjuvant treatments such as radiation therapy (RT) and/or systemic therapy. While a subset of patients may not derive significant benefits from lymphadenectomy, preoperatively identifying these specific cases can be challenging. The National Comprehensive Cancer Network (NCCN) panel recommends nodal evaluation for patients with endometrial carcinoma, advocating for para-aortic lymphadenectomy in high-risk patients [15].

17.3.1 Advantages of SLN Mapping

1. It is a more targeted method of assessing the spread of apparent early-stage endometrial cancer, compared with systematic lymph node dissection,
2. It improves staging accuracy and enables appropriate selection of adjuvant radiotherapy or chemotherapy
3. It avoids overtreatment.
4. The nodes undergo ultra-staging and this increases detection of lymph node metastasis.
5. Standard histopathological report will miss micro metastases.
6. It reduces morbidity associated with complete lymphadenectomy
7. It allows for node ultra-staging on limited number of nodes.

17.3.2 ICG

Fluorescent SLN localization with ICG is currently the preferred mapping method. ICG is a water-soluble tricarbocyanine dye known for emitting a fluorescent signal in the near-infrared (NIR) light range. Near-infrared (NIR) imagers, designed to receive the 830 nm wavelength emitted by ICG, enable the visualization of the dye during surgery (Fig. 17.1). These imagers are adaptable to various surgical approaches, including laparotomy, laparoscopy, and robotic surgery. One of the significant advantages of ICG is its real-time visualization capabilities during dissection, offering a combination of colorimetric and radionuclear techniques. In comparison to blue dyes, ICG has demonstrated superiority in detection, particularly in obese patients [16]. Despite its advantages, the main drawback of ICG is the requirement for specialized NIR imaging equipment. However, the risk of adverse events associated with ICG is extremely low, with a reported incidence of anaphylaxis being 1 in 42,000 cases. It is important to note that ICG should be avoided in patients with severe iodine allergy or liver failure, as the dye is excreted entirely by the liver. The main contraindication is iodine allergy, which the current US-available product contains. The SLN detection rates with ICG and the bilateral SLN detection rates appear comparable or better than those of blue dye only or radiocolloid. Various laparoscopic systems have an inbuilt NIR system for ICG mapping. The preferred site of ICG injection is at the cervix at 3 o'clock and 9 o'clock position [6]. Injecting dye into the uterine cervix proves effective in achieving excellent dye penetration into the uterine vessels and the primary uterine lymphatic trunks.

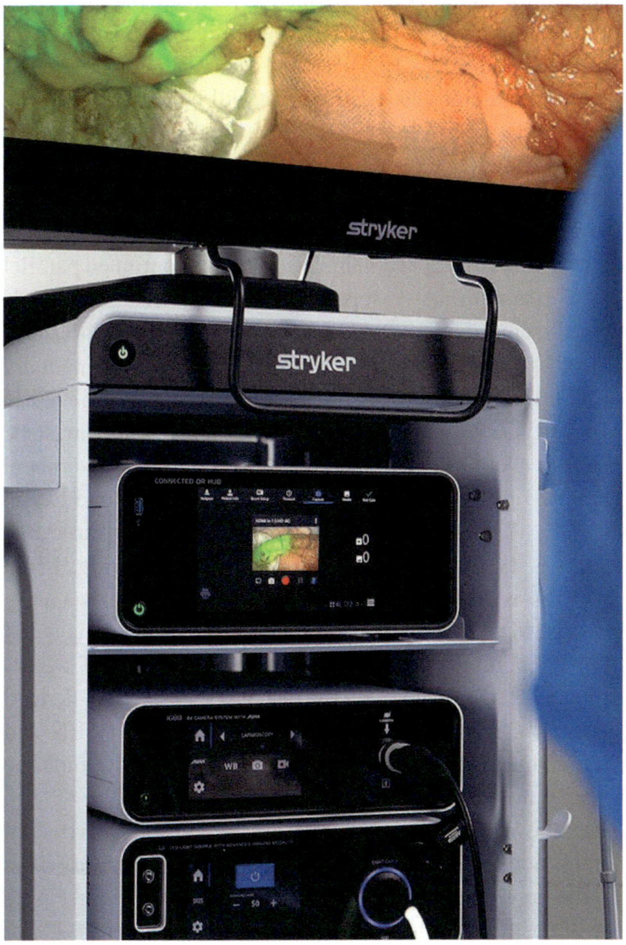

Fig. 17.1 Stryker 1688 Advanced Imaging Modalities (AIM) 4K Platform enables the visualization of sentinel lymph nodes through ICG mapping

17.3.3 Sentinel Lymph Node Biopsy Algorithm

A surgical algorithm for Sentinel Lymph Node (SLN) mapping is proposed to reduce the false-negative rate in patients with apparent uterine-confined disease. SLN mapping may be particularly suitable for individuals at low to intermediate risk for metastases or those who may not tolerate a standard lymphadenectomy [17]. It is recommended that SLN identification should be performed before hysterectomy, except in cases where the removal of a bulky uterus is necessary for accessing iliac vessels and lymph nodes. The surgeon's expertise and attention to technical details are crucial during SLN mapping, as it can potentially spare patients from the morbidity associated with a standard lymphadenectomy. Since SLNs identify the primary lymphatic pathway, they enhance the likelihood of detecting metastatic disease during the mapping process. In cases of failed SLN mapping, re-injection of the cervix may be considered. However, if SLN mapping is unsuccessful, a reflex side-specific nodal dissection should be performed, and any suspicious or grossly enlarged nodes should be removed, irrespective of mapping results.

The Society of Gynecologic Oncology (SGO) conducted a literature review and released consensus recommendations for SLN mapping in endometrial cancer [18]. Adhering closely to the National Comprehensive Cancer Network (NCCN), SLN surgical algorithm was found to result in accurate prediction of pelvic lymph node metastasis with a false-negative rate of less than 5% [19]. It is emphasized that SLN mapping should be performed in institutions with expertise in this procedure.

Historically, SLN mapping was controversial in patients with high-risk histology (e.g., serous carcinoma, clear cell carcinoma, carcinosarcoma) [20]. However, recent reports suggest promising results for SLN mapping in patients with high-risk histologies, serving as a potential alternative to complete lymphadenectomy [21]. A multi-institutional retrospective study concluded that SLN mapping versus SLN mapping with lymphadenectomy in high-risk endometrial cancer did not impact survival outcomes [22]. A prospective, multicenter cohort study (SENTOR-trial) demonstrated the acceptable accuracy of SLN mapping in high-grade endometrial cancer, further supporting its value for surgical staging in this patient population [23].

We at our center follow the SLNB(sentinel lymph node biopsy) algorithm which refers to.

1. peritoneal and serosal inspection and peritoneal washings.
2. retroperitoneal evaluation localization of stained lymphatic channels from the parametria to the primary nodal basin, and removing all SLNs and any suspicious large sized nodes
3. retroperitoneal dissection up to common iliac region, presacral region and/or para-aortic region to look for rare, isolated para-aortic lymph nodes especially when no pelvic SLN is found
4. a side-specific systematic lymph node dissection, if SLN is not detected on the ipsilateral hemipelvis.

It has been shown that the rate of systematic lymph node dissection was reduced from 65% to 23% since the introduction of such SLNB algorithm [9].

17.4 Surgical Technique of Sentinel Lymph Node Biopsy in Endometrial Cancer

The success of sentinel lymph node mapping depends on various factors, such as patient's age, depth of myometrial invasion, risk of lymphatic infiltration [24], surgical expertise [25]and the algorithm in sentinel lymph node mapping failure [26].

To optimize the detection of sentinel lymph nodes, we prepare ICG solution in the operating room by dissolving 25 mg of sterile amorphous ICG in 10 mL of distilled water (concentration of 2.5 mg/mL). Two milliliters of this solution is taken and further diluted in 10 ml of distilled water (concentration around 0.5 mg/mL). Patient position to be kept in low lithotomy. Following general anesthesia, inject 1 ml of ICG at two points, precisely at 03:00 and 09:00 o'clock positions in the cervical stroma (approximately at a depth of 1–2 centimeters). 1 mL is also injected into the submucosa (approximately at a depth of 1–3 mm) (Fig. 17.2a, b. Care is taken to prevent excess amount of ICG, otherwise most of the surgical field turns green.

Once the ICG is injected, ports are made and pneumoperitoneum is created. By this time, ICG dye would have well reached its destination in the SLN, turning it as fluorescent green. Alternatively, pneumoperitoneum can be created initially followed by port placement and thereafter injection of ICG dye can be done in the cervix. This could also help us in visualization of the lymphatic tracts and accumulation of dye in the sentinel node in real time. We may use two modes, either the NIR (near infrared imaging), or the ONLAY mode. ONLAY mode is easy to use, as the normal laparoscopic picture has a super added fluorescent green image of SLN. For the NIR image, we have to change over the camera system to NIR image setting and then see the fluorescent green lymph nodes (Fig. 17.3). Slight modifications are to be done when SLN mapping is done as retroperitoneal dissection would be difficult with normal port positions of laparoscopic hysterectomy. We prefer to place the camera at supraumbilical port, at least 2 cm above; to have a better lateral view and ease of performing laterally. We have been doing SLN mapping for last seven years and found good co-relation of the entire system of injecting ICG, staining the lymph nodes, their removal and sending for HPE; closely correlating with patient's clinical and oncological outcomes. A close adherence to the algorithm is needed, to ensure complete benefits of SLN mapping.

Bipolar forceps and energy sources like HARMONIC ACE™ (Ethicon Johnson &Johnson surgical, USA) are the most common instruments used while performing the SLN mapping and dissection. We begin with an incision in the triangle which has been described to be made parallel to the infundibulopelvic ligament, the round ligament and the pelvic side wall (Fig. 17.4). Round ligament could also be divided as laterally as possible that will help in opening the space (Fig. 17.5). Anterior leaf of broad ligament is then opened caudally upto the parietal origin of round ligament and cephalically upto the point where gonadal vessels cross the external iliac vessels. This aids in visualization of the external iliac artery and vein. Dissection is continued parallel to the external iliac vessels. Caudally the dissection is made upto the umbilical artery and the paravesical fossa, inferiorly upto the obturator fossa. Further dissection is made medially to identify the ureter (Fig. 17.6). Dissection is continued to expose the internal iliac vessels (Fig. 17.7). Care must be taken to avoid injury to the veins. The obliterated umbilical artery divides the para-vesical space into medial and lateral (Fig. 17.8). Internal iliac artery must be carefully dissected as this is the most common location of the SLN (Fig. 17.9). Once this is done, inferiorly obturator nerve, which is a whitish cord like structure is visible [27]. Now our field is ready for harvesting the SLN. One must be curious that if we are doing SLN, then why to go for such an extensive full-fledged dissection; reason being to harvest all the green SLN and avoid injury to vessels and ureter. Dissection should be directly over the fluorescent green lymph node (Fig. 17.10). The site of dissection is inspected to confirm no residual lymph nodes (Fig. 17.11). Similar dissection is carried out on the contralateral side (Fig. 17.12a–i). So, we start doing the dissection and the lymph node is excised out and we take two endo bags, one for the right side and one for the left side (Fig. 17.13). Usually, the most common draining sites for cancer endometrium are the internal iliac, external iliac groups and the obturator group of lymph nodes. However,

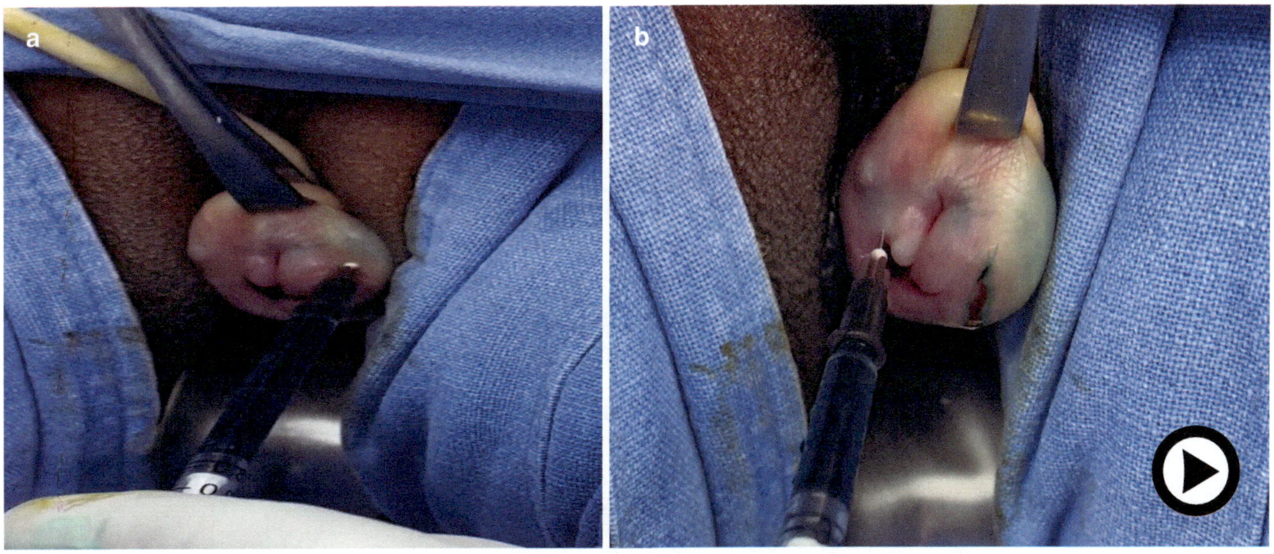

Fig. 17.2 **a** Injecting ICG dye on right side of cervix at 3 o' clock position (Video 17.2a Sentinel Node Sampling in TLH) (▶ https://doi.org/10.1007/000-c9b). **b** Injecting ICG dye on left side of cervix at 9 o' clock position

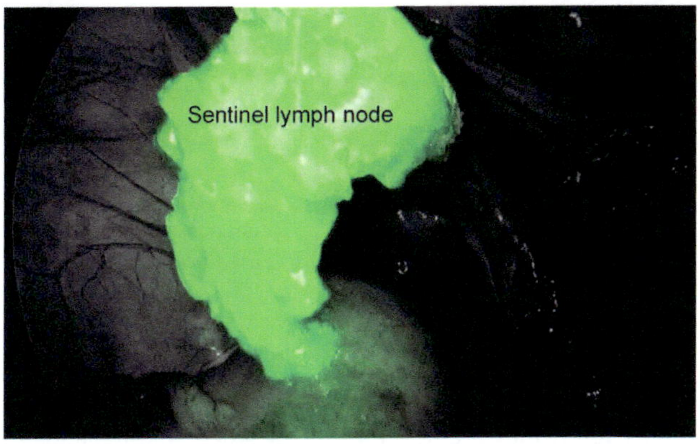

Fig. 17.3 The NIR view helps in distinguishing the sentinel lymph node from lymphatic channels and fat

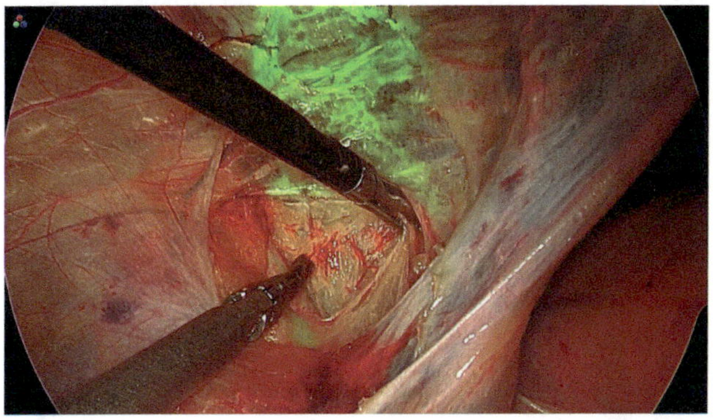

Fig. 17.5 Coagulation and cutting the left round ligament allows access into the retroperitoneal space which will aid in visualization of the ICG mapping

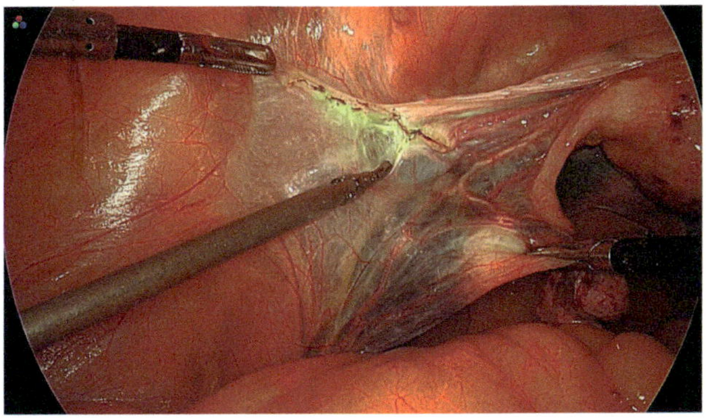

Fig. 17.4 Making incision parallel to the left infundibulopelvic ligament

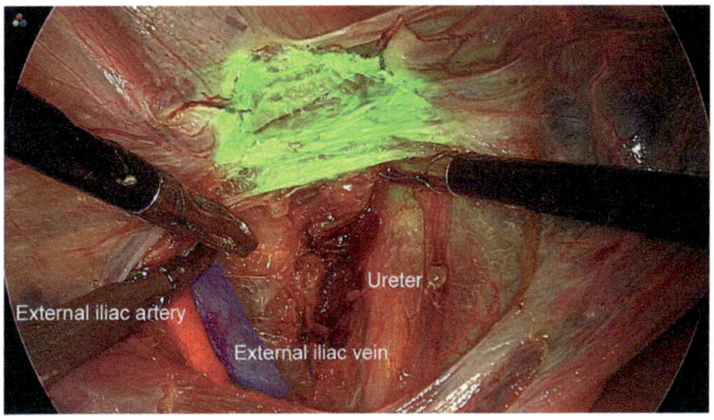

Fig. 17.6 The left paravesical and pararectal spaces are opened up and the ureter is identified to avoid injury

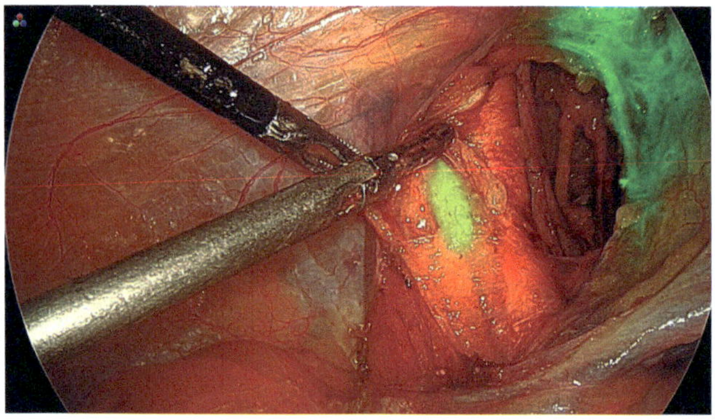

Fig. 17.7 Dissection proceeds anterior to the node

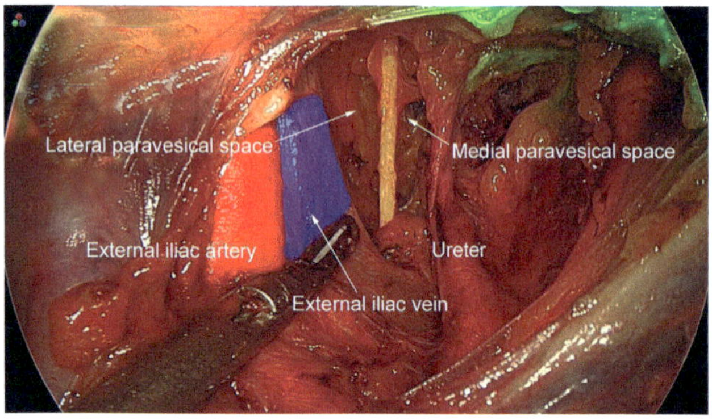

Fig. 17.8 The obliterated umbilical artery divides the paravesical space into medial and lateral

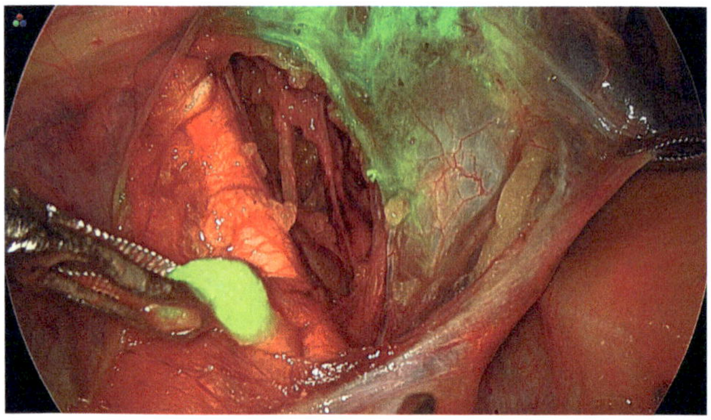

Fig. 17.9 Most common location of sentinel lymph node is lateral paravesical space near the external and internal iliac artery

any lymph nodes could be involved and whichever lymph node appears to be fluorescent green; is taken up for removal and put in respective bags.

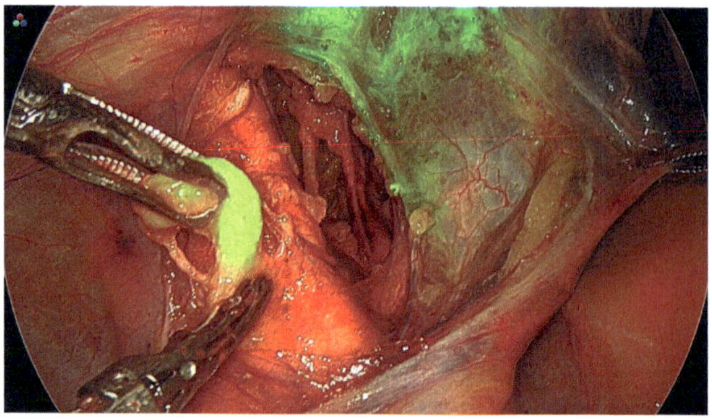

Fig. 17.10 The left sentinel lymph node is carefully dissected away from the underlying left external iliac artery

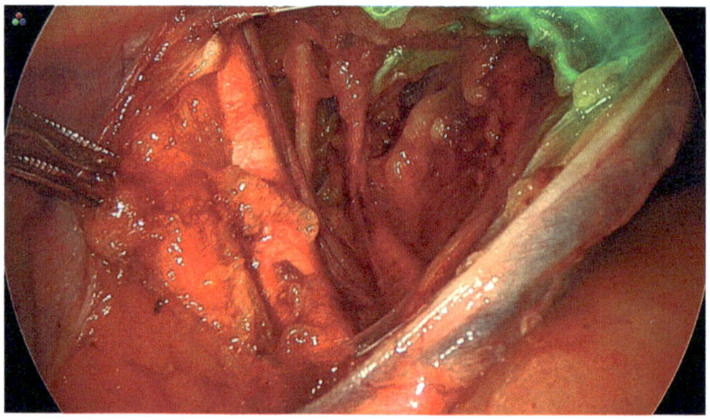

Fig. 17.11 The site of dissection is inspected to confirm no residual lymph nodes

It is important to note that if any enlarged lymph node is seen, even if they are not fluorescent green, and look suspicious, they must be removed along with SLN mapping. Complete ureteral dissection is not mandatory, but in most cases, will be needed while doing a sentinel lymph node mapping, else there is high chance of injury to ureter and iliac vessels. Hence it is advisable to do a ureteric dissection initially before dissecting and removing SLN. If no SLN is identified, then ipsilateral pelvic lymphadenectomy is to be performed [17, 19, 28].

After SLN mapping, we proceed with laparoscopic hysterectomy. If the tumor involves the lower uterine segment, where parametrial clearance is needed, TYPE II radical hysterectomy is indicated. TLH is completed in the usual manner.

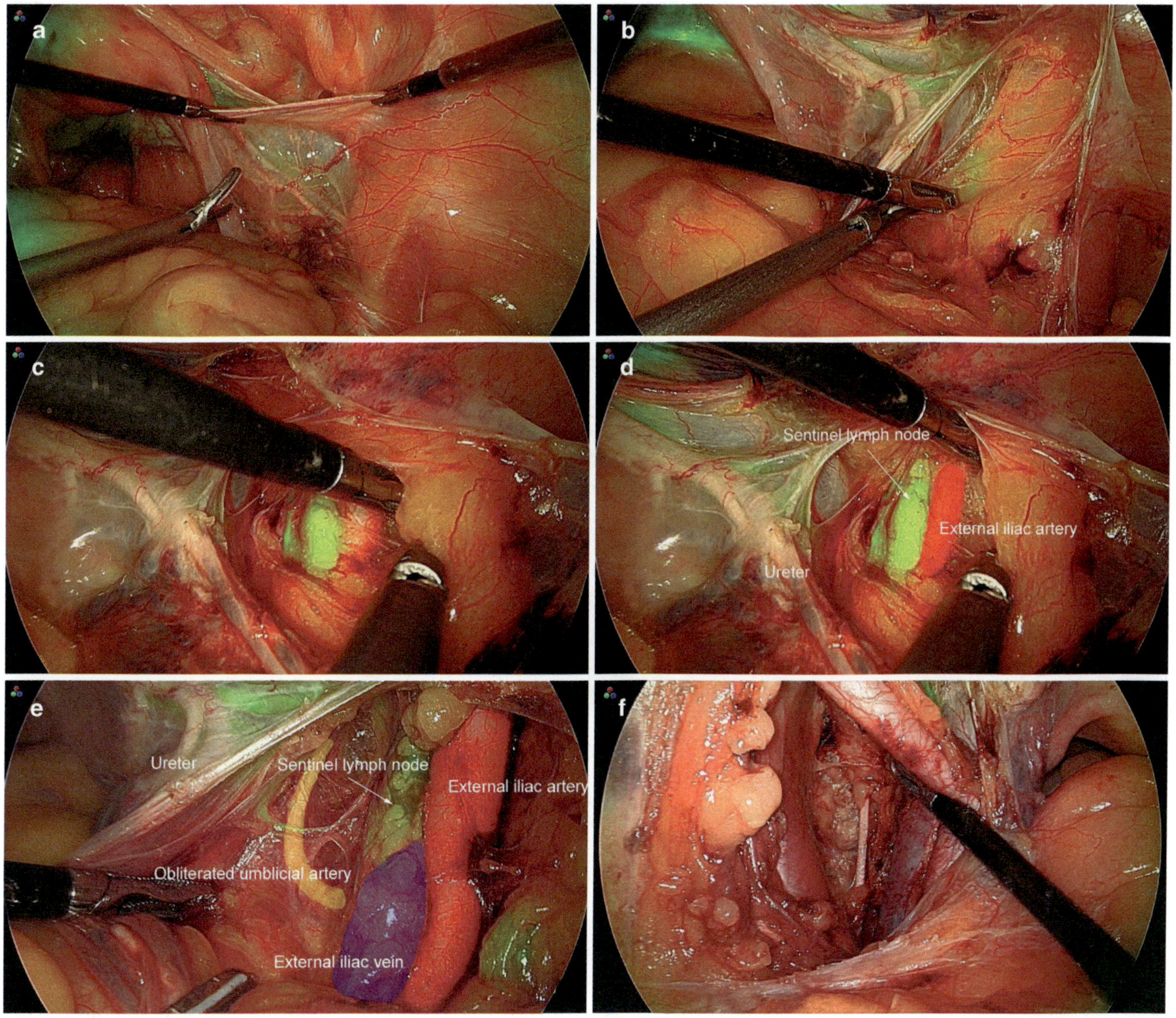

Fig. 17.12 **a** Dissection is then proceeded to the right side. **b** The right broad ligament is dissected parallel to the infundibulopelvic ligament in order to make entry into the right retroperitoneal space. **c** The right pararectal and paravesical spaces are opened to identify the right sentinel lymph node and avoid injury to critical structures. **d** The ICG channels are identified crossing across the obliterated umbilical artery to the sentinel lymph node located near the right external iliac artery. **e** The right ureter is deflected medially to avoid injury. **f** When dissecting the paravesical space, the median umbilical ligament and obturator nerve are the two important landmarks to identify the sentinel lymph nodes. **g** the right sentinel lymph node excised from right external iliac vein. **h** the right sentinel lymph node is excised under direct visualization. **i** At the end of dissection, the ureter is inspected for peristalsis. No further lymph nodes are identified in the area of dissection

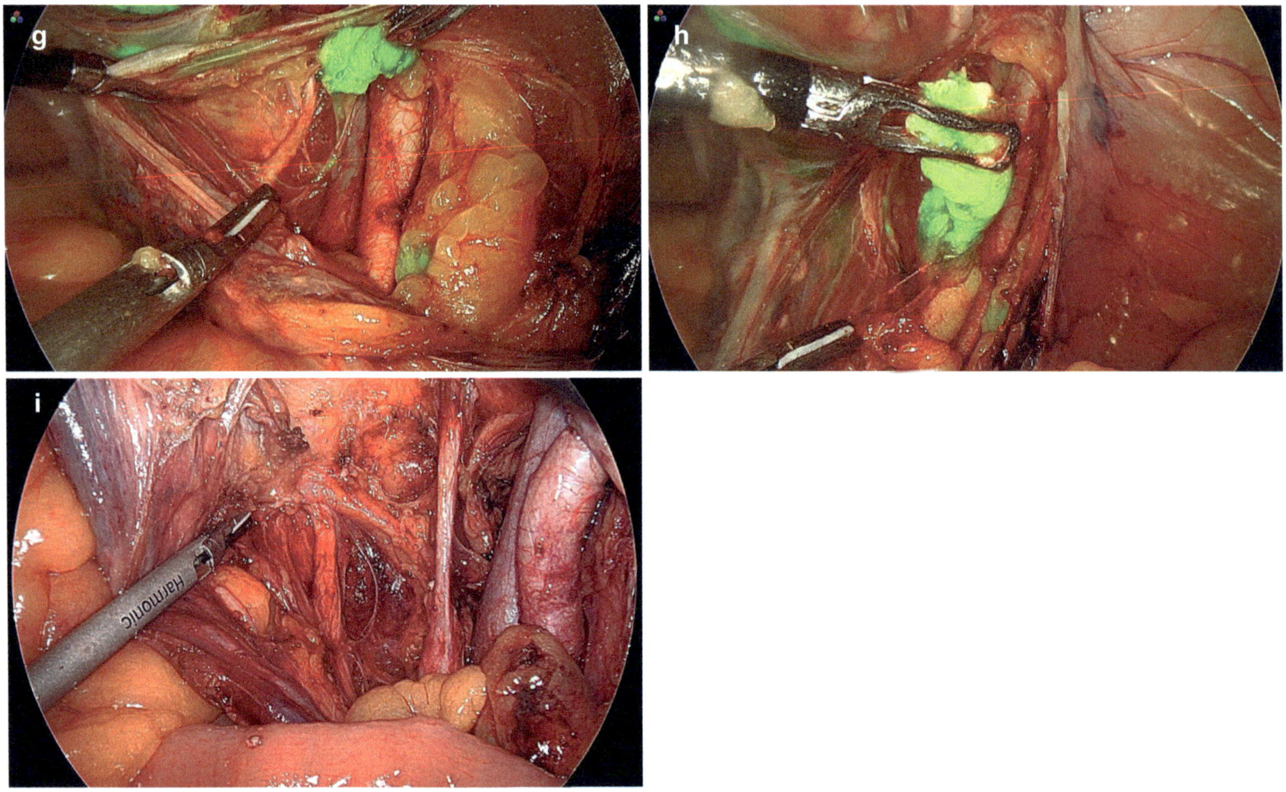

Fig. 17.12 (continued)

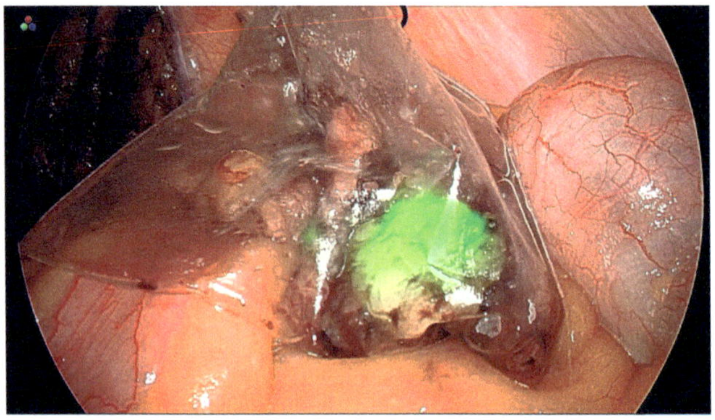

Fig. 17.13 The respective sentinel lymph nodes are kept in separate labelled endobags and removed

17.5 SLN Ultra Staging Protocol

A crucial aspect of the added value of Sentinel Lymph Node (SLN) procedures in endometrial cancer is the implementation of enhanced pathology, often referred to as ultra staging. Sentinel lymph nodes (SLNs) in endometrial cancer cases should undergo ultra staging to detect low-volume metastasis. Ultra staging typically involves deeper serial sectioning of the gross SLN and the review of multiple haematoxylin and eosin (H&E)stained sections, with or without cytokeratin immunohistochemical (IHC) staining [9].

- The initial examination is performed using hematoxylin and eosin (H&E) staining.
- If the H&E assessment is negative, 2 adjacent 5-mcg sections are cut in a bread loaf fashion from each paraffin block at each of 2 levels, 50 mcg apart.
- At each level, one slide is stained with H&E and the other is reserved for immunohistochemistry staining (IHC) using the anti-cytokeratin AE1:AE3 for a total of 4 slides per block.

17.6 Conclusion

Sentinel Lymph Node (SLN) mapping provides enhanced intraoperative surgical precision, enabling the identification of nodes more likely to harbor metastasis. It also avoids unnecessary pelvic lymphadenectomy for all cases, reducing the cost of treatment, reducing hospital stay and morbidities like lymphocele, vessel & ureteric injury. This, coupled with improved pathology protocols, has demonstrated an increase in the detection of nodal metastasis. The heightened sensitivity in detecting metastasis through SLN mapping has the potential to influence the staging of the disease and may lead to alterations in adjuvant therapy recommendations. This approach contributes to a more refined and individualized management of patients, facilitating a more targeted response based on the specific characteristics of the disease.

Learning Points

- Surgical approaches for endometrial cancer have shifted from traditional to minimally invasive methods, aiming to reduce morbidity.
- Surgical management has evolved to a more selective approach based on preoperative imaging, grade and depth of myometrial invasion.
- Sentinel lymph node mapping is an acceptable alternative to complete lymphadenectomy in early-stage endometrial cancer, to reduce morbidity.
- SLN mapping helps in identifying and taking a biopsy of initial lymph nodes likely to contain cancer cells.
- The role of SLN mapping lies in providing enhanced surgical precision, accurate staging, individualized management, and influencing adjuvant therapy decisions.

Competing Interest The author declares no conflict of interest that are relevant to content of this chapter.

Ethical Approval Informed consent was obtained from individual participants and patients regarding publication and documentation without disclosing their identity.

References

1. World Health Organization (WHO). Global health estimates 2020: deaths by cause, age, sex, by country and by region, 2000–2019, vol. 2020. WHO. Accessed December 11, 2020.
2. Sung H, Ferlay J, Siegel RL, Laversanne M, Soerjomataram I, Jemal A, Bray F. Global cancer statistics 2020: GLOBOCAN estimates of incidence and mortality worldwide for 36 cancers in 185 countries. CA Cancer J Clin. 2021;71(3):209–49. https://doi.org/10.3322/caac.21660. Epub 2021 Feb 4. PMID: 33538338.
3. Henley SJ, Ward EM, Scott S, Ma J, Anderson RN, Firth AU, Thomas CC, Islami F, Weir HK, Lewis DR, Sherman RL, Wu M, Benard VB, Richardson LC, Jemal A, Cronin K, Kohler BA. Annual report to the nation on the status of cancer, part I: National cancer statistics. Cancer. 2020;126(10):2225–49. https://doi.org/10.1002/cncr.32802. Epub 2020 Mar 12. PMID: 32162336; PMCID: PMC7299151.
4. Lortet-Tieulent J, Ferlay J, Bray F, Jemal A. International patterns and trends in endometrial cancer incidence, 1978–2013. J Natl Cancer Inst. 2018;110(4):354–61. https://doi.org/10.1093/jnci/djx214. PMID: 29045681.
5. Abu-Rustum NR, Alektiar K, Iasonos A, et al. The incidence of symptomatic lower-extremity lymphedema following treatment of uterine corpus malignancies: a 12-year experience at Memorial Sloan-Kettering Cancer Center. Gynecol Oncol. 2006;103:714–8.
6. Abu-Rustum N, Yashar C, Arend R, Barber E, Bradley K, Brooks R, Campos SM, Chino J, Chon HS, Chu C, Crispens MA, Damast S, Fisher CM, Frederick P, Gaffney DK, Giuntoli R, Han E, Holmes J, Howitt BE, Lea J, Mariani A, Mutch D, Nagel C, Nekhlyudov L, Podoll M, Salani R, Schorge J, Siedel J, Sisodia R, Soliman P, Ueda S, Urban R, Wethington SL, Wyse E, Zanotti K, NR MM, Aggarwal S. Uterine neoplasms, version 1.2023, NCCN Clinical Practice Guidelines in oncology. J Natl Compr Canc Netw. 2023;21(2):181–209. https://doi.org/10.6004/jnccn.2023.0006. PMID: 36791750.
7. Oaknin A, Bosse TJ, Creutzberg CL, Giornelli G, Harter P, Joly F, Lorusso D, Marth C, Makker V, Mirza MR, Ledermann JA, Colombo N; ESMO Guidelines Committee. Electronic address: clinicalguidelines@esmo.org. Endometrial cancer: ESMO Clinical Practice Guideline for diagnosis, treatment and follow-up. Ann Oncol 2022;33(9):860–877. doi: https://doi.org/10.1016/j.annonc.2022.05.009. Epub 2022 Jun 8. PMID: 35690222.
8. Hari AY, Tewari KS. Sentinel lymphatic mapping for gynecologic malignancies. Curr Opin Obstet Gynecol. 2023;35(1):43–53. https://doi.org/10.1097/GCO.0000000000000841. PMID: 36595648.
9. Abu-Rustum NR. Sentinel lymph node mapping for endometrial cancer: a modern approach to surgical staging. J Natl Compr Cancer Netw. 2014;12(2):288–97. https://doi.org/10.6004/jnccn.2014.0026. PMID: 24586087.
10. Kumar S, Podratz KC, Bakkum-Gamez JN, Dowdy SC, Weaver AL, McGree ME, Cliby WA, Keeney GL, Thomas G, Mariani A. Prospective assessment of the prevalence of pelvic, paraaortic and high paraaortic lymph node metastasis in endometrial cancer. Gynecol Oncol. 2014;132(1):38–43. https://doi.org/10.1016/j.ygyno.2013.10.002. Epub 2013 Oct 9. PMID: 24120926; PMCID: PMC4381544.
11. Abu-Rustum NR, Khoury-Collado F, Pandit-Taskar N, et al. Sentinel lymph node mapping for grade 1 endometrial cancer: is it the answer to the surgical staging dilemma? Gynecol Oncol. 2009;113:163–9.
12. Creasman WT, Odicino F, Maisonneuve P, et al. Carcinoma of the corpus uteri. J Epidemiol Biostat. 2001;6:47–86.
13. Milam MR, Java J, Walker JL, et al. Nodal metastasis risk in endometrioid endometrial cancer. Obstet Gynecol. 2012;119:286–92.
14. Mariani A, Dowdy SC, Cliby WA, et al. Prospective assessment of lymphatic dissemination in endometrial cancer: a paradigm shift in surgical staging. Gynecol Oncol. 2008;109:11–8.
15. NCCN, Uterine Neoplasms, Version 3.2021-JUNE 03 2021. NCCN clinical practice guidelines in oncology. J Natl Compr Cancer Netw 2021:26–29.
16. Martínez Bravo WR, García Vicente AM, Noriega Álvarez E, González García B, López-de la Manzanara C, Cordero García JM, Soriano Castrejón Á. Failure of scintigraphy lymphatic mapping in endometrial cancer. Causes and solutions. Rev Esp Med Nucl Imagen Mol (Engl Ed). 2022;41(2):78–85. https://doi.org/10.1016/j.remnie.2021.04.004. Epub 2021 Apr 14. PMID: 35292142.
17. Soliman PT, Westin SN, Dioun S, et al. A prospective validation study of sentinel lymph node mapping for high-risk endometrial cancer. Gynecol Oncol. 2017;146:234–9.
18. Holloway RW, Abu-Rustum NR, Backes FJ, et al. Sentinel lymph node mapping and staging in endometrial cancer: a Society of Gynecologic Oncology literature review with consensus recommendations. Gynecol Oncol. 2017;146:405–15.
19. Barlin JN, Khoury-Collado F, Kim CH, et al. The importance of applying a sentinel lymph node mapping algorithm in endometrial cancer staging: beyond removal of blue nodes. Gynecol Oncol. 2012;125:531–5.
20. Naoura I, Canlorbe G, Bendifallah S, et al. Relevance of sentinel lymph node procedure for patients with high-risk endometrial cancer. Gynecol Oncol. 2015;136:60–4.
21. Lecointre L, Lodi M, Faller E, et al. Diagnostic accuracy and clinical impact of sentinel lymph node sampling in endometrial cancer at high risk of recurrence: a meta-analysis. J Clin Med. 2020;9:3874.

22. Bogani G, Papadia A, Buda A, et al. Sentinel node mapping vs sentinel node mapping plus back-up lymphadenectomy in high-risk endometrial cancer patients: results from a multi-institutional study. Gynecol Oncol. 2021;161:122–9.
23. Cusimano MC, Vicus D, Pulman K, et al. Assessment of sentinel lymph node biopsy vs lymphadenectomy for intermediate- and high-grade endometrial cancer staging. JAMA Surg. 2021;156:157–64.
24. Capozzi VA, Valentina C, Giulio S, Alessandra C, Giulia G, Giulia A, Vito C, Roberto B. Sentinel node mapping in endometrial cancer: tips and tricks to improve bilateral detection rate. The sentitricks study, a monocentric experience. Taiwan J Obstet Gynecol. 2021;60(1):31–5. https://doi.org/10.1016/j.tjog.2020.11.006. PMID: 33495004.
25. Koskas M, Amant F, Mirza MR, Creutzberg CL. Cancer of the corpus uteri: 2021 update. Int J Gynaecol Obstet. 2021;155(Suppl 1(Suppl 1)):45–60. https://doi.org/10.1002/ijgo.13866. PMID: 34669196; PMCID: PMC9297903.
26. Holloway RW, Ahmad S, Kendrick JE, Bigsby GE, Brudie LA, Ghurani GB, Stavitzski NM, Gise JL, Ingersoll SB, Pepe JW. A prospective cohort study comparing colorimetric and fluorescent imaging for sentinel lymph node mapping in endometrial cancer. Ann Surg Oncol. 2017;24(7):1972–9. https://doi.org/10.1245/s10434-017-5825-3. Epub 2017 Mar 6. PMID: 28265777.
27. Guan J, Xue Y, Zang RY, Liu JH, Zhu JQ, Zheng Y, Wang B, Wang HY, Chen XJ. Sentinel lymph Node mapping versus systematic pelvic lymphadenectomy on the prognosis for patients with intermediate-high-risk Endometrial Cancer confined to the uterus before surgery: trial protocol for a non-inferiority randomized controlled trial (SNEC trial). J Gynecol Oncol. 2021;32(4):e60. https://doi.org/10.3802/jgo.2021.32.e60. PMID: 34085796; PMCID: PMC8192227.
28. Int J Gynecol Cancer: first published as 10.1136/ijgc-2019 000847 on 18 December 2019.Downloaded from http://ijgc.bmj.com/ on December 19, 2019 at Ankara Univ.

18 Laparoscopic Radical Hysterectomy: Pune Technique

Shailesh Puntambekar, Madhavi Patil, Mangesh Panse, Seema Puntambekar, Ravindra M. Sathe, Mihir Chitale, Kshitij Manerikar, and Aishwarya Puntambekar

18.1 Introduction

Uterine corpus cancer ranked as the sixth most frequently identified cancer in women, witnessing 417,000 new cases and 97,000 fatalities in 2020 [1]. Notably, birth cohort effects were prominently observed in several countries, including Japan, the Philippines, Belarus, Singapore, India, Lithuania, Costa Rica, and New Zealand. This trend may be attributed, at least in part, to the growing prevalence of risk factors such as excess body weight and physical inactivity in more recent generations [2]. The reported increase in incidence in recent years is likely due to heightened awareness and improved screening practices [3].

Cervical cancer ranks as the fourth most commonly identified cancer and the fourth primary contributor to cancer-related fatalities among women. In 2020, there were approximately 604,000 new cases and 342,000 deaths globally associated with this disease [4]. It stands out as the most prevalent cancer in 23 nations and holds the position of the primary cause of cancer-related deaths in 36 countries [5]. Due to inadequate screening initiatives and a lack of awareness, a significant majority- 70% or more of patients are diagnosed at stage III or beyond when seeking medical attention [6]. The treatment options available to these patients are limited because they present with advanced diseases [7].

The primary and most widely accepted method for treating uterine cancer is a radical hysterectomy. Since the first radical hysterectomy performed by Clark in 1895 and the advent of Wertheim's technique of radical hysterectomy in 1898, radical hysterectomy has evolved into a simpler procedure and the surgical approach has also transformed over a period of time into a highly specialised and minimally invasive modality [8]. With technological advances, we can now perform the radical hysterectomy with minimally invasive techniques, such as laparoscopy and robotics [9]. After the first total laparoscopic radical hysterectomy with pelvic and paraaortic lymphadenectomy which was performed by Nezhat et al in June of 1989, in the last two decades minimally invasive endoscopic surgery has become an acceptable alternative for open method [10].

The mainstay of these procedures is less post-operative pain, an early recovery of the patient due to smaller incisions, allowing the patient to take up adjuvant treatment as early as possible and overall, 'a good quality of life of the patient' [11]. Thus, the acceptance of minimally access surgeries in recent years has increased [12].

In this chapter, the **"Pune technique"** of laparoscopic radical hysterectomy is described by the authors with operative steps that are standardised. This method becomes widely embraced due to its ease of replication. Its application in robotic radical hysterectomy, pelvic exenterations and single- port surgeries are also covered.

18.2 Laparoscopic Radical Hysterectomy

18.2.1 Indications

1. Cervical cancer ranging from stage 1A2 to stage 2A is encompassed in this category. Additionally, instances of stage 1A1 exhibiting a heightened risk of lymph node dissemination are also considered within this group.
2. Laparoscopic surgery is not contraindicated for endometrial cancer up to stage 2, even in cases where pre-operative irradiation has been administered.

Supplementary Information The online version contains supplementary material available at https://doi.org/10.1007/978-981-97-3226-5_18. The videos can be accessed individually by clicking the DOI link in the accompanying figure caption or by scanning this link with the SN More Media App.

S. Puntambekar (✉) · M. Patil · M. Panse · S. Puntambekar · R. M. Sathe · M. Chitale · K. Manerikar · A. Puntambekar
Galaxy Care Hospital, Pune, Maharashtra, India

N. Jain (ed.), *Complex Total Laparoscopic Hysterectomy (TLH) with Newer Approaches in Bladder Dissection*,
https://doi.org/10.1007/978-981-97-3226-5_18

18.2.2 Contraindications

1. Tumor size of more than 4 cm at the largest diameter.
2. Evidence of peritoneal carcinomatosis or distant metastatic disease
3. Evidence of grossly involved lymph nodes.

18.2.3 Preoperative Preparation

Liquid diet one day prior to surgery. Polyethylene glycol the night before the operation to clear the bowels so as to keep them away from the operative field. Enema and bowel wash should be avoided as this leads to dilatation of sigmoid colon.

18.2.4 Anaesthesia

A combined Regional and General Anaesthesia is administered. Regional anaesthesia—blocking the sympathetic activity, contracts the small bowel and keeps it away from the operative field.

18.2.5 Patient Position

Patient is placed in a "Modified Lloyd Davis position". A bolster is placed at the level of the anterior superior iliac spine, which causes elevation of the pelvis results in a drop of the intestines cephalad. A gauze piece is kept in the vagina to prevent loss of peritoneum after colpotomy (Fig. 18.1).

A total of five ports are used:

Camera port (10 mm) at infra-umbilical.

Working port (10 mm) at McBurney's point on right side.

(5 mm)-Port para-rectally at midclavicular line at the level of umbilicus.

A set of two 5 mm ports are inserted as mirror image on left side.

The surgeon stands on the right side, the assistant and camera surgeon on the left side.

The surgeon does not change his position during the contralateral dissection.

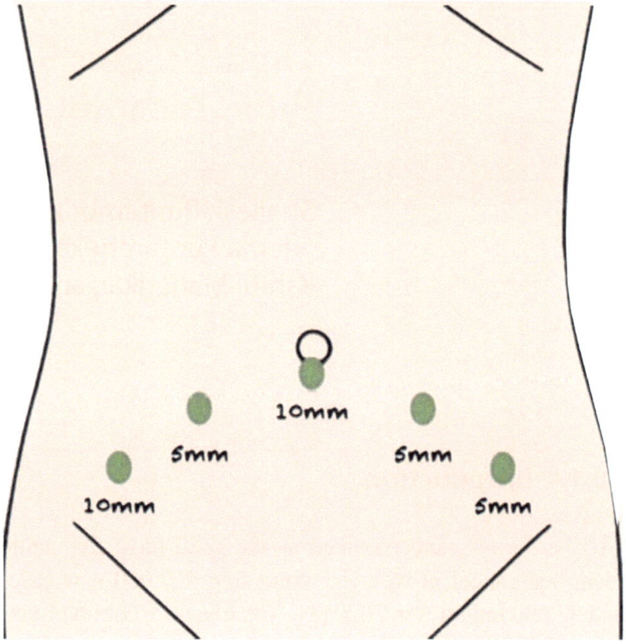

Fig. 18.1 Port positions

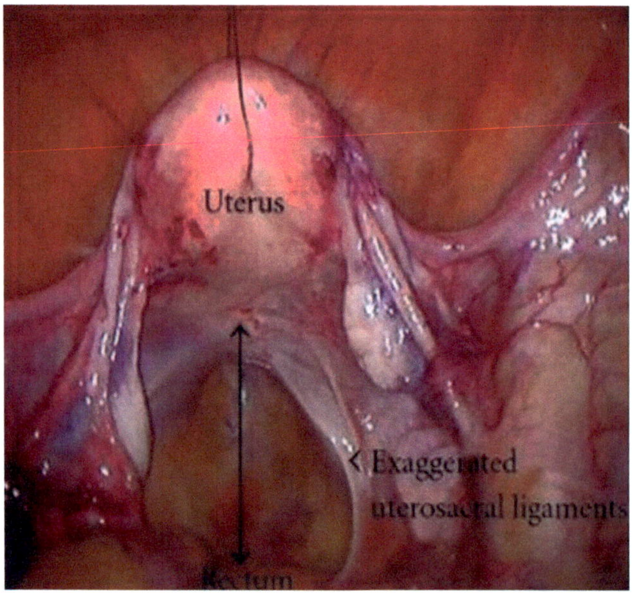

Fig. 18.2 Uterine hitched

18.2.6 Procedure

In order to manipulate the uterus in endometrial & cervical cancers uterus is hitched. Hitching the uterus is done with Monofilament polyamide suture on needle. The suture is passed through the uterine fundus antero-posteriorly and brought out to the exterior through the anterior abdominal wall (Fig. 18.2). Tenaculum forceps may be used in cervical cancers for uterine manipulation.

Step 1: Posterior U Cut (Fig. 18.3)

Uterus is anteverted. At the level of Sacral Promontory, the right ureter is identified below the peritoneum. With the help of harmonic shears, the peritoneum was able to excise medial to the ureter in order to expose the ureter. This cut is extended down upto the pouch of Douglas keeping the ureters laterally and constantly under vision. On the left side, these steps are repeated and both peritoneal cuts join to POD forming a posterior U cut (Figs. 18.3 and 18.4).

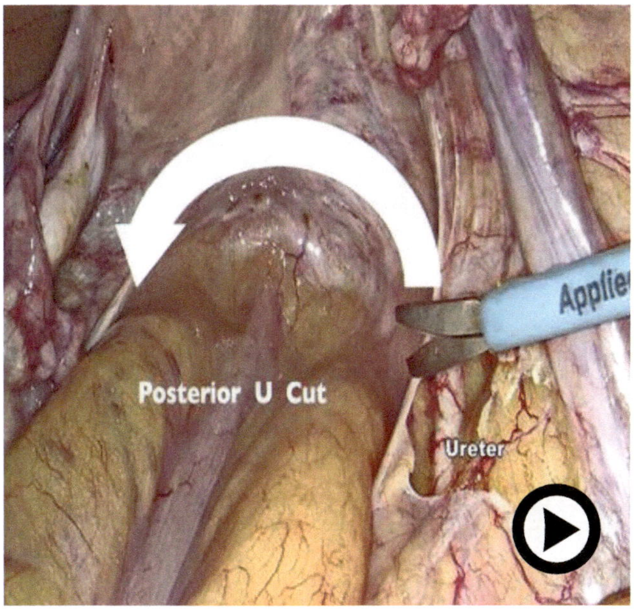

Fig. 18.3 Posterior U-cut (Video.18.3. Laparoscopic Radical Hysterectomy -Pune Technique) (▶ https://doi.org/10.1007/000-c9c)

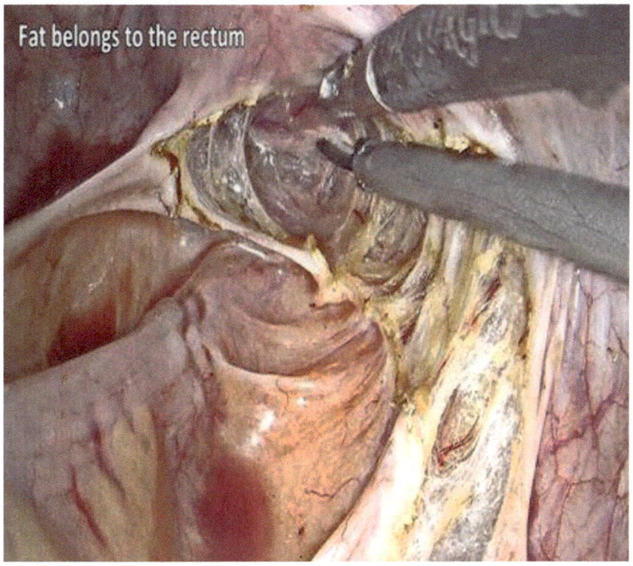

Fig. 18.4 Posterior U-cut extended

Step 2: Dissection of Rectovaginal Space (Figs. 18.5 and 18.6)
In order to stretch the peritoneum in the Pouch of Douglas, the assistant should draw the rectum cranially. The peritoneum is then cut open using harmonic shear. The insufflation of CO_2 gas opens the loose areolar planes between the 2 layers of Denonvillier's fascia. The dissection is carried out between the two layers of Denon-Villier's fascia (Fig. 18.5). Keeping in mind that **"fat belongs in the rectum,"** the plane between the fat and the posterior vaginal wall is dissected (Fig. 18.6). The rectum is dissected off the posterior vaginal wall up to the levator ani muscle.

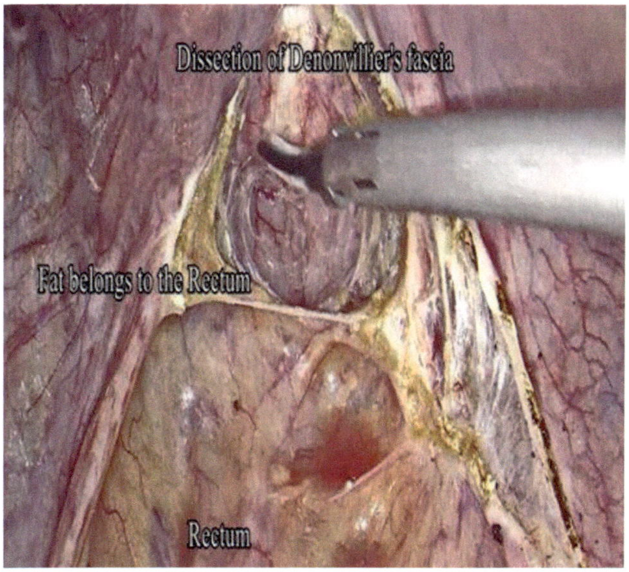

Fig. 18.5 Two layers of Denonvillers fascia

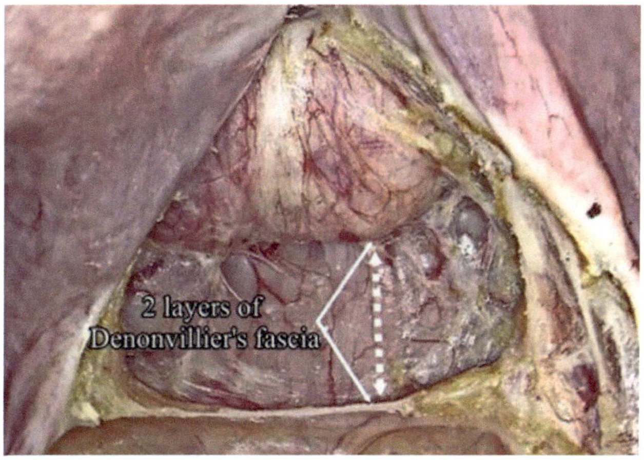

Fig. 18.6 Dissection in POD fat belongs to rectum

Step 3: Dissection of the Pararectal Space (Fig. 18.7)
The posterior leaf of broad ligament is cut above the ureter, and the left ureter is retracted medially. The incision was extended downwards, reaching the bladder and resulting in the formation of a window in the broad ligament. The pararectal space was exposed by moving the ureter medially once more and using the Harmonic Shear in a parallel and lateral motion to the ureter. Immediately evident was the internal iliac artery, which marked the lateral boundary of para-rectal space. The only structure crossing pararectal space transversely is the uterine artery.

Subsequently, the uterine artery underwent either clipping or ligation, followed by cutting; a process executed using Harmonic Shears. Within the pararectal space, the ureter demarcates both medial, also referred to as "**Okabayashi Space**," and lateral sections, commonly known as **"Latzko Space**." The ureter is pulled inward, and the dissection is carried out alongside it to expose the pararectal space. The

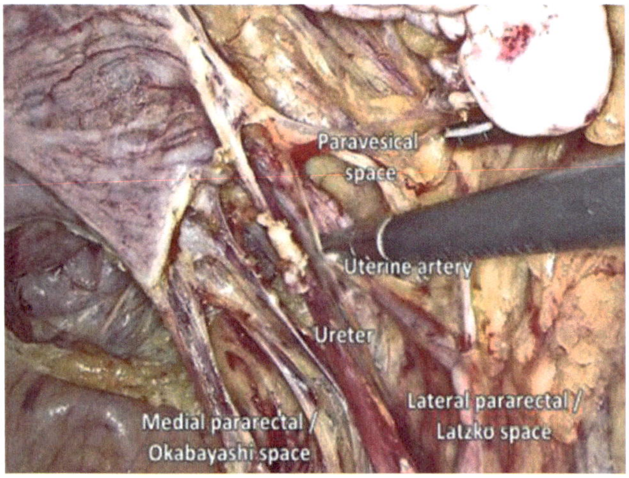

Fig. 18.7 Para-rectal space dissection

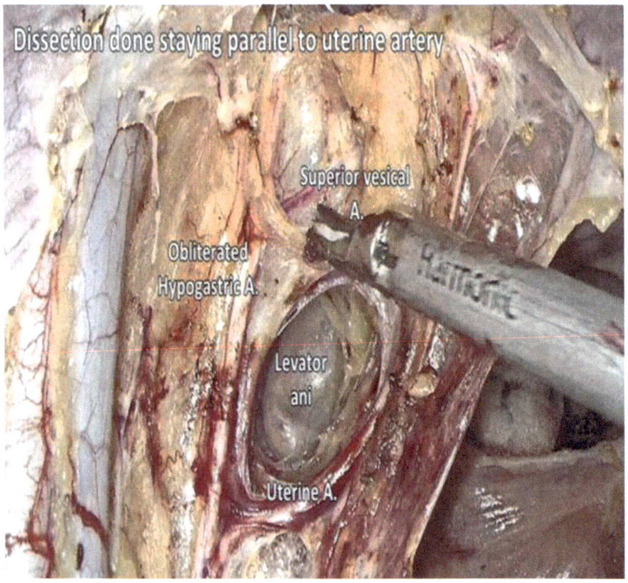

Fig. 18.8 Left para-vesical space

medial pararectal space contains the hypogastric nerves, crucial for nerve-sparing radical hysterectomy. On the other hand, the lateral pararectal space accommodates the pelvic splanchnic nerves and the uterine artery. Perfect location for clamping the uterine artery, a necessary step in any hysterectomy procedure.

The uterine artery traverses the para-rectal space in a horizontal direction. The area located in front of the uterine artery and toward the inner side of the obliterated hypogastric artery is explored & called as the para-vesical space (Fig. 18.8). This exploration extends through the para-vesical space until reaching the levator ani. Within the Para-Vesical space, one finds the umbilical artery, superior vesical artery, the neurovascular bundle of the obturator, lymphatic tissue, and accessory obturator vessels. The obliterated hypogastric

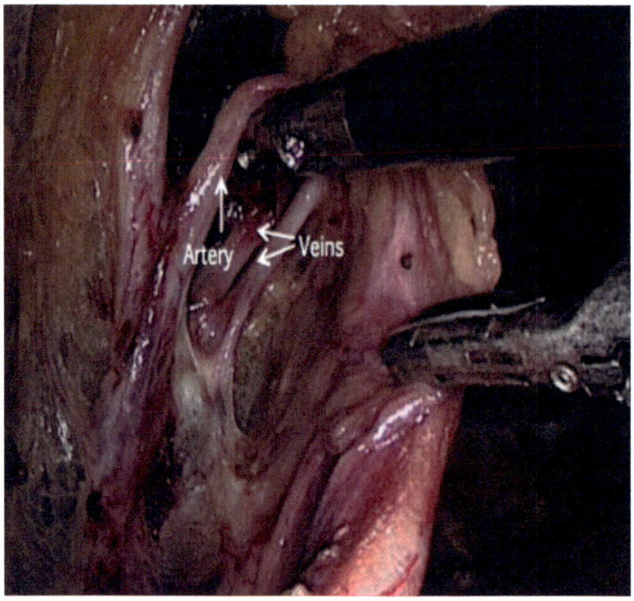

Fig. 18.9 Uterine artery-vein-ureter complex

artery divides this space into lateral paravesical space (LPS), and medial paravesical space. (MPS).

This dissection provides best acess to lateral pelvic Wall for optimal oncological clearance & Lymph Node dissection. The uterine vein is seen below the artery (Fig. 18.9). Both the artery and the vein are individually clipped or ligated and then cut.

The uterine vein ligated medial to ureter which facilitates nerve preservation, help in prevention of bladder innervation. The ureter is retracted medially to expose the uterosacral's and Mackenrodt's ligaments. They are then cut with the harmonic shears in the downward direction toward the levator ani. The identical procedures are replicated on the right-hand side.

Step 4: Anterior U-Cut (Figs. 18.10 and 18.11)

The uterus is retroverted and a peritoneal cut (anterior U cut) is taken starting from the round ligament on the right side with harmonic shears (Fig. 18.10). This cut is extended into the uterovesical fold. The uterus is pulled cranially and the assistant lifts the bladder. The fascial plane between the bladder and the uterus is developed. The bladder is dissected with scissors (Fig. 18.11). This dissection is facilitated by the carbon dioxide gas insufflation that penetrates into and separates the spaces. The peritoneal cut is extended on the left side to cut the round ligament using the harmonic shears.

Step 5: Dissection of Ureteric Tunnel (Figs. 18.12 and 18.13)

The uterus is pulled upwards and towards the right, while the entire length of the left ureter is carefully followed towards the bladder. The peritoneum covering the bladder is

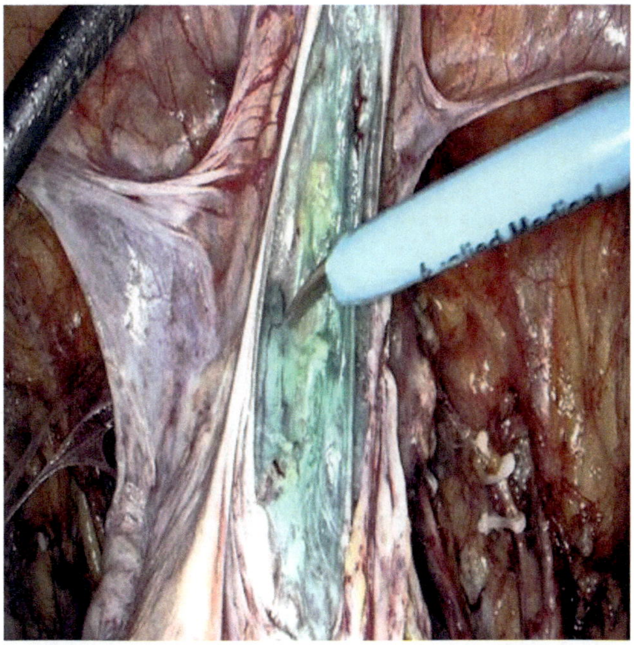

Fig. 18.10 Anterior U-cut

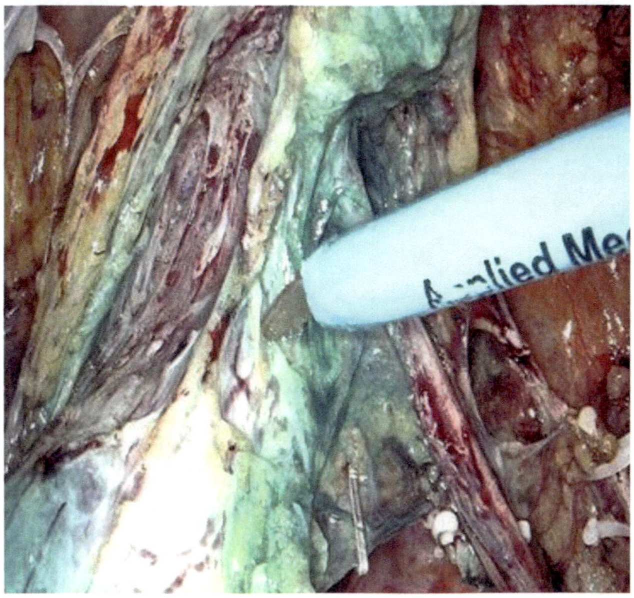

Fig. 18.11 Dissection of bladder piller

grasped, and the bladder is lifted upwards by the assisting surgeon. This maneuver allows for clear visualization of the ureteric tunnel, revealing small veins. The tunnel is dissected using Maryland's forceps, and within its roof, two veins are identified, clipped, and subsequently cut (refer to Figs. 18.12 and 18.13). This process facilitates the lateral movement of the ureter. The point where the ureter enters the bladder at the utero-vesical junction becomes visible. To achieve a well-formed vaginal cuff below the growth, the bladder is further pushed downwards. Understanding of

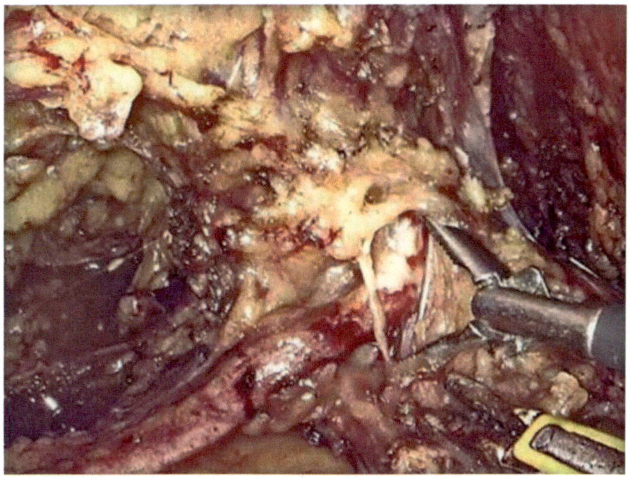

Fig. 18.12 Dissection of the ureteric tunnel left side

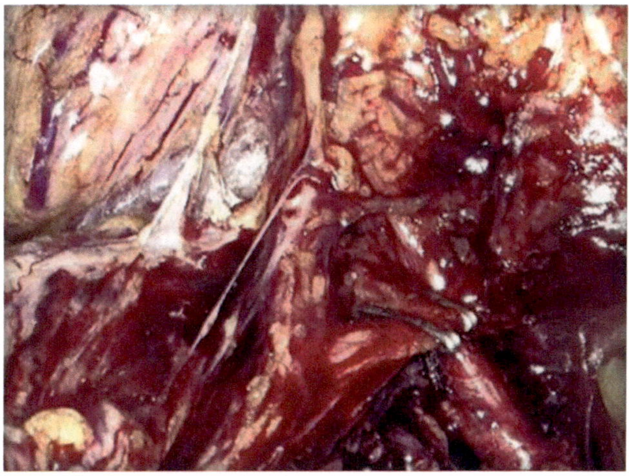

Fig. 18.13 Right ureteric tunnel dissection

anterior parametrectomy—Answer to "LACC TRAIL" as complete parametrium dissection help in prevention of local or pelvic recurrence of cervical cancers (Fig. 18.14). The paracolpos is then cut as laterally as possible. These procedures guarantee the attainment of the maximum paracolpos and visibility of the vaginal margin. The identical steps are repeated on the right side to expose the trigonal area. Purse string suturing taken above colpotomy to prevent spillage. A colpotomy is performed beyond this point using harmonic shears (Figs. 18.15, 18.16, and 18.17). The infundibulopelvic ligaments are subsequently incised, and the complete specimen is then isolated and placed inside an endobag (Fig. 18.18).

Step 6: Lymph Node Excision (Fig. 18.19)

The dissection of lymph nodes begins at the common iliac artery bifurcation. The ideal tool for dissection is a suction cannula due to its very mild approach. Using the suction cannula, the fibrofatty tissue along the external iliac vein is carefully

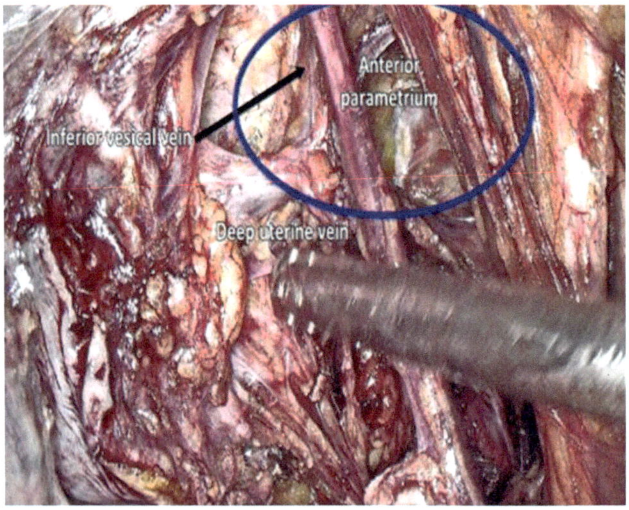

Fig. 18.14 Dissection of anterior parametrium

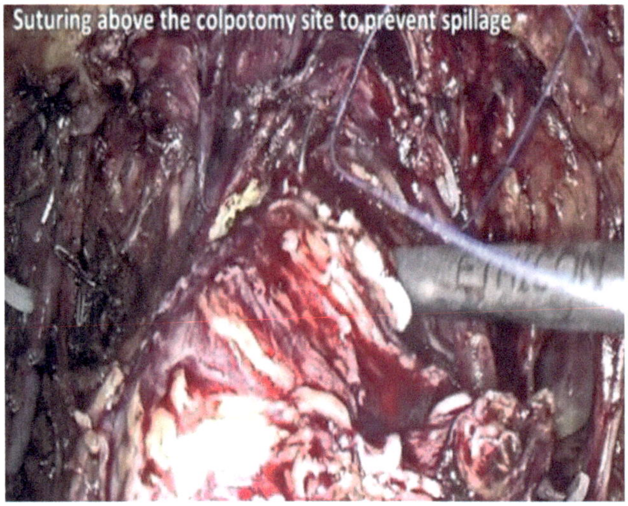

Fig. 18.15 Purse string suturing above colpotomy to prevent spillage

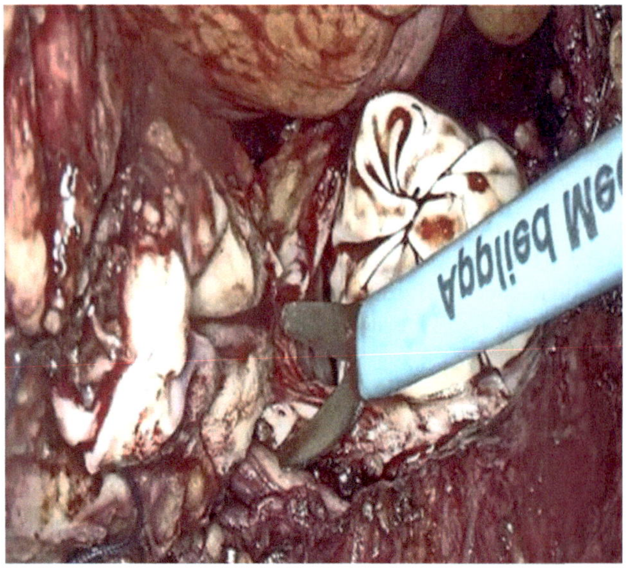

Fig. 18.16 Complete colpotomy

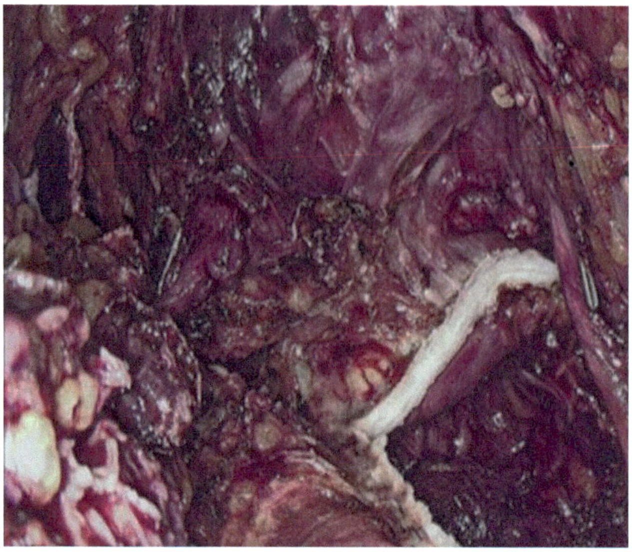

Fig. 18.17 Use of stapler for colpotomy

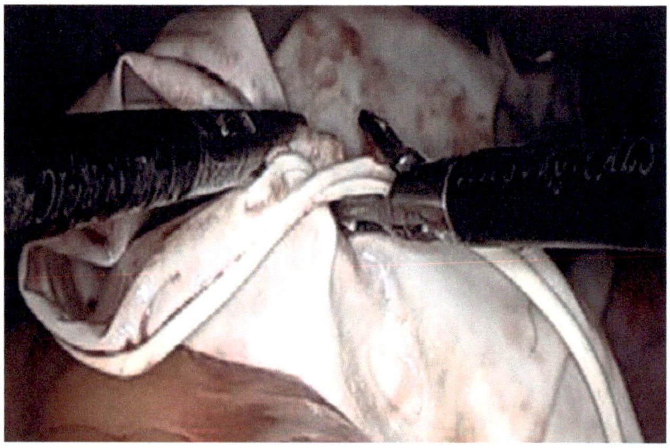

Fig. 18.18 In bag specimen retrieval

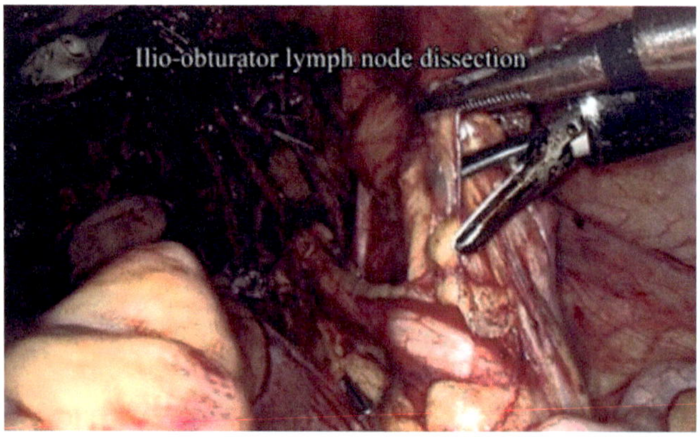

Fig. 18.19 Dissection of the lymph nodes in the right ilio-obturator region

dissected, passing parallel to the arteries and up to the iliac bone, which acts as the lateral border of the dissection.

To visualize nodes in the obturator fossa, the peritoneum is stretched by the assistant, and the nodes are systematically cleared from the pubic bone in a cranial direction. Exposure of the obturator nerve occurs, and all nodes situated above the nerve are meticulously removed. The medial limit is defined by the internal iliac artery, while the lower limit is determined by the obturator nerve (Fig. 18.20).

Be aware of **"corona mortis",** an anastomosis between the obturator & external iliac vein (Fig. 18.21) and dissection around the hypogastric nerve. Keep in mind the preservation of the hypogastric nerve to avoid complications of urinary incontinence, erectile dysfunction and vaginal dryness (Fig. 18.22). A comparable analysis is conducted on both sides, as illustrated in Fig. 18.19. The complete nodal tissue extracted is placed inside the endobag. The endobag is removed vaginally. Complete plane of retroperitoneal anatomy is illustrated (Fig. 18.23) Haemostasis is achieved. The wound is irrigated with normal saline. The enclosure is securely shut by employing a consistent internal stitching technique using Vicryl 2-0, threaded through the 10 mm operational opening. The utilization of intra-abdominal drainage is deemed unnecessary. The removal of ports is conducted under visual guidance, followed by the closure of the port sites.

The sample: This method accomplishes a Pivers type III radical hysterectomy (Type C2 Querleu and Morrow) with a paracervical clearance exceeding 3 cm. It also ensures a distal vaginal margin of over 2.5–3 cm and a retrieval of at least 18–20 nodes, as illustrated in Fig. 18.17.

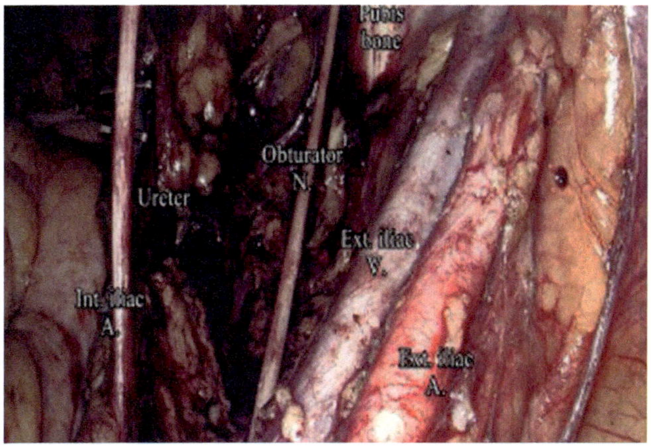

Fig. 18.20 Ilio-obturator lymph node dissection

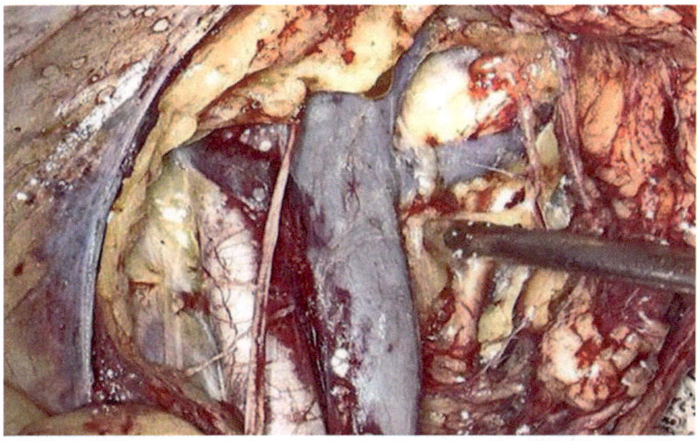

Fig. 18.21 Corona mortis

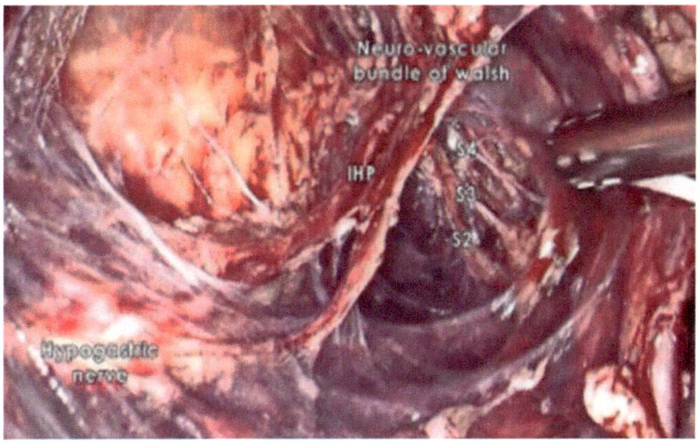

Fig. 18.22 Hypogastric nerve preservation

18.2.7 Complications

1. Haemorrhage
2. Bladder injury
3. Ureteric injury
4. Bowel injury
5. Fistulas

18.2.8 After Surgery

After 24–48 hours, the Foley catheter is taken out. Every 7 days, the patient is reviewed.

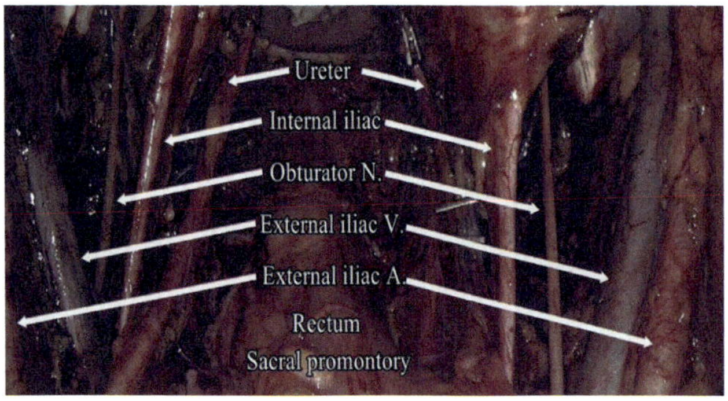

Fig. 18.23 Post dissection, there is a plan or a course of action laid out to guide the subsequent steps or directions

18.3 Conclusion

In conclusion, we would like to stress that laparoscopic radical hysterectomy, when itcomes to margins, lymph node clearing, parametrium resection, shows oncological outcomes that are similar to those of open surgery, thereby leading to successful type III radical hysterectomy. Comparing this technique to the abdominal method, it shows less morbidity and fewer postoperative problems, making it both technically and financially favorable. In addition, patients will have less bladder or bowel dysfunction, return to work sooner, walk after surgery with less discomfort, ambulate earlier. Additionally, this strategy makes it possible to start adjuvant therapy earlier. The standard multiport laparoscopic radical hysterectomy steps can be duplicated using other minimal access modalities (LESS, OASIS, Robotic) [13].

Learning Points

- Laparoscopic radical hysterectomy is suitable for patients with early-stage cervical cancer (FIGO stage IA1 and IB2), and cases of endometrial cancer up to stage 2.
- Prior to surgery, thorough clinical examination, cervical punch biopsy, and histopathological evaluation are essential for accurate diagnosis and treatment planning.
- The "Pune-Technique" involves meticulous port placement and standardized steps for systematic dissections of pelvic structures, guided by anatomical landmarks.
- The dissection of rectovaginal space is carried out between the two layers of Denonvillier's fascia keeping in mind that **"fat belongs in the rectum"**.
- Early mobilization, initiation of oral feeds, and urinary catheter removal within 4–7 days contribute to a quicker recovery and shorter hospital stay for patients undergoing laparoscopic radical hysterectomy.
- Surgeons should undergo specialized training and gain experience in laparoscopic techniques to ensure proficiency in performing laparoscopic radical hysterectomy and managing potential intraoperative complications effectively.

Competing Interest The author declares no conflict of interest that are relevant to content of this chapter.

Ethical Approval Informed consent was obtained from individual participants and patients regarding publication and documentation without disclosing their identity.

References

1. Ferlay J, Colombet M, Soerjomataram I, Mathers C, Parkin DM, Piñeros M, et al. Estimating the global cancer incidence and mortality in 2018: GLOBOCAN sources and methods. Int J Cancer. 2019;144(8):1941–53. Available from: https://onlinelibrary.wiley.com/doi/full/10.1002/ijc.31937
2. Bray F, Ferlay J, Soerjomataram I, Siegel RL, Torre LA, Jemal A. Global cancer statistics 2018: GLOBOCAN estimates of incidence and mortality worldwide for 36 cancers in 185 countries. CA Cancer J Clin. 2018;68(6):394–424. Available from: https://acsjournals.onlinelibrary.wiley.com/doi/full/10.3322/caac.21492
3. World Health Organization (WHO). Global health estimates 2018: disease burden by cause, age, sex, by country and by region, 2000–2016. Geneva: WHO; 2018. Available from: https://www.who.int/healthinfo/global_burden_disease/estimates/en/
4. Omran AR. The epidemiologic transition. A theory of the epidemiology of population change. Milbank Mem Fund Q. 1971;49(4):509–38.
5. Piver MS, Rutledge F, Smith JP. Five classes of extended hysterectomy for women with cervical cancer. Obstet Gynecol. 1974;44(2):265–72.
6. Nandakumar A, Anantha N, Venugopal TC. Incidence, mortality and survival in cancer of the cervix in Bangalore. India Br J Cancer. 1995;71(6):1348–52.
7. Morrow CP, Curtin J. Gynecologic cancer surgery. Philadelphia: Churchill Livingstone; 1996.
8. Canis M, Mage G, Wattiez A, Ponly JL, Manhes H, Bruhat MA. Does endoscopic surgery have a role in radical surgery of cancer of the cervix uteri? [in French]. J Gynecol Obstet Biol Reprod (Paris). 1990;19:921.
9. Shoup M, Brennan MF, Karpeh MS, Gillern SM, McMahon RL, Conlon KC. Port site metastasis after diagnostic laparoscopy for upper gastrointestinal tract malignancies: an uncommon entity. Ann Surg Oncol. 2002;9(6):632–6.
10. Nezhat CR, Burrell MO, Nezhat FR, Benigno BB, Welander CE. Laparoscopic radical hysterectomy with para aortic and pelvic node dissection. Am J Obstet Gynecol. 1992;166(3):864–5. [PubMed] [Google Scholar]
11. Abu-Rustum NR, Rhee E, Chi DS, Sonoda Y, Sonoda Y, Gemignani M, Barakat RR. Subcutaneous tumor implantation after lapa-

roscopic procedures in women with malignant disease. Obstet Gynecol. 2004;103(3):480–7.
12. Abu-Rustum NR, Gemignani ML, Moore K, et al. Total laparoscopic radical hysterectomy with pelvic lymphadenectomy using the argon-beam coagulator: pilot data and comparison to laparotomy. Gynecol Oncol. 2003;91(2):402–9. Erratum in Gynecol Oncol. 2004;93(2):275.
13. Puntambekar SP, Katakdhond SS, Galgali S, Iche A, Barik S, Puntambekar AS. Duplication of conventional multiport laparoscopic radical hysterectomy steps with other minimal access modalities (LESS, OASIS, Robotic). Available from: https://www.researchgate.net/publication/272028069_Duplication_of_Conventional_Multiport_Laparoscopic_Radical_Hysterectomy_Steps_with_Other_Minimal_Access_Modalities_LESS_OASIS_Robotic

Part IV

Complications

Urological Complications in Total Laparoscopic Hysterectomy (TLH)

19

Andrea Tinelli, Gaetano Panese, and Giovanni Pecorella

Acronyms

TLH	Total Laparoscopic Hysterectomy
LASH	Laparoscopic Assisted Supracervical Hysterectomy
LAVH	Laparoscopic-Assisted Vaginal Hysterectomy
BUN	Blood Urea Nitrogen

19.1 Introduction

Hysterectomy is the most common major gynecological surgery [1], and the Total Laparoscopic Hysterectomy (TLH) is nowadays no longer, a revolution but rather a milestone in the gynecological surgery. The spectrum of the treatable pathology ranges from the benign pathology (Adenomyosis, Uterine fibromatosis, Hypermenorrhea, Prolapse Uteri), to the malignant entity (endometrial carcinoma, uterine sarcomas, cervical cancer, ovarian cancer, borderline tumor). It is a relatively flexible procedure which allows for the removal of large masses, as fibroids or the uterine supracervical tract in case of a Laparoscopic Supracervical Hysterectomy (LASH), through an ancillary 12 mm laparoscopic incision, thanks to morcellation in cases of proven benign pathology [2].

TLH allows complex oncological debulking with the opportunity to access lymph nodes and stage various intraabdominal structures under direct visualization [3]. Furthermore, TLH also allows traditional urogynecological procedures, with or without mesh implantation [4]. The main advantages of the laparoscopic approach is shorter hospital stay [5], lower cost for the health system (comparable just to the vaginal approach, which, however, shows several limitation) [6], a faster recovery of the patient because of the smaller incision, less pain and bleeding, and reduced risk of infections [7]. On the other side, the TLH needs expertise, trained and skilled surgeons to avoid early and late complications. In this chapter we will discuss about the urological complications, which could occur after a TLH.

19.2 Urological Complications

The rate of urological complications ranges from 0.3% in case of simple laparoscopic surgery, to 8% by laparoscopic radical hysterectomy with debulking and lymphonodectomy, in case of oncological treatment [8–11]. Of course, these rates increase in case of previous abdominal surgery. The complication rate decreased with the increasing experience over time. One principle of the modern safe laparoscopy is the nerve sparing approach [12]. Standardizing the surgical procedures is crucial in order to reduce difficulties in TLHs. This includes the gradual opening of the cervicorectal and cervico-vesical spaces, the identification and separation of the ureter (Fig. 19.1), as well as the recognition and sparing of neural structures (Fig. 19.2) [13]. As previously stated, the risk rates are higher with TLH due to the radical nature of oncological surgery [14].

The incidence of bladder and ureteral injuries during or after a TLH ranges from 0.3 to 1.3% and from 2.5 to 12.1% respectively [15, 16]. The intraoperative identification of bladder (Fig. 19.3) and ureter (Fig. 19.4) injuries varies from 51.1% to 84.4% of cases [17].

Contributing factors included caesarian section, associated with 4.33-fold increased risk of bladder injury (with a 95% confidence interval ranging from 1.53 to 12.30) (Fig. 19.5), and previous laparotomy, which was linked to a 4.69-fold higher risk (with a 95% confidence interval ranging

A. Tinelli (✉) · G. Panese
Department of Obstetrics and Gynecology, and CERICSAL (CEntro di RIcerca Clinico SALentino), Veris delli Ponti Hospital, Lecce, Italy

G. Pecorella
Department of Gynecology, Obstetrics and Reproduction Medicine, Saarland University, Homburg, Germany

N. Jain (ed.), *Complex Total Laparoscopic Hysterectomy (TLH) with Newer Approaches in Bladder Dissection*,
https://doi.org/10.1007/978-981-97-3226-5_19

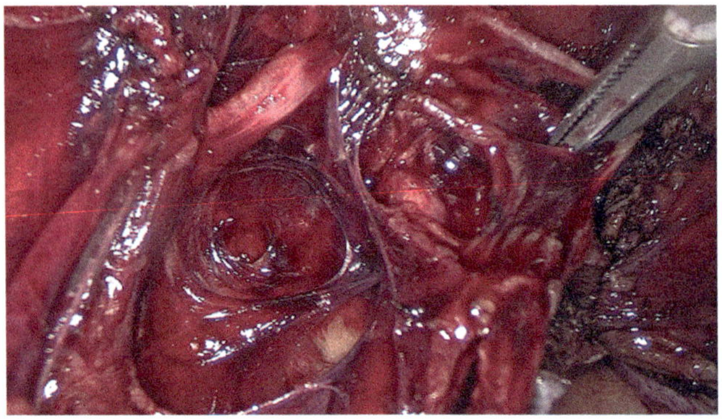

Fig. 19.1 Laparoscopic gradual opening of the cervicorectal and cervicovesical spaces, and identification of ureter

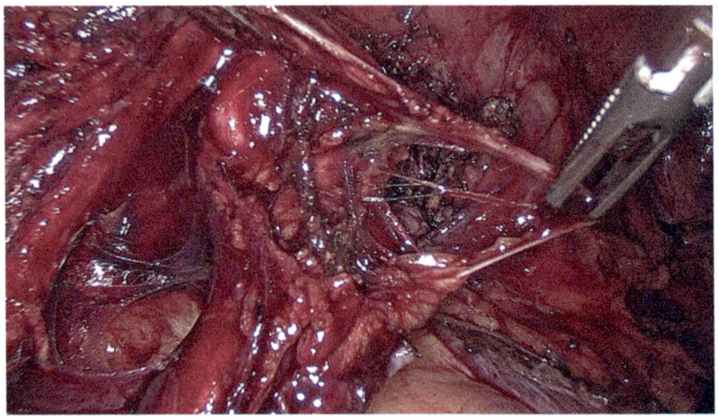

Fig. 19.2 Laparoscopic recognition and sparing of neural structures, after ureter identification

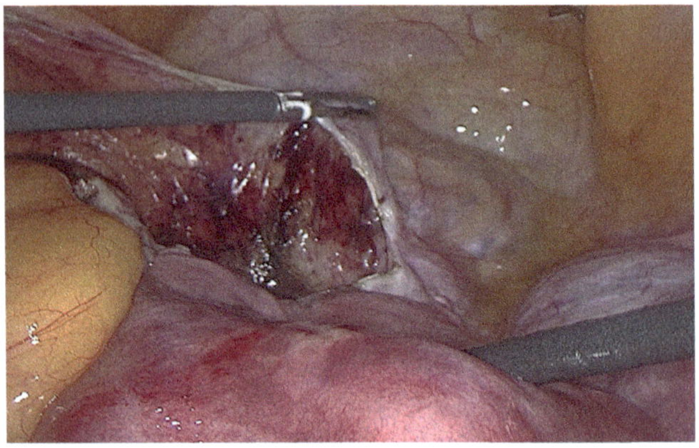

Fig. 19.3 Laparoscopic lateral incision of the vesico-uterine plica, with recognition of bladder during detachment

from 1.59 to 13.8). The experience of the surgeon allows for a decrease in injuries rate, reaching a plateau to 0.4% every 100 hysterectomies [18–20].

A Delphi Survey was conducted by Hasson et al. to collect recommendations about how to avoid urological injury during a laparoscopic hysterectomy [21]. Many statements from experts were obtained from this questionnaire, includ-

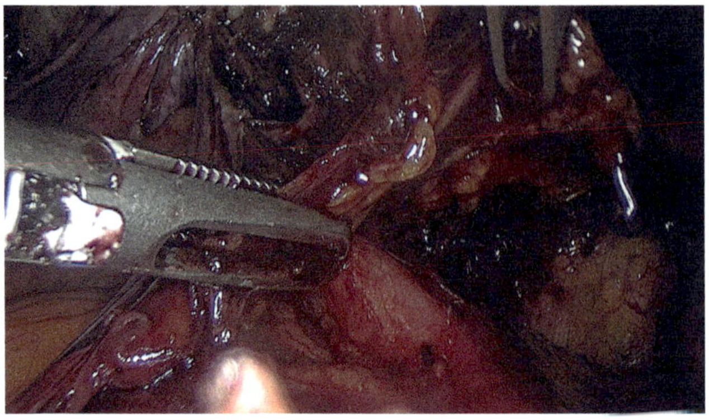

Fig. 19.4 Laparoscopic identification of ureter under the surgical forceps before entering the parametrium

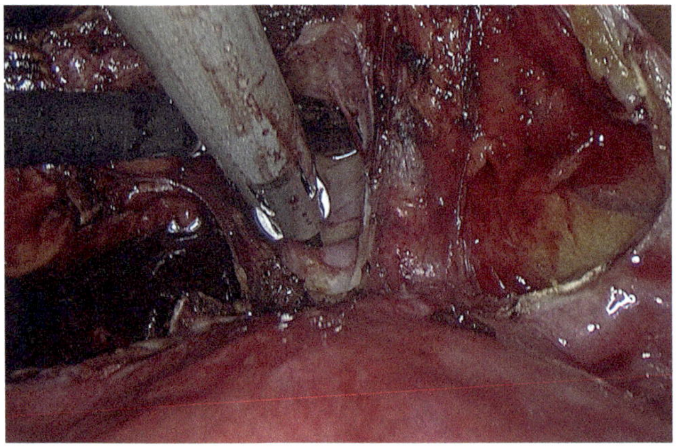

Fig. 19.5 Laparoscopic identification of vesico-uterine space, with the surgical instrument entering this space, in a patient with previous cesarean section and many adhesions between the anterior uterine wall and the bladder

ing the significance of the surgeon's education and training, the necessity of using a vaginal manipulator as an essential surgical tool, the restoration of abnormal anatomy, the use of diagnostic tools to identify urinary structures, and the training of surgeons with laparoscopy simulators and under supervision [22].

19.3 Bladder Injuries

Adelman et al. revised 37 articles, in which 252 bladder injuries were described. The 80.6% were recognized intraoperatively (Fig. 19.6), and 7.5% postoperatively, 11.9% were uncategorized [17]. 11.1% of the bladder injuries was repaired which required a conversion to laparotomy, the rest have been treated laparoscopically or transvaginally. Of the 7.5% recognized postoperative injuries, the 84% required a secondary surgery, 10 of them with a laparotomic, 6 with a laparoscopic or vaginal approach [17]. Statistical representative risk factors are represented by: (1) BMI ($\leq$25 kg/m^2

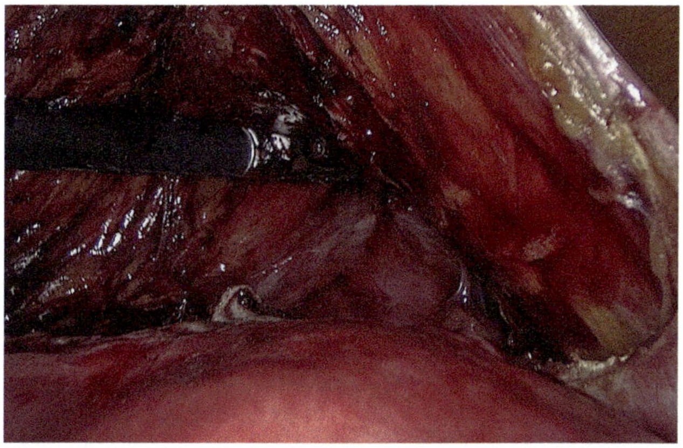

Fig. 19.6 Laparoscopic recognition of a small bladder lesion during detachment of the bladder from the vesico-uterine space, after an intraoperative cystoscopy; the assistant lifts the vesico-uterine fold and the surgeon highlights the lesion on the posterior wall of the bladder with atraumatic laparoscopic forceps

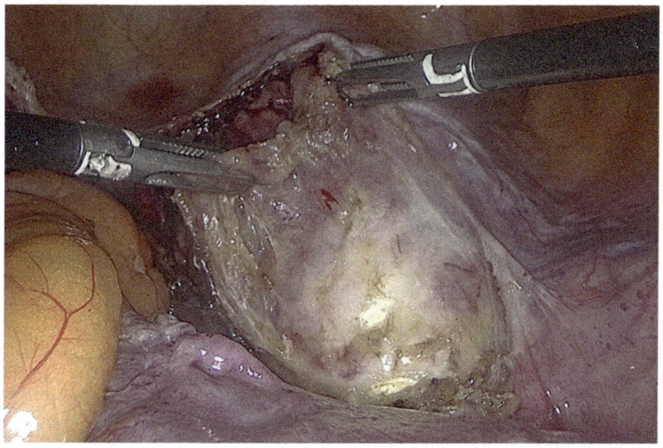

Fig. 19.7 Laparoscopic sharp and a bunt approach of the posterior bladder wall during the vescico-uterine space dissection; the surgeon lifts the vesico-uterine fold with two atraumatic forceps and highlights the loose tissue present on the posterior uterine wall

p-value 0.06); (2) smoking status (p-value 0.04); (3) vaginal deliveries (nullipara p-value <0.01); (4) transvaginal morcellation (p-value 0.10); (5) endometriosis (P-value < 0.01). On the contrary, age, history of caesarean section or pelvic surgery, method of colpotomy or cervical amputation, uterine weight are not strong predictive factors. Inan et al. performed a study analyzing 547 total laparoscopic hysterectomies performed at a technique training and research hospital in Izmir, Turkey, providing valuable information to the scientific community. Among the 547 included patients, only 7 bladder injuries were recorded. All of them were on the posterior bladder wall during the dissection (Fig. 19.7) of the vesico-uterine space (the author tried a sharp and a bunt approach without showing a substantial difference in the results). Six were detected and treated intraoperatively, and one on the first postoperative day. The rate of diagnosticated endometriosis and previous cesarean sections in the women with injuries was definitely higher compared with the other (p < 0.001 and p < 0.001, respectively) [23].

19.4 Surgical Treatment of Iatrogenic Injury

The detection of the bladder damage is the first step in the management. The most of the perforation are noted intraabdominal with or without Methylene blue or indigo carmine bladder filling, some need an intraoperative cystoscopy [24]. The bladder was repaired with double layer interrupted suture using 3/0 VICRYL™ (polyglactin 910) and/or 4/0 VICRYL™ (polyglactin 910). After suturing, patients underwent leakage control using diluted methylene blue solution or normal saline testing. The urethral Foley catheter was left 5–7 day to support the bladder recovery [25].

19.5 Ureteral Injuries

Ureteral injury could cause a range of sequelae, leading to acute or chronic kidney failure, with the necessity of unilateral nephrectomy [26]. The most common location of ureteral injury is at level of the uterine artery (Fig. 19.8) or at level of the vaginal stump (Fig. 19.9), 2–4 cm from the ureteral ostium [27]. The ureter which runs in Mackenrodt's ligament (Fig. 19.10) before his insertion into the bladder is hard to be palpated and demarked. The second most common localization is at the vaginal stump (Fig. 19.11), during its closure in case of TLH [28, 29].

According to the evaluation by İnan AH et al., in their retrospective analysis of 547 TLH cases, 4 ureteral injuries were recorded. Of these, 75% occurred on the right side at

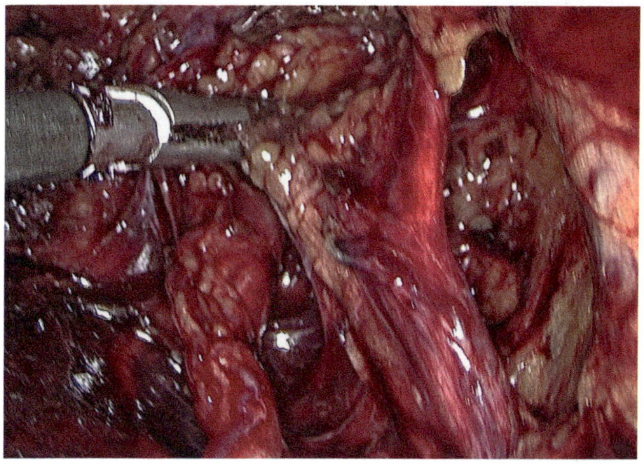

Fig. 19.8 Laparoscopic identification of ureter (left) at level of the uterine artery, raised by the surgeon with atraumatic forceps

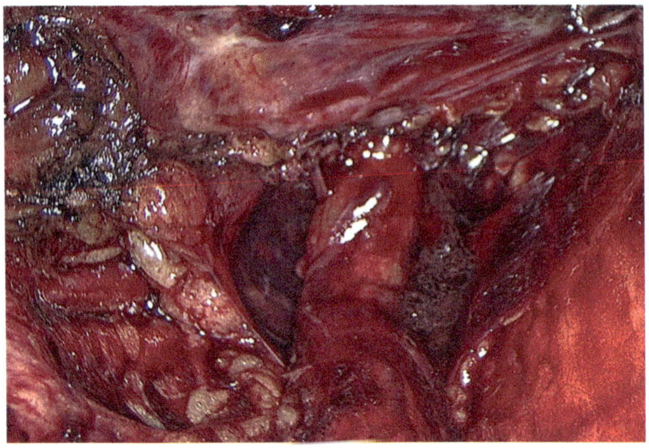

Fig. 19.9 Laparoscopic identification of the ureter (center) at level of the vaginal stump

the level of the uterine artery, 3 cm from the point of entry to the bladder [23].

It is important to note that ureteral injuries are not limited to burn (Fig. 19.12) or cut wounds; kinking injuries (Fig. 19.13) have also been documented in literature [26]. Risk factors includes age (≤ 40 yrs. p-value 0.76), parity, uterus weight (> 200 g p-value 0.03), pelvic surgical history (p-value 0.26), history of caesarean section (p-value 0.44), adhesions, endometriosis (p-value 0.42) [16, 27]. Uterine weight itself shows shows a weak association with urethral injuries (p-value = 0.07). In the multivariable logistic model, having a BMI in the range of 26–30 kg/m^2 (as opposed to having a BMI greater than 30 kg/m^2) was linked to a higher likelihood of experiencing ureteral injury. Additionally, individuals of African American ethnicity (in contrast to those of White ethnicity) displayed a tendency

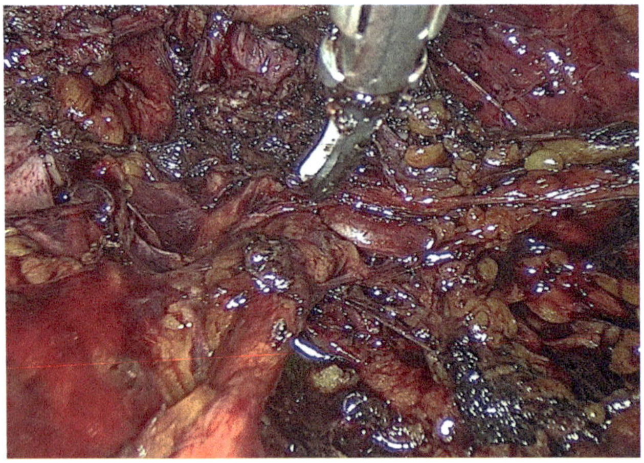

Fig. 19.10 Laparoscopic identification of the ureter (center) at the level of the entrance to the Mackenrodt ligamentum, highlighted by the surgical instrument

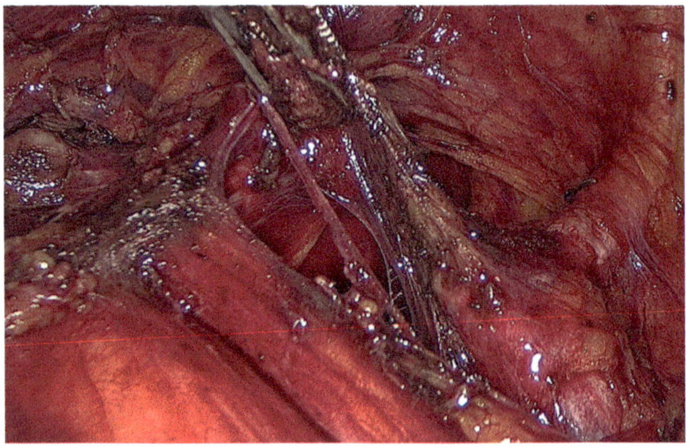

Fig. 19.12 Laparoscopic identification of ureter on the left and origin of the coagulated and cut uterine artery on the right (raised by the surgeon with atraumatic forceps) with bipolar coagulation performed very close to the ureteral surface

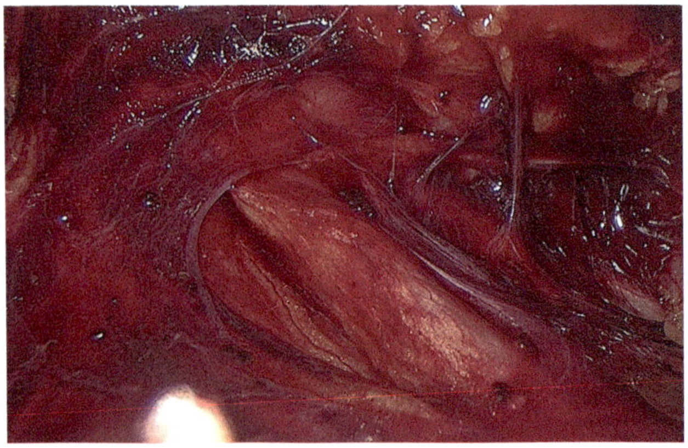

Fig. 19.11 The second most common laparoscopic localization of the ureter (center) is at level of the vaginal stump

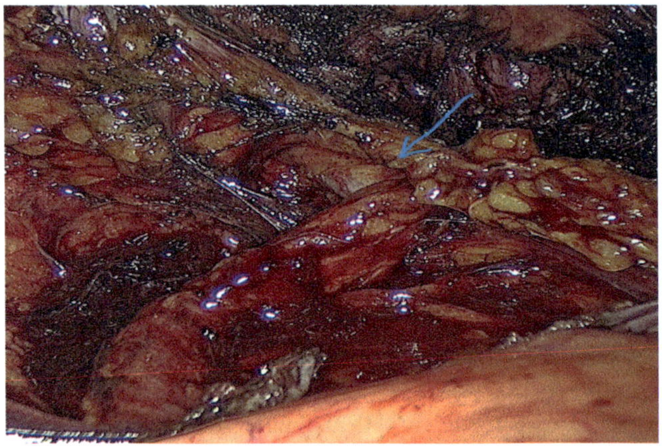

Fig. 19.13 Laparoscopic identification of ureter with kinking (highlighted by a blue arrow), during dissection with atraumatic forceps

towards an elevated risk of ureteral injury, although this trend did not attain statistical significance (with a p-value of 0.05) [27].

19.6 Surgical Treatment of Iatrogenic Injury

The 54% of the intraoperative recognized injuries were treated through stent insertion, 13.5% treated with an end-to-end anastomosis, 18% with ureter neo implantation, 13.5% received an uncategorized surgical treatment. In the group with delayed presentation, medical interventions included the placement of 22 stents and 4 percutaneous nephrostomy tubes, 4 end-to-end ureteral reconnections, 27 ureteral replantations, 2 unspecified reparative surgeries, and 1 nephrectomy. Thus, a total of 34 surgical procedures were performed for delayed cases, accounting for 60.7% of the cases. Among the 79 unclassified ureteral injuries, documentation indicated 43 ureteral reimplantation, but there was no reference to the timing of the reparative procedures [17].

The Koh Technique is a simple procedure designed to prevent ureteral injury during a laparoscopic-assisted vaginal hysterectomy (LAVH) This technique is perfectly suitable to TLH as well [30]. The procedure commences following a thorough inspection of the entire abdominal cavity. First, after coagulating with bipolar forceps, the left round ligament is cut approximately two-thirds of the way from the uterus. The uterus is then moved to the right, and dissection of the left anterior broad ligament is carried out up to the vesico-uterine junction (Fig. 19.14). To aid in this, a mini-retractor is placed on the left posterior broad ligament, just behind the ovarian ligament, creating an opening in the anterior broad ligament. This opening is then widened using two atraumatic forceps applying opposing pressure.

If an oophorectomy is anticipated, the left suspensory ligament is either ligated with endo ligatures or cauterized using a bipolar instrument before being severed. This process is repeated on the right side. To aid in separating the bladder from the lower uterine segment and cervix, 5–10 mL of saline solution is injected into the vesico-uterine peritoneum. Subsequently, an incision is carefully made at the vesico-uterine peritoneal reflection using monopolar scissors with a 40 W coagulating current. The bladder is then dissected away from the anterior aspect of the cervix (Fig. 19.15). Following the shift of the uterus to the right, atraumatic forceps grasp the uterine margin of the left posterior broad ligament. With care, the tissue on the ligament, including the ureter and uterine vessels, is gently maneuvered anterolaterally using the blunt posterior aspect of an endoscissors. When encountering highly vascular areolar tissue surrounding the ureter and uterine artery prone to bleeding during blunt dissection, cauterization is meticulously conducted using bipolar forceps. Subsequently, the posterior broad ligament is incised with care towards the vagina until reaching the uterosacral ligament, which is then desiccated with bipolar forceps and partially transected. The cardinal ligament remains is not dissected and remains intact. This procedure is then repeated on the right posterior broad ligament. After coagulating both ascending uterine arteries with bipolar forceps, anterior and posterior colpotomy are executed using monopolar diathermy. The subsequent stages of the surgery, encompassing dissection of the cardinal ligaments, ligation of the uterine arteries, extraction of the uterus, and closure of the vaginal cuff, are performed laparoscopically. A No.18 Foley catheter is inserted into the vaginal cuff to function as a drain for 24–48 hours, the duration depends upon the degree of bleeding. Thorough irrigation and suction of the pelvis are meticulously conducted to ensure proper hemostasis. Instead of employing the conventional peritonization approach, the peritoneal edge is cauterized using bipolar forceps to prevent [30].

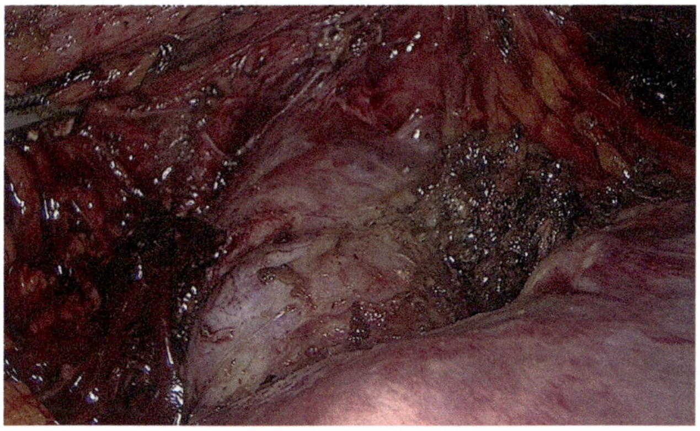

Fig. 19.14 Laparoscopic dissection of the vesico-uterine junction and exposure of the uterine cervix during a LASH, at the point where it meets the left anterior broad ligament (on the right)

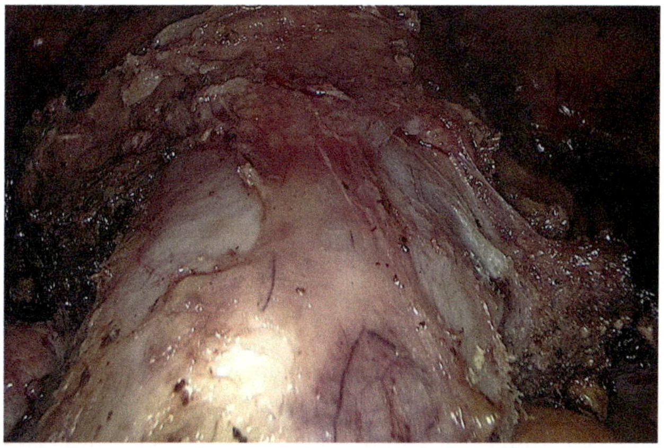

Fig. 19.15 After the incision made at the vesico-uterine peritoneal reflection, the cervix is delicately exposed as the bladder is dissected away from the anterior aspect of the cervix. In the center of the cervix, a strip of loose connective tissue of the vesical-uterine space is highlighted

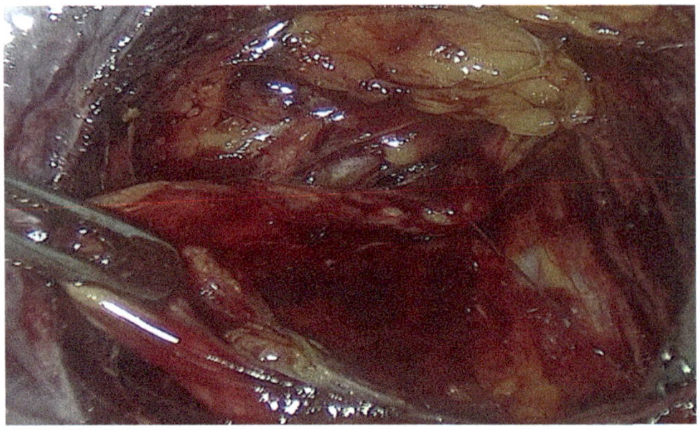

Fig. 19.16 Laparoscopic image of a duplex ureter, already reported by radiological imaging before the laparoscopic operation; on the left the atraumatic forceps lifts the left ureter to highlight it, leaving the other ureter on the right

The prevention of the complications is surely the most important prerequisite, but if unpreventable the complication has to be recognized prompt. The regression of the postoperative discomfort has to be gradual but constant. In case of postoperative pain increase (pain in the renal lodge, peritonismus and dynamic ileus) or plateau, an imaging with contrast media is supposed to be indicated [26].

The typical biochemical alteration of the vesical/ureteral injury is the increase if creatinine and blood urea nitrogen (BUN) in serum, however the increase in not pathognomonic and the imaging diagnostic remains the gold standard [31].

What every surgeon should keep in mind is the ureter anatomical alteration, which involve a customization of the surgery. One woman in 400–666 shows a horseshoe kidney, while a duplex ureter (Fig. 19.16) shoes an incidence from 0.5 to 0.7%, mega-ureter shows an incidence from 1/10,000, ectopic ureter with an occurrence of ectopic ureters is 1/2000 in newborns and 1/2000–4000 in general population, and ureterocele 1 in every 4000 children and are most common in whites [32, 33].

19.7 Fistulas

Hysterectomy is widely considered the most frequent cause of genital fistula disease [34]. A Swedish study tried to establish, through a cohort study, the overall prevalence of the fistulas in women who underwent to hysterectomy. The pool of analyzed patients was 182.1641 hysterectomized women and 524.826 as control group, who didn't undergo to this kind of surgery. During the follow-up phase, 469 (0.26%) fistula cases were identified in the post-hysterectomy groups and 384 in the control group. The data arising from this study are that the patients undergoing to hysterectomy have a four times higher risk of developing. Among the different hysterectomy approaches (abdominal, vaginal and laparoscopic), TLH has 3 times higher rates of fistula formation as compared to abdominal approoach. The overall most common fistulae were urogenital fistulae (vesicovaginal most commonly) and intestine-genital (rectovaginal most commonly). The source of urogenital fistulae was often a too-deep suture invading the bladder wall or cavity, or direct damage to the lower urinary tract [35, 36]. Another similar study was also conducted in Finland, where from the 62.379 investigated patients, the overall prevalence was of 1 on 1200 operations (0.08%) [37]. Among the recognized risk factors for developing a fistula, cigarette smoking is notable due to its impact on wound healing [38]. Overweight is a general risk factor for surgery, but its specific association with fistula development has not been proven [39]. Diverticulitis appears to be a predisposing factor, with an increased fistula rate (51.7 compared with 22.0 per 100,000 women-years). Other proven risk factors include diabetes, postoperative infections, and radiation therapy for cervical cancer [40].

19.8 Neurological Injuries (Pudendum Incontinence)

Pudendal neuropathy or pudendal damage may not be directly linked with urogynecological complication after a TLH, but the consequences linked to the malfunctioning of the nerve, affect surely the urogynecological sphere. The pudendal nerve is a peripheral nerve arising from the ventral rami of the S2, S3, and S4 spinal nerve roots within the sacral plexus. It traverses between the piriformis and coccygeus muscles, heading towards the pelvic cavity, passing through the greater sciatic foramen ventral to the sacrotuberous ligament. Although the pudendal nerve is not typically disrupted, its intrapelvic course is still susceptible to injury during a TLH, making it relevant to this discussion [41].

The typical nerve disturbances are consequences of compression due to hematomas or tissue scarring following a Total Laparoscopic Hysterectomy (TLH). Beyond the common neurological symptoms, such us numbness, pain, it can cause a dysfunction of the anatomical structures supplied from the nerve, such us genitalia, perineum, rectum, and lower urinary tract. Focusing on the urine incontinence, a pudendal dysfunction could cause urinary issues, such as urgency and frequency, causing pain a full bladder. The diagnosis is manly clinic, according to the "Nantes" criteria and its treatment could be conservative, pharmacologic and surgical, to reach a mechanic decompression or the pharmacologic decongestion [42].

19.9 Final Considerations

Bladder injuries are more frequent than ureteral injuries in case of TLH. The most of the bladder injuries occur on the posterior bladder wall during the vesico-uterine dissection. In contrast, ureteral injuries are predominantly found on the right side, typically occurring about 3 cm from the ureter's insertion into the bladder [27]. It might be logical to assume in the proximity of the bladder it can increase the bladder injury rate. That's why tumors located in the lower uterine area might be expected to cause more injuries. However, Inan et al. found no statistical association between bladder injuries and tumor proximity. Despite this, the lower segment of the ureter is associated with a higher risk of ureteral injuries [23]. Bladder injuries can also occur during the insertion of Verres' needle or a suprapubic trocar, particularly in patients with a history of extensive prior surgeries, including multiple cesarean sections ($p < 0.005$) [43–45]. In addition to history of previous surgery, endometriosis is an important risk factor for both ureteral and bladder injuries ($p < 0.001$), because of the loss of the anatomic layer and the fibrosis due to the chronic inflammation [27, 44]. These injuries exhibit several differences, with the most notable being in their detection timing. Bladder injuries demonstrate an intraoperative detection rate of 85.7%, whereas 75% of ureteral injuries are identified during the postoperative period [23, 46]. The importance of the insertion of a preoperatively ureteral catheter for a better visualization of anatomical course of the ureter, as prevention, was widely discussed [47, 48]. The different injuries show different etiology and risk factors. Bladder injuries are mainly associated with a high BMI (≤25 kg/m^2, p-value 0.06), nicotine abuse (p-value <0.01), and endometriosis (p-value <0.01). In contrast, potential ureteral injuries are linked with age (≤40 yrs., p-value 0.76), parity, uterine weight (>200 g, p-value 0.03), pelvic surgical history (p-value 0.26), history of cesarean section (p-value 0.44), adhesions, and endometriosis (p-value 0.42). Cigarette smoking, known to impair wound healing, is associated with an increased risk of both ureteral and bladder fistulas. Also, diverticulosis is a predisposing factor increasing the fistula's rate. Diabetes postoperative infections and, last but not least, radiation therapy for cervical cancer play an important role in fistulas development [40]. The prevention of the urological complication is surely the most important prerequisite, but if unpreventable, the complication has to be recognized promptly. After TLH, there must be a gradual but steady decrease of the postoperative discomfort associated with urological problems. Imaging using contrast media is meant to be recommended in the event that postoperative discomfort (such as pain in the renal lodge, peritonismus, and dynamic ileus) increases or plateaus [26]. Typical signs of a possible vesical and ureteral injury is the increase or alteration of biochemical parameters, as creatinine and blood urea nitrogen (BUN) in serum; however the increase in not pathognomonic and the imaging diagnostic remains the gold standard [31]. Every surgeon should avoid overconfidence in their abilities, even after performing hundreds of operations, as the risk of intraoperative and postoperative damage is always present. Preoperative imaging is valuable but does not eliminate the risks associated with altered surgical anatomy, particularly in patients with known risk factors. Therefore, it is essential to remain vigilant about potential anatomical variations of the ureter or bladder and to customize the surgical approach according to the patient's unique characteristics.

Learning Points

1. TLH brings significant benefits such as shorter hospital stays and faster recovery, transforming gynecological surgery.
2. TLH poses a 0.3–8% risk of urological complications, necessitating skilled surgeons and standardized procedures.
3. TLH complications can be reduced through precise understanding of the retroperitoneal anatomy, identifying the ureter correctly and dissection whenever necessary.
4. Complication rate can be decreased with better understanding of anatomical variations, ongoing surgical training and sharpening surgical skills on simulator.
5. Urological injury is influenced by factors like prior surgeries, especially caesarean sections, previous history of laparotomy, smoking, higher BMI. Hence focus on individual patient factors is necessary.
6. Early identification of injury is critical to outcome; knowledge of nerve sparing surgery, Koch's technique and treatment tailored to the patient will help to reduce the incidence of urological complications in TLH.

Acknowledgments None.

Funding This research received no external funding.

Competing Interest The author declares no conflict of interest that are relevant to content of this chapter.

Ethical Approval Informed consent was obtained from individual participants and patients regarding publication and documentation without disclosing their identity.

References

1. Manandhar T, Sitaula S, Thapa BD, Agrawal A, Thakur A. Prevalence of hysterectomy among gynecological surgeries in a tertiary care hospital. JNMA J Nepal Med Assoc. 2020;58(232):965–70.
2. Denschlag D, Ackermann S, Battista MJ, Cremer W, Egerer G, Follmann M, et al. Sarcoma of the uterus. Guideline of the DGGG and OEGGG (S2k level, AWMF register number 015/074, February 2019). Geburtshilfe Frauenheilkd. 2019;79(10):1043–60.

3. Brodowski L, Jentschke M, Hertel H, Hillemanns P, Kohls F. Abdominal and laparoscopic cervical carcinoma therapy—a comparative economic assessment. Geburtshilfe Frauenheilkd. 2021;81(10):1154–60.
4. Mereu L, Tateo S, D'Alterio MN, Russo E, Giannini A, Mannella P, et al. Laparoscopic lateral suspension with mesh for apical and anterior pelvic organ prolapse: a prospective double center study. Eur J Obstet Gynecol Reprod Biol. 2020;244:16–20.
5. Antoun L, Smith P, Afifi Y, Cullis K, Clark TJ. Short stay laparoscopic hysterectomy: an evaluation of feasibility and patient satisfaction. Facts Views Vis Obgyn. 2021;13(4):377–85.
6. Sculpher M, Manca A, Abbott J, Fountain J, Mason S, Garry R. Cost effectiveness analysis of laparoscopic hysterectomy compared with standard hysterectomy: results from a randomised trial. BMJ. 2004;328(7432):134.
7. Sokol AI, Green IC. Laparoscopic hysterectomy. Clin Obstet Gynecol. 2009;52(3):304–12.
8. Capozzi VA, Monfardini L, Scarpelli E, Barresi G, Rotondella I, De Finis A, et al. Urologic complication after laparoscopic hysterectomy in gynecology oncology: a single-center analysis and narrative review of the literature. Medicina (Kaunas). 2022;58(12):1869.
9. Likić-Ladević I, Kadija S, Ladević N, Stefanović A, Argirović R, Petković S, et al. Urological complications after radical hysterectomy: incidence rates and predisposing factors. Vojnosanit Pregl. 2007;64(6):381–4.
10. Uccella S, Laterza R, Ciravolo G, Volpi E, Franchi M, Zefiro F, et al. A comparison of urinary complications following total laparoscopic radical hysterectomy and laparoscopic pelvic lymphadenectomy to open abdominal surgery. Gynecol Oncol. 2007;107(1 Suppl 1):S147–9.
11. Hwang JH, Lim MC, Joung JY, Seo SS, Kang S, Seo HK, et al. Urologic complications of laparoscopic radical hysterectomy and lymphadenectomy. Int Urogynecol J. 2012;23(11):1605–11.
12. Naveiro-Fuentes M, Rodríguez-Oliver A, Fernández-Parra J, González-Paredes A, Aguilar-Romero T, Mozas-Moreno J. Effect of surgeon's experience on complications from laparoscopic hysterectomy. J Gynecol Obstet Hum Reprod. 2018;47(2):63–7.
13. Magrina J, Yang J, Yi J, Wasson M. Nerve-sparing in gynecology. J Minim Invasive Gynecol. 2021;28(3):387.
14. Torres-Lobaton A, Rueda-Mesias M, Román-Bassaure E, Guadaluperojo H, Barra-Martínez R. Complications of radical hysterectomy during management of stage Ib and IIa cervix uteri cancer. Experience with 145 patients. Ginecol Obstet Mex. 1996;64:265–71.
15. Api M, Boza A, Kayataş S, Boza B. Laparoscopic repair of ureter damaged during laparoscopic hysterectomy: presentation of two cases. Turk J Obstet Gynecol. 2017;14(3):191–4.
16. Chang EJ, Mandelbaum RS, Nusbaum DJ, Violette CJ, Matsushima K, Klar M, et al. Vesicoureteral injury during benign hysterectomy: minimally invasive laparoscopic surgery versus laparotomy. J Minim Invasive Gynecol. 2020;27(6):1354–62.
17. Adelman MR, Bardsley TR, Sharp HT. Urinary tract injuries in laparoscopic hysterectomy: a systematic review. J Minim Invasive Gynecol. 2014;21(4):558–66.
18. Lafay Pillet MC, Leonard F, Chopin N, Malaret JM, Borghese B, Foulot H, et al. Incidence and risk factors of bladder injuries during laparoscopic hysterectomy indicated for benign uterine pathologies: a 14.5 years experience in a continuous series of 1501 procedures. Hum Reprod. 2009;24(4):842–9.
19. Blackwell RH, Kirshenbaum EJ, Shah AS, Kuo PC, Gupta GN, Turk TMT. Complications of recognized and unrecognized Iatrogenic ureteral injury at time of hysterectomy: a population based analysis. J Urol. 2018;199(6):1540–5.
20. Pal DK, Wats V, Ghosh B. Urologic complications following obstetrics and gynecologicai surgery: our experience in a tertiary care hospital. Urol Ann. 2016;8(1):26–30.
21. Hasson F, Keeney S, McKenna H. Research guidelines for the Delphi survey technique. J Adv Nurs. 2000;32(4):1008–15.
22. Janssen PF, Brölmann HA, Huirne JA. Recommendations to prevent urinary tract injuries during laparoscopic hysterectomy: a systematic Delphi procedure among experts. J Minim Invasive Gynecol. 2011;18(3):314–21.
23. İnan AH, Budak A, Beyan E, Kanmaz AG. The incidence, causes, and management of lower urinary tract injury during total laparoscopic hysterectomy. J Gynecol Obstet Hum Reprod. 2019;48(1):45–9.
24. Kang L, Geube A. Bladder trauma. StatPearls. Treasure Island: StatPearls Publishing. Copyright © 2023, StatPearls Publishing LLC; 2023
25. Aydin C, Mercimek MN. Laparoscopic management of bladder injury during total laparoscopic hysterectomy. Int J Clin Pract. 2020;74(6):e13507.
26. Jacob GP, Vilos GA, Al Turki F, Bhangav G, Abu-Rafea B, Vilos AG, et al. Ureteric injury during gynaecological surgery—lessons from 20 cases in Canada. Facts Views Vis Obgyn. 2020;12(1):31–42.
27. Tan-Kim J, Menefee SA, Reinsch CS, O'Day CH, Bebchuk J, Kennedy JS, et al. Laparoscopic hysterectomy and urinary tract injury: experience in a health maintenance organization. J Minim Invasive Gynecol. 2015;22(7):1278–86.
28. Ibeanu OA, Chesson RR, Echols KT, Nieves M, Busangu F, Nolan TE. Urinary tract injury during hysterectomy based on universal cystoscopy. Obstet Gynecol. 2009;113(1):6–10.
29. Utrie JW Jr. Bladder and ureteral injury: prevention and management. Clin Obstet Gynecol. 1998;41(3):755–63.
30. Koh LW, Koh PH, Lin LC, Ng WJ, Wong E, Huang MH. A simple procedure for the prevention of ureteral injury in laparoscopic-assisted vaginal hysterectomy. J Am Assoc Gynecol Laparosc. 2004;11(2):167–9.
31. Vilos GA, Haebe J, Crumley TL, Maruncic MA, King JH, Denstedt JD. Serum biochemical changes after laparoscopy may be indicators of bladder injury. J Am Assoc Gynecol Laparosc. 2001;8(2):285–90.
32. Duicu C, Kiss E, Simu I, Aldea C. A rare case of double-system with ectopic ureteral openings into vagina. Front Pediatr. 2018;6:176.
33. Schultza K, Todab LY. Genetic basis of Ureterocele. Curr Genomics. 2016;17(1):62–9.
34. Medlen H, Barbier H. Vesicovaginal fistula. StatPearls. Treasure Island: StatPearls Publishing Copyright © 2023, StatPearls Publishing LLC; 2023.
35. Eilber KS, Kavaler E, Rodríguez LV, Rosenblum N, Raz S. Ten-year experience with transvaginal vesicovaginal fistula repair using tissue interposition. J Urol. 2003;169(3):1033–6.
36. Forsgren C, Altman D. Risk of pelvic organ fistula in patients undergoing hysterectomy. Curr Opin Obstet Gynecol. 2010;22(5):404–7.
37. Härkki-Sirén P, Sjöberg J, Tiitinen A. Urinary tract injuries after hysterectomy. Obstet Gynecol. 1998;92(1):113–8.
38. Duong TH, Gellasch TL, Adam RA. Risk factors for the development of vesicovaginal fistula after incidental cystotomy at the time of a benign hysterectomy. Am J Obstet Gynecol. 2009;201(5):512.e1–4.
39. Chopin N, Malaret JM, Lafay-Pillet MC, Fotso A, Foulot H, Chapron C. Total laparoscopic hysterectomy for benign uterine pathologies: obesity does not increase the risk of complications. Hum Reprod. 2009;24(12):3057–62.
40. Perez CA, Grigsby PW, Lockett MA, Chao KS, Williamson J. Radiation therapy morbidity in carcinoma of the uterine cervix:

dosimetric and clinical correlation. Int J Radiat Oncol Biol Phys. 1999;44(4):855–66.
41. Kinter KJ, Newton BW. Anatomy, abdomen and pelvis, pudendal nerve. StatPearls. Treasure Island: StatPearls Publishing Copyright © 2023, StatPearls Publishing LLC; 2023.
42. Kaur J, Leslie SW, Singh P. Pudendal nerve entrapment syndrome. StatPearls. Treasure Island: StatPearls Publishing Copyright © 2023, StatPearls Publishing LLC; 2023.
43. Wohlrab KJ, Sung VW, Rardin CR. Management of laparoscopic bladder injuries. J Minim Invasive Gynecol. 2011;18(1):4–8.
44. Minas V, Gul N, Aust T, Doyle M, Rowlands D. Urinary tract injuries in laparoscopic gynaecological surgery; prevention, recognition and management. Obstet Gynaecol. 2014;16 https://doi.org/10.1111/tog.12073.
45. Wang L, Merkur H, Hardas G, Soo S, Lujic S. Laparoscopic hysterectomy in the presence of previous caesarean section: a review of one hundred forty-one cases in the Sydney west advanced pelvic surgery unit. J Minim Invasive Gynecol. 2010;17(2):186–91.
46. Wong JMK, Bortoletto P, Tolentino J, Jung MJ, Milad MP. Urinary tract injury in gynecologic laparoscopy for benign indication: a systematic review. Obstet Gynecol. 2018;131(1):100–8.
47. Tanaka Y, Asada H, Kuji N, Yoshimura Y. Ureteral catheter placement for prevention of ureteral injury during laparoscopic hysterectomy. J Obstet Gynaecol Res. 2008;34(1):67–72.
48. Chou MT, Wang CJ, Lien RC. Prophylactic ureteral catheterization in gynecologic surgery: a 12-year randomized trial in a community hospital. Int Urogynecol J Pelvic Floor Dysfunct. 2009;20(6):689–93.

Cystoscopy and Guided Procedures for a Gynecologists

20

Prateek Gupta, Parima Jain, and Nutan Jain

20.1 Introduction

All gynecologists should consider themselves a urologist for a basic procedure called cystoscopy. Female urethra is hospitable even for beginners, beginning short and wide.

Cystoscopy (Cystourethroscopy) is a minimally invasive telescopic inspection of the bladder and the urethra used to investigate, diagnose, or treat any urological problem. It is a day-care procedure which is like a stethoscope for urologist.

There are innumerable indications of cystoscopy in scope of urology like **diagnostic indications**—diagnosis of lower urinary tract symptoms (obstructive/irritative), evaluation of hematuria, evaluation of recurrent urinary tract infections, assessment of genitourinary fistulas, evaluation of congenital anomalies, taking material for cytological or histological examination etc. and **therapeutic indications**—removal of stones, treating neoplastic conditions of bladder, treating urethral strictures, bladder neck problems, chronic pelvic pain [1] etc.

Though not a part of routine curriculum for a gynecologist, cystoscopy is a valuable tool as an adjunct to gynecological procedures:

1. After Laparoscopic/Open Hysterectomy for evaluating bladder and ureteric orifice
2. Along with TVT/TOT sling procedures as a guide

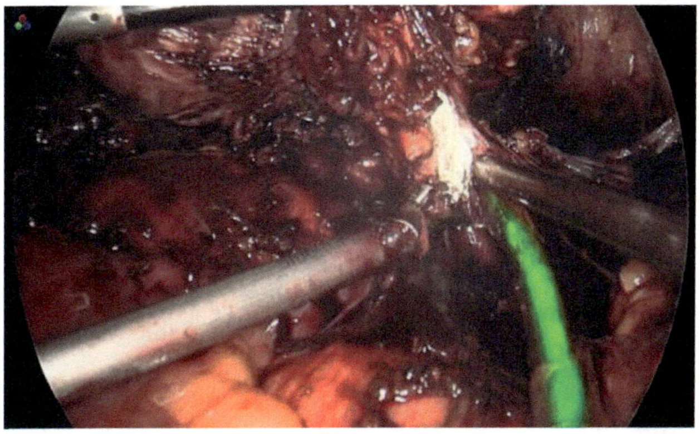

Fig. 20.1 Ureteric catheter guiding in endometriosis

3. Along with all pelvic floor procedures viz. Burch colposuspension, uterosacral ligament suspension and sacrocolpopexy
4. Preoperatively for placing ureteric catheters as a guide for ureters (additionally using indocyanine green or lighted ureteric stents) in difficult pelvic surgeries like severe endometriosis (Fig. 20.1).
5. Confirming any ureteric injury by performing on table retrograde pyelography
6. For placing double J stents in cases of suspected or confirmed ureteric injury or while re-implanting ureters (Fig. 20.2).

P. Gupta (✉) · P. Jain
City Nursing Home and Surgical Center, Bhiwani, Haryana, India
e-mail: parima.jain89@gmai.com

N. Jain
Obstetrics and Gynecology, GSVM Medical College, Affiliated by Kanpur University, Kanpur, Uttar Pradesh, India

Department of Obstetrics and Gynecology, Vardhman Trauma and Laparoscopy Centre Pvt. Ltd., Muzaffarnagar, Uttar Pradesh, India

N. Jain (ed.), *Complex Total Laparoscopic Hysterectomy (TLH) with Newer Approaches in Bladder Dissection*,
https://doi.org/10.1007/978-981-97-3226-5_20

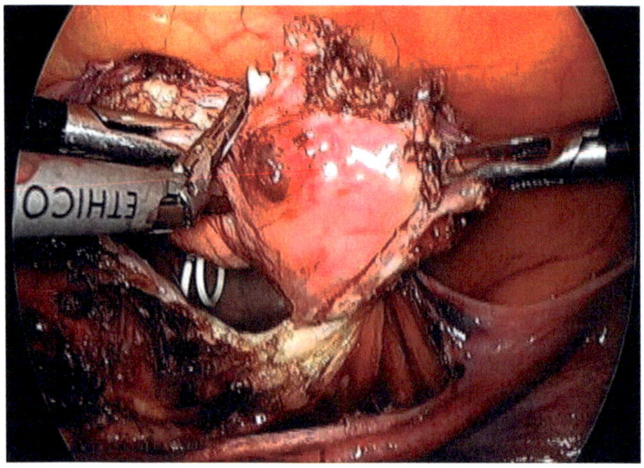

Fig. 20.2 DJ stent while reimplanting ureter

20.2 Types of Cystoscopes [2, 3]

1. **Rigid cystoscope** is a solid straight telescope used with a high intensity light source.
2. **Flexible cystoscope** is a fiberoptic instrument that can bend easily and has a maneuverable tip.

Flexible cystoscope is an office procedure used particularly for diagnosis and for the follow-up in urology [4].

Intraoperative cystourethroscopy can be performed with either rigid or flexible endoscopes.

Flexible cystoscope is mostly advantageous for patients comfort as procedure is easily performed under local anaesthesia.

There are many advantages to the use of the rigid endoscope for cystourethroscopy:

1. **Better optics** because of the use of a rod-lens system in rigid instruments in contrast to the fiber optic system in flexible instruments
2. **A larger working channel** that allows the endoscopist greater versatility in passage of accessory instruments like ureteric catheters, stents etc.
3. **A larger lumen** for water flow, thus improving visualization
4. **Ease of manipulation** and maintaining orientation during inspection within the bladder as flexible scopes require long learning curve for gynecologists.

As gynecologists majorly perform cystoscopy intraoperatively under anesthesia, rigid cystoscope is a better tool (Fig. 20.3). More so they can use their hysteroscope in place of cystoscope (slightly small caliber similar optics scope) thus saving additional expenses [5].

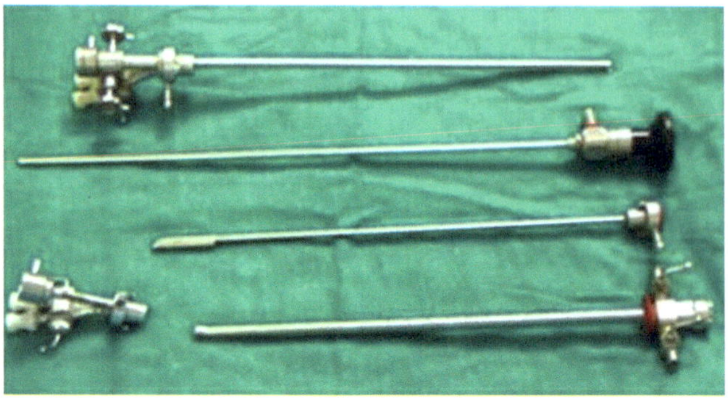

Fig. 20.3 Rigid cystoscope consist of metal sheath, obturator, telescope and bridge

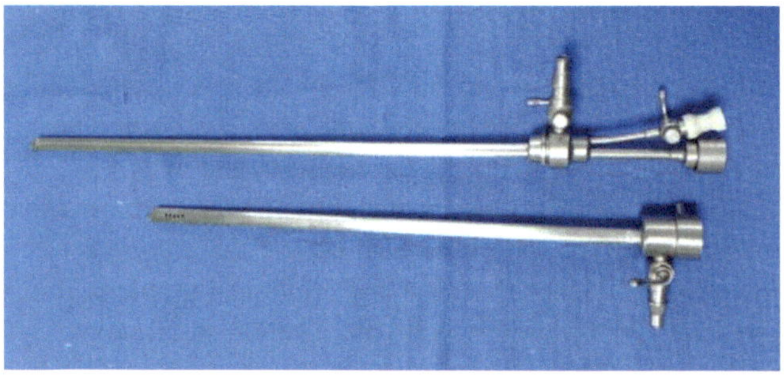

Fig. 20.4 Hysteroscope consists of inner and outer sheath with channels

Commonly used hysteroscopes are 2.9 mm 30 degree as compared to conventional cystoscopes which are 4 mm 30 degree. (diameters and sizes vary from 1.2 mm to 4 mm, 0 degree, 30, 70 or 90 degree). Hysteroscopes comes with inner and outer sheath where inner sheath contains inlet and working channel while outer sheath consist of outlet channel [5, 6] (Fig. 20.4).

Cystoscopes consist of a sheath with obturator, bridge, and telescopes. Sheath sizes vary from 16 to 25 Fr.

20.3 Cystoscopy Procedure [6, 7]

20.3.1 Making Attachments

Firstly bridge is attached to the sheath as per 'zero' markings and locked. Then telescopic lens is placed through the sheath gently. On a bridge, there is inlet and outlet for attaching irrigation fluid. One or two working channels for passing instruments, catheters or stents (Fig. 20.5). Similarly, in hysteroscopes inner sheath is introduced inside outer sheath as per markings. The irrigating fluid is connected to the sheath, and the fiber optic light source connects directly to the telescope (Fig. 20.6). Finally attaching telescope to camera head provides magnified quality image.

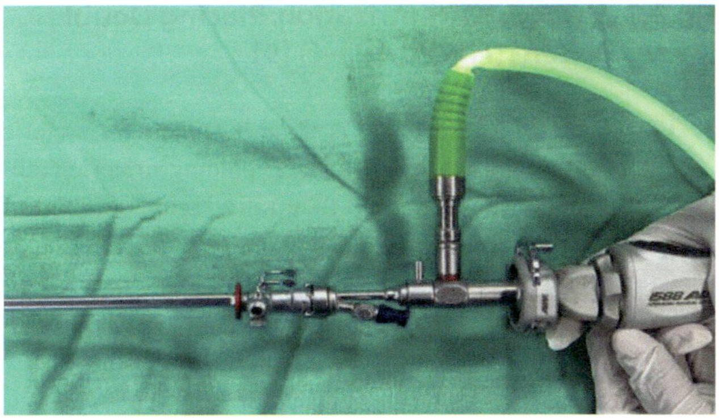

Fig. 20.5 Cystoscope attached

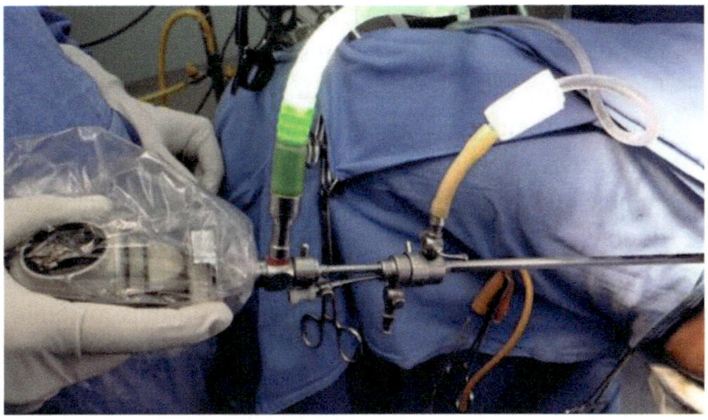

Fig. 20.6 Hysteroscope attached

20.3.2 Introduction and Inspection

- Lubricate the sheath of the cystourethroscope generously with water soluble anesthetic-lubricant, commonly used is lidocaine jelly.
- Inspection of urethral meatus, if the meatal size appears inadequate to accept the endoscope, it can be dilated with metal sounds.
- Introduction of scope in urethra by directing the instrument cephalad towards the umbilicus.
- Systematic inspection of the entire urethra and bladder should be performed.
- Urethral inspection includes looking for any narrowing (stricture), diverticula, caruncle, polyp fistulous opening etc [8] (Fig. 20.7).
- Cystoscopy should begin with filling the bladder at a low pressure (30–40 cm of water) with sterile water or saline solution.
- Bladder inspection includes a systematic evaluation of entire bladder surface sector-wise from 7 to 12 o' clock position and from 5 to 1 o' clock position. Each sector must include the entire length of urinary bladder. Any abnormalities such as vesical calculi, granulations, foreign bodies, diverticula, trabeculae, saccules, neoplasms etc. are carefully noted (Fig. 20.8).
- Identifying both ureteric orifices by filling bladder slightly and identifying a raised horizontal bar (inter ureteric ridge/Mercier's bar) just inside the bladder neck along the trigone (Fig. 20.9). Following interureteric ridge laterally can help in locating an opening with efflux of urine.

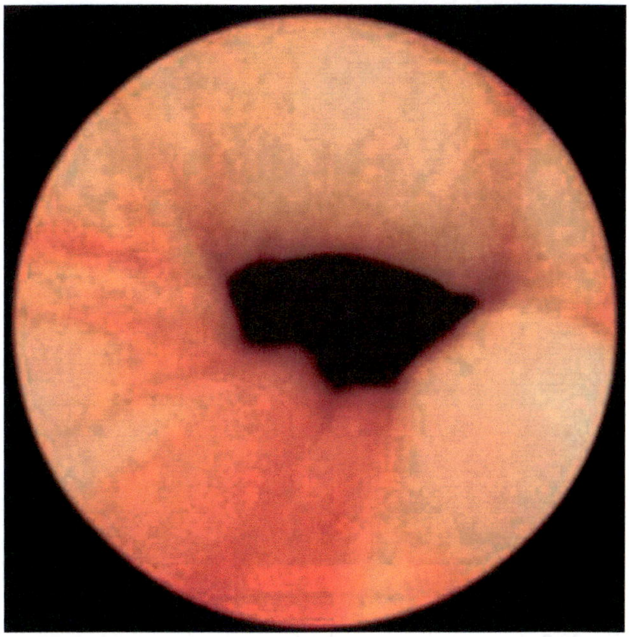

Fig. 20.7 Female urethra

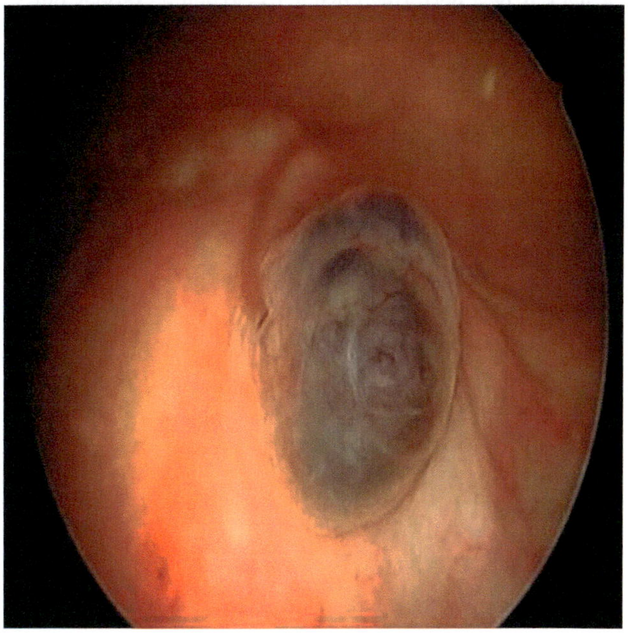

Fig. 20.8 Incidentally detected mass in bladder

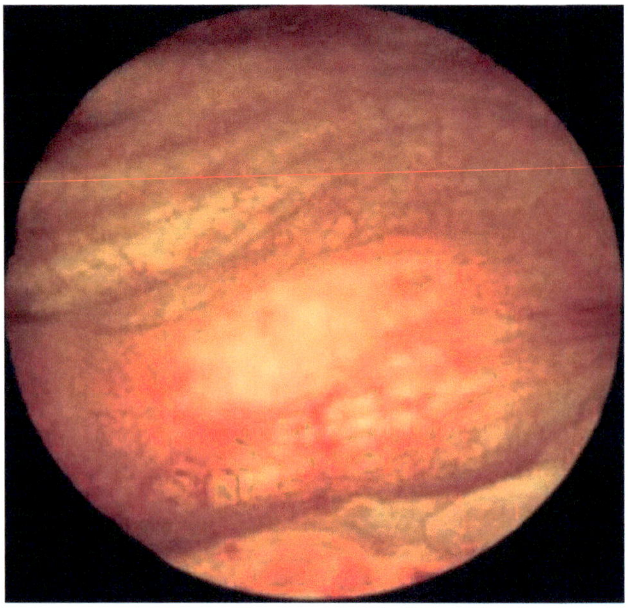

Fig. 20.9 Interureteric ridge with left ureteric orifice visible

- Inspecting lateral walls, dome, anterior wall and bladder neck is best performed using 70–90 degree scopes but 30 degree scope can also be used for careful inspection.
- Finally, bladder capacity should be measured by fully distending the bladder and then removing telescope thus emptying entire bladder in a container.

20.3.3 Ureteric Cathetrization/Placing Double J Stent (Fig. 20.10a–f) [9]

- Introduction of guide wire is done by placing a ureteric catheter through working channel, placing ureteric catheter at ureteric opening and then introducing soft end of guide wire preferably under fluoroscopic guidance Commonly used guide wire is Terumo Radiofocus™ (Nitinol covered with a polyurethrane containing tungsten and a hydrophylic polymer coating- M Coat in varying sizes 0.025/0.032/0.035).
- Guide wire should never be inserted forcefully, if any resistance is felt—it should be withdrawn, and retrograde pyelography should be done via ureteric catheter to confirm cause of resistance. Many a times injuries have been reported due to strictures, kinks, or stones inside ureter.
- Introduction of ureteric catheter should be done till renal pelvis over guide wire after confirming proper coiling of guide wire in pelvicalyceal system of kidney. Ureteric catheter can be used for intraoperative ICG or replaced by double j stent when needed.
- Double J stent is placed by gradually withdrawing ureteric catheter while pushing guide wire in thus maintaining guide wire coiled in pelvicalyceal system. Now over this guide wire appropriate size double j stent is placed with the help of a pusher and finally withdrawing guide wire out.

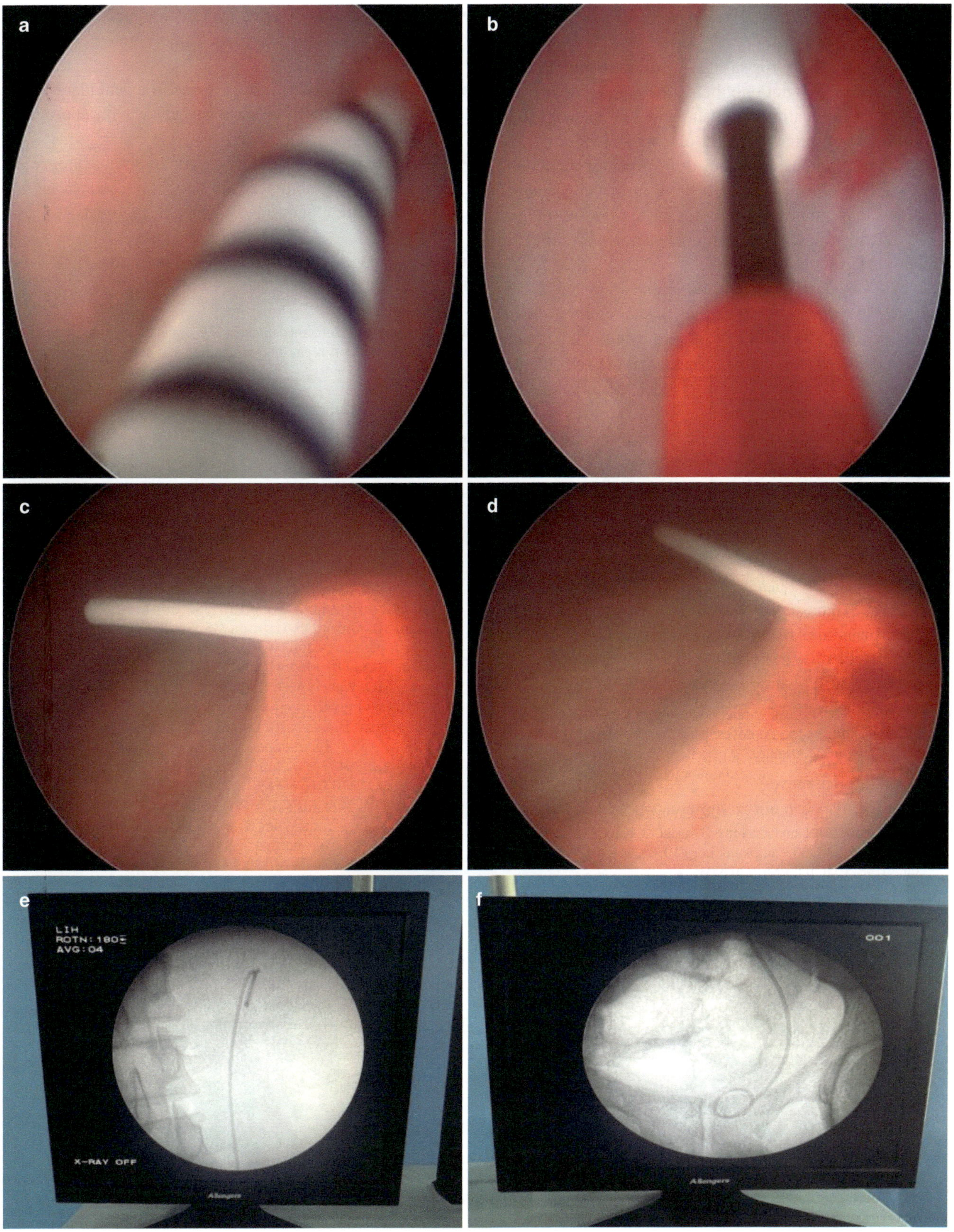

Fig. 20.10 **a** Stent being pushed (marking at 20 cm). **b** Stent pushed till end. **c** Guide wire pulled out. **d** Proper coiling of stent lower end. **e** Coiled upper end of stent (on c-arm). **f** Coiled lower end of stent (on c arm)

20.4 Discussion

Learning cystoscopy for safe gynecological practice is a must now a days. It not only helps in diagnosing any intra operative complication, it also helps in managing the same. Latest advancements by placing preoperative ureteric catheters and using indocyanine green or lighted ureteric stents has proved to be a boon in difficult cases of endometriosis. Incidental findings of tumors in bladders, stones, fistulae has helped patients seek timely intervention [10, 11].

Like any other invasive procedure cystoscopy has its complications like infection, hematuria, bladder perforation, urethral injury etc. which can be managed by antibiotic therapy or continuous bladder drainage. Rare complications like ureteric injury or intraperitoneal bladder perforations may require urologic interventions.

Thus a basic understanding of lower urinary tract anatomy and availability of instruments can make cystoscopy a safe and successful procedure for gynecologists.

Learning Points

- Cystoscopy, essential for gynecologists, is a telescopic inspection of the bladder and urethra.
- It serves diagnostic purposes for lower urinary tract symptoms, hematuria, recurrent infections, and more.
- Therapeutically, cystoscopy addresses conditions like stone removal, treating bladder neoplasms, urethral strictures, and chronic pelvic pain.
- Flexible cystoscopes offer patient comfort, often used under local anesthesia, while rigid cystoscopes are preferred intraoperatively.
- Gynecologists can utilize hysteroscopes as an alternative to cystoscopes, saving cost and maintaining effectiveness.
- Learning cystoscopy is crucial for safe gynecological practices, aiding in diagnosis and management of intraoperative complications.
- Advancements, such as preoperative ureteric catheters and lighted ureteric stents, prove beneficial in challenging cases like severe endometriosis.
- Incidental findings during cystoscopy, including bladder tumors and stones, facilitate timely intervention and patient care.
- Complications like infection, hematuria, and bladder perforation can occur but are manageable with appropriate measures.
- A basic understanding of lower urinary tract anatomy and instrument availability ensures the safe and successful implementation of cystoscopy by gynecologists.

Competing Interest The author declares no conflict of interest that are relevant to content of this chapter.

Ethical Approval Informed consent was obtained from individual participants and patients regarding publication and documentation without disclosing their identity.

References

1. Partin AW, Wein AJ, Kavoussi LR, editors. Campbell walsh urology, 3 vol set. 12th ed. Philadelphia: Elsevier; 2020. p. 117–9. ISBN: 9780323672269.
2. Chou DS, McDougall EM. Advanced endourology. In: Nakada SY, Pearle MS, editors. Springer; 2006 . p. 1–17.
3. Albala DM, Grasso M. Atlas of endourology. CBS publishers and distributors Pvt Ltd; 2021: 3–10.
4. Fozard JB, Green DF, Harrison GS, Smith PH, Zoltie N. Asepsis and out-patient cystoscopy. Br J Urol. 1983;55(6):680–3. https://doi.org/10.1111/j.1464-410x.1983.tb03403.x.
5. Barber MD, Walters MD, Karram MM, Bradley C, editors. Walters & Karram urogynecology and reconstructive pelvic surgery. 5th ed. Philadelphia: Elsevier; 2021. p. 111–20. ISBN: 9780323697835.
6. Fowler CG. Fibrescope urethrocystoscopy. Br J Urol. 1984;56(3):304–7. https://doi.org/10.1111/j.1464-410X.1984.tb05392.x. PMID: 6544615.
7. Parsons DW, Nina LRN, Lee RN, Preminger GM. Smiths' textbook of endourology. John Wiley & Sons Ltd; 2018. 1:4–10,12–20.
8. Uehling DT. The normal caliber of the adult female urethra. J Urol. 1978;120(2):176–7. https://doi.org/10.1016/s0022-5347(17)57092-5.
9. Leslie SW, Sajjad H. Double J placement methods comparative analysis. [Updated 2023 May 30]. In: StatPearls [Internet]. Treasure Island: StatPearls Publishing; 2024.
10. Hamblin JE, Assimos DG, Kroovand RL. Pediatric urology. Prim Care. 1989;16(4):889–904. ISSN 0095-4543. https://doi.org/10.1016/S0095-4543(21)01352-X.
11. Rajamaheswari N. Urogynaecology: an Indian focus. 2003.

Prevention of Ureteric Injuries in Total Laparoscopic Hysterectomy: Use of Indocyanine Green

21

Nutan Jain, Suksham Sharma, and Priyanka Sureddi

Abbreviation

ICG IndoCyanine Green

21.1 Introduction

The integration of laparoscopy into gynecological surgery has brought forth not only innovative advancements but also new challenges in the field. As the complexity of laparoscopically approached gynecological cases rises, it becomes crucial for surgeons to be aware of the risk of ureteral injury. Regarding the incidence of ureteral injury during operative gynecologic laparoscopy, several extensive cohort studies have been conducted, estimating the occurrence rate of ureteral injury during various procedures to be approximately 0.35–1.5% [1, 2]. Multiple studies have highlighted an increased risk of ureteral injury associated with laparoscopic hysterectomy compared to abdominal or vaginal approaches [3–5]. This risk escalates further during hysterectomy for severe endometriosis or high-risk reconstructive pelvic surgery for pelvic organ prolapse, potentially resulting in serious complications and legal ramifications if undetected during surgery. Engel and colleagues documented the first case of ureteral injury during laparoscopic tubal ligation in 1971, where the patient subsequently presented with postoperative flank pain and was diagnosed with right ureteral obstruction, necessitating ureteroneocystostomy and Boari flap repair. Since then, considerable research efforts have been directed towards the prevention and management of ureteral injury during gynecologic surgery. Despite their rarity, ureteral complications arising from gynaecological procedures can be highly morbid. Thus, comprehensive understanding of their prevention, diagnosis, and management is paramount.

Employing meticulous surgical technique and paying close attention to pelvic anatomy are essential in the endeavour to reduce the incidence of ureteral injury. It's crucial for surgeons performing gynaecological surgeries to be aware of the anatomy and potential sites of ureteral injury.

21.2 Sites of Injury

The lower third of the ureter is most prone to injury [6]. The common locations where it is most susceptible to injury in pelvic surgery are:

1. At the pelvic brim, the ureters are situated beneath the insertion point of the infundibulopelvic (IP) ligament.

Supplementary Information The online version contains supplementary material available at https://doi.org/10.1007/978-981-97-3226-5_21. The videos can be accessed individually by clicking the DOI link in the accompanying figure caption or by scanning this link with the SN More Media App.

N. Jain (✉)
Obstetrics and Gynecology, GSVM Medical College, Affiliated by Kanpur University, Kanpur, Uttar Pradesh, India

Department of Obstetrics and Gynecology, Vardhman Trauma and Laparoscopy Centre Pvt. Ltd., Muzaffarnagar, Uttar Pradesh, India

S. Sharma
Obstetrics and Gynecology, Government Medical College, Affiliated by Jammu University, Jammu, Jammu and Kashmir, India

Gynae Endoscopy, Vardhman Trauma and Laparoscopy Centre Pvt. Ltd., Muzaffarnagar, Uttar Pradesh, India

P. Sureddi
Gynaecology Endoscopy, Vardhman Trauma and Laparoscopy Centre Pvt. Ltd., Muzaffarnagar, Uttar Pradesh, India

Obstetrics and Gynecology, Seth GS Medical College and KEM Hospital, Affiliated by Maharashtra University of Health Sciences, Mumbai, Maharashtra, India

N. Jain (ed.), *Complex Total Laparoscopic Hysterectomy (TLH) with Newer Approaches in Bladder Dissection*,
https://doi.org/10.1007/978-981-97-3226-5_21

2. At the cardinal ligament, at the level of the internal cervical os, where the ureter passes inferior to the uterine vessels.
3. At the anterolateral fornix of the vagina where the ureter enters the bladder.

In laparoscopic surgery specifically for deep infiltrating endometriosis, the ureter is at greatest risk of injury during dissection of the parametrium and excision of DIE nodules [7].

During surgery, intraoperative ureteral injury can occur due to various factors such as ligation, kinking, or angulation, as well as complete or partial transection, laceration, crush injury, devascularization, or injury related to diathermy. Avascular necrosis may develop subsequent to extensive dissection of periureteric tissue, leading to compromised blood supply to the anastomotic region during the postoperative phase.

21.3 Risk Factors

Preoperative assessment plays a crucial role in identifying patients at increased risk of ureteral injury. While many ureteral injuries occur without discernible risk factors, certain conditions elevate the likelihood of such injuries, particularly those that disrupt the normal anatomy and architecture of the ureters [8]. These conditions include an enlarged uterus, endometriosis, sizable ovarian masses, pelvic inflammatory disease, prior pelvic surgery, cervical and broad ligament fibroids, historical pelvic radiation, and malignancies.

Less common factors contributing to ureteral injury include TLH in patients with congenital abnormalities such as ureteral duplication, megaureter, ectopic ureter, or kidney, as well as in patients with varying degrees of complexity of Mullerian anomalies. However, it is notable that half of all ureteral injuries occur without identifiable predisposing factors.

21.4 Pre-operative Workup

Numerous preoperative and intraoperative measures can be implemented to mitigate the risk of ureteric injury. Appropriate and adequate imaging to be done preoperatively so as to identify the above mentioned high risk conditions and plan the proposed surgery.

Practical Tip- is to always do imaging of the kidneys as a part of pelvic sonography when evaluating patients preoperatively.

As is the dictum, *"**Anatomy is the mother and Exposure is the father of a good surgery**"*. Therefore, precise intraoperative identification of the ureters stands as the paramount step in preventing iatrogenic ureteral injuries. A comprehensive understanding of ureteral anatomy coupled with meticulous surgical dissection is imperative. Neuman et al. [9] observed that accurate identification and dissection of the ureter during abdominal hysterectomy led to a notable decrease in the rate of iatrogenic ureteral injuries, ranging from 0.2% to 0.7%.

Gynaecologists have utilized various techniques like cystoscopy-directed ureteral catheters and lighted ureteral catheters to avert ureteral injuries. Nevertheless, the rising occurrence of surgeries for severe stages of endometriosis and other intricate conditions mandates a re-evaluation of the efficacy of these techniques and the development of new ones.

21.5 Intraoperative Cystoscopy

While intraoperative cystoscopy is utilized to identify ureteral injuries, it's important to note that a normal cystoscopy doesn't necessarily rule out ureteral injury. Ureteral injuries leading to partial obstruction can be challenging to detect via cystoscopy. Additionally, thermal damage to the ureter may take days for the full extent of injury to become apparent and may not be visible during intraoperative cystoscopy [10]. Hence, there is a need to mark the ureters with illuminated stents and ICG for enhanced visualization and detection.

21.6 Intraoperative Lighted Ureteral Stents

Lighted ureteral stents have been suggested as an innovative approach to maintain awareness of ureteral location throughout the procedure. They aid the surgeon by visually delineating the ureters as a pink glowing line [11–13]. Concerns have been raised regarding potential urothelial injury and stricture formation due to the heat generated by illuminated lighted ureteral stents within the ureteral lumen. Additionally, this technique is costly and may pose challenges in terms of implementation for gynaecologists.

21.7 Intraureteric Indocyanine Green (ICG)

This technique involves injecting indocyanine green (ICG) retrograde into ureteral catheters, which are then visualized under a near-infrared fluorescence (NIRF) imaging system, enabling easier identification of the ureters.

21.8 History and Pharmacokinetics

Indocyanine Green (ICG) is an approved dye for near-infrared fluorescence (NIRF) imaging in clinical practice.

ICG, a tricarbocyanine dye weighing 751.4 Da, is a negatively charged ion belonging to the cyanine dye family. Pharmaceutically available ICG is stable in its dry form at room temperature [14, 15]. Each vial of ICG contains 25 mg of ICG as a sterile lyophilized powder, with less than 5% of sodium iodide. While ICG is soluble in water, it is not readily soluble in saline. ICG fluoresces at approximately 800 nm and longer wavelengths [16].

In 1955, Kodak laboratories pioneered the development of ICG dye for near-infrared (NIR) photography. Initially, the ICG-NIRF technique found clinical use in measuring hepatic function, cardiac output, and ophthalmic angiography after FDA approval for intravenous administration in 1959. Its application has since expanded to include the real-time assessment of tissue and organ perfusion. Presently, NIRF-ICG is utilized to evaluate blood flow in colorectal anastomoses and various urologic surgeries, among other medical procedures. Moreover, fluorescence-guided surgery has been increasingly explored and applied in robotic or laparoscopic gynecologic procedures, including sentinel lymph node biopsy in gynecologic cancers, mapping of endometriosis, and assessment of vascular perfusion in structures like the ureters, vagina, or ovaries [17–19]. When administered systemically, ICG is initially processed by the liver, bile duct, and intestines rather than the kidneys. Therefore, retrograde instillation via a ureteral catheter is necessary for intraoperative visualization of the ureters [20].This dye possesses the unique capability of binding to and staining the proteins of the ureteral epithelium throughout the entire procedure, (although reversibly) [21]. The risk of adverse events is extremely low for ICG, however, it should be avoided in patients with severe Iodine allergy, in patients with liver failure and in patients with uraemia.

21.9 Properties

ICG exhibits numerous clinically valuable properties that have been extensively validated over its prolonged clinical utilization [22]:

(i) Excellent patient safety: nontoxic and non-ionizing,
(ii) It has a short lifespan in blood circulation, enabling repeated applications.
(iii) High signal-to-noise ratio (SNR): There is minimal near-infrared auto fluorescence in tissue, resulting in a low-noise background.
(iv) Deep imaging and tissue penetration: ICG operates within the tissue optical window (NIR), allowing for deep imaging and penetration into tissues.
(v) Needs special camera system for NIR imaging.

21.10 Procedure of Intraoperative ICG Instillation

Cystoscopy for ICG instillation is carried out by either a targeted cystoscope or with a 30 degree hysteroscope readily available in the gynaecology O.T (Fig. 21.1). Ensure the patient is lying supine, in lithotomy position (on their back with the leg in stirrups). Prior to insertion of the instrument, the external urethral meatus is inspected and lubricated well with a local anaesthetic jelly. Then the scope is gently introduced into the urethra under vision. It is further advanced through the urethra into the bladder. Once inside the bladder, a systematic examination of the entire bladder surface is performed. Any abnormalities such as vesical calculi, diverticulae, granulations, trabeculae, neoplasms, endometriotic implants etc. are carefully noted. The ureteral orifices are also assessed for any signs of obstruction or abnormality. A Terumo Radifocus™ guide wire (0.035″, 150 cm) is then placed through the scope, into the ureteric orifice. Over the guide wire, a 5F ureteric catheter is introduced upto the mid ureters (Figs. 21.2 and 21.3).

ICG is prepared in the operating room by dissolving 25 mg of sterile amorphous ICG in 10 mL of distilled water, resulting in a concentration of 2.5 mg/mL. Two millilitres of this solution is taken and further diluted in 10 mL of distilled water. 5 mL of ICG is injected retrograde into the lumen of each ureter, typically up to approximately 10 cm in the ureter, through the catheter, after which the catheter is slowly withdrawn (Figs. 21.4 and 21.5).

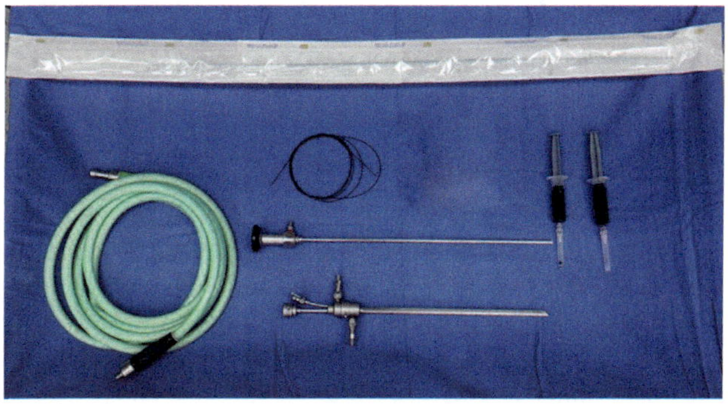

Fig. 21.1 Trolley for ICG instillation: hysteroscope with light cable, ureteric catheter, guide wire, and diluted ICG

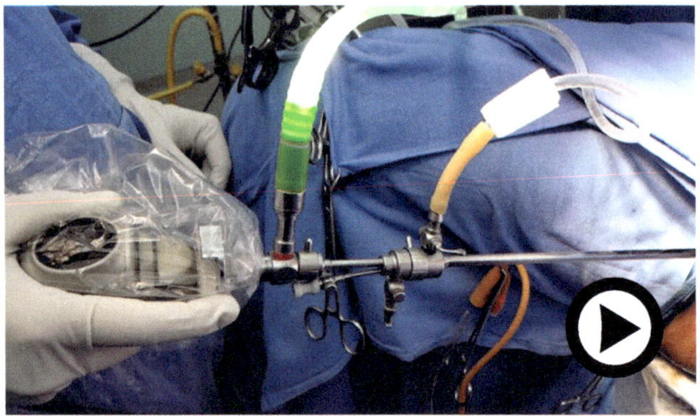

Fig. 21.2 Cystoscopy procedure being initiated (Video.21.2 Cystoscopy and injection of ICG by Ureteric catheter) (▶ https://doi.org/10.1007/000-c9d)

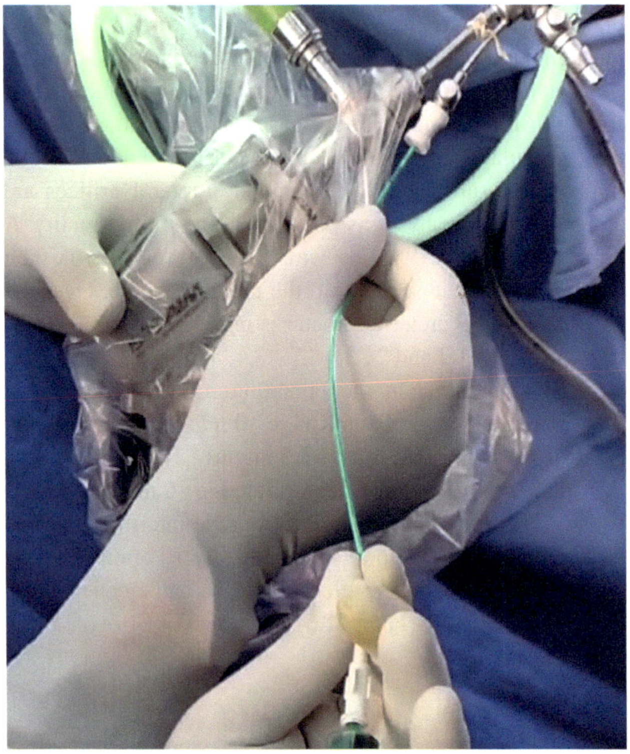

Fig. 21.3 5-F ureteric catheter being inserted cystoscopically for ICG instillation

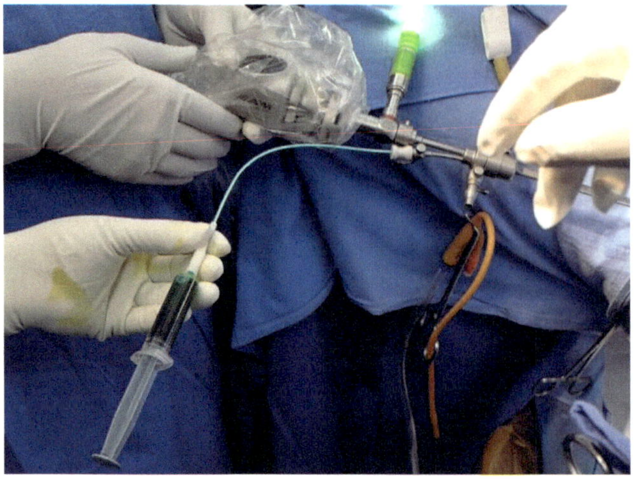

Fig. 21.4 ICG being injected through ureteric catheter

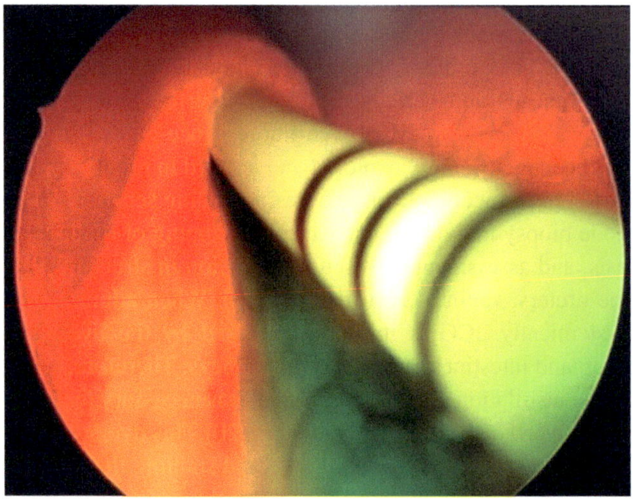

Fig. 21.5 Cystoscopic view: intraureteral 5-fr open-ended catheter insertion into the left ureteral orifice for indocyanine green (ICG) instillation

The ureteral catheters are clamped to minimize leakage of ICG, and then a Foley's catheter is inserted. ICG quickly stains the epithelial lining of the ureter and the bladder by binding to the urothelial proteins. Fluorescence becomes visible approximately 5 minutes after intraureteric injection and typically persists for over 5 hours. On average, the procedure for cystoscopic intraureteric ICG instillation takes around 15 minutes. Our setup utilizes a special camera system with onlay mode, which displays NIR images superimposed on white light images in real-time. Once the ureter is identified, NIRF is intermittently used to safely track the course of the ureter and perform effective ureterolysis, including excising endometriosis (Fig. 21.6a–f).

Lee et al. [23] reported on the intraureteric injection of ICG to localize ureteral stenosis during ureteroureterostomy cases. They found this technique to be beneficial for guiding ureter repair.

Sam Siddhigi et al. [24] used intraureteric injection of diluted ICG for localising ureters during robot assisted laparoscopic sacrocolpopexy. No intraoperative or postoperative adverse effects related to ICG administration were observed during the 2-month follow-up period.

Mandrova et al. [25] used cystoscopic-guided intraureteric ICG immediately before the laparoscopic pelvic surgery. The utilization of ICG enabled the localization of

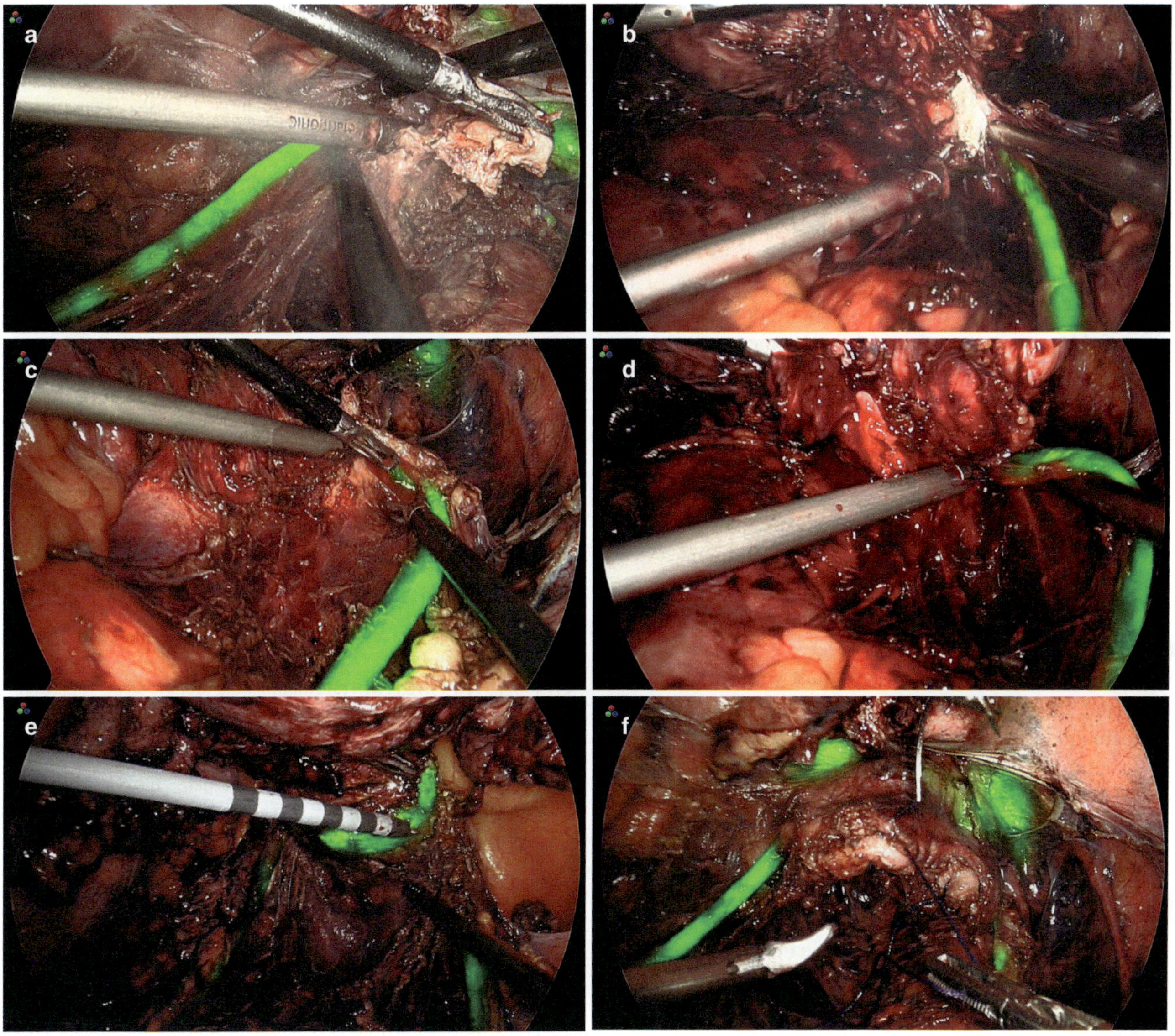

Fig. 21.6 **a** A case of extensive parametrial endometriosis: endometriotic nodule being excised close to the ICG tagged left ureter. **b** Right ureter completely engulfed by severe fibrotic endometriotic tissue. **c** Meticulous ureterolysis being performed with the aid of ICG fluorescence. **d** Navigating extensive endometriosis with ureteric dissection under ICG NIRF imaging. **e** ICG tagged ureters well visualized at the time of colpotomy. **f** Laparoscopic bilateral ureteral visualization under ICG and near-infrared fluorescence (NIRF) imaging during vault closure in TLH

ureters in situations where conventional white light mode failed to visualize them, demonstrating ICG as a safe and viable method that offers real-time ureteral demarcation.

Cabanes et al. [26] described the utilization of this method to aid in intraoperative ureteral dissection and to precisely locate the ureteral pathway in real-time during gynecological oncology surgery. Their study included sixteen patients, and the surgeons were able to visualize both ureters, successfully avoiding ureteral injury in all cases.

In a study conducted by Ramiond et al. [19] 31 cases of ureters were examined during conservative ureteral endometriosis surgery. Among them, five cases showed suspected local ischemia under white light. Upon examination with NIRF-ICG, two cases exhibited regular fluorescence, while three cases showed irregular or absent fluorescence. Consequently, ureteral stent placement was necessary in these cases. This suggests that NIRF-ICG can effectively assess ureteral perfusion and assist in making surgical decisions.

In our experience as well, this innovative approach of intraureteric ICG injection has proven to be immensely beneficial in identifying the entire course of the ureter, thereby aiding in injury prevention during complex gynecologic cases. We have consistently employed this technique for such purposes.

The illuminative identification of ureters via intraureteric ICG instillation and near-infrared fluorescence (NIRF) imaging has been reported to be beneficial in both robotic and laparoscopic surgeries [7, 27–29]. The European Association for Endoscopic Surgery consensus indicated that ICG fluorescence-guided surgery can be regarded as a safe and effective technology [30]. Therefore, with the use of this adjuvant technological imaging system for precise visualization of the retroperitoneal ureter, iatrogenic ureteral injury can be avoided, making surgery safer. Additionally, even beginners can diminish the learning curve through ureteral navigation [31].

Learning Points

- Laparoscopy in gynecology introduces innovations and challenges, heightening the risk of ureteral injury.
- Ureteral injury during gynecologic laparoscopy is estimated at 0.35–1.5%, with increased risks in severe endometriosis hysterectomy.
- The lower third of the ureter is most vulnerable, emphasizing the need for surgeon awareness and meticulous techniques.
- Conditions like an enlarged uterus and endometriosis increase the likelihood of ureteral injuries, necessitating preoperative imaging for risk identification.
- Surgical techniques, including cystoscopy-directed catheters and intraureteric Indocyanine Green (ICG), improve ureteral identification and reduce injury risks.
- ICG with near-infrared fluorescence imaging is a safe and effective tool for real-time ureter visualization during surgery.
- These technologies have a transformative impact on gynecologic surgeries, enhancing safety and potentially aiding surgeon learning curves.

Competing Interest The author declares no conflict of interest that is relevant to content of this chapter.

Ethical Approval Informed consent was obtained from individual participants and patients regarding publication and documentation without disclosing their identity.

References

1. Liapis A, Bakas P, Giannopoulos V, Creatsas G. Ureteral injuries during gynecological surgery. Int Urogynecol J Pelvic Floor Dysfunct. 2001;12(5):391–393; discussion 394. https://doi.org/10.1007/PL00004045.
2. Saidi M, Kentsadler R, Vancaillie T, et al. Diagnosis and management of serious urinary complications after major operative laparoscopy. Obstet Gynecol. 1996;87(2):272–6.
3. Tamussino K, Lang P, Breinl E. Ureteral complications with operative gynecologic laparoscopy. Am J Obstet Gynecol. 1998;178(5):967–70.
4. Ostrzenski A, Radolinski B, Ostrzenska KM. A review of laparoscopic ureteral injury in pelvic surgery. Obstet Gynecol Surv. 2003;58(12):794–9.
5. Manoucheri E, Cohen SL, Sandberg EM, et al. Ureteral injury in laparoscopic gynecologic surgery. Rev Obstet Gynecol. 2012;5:106–11.
6. Brandes S, Coburn M, Armenakas N, McAninch J. Diagnosis and management of ureteric injury: an evidence-based analysis. BJU Int. 2004;94(3):277–89. https://doi.org/10.1111/j.1464-410X.2004.04978.x.
7. Thigpen B, Koythong T, Guan X. Robotic-assisted laparoscopic ureterolysis for deep infiltrating endometriosis using indocyanine green under near-infrared fluorescence. J Minim Invasive Gynecol. 2022;29(5):586–7. https://doi.org/10.1016/j.jmig.2022.01.018.
8. Abboudi H, Ahmed K, Royle J, Khan MS, Dasgupta P, N'Dow J. Ureteric injury: a challenging condition to diagnose and manage. Nat Rev Urol. 2013;10(2):108–15. https://doi.org/10.1038/nrurol.2012.254.
9. Neuman M, Eidelman A, Langer R, Golan A, Bukovsky I, Caspi E. Iatrogenic injuries to the ureter during gynecologic and obstetric operations. Surg Gynecol Obstet. 1991;173(4):268–72.
10. Lee Z, Kaplan J, Giusto L, Eun D. Prevention of iatrogenic ureteral injuries during robotic gynecologic surgery: a review. Am J Obstet Gynecol. 2016;214(5):566–71. https://doi.org/10.1016/j.ajog.2015.10.150.
11. Phipps JH, Tyrrell NJ. Transilluminating ureteric stents for preventing operative ureteric damage. Br J Obstet Gynaecol. 1992;99:81–2.
12. Redan JA, McCarus SD. Protect the ureters. JSLS. 2009;13:139–41.
13. Siddighi S, Carr KR. Lighted stents facilitate robotic-assisted laparoscopic ureterovaginal fistula repair. Int Urogynecol J. 2013;24:515–7.
14. Ebert B, Riefke B, Sukowski U, Licha K. Cyanine dyes as contrast agents for near-infrared imaging in vivo: acute tolerance, pharmacokinetics, and fluorescence imaging. J Biomed Opt. 2011 Jun;16(6):066003. https://doi.org/10.1117/1.3585678.
15. Mishra A, Behera RK, Behera PK, Mishra BK, Behera GB. Cyanines during the 1990s: a review. Chem Rev. 2000;100(6):1973–2011.
16. Landsman ML, Kwant G, Mook GA, Zijlstra WG. Light absorbing properties, stability, and spectral stabilization of indocyanine green. J Appl Physiol. 1976;40(4):575–83.
17. Cacciamani GE, Shakir A, Tafuri A, et al. Best practices in near-infrared fluorescence imaging with indocyanine green (NIRF/ICG)-guided robotic urologic surgery: a systematic review-based expert consensus. World J Urol. 2020;38:883–96.
18. Rossi EC, Jackson A, Ivanova A, Boggess JF. Detection of sentinel nodes for endometrial cancer with robotic assisted fluorescence imaging: cervical versus hysteroscopic injection. Int J Gynecol Cancer. 2013;23:1704–11.
19. Raimondo D, Borghese G, Mabrouk M, et al. Use of indocyanine green for intraoperative perfusion assessment in women with ureteral endometriosis: a preliminary study. J Minim Invasive Gynecol. 2021;28:42–9.
20. Mahalingam SM, Dip F, Castillo M, et al. Intraoperative ureter visualization using a novel near-infrared fluorescent dye. Mol Pharm. 2018;15:3442–7.
21. Alander JT, Kaartinen I, Laakso A, et al. A review of indocyanine green fluorescent imaging in surgery. Int J Biomed Imaging. 2012;2012:940585.
22. Miwa M, Shikayama T. ICG fluorescence imaging and its medical applications. In: Proceedings of the 2008 international conference on optical instruments and technology: optoelectronic measurement technology and applications. SPIE-7160. The International Society for Optical Engineering; 2009.

23. Lee Z, Simhan J, Parker DC, et al. Novel use of indocyanine green for intraoperative, real-time localization of ureteral stenosis during robot-assisted ureteroureterostomy. Urology. 2013;82:729–33.
24. Siddighi S, Yune JJ, Hardesty J. Indocyanine green for intraoperative localization of ureter. Am J Obstet Gynecol. 2014;211(4):436.e1–2.
25. Mandovra P, Kalikar V, Patankar RV. Real-time visualization of ureters using indocyanine green during laparoscopic surgeries: can we make surgery safer? Surg Innov. 2019;26(4):464–8.
26. Cabanes M, Boria F, Hernández Gutiérrez A, Zapardiel I. Intraoperative identification of ureters using indocyanine green for gynecological oncology procedures. Int J Gynecol Cancer. 2020;30:278.
27. Polom J, Kalinowski L, Diana M, et al. Comprehensive review of fluorescence applications in gynecology. J Clin Med. 2021;10:4387.
28. Lee Z, Moore B, Giusto L, Eun DD. Use of indocyanine green during robot-assisted ureteral reconstructions. Eur Urol. 2015;67:291–8.
29. Raffone A, Raimondo D, Oliviero A, et al. The use of near infra-red radiation imaging after injection of indocyanine green (NIR-ICG) during laparoscopic treatment of benign gynecologic conditions: towards minimalized surgery. A systematic review of literature. Medicina. 2022;58:792.
30. Cassinotti E, Al-Taher M, Antoniou SA, et al. European Association for Endoscopic Surgery (EAES) consensus on indocyanine green (ICG) fluorescence-guided surgery. Surg Endosc. 2023;37(3):1629–48. https://doi.org/10.1007/s00464-023-09928-5.
31. Shibata R, Goldman T, Acholonu U Jr. Intraoperative dyes, fluorescence and enhanced imaging in benign gynaecologic surgery. Curr Opin Obstet Gynecol. 2022;34:237–43.

Management of Bladder Injury in Total Laparoscopic Hysterectomy

22

Nutan Jain, Sakshi Srivastava, and Suksham Sharma

22.1 Introduction

This chapter delves into the various nuances of avoiding bladder injury. During the various complex scenarios where TLH is being carried out, despite one's best efforts and precautions still, sometime or the other bladder injuries may be encountered. So, now we present a text of careful per operative identification of bladder injury, steps of closure of the bladder injury and the follow up of these patients after a vesical injury repaired during the surgery.

The incidence of urological complications varies depending on the type of laparoscopic surgery performed. The rate of urinary tract injuries is 0.3–1% during pelvic surgery, 0.33% in gynaecological laparoscopic surgery, and 1.3% in LH [1–3]. During LH, bladder injury occurs 3 times as common as ureter injuries [1, 4]. Nezhat et al. reported the incidence of bladder injury during laparoscopic procedures ranging from 0.02% to 8.3% of cases. The bladder dome is the most common site of injury [5].

N. Jain (✉)
Obstetrics and Gynecology, GSVM Medical College, Affiliated by Kanpur University, Kanpur, Uttar Pradesh, India

Department of Obstetrics and Gynecology, Vardhman Trauma and Laparoscopy Centre Pvt. Ltd., Muzaffarnagar, Uttar Pradesh, India

S. Srivastava
Obstetrics and Gynecology, Rohilkhand Medical College and Hospital, Affiliated by Bareilly International University, Bareilly, Uttar Pradesh, India

Gynae Endoscopy, Vardhman Trauma and Laparoscopy Centre Pvt. Ltd., Muzaffarnagar, Uttar Pradesh, India

S. Sharma
Gynae Endoscopy, Vardhman Trauma and Laparoscopy Centre Pvt. Ltd., Muzaffarnagar, Uttar Pradesh, India

Obstetrics and Gynecology, Government Medical College, Affiliated by Jammu University, Jammu, Jammu and Kashmir, India

22.1.1 Bladder Injuries

Bladder injuries mainly occur at the dome as a result of suprapubic trocar insertion or dissection of the vesico-uterine peritoneal fold. Prevention of these injuries may be accomplished by:

1. Catheterization of the bladder prior to Trendelenburg positioning.
2. Indwelling catheters in any case longer than 30 minutes or insertion if the procedure inadvertently lasts longer than 30 minutes.
3. Directing the suprapubic trocar away from the retropubic space on insertion.
4. Careful dissection of the vesico-uterine peritoneal fold.

Many times, the dissection of vesico-uterine space can be difficult if the patient has a surgical history of previous caesarean sections or pelvic surgery. The procedure with the highest frequency of bladder injury is the laparoscopic hysterectomy, and occurs mostly with blunt or sharp electrosurgical dissection [6], in the utero vesical plane.

These injuries may be recognized intra-operatively by the following signs:

1. Presence of gas in the Foley catheter bag.
2. Appearance of the Foley's catheter tip & bulb in the laparoscopic field.
3. Development of hematuria during the case.
4. Leakage of indigo carmine or methylene blue from the bladder injury site.
5. Movement of the bladder with manipulation of the accessory trocar.
6. Formation of a suprapubic mass during the case.

When these injuries are recognized, the site and extent of the injury should be recognized. Transurethral injection of indigo carmine or methylene blue can be done to confirm

N. Jain (ed.), *Complex Total Laparoscopic Hysterectomy (TLH) with Newer Approaches in Bladder Dissection*,
https://doi.org/10.1007/978-981-97-3226-5_22

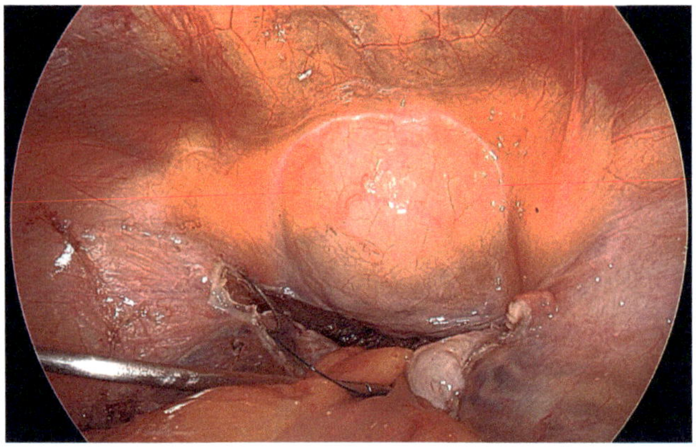

Fig. 22.1 Bladder visualised after cystosufflation done to recognize the bladder limits in case of difficult dissection

the diagnosis. Cystosufflation [7], i.e. (Fig. 22.1) connecting the CO2 insufflation pipe to the Foley's catheter and allowing bladder to distend and show its margins in an adherent uterus. This has the benefit over saline injection that filling and emptying of CO2 from bladder is much faster. This approach can be used for checking bladder integrity in an expedited manner. A surgical bougie can also be used to identify the limits of the bladder in densely adherent bladder and uterus with multiple previous caesarean sections (Fig. 22.2a, b).

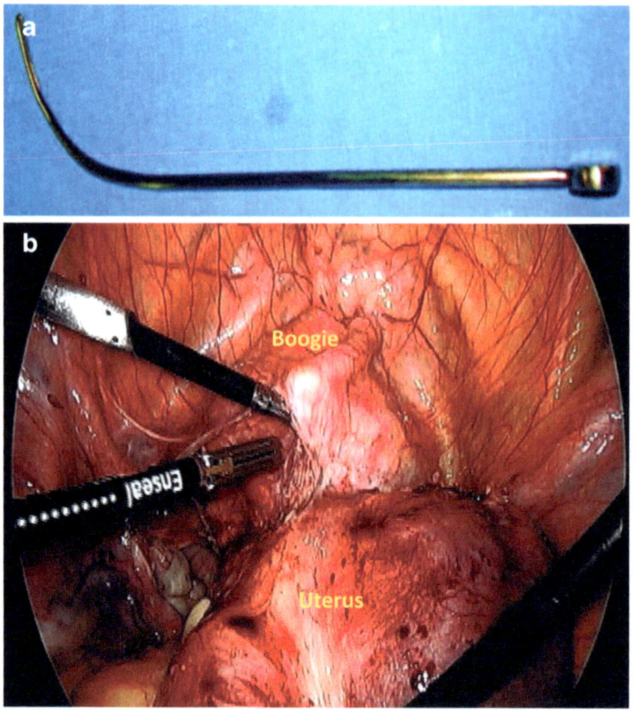

Fig. 22.2 **a** Surgical bougie. **b** Surgical bougie delineating margin of bladder

22.1.2 Bladder Injury Detection

If injury is suspected, then on performing a check for bladder integrity, leakage of methylene blue or indigo carmine can be seen from bladder rent laparoscopically or it can be detected during check cystoscopy.

22.1.2.1 Surgical Technique

In cases of dense adhesions obliterating the anterior cul-de-sac, risk of bladder injury is high (Fig. 22.3a, b). The first sign of bladder injury is that the urobag fills up with air. The moment the pelvic assistant mentions this, we should make an endeavor to find out from where the bladder injury has occurred. Secondly, the Foley's bulb can be visualized in its full view from the bladder rent, as the yellow bulb can never be missed from the laparoscopic view. Thirdly, there could be bleeding, however, usually vesical injuries do not bleed. After identification of the site of injury one must proceed to close the vesical rent (Fig. 22.4a–i) before the colpotomy. This is because when the manipulator cup is pushed cephalad, we can see the bladder in its full anatomical configuration and then identifying both the edges of the rent and doing a good single or a double layer closure is very easy. Hence, this point should be remembered at all costs, that uterus removal should be done after the bladder injury site has been duly repaired. The suture material, used for the bladder injury at our setup is 2-0 or a 3-0 VICRYL™ (polyglactin 910), though many centers have now changed over to barbed sutures, which are easy, knotless, and a simple 15-centimeter barbed suture length can easily tide over the vesical injury. When injury occurs during adhesiolysis bladder injuries usually tend to be small, just about a centimeter or two, while, when they are encountered during the entry by a trocar the injury would be just 5 mm in size. Since the injury usually tends to be small so one must actively lookout for the early warning symptoms. We start with suturing from one end of the bladder rent, and each bite is taken 1 cm away from the edge of the rent in the bladder, done in a non-locking continuous manner. As we finish the first layer, we instill the bladder with saline and check if there is any leakage from the anastomotic site. If there is any leakage of urine or saline

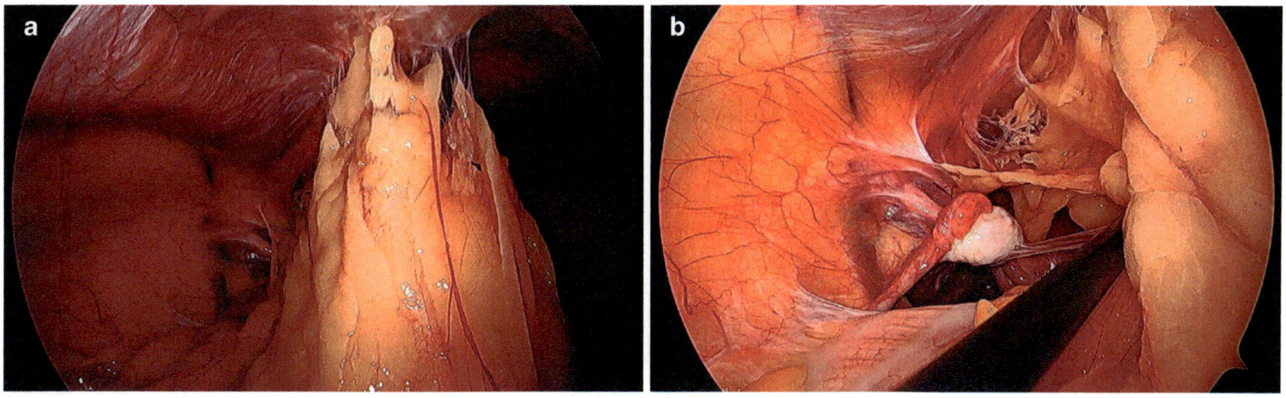

Fig. 22.3 **a** Dense omental adhesions. **b** Dense omental adhesions

then, we then continue back with a second layer closure and then tie the knot at the starting point. Once the suture has been completely done in two layers, we again re-fill the bladder with saline and see that the closure is watertight. The same can be achieved with barbed sutures in a single or double layer. In suturing it is important to incorporate mucosa in full thickness and to ensure a watertight closure, but it should not be under undue tension. Finally, it is very important to put an omental patch to give more support and increase the blood supply to the anastomotic site. This is done by bringing down an omental patch.

For this, the patient is readjusted, from steep Trendelenburg position, we bring the patient slightly head up so that the omentum can be brought down without any tension. Two bites are taken in the omentum and another two or three bites over the bladder sutured site, in this manner the omentum is hitched to the bladder. Hence, this gives reinforcement and a good blood supply to the anastomotic site.

At end of the procedure a low pressure cystoscopy is recommended. Identification of the ureteral orifices and insertion of ureteral stents are recommended when the injuries are close to the ureteral orifices. These patients usually fare very well in the post-operative phase and the follow -up of these patients is carefully done. The Foley's catheter is left in situ for 7–10 days. Before removal of the Foley's catheter a cystogram [8] may be considered to confirm bladder healing. It has become standard of care to keep Foley's catheter for only 7–10 days. Bladder is a perfect gentleman and heals well in 1 week. Hence, the patient can be called for removal of the sutures and Foleys in the same sitting.

Bladder repair usually does not cause any concern. But it is important to be aware of an occasional vesicovaginal fistula. So, the closure should not be under tension and applying an omental patch is a good move. A complete evaluation of the bladder dome, trigone and ureteral orifices should be done before concluding the procedure by conducting a cystoscopy and a tension free closure of injury site. Patients receive prophylactic antibiotic cover.

Oral Pyridium tablets could be prescribed to the patient night before the surgery in all cases, so that urine turns orange in colour and can be promptly seen in the advent of any injury intra-operatively. We have extensively used this technique and this step also helps to recognize the ureteric spurt during cystoscopy (Fig. 22.5).

22.1.3 Pitfalls [1]

1. Bladder injury which is missed intra-operatively may present postoperatively as decreased urine output, prominent suprapubic mass, azotaemia (Sr.Creatinine >1.2). Hence, it is very important to recognize the site of injury by instilling methylene blue dye from catheter below or indigo carmine on the slightest suspicion of injury.
2. The development of fistulas is a consequence of inadequately repaired bladder injuries or premature removal of the Foley catheter before the completion of the bladder healing process. It is crucial to ensure proper drainage and assess the cystotomy repair through a cystogram before discontinuing the Foley catheter.

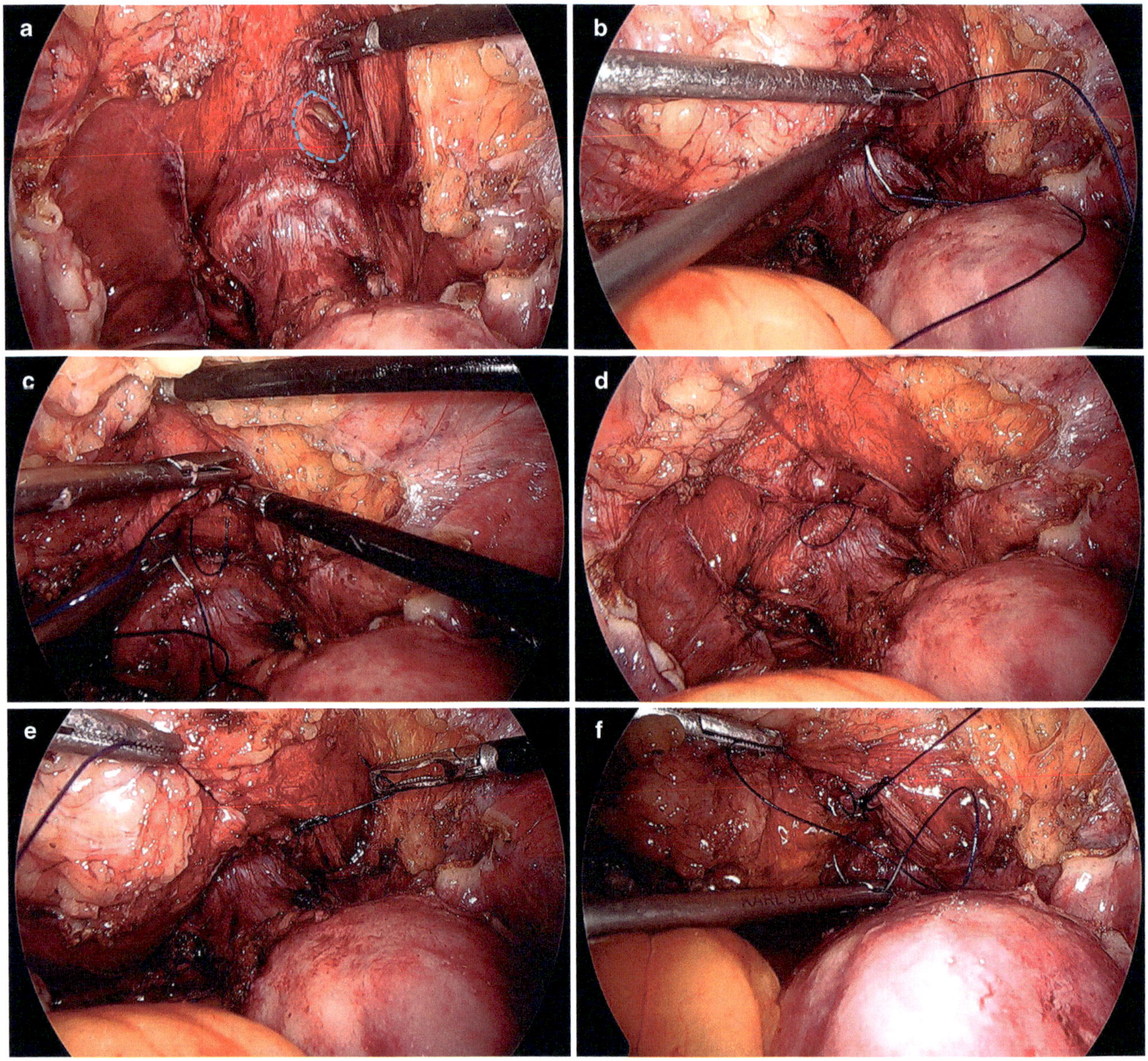

Fig. 22.4 **a** A rent in the dome of bladder noted. **b** Suturing started with 2-0 polyglactin suture. **c** First layer closure with Vicryl 2.0. **d** First layer completed. **e** Filling the bladder with saline to see for integrity of first layer. **f** Slight leak seen from the sutured site after first layer closure. **g** Second layer of suturing started. **h** Second layer completed. **i** Checking for the water tight closure. **j** Bladder rent to be closed before the colpotomy. **k** Putting an omental patch. **l** Completed picture of bladder repair with omental patch

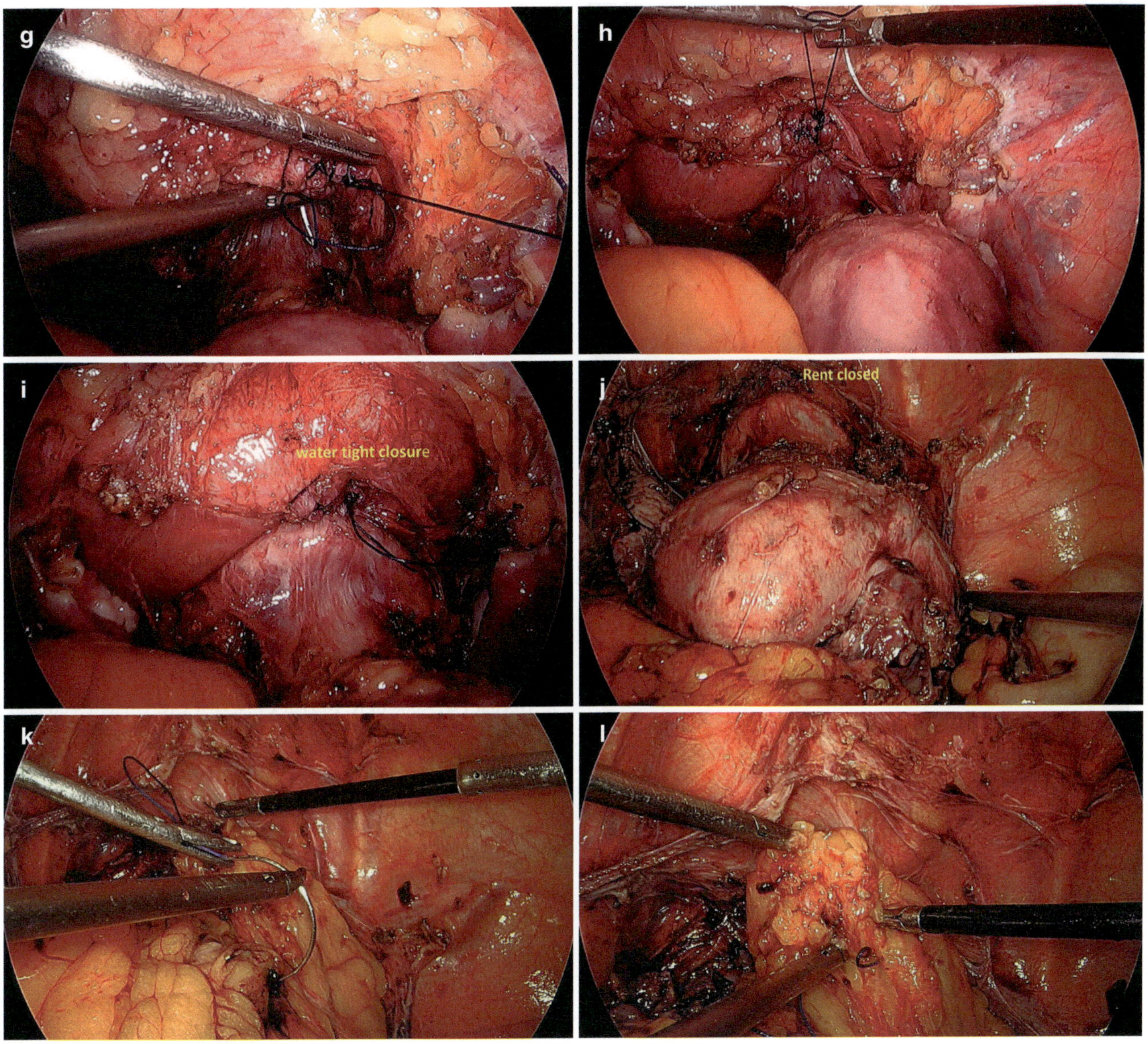

Fig. 22.4 (continued)

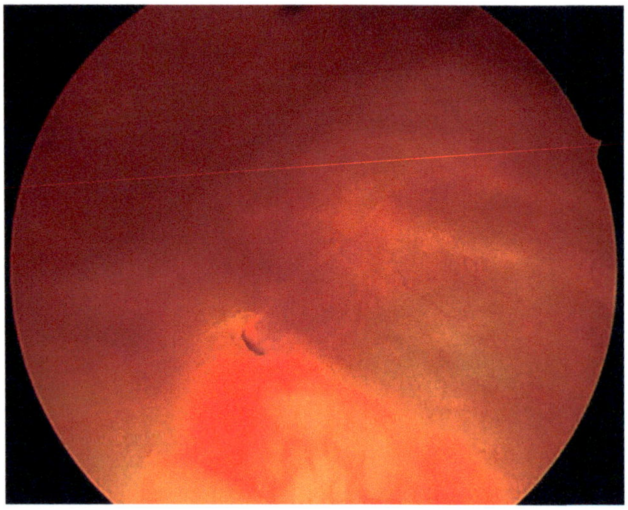

Fig. 22.5 Ureteric peristalsis & reflux noted in cystoscopy

Learning Points to Avoid a Bladder Injury

- Always catheterize the bladder prior to Trendelenburg position.
- Indwelling catheter should be used in any prolonged surgery.
- Careful sharp and blunt dissection of the pubo-vesico-cervical fascia in the uterovesical pouch should be done during laparoscopic hysterectomy.
- Try lateral approach or the novel, Comprehensive Canopy Concept- 'The 3 Step Technique' of bladder dissection.
- Suprapubic trocar insertion, if required should be careful, under direct vision and directed away from retropubic space.
- Use of a surgical bougie to find the limits of bladder in difficult and complex bladder adhesions.
- Cystosufflation can be tried, with CO2 pneumoperitoneum tubing attached to Foley's catheter.
- Pyridium tablet the night before to stain urine orange for easy detection.

Competing Interest The author declares no conflict of interest that are relevant to content of this chapter.

Ethical Approval Informed consent was obtained from individual participants and patients regarding publication and documentation without disclosing their identity.

References

1. Teeluckdharry B, Gilmour D, Flowerdew G. Urinary tract injury at benign gynecologic surgery and the role of cystoscopy: a systematic review and meta-analysis. Obstet Gynecol. 2015;126:1161–9.
2. Blackwell RH, Kirshenbaum EJ, Shah AS, Kuo PC, Gupta GN, Turk TM, et al. Complications of recognized and unrecognized iatrogenic ureteral injury at time of hysterectomy: a population based analysis. J Urol. 2018;199:1540–5.
3. Lee JS, Choe JH, Lee HS, Seo JT. Urologic complications following obstetric and gynecologic surgery. Korean J Urol. 2012;53:795–9.
4. Wong JM, Bortoletto P, Tolentino J, Jung MJ, Milad MP. Urinary tract injury in gynecologic laparoscopy for benign indication: a systematic review. Obstet Gynecol. 2018;131:100–8.
5. Nezhat FR, Apostol R, Nezhat C, Nezhat CR. Ureteric and bladder injury and repair. In: Nezhat CR, editor. State-of-the-art atlas and textbook of laparoscopic suturing in gynecology. Jaypee Brothers Medical Publishers; 2015. p. 203–11.
6. Jain N, Sahni P. Laparoscopic surgery in infertility and gynecology. In: Prevention and management of complications, Jaypee Gold Standard Mini Atlas Series®. Jaypee Brothers Medical Publishers; 2011. p. 249–81.
7. O'Hanlan KA. Cystosufflation to prevent bladder injury. J Minim Invasive Gynecol. 2009;16(2):195–7.
8. Rödder K, Olianas R, Fisch M. Das Blasentrauma. Diagnostik und Behandlung [Bladder injury. Diagnostics and treatment]. Urologe A. 2005;44(8):878–82. German. https://doi.org/10.1007/s00120-005-0853-1. PMID: 15959610.

Vesico Vaginal Fistula

23

Hrishikesh Pandit, Amit Tajane, Hrishikesh Wagholika, and Ambreen Shaikh

23.1 Introduction

Persistent urinary leakage, dampness, and odor contribute to the social ostracism experienced by individuals with vesicovaginal fistula (VVF), significantly impacting their quality of life [1].

In the developed countries, the most common cause of vesicovaginal fistula is gynecological surgery [2].

Vesicovaginal fistulas primarily result from obstructed labor in developing countries, causing pressure necrosis. A comprehensive diagnostic workup is essential, given that most cases necessitate definitive surgical management. Achieving successful outcomes mainly depends on optimizing the timing, approach, graft utilization, postoperative care, and surgical proficiency.

23.2 Etiology

This condition's etiology exhibits variations and falls into two main categories: congenital or acquired. Acquired vesicovaginal fistula are further categorized into obstetric, surgical, malignant, radiation and miscellaneous categories. Although congenital vesicovaginal fistula is very rare, the acquired variant mainly occurs following obstetric and gynaecological trauma. Particularly in developed regions, gynaecological surgeries emerge as the primary causative factor, with bladder injury during hysterectomy being the most prevalent cause.

In developing countries, obstructed labour and the resulting pressure necrosis is the most common cause of vesicovaginal fistulas. Poor socioeconomic status, malnourishment, low literacy rate, early marriage, childbearing and inadequate obstetrical care are important risk factors for developing a vesicovaginal fistula in the developing world [1].

Additional acquired factors contributing to this condition include retroperitoneal, vascular, or pelvic surgeries, urologic or gynaecological procedures, infectious and inflammatory diseases, sexual trauma, vaginal laser interventions, external violence, and the presence of vaginal foreign bodies [3]. Furthermore, locally advanced malignancies, particularly cervical, vaginal, and endometrial carcinomas, contribute to approximately 3–5% of VVF cases in industrialized nations [4].

Etiology of Vesicovaginal Fistula

1. Post-surgical:
   (a) Abdominal hysterectomy
   (b) Vaginal hysterectomy
   (c) Anti-incontinence surgery
   (d) Anterior vaginal wall prolapse surgery (e.g. colporrhaphy)
   (e) Vaginal biopsy
   (f) Other pelvic surgery (e.g., vascular, rectal)
   (g) Bladder biopsy/endoscopic resection/laser
2. Obstetric causes:
   (a) Obstructed labour
   (b) Forceps laceration
   (c) Uterine rupture
   (d) Caesarean section injury to bladder

Supplementary Information The online version contains supplementary material available at https://doi.org/10.1007/978-981-97-3226-5_23. The videos can be accessed individually by clicking the DOI link in the accompanying figure caption or by scanning this link with the SN More Media App.

H. Pandit (✉)
Pandit Hospital and 3D Laparoscopic Center, Ahmednagar, Maharashtra, India

A. Tajane
Archit Hospital, Sangamner, Maharashtra, India

H. Wagholika
Wagholikar Hospital, Sangamner, Maharashtra, India

A. Shaikh
Department of Obstetrics and Gynaecology, Seth G S Medical College and Kem Hospital, Mumbai, Maharashtra, India

N. Jain (ed.), *Complex Total Laparoscopic Hysterectomy (TLH) with Newer Approaches in Bladder Dissection*, https://doi.org/10.1007/978-981-97-3226-5_23

3. Traumatic:
   External trauma (e.g., penetrating, pelvic fracture, sexual)
4. Others:
   (a) Radiation therapy
   (b) Advanced pelvic malignancy
   (c) Infectious/inflammatory
   (d) Foreign body

23.3 Epidemiology

The occurrence of vesicovaginal fistula is uncommon in developed nations. However, its prevalence is significantly higher in developing and underdeveloped countries [5]. Determining the precise incidence and prevalence among females globally is challenging due to substantial stigma within many populations.

Hysterectomy stands as the most common gynaecological surgery leading to vesicovaginal fistula formation, contributing to 80% of the yearly incidence in developed nations. The occurrence of vesicovaginal fistula formation varies depending on the surgical approach. Laparoscopic procedures exhibit the highest incidence (2.2 in 1000), followed by transabdominal (1 in 1000), with the transvaginal approach showing the lowest incidence (0.2 in 1000) [6].

Causes of VVF

- Suture passes through the bladder at the time of vault closure. This happens because of inadequate bladder dissection at the time of TLH /TAH/VH or inadequate retraction of bladder.
- Thermal injury is most common cause. It happens more frequently while bladder dissection in cases of previous LSCS. Use of Bipolar Clamp in open surgery after the uterine artery clamp may lead to thermal injury.

23.3.1 History and Clinical Presentation

In historical context, a patient commonly presents with persistent urinary incontinence following recent pelvic surgery, which is the classic clinical manifestation of a vesicovaginal fistula. The severity and timing of symptoms can vary. Diagnosis is often straightforward in postoperative cases, with patients typically reporting urine leakage through the vagina around 7–12 days after gynaecological or pelvic surgery. The onset of symptoms is likely related to tissue necrosis caused by obstructed prolonged labor or sutures leading to tissue strangulation during pelvic surgery. Patient may show decreased urine output with development of urinary leak per vaginum if direct rent has occurred at the time of surgery. The hallmark presentation sign involves persistent (day and night) incontinence following a recent pelvic operation. In cases of small fistulas, the sole symptom might be a watery discharge from the vagina alongside normal voiding. Notably, a fistula induced by radiation therapy can manifest even up to 20 years after the initial insult [7].

23.3.2 Physical Examination and Evaluation

In the assessment and examination process, a tampon dye test can confirm the diagnosis. This procedure involves inserting a regular tampon or gauze into the vagina, followed by filling the bladder with dilute methylene blue. The patient is then asked to ambulate.

To prevent contamination, it is recommended to insert the gauze or tampon before filling the bladder. After removal and inspection, the presence of blue dye near the apex of the gauze confirms a vesicovaginal fistula. If the dye is only found on the distal end of the tampon, it may indicate spillage during filling or other types of urinary incontinence.

In an outpatient clinical setting, diagnosing a vesicovaginal fistula requires a comprehensive evaluation of its size, number and location before considering curative surgery. A crucial part of this assessment is a thorough physical examination. This examination is crucial to evaluate for acute inflammation, infection, edema, necrosis, or any other bladder or vaginal pathology. If necessary, surgical correction can be postponed for 2–3 months to allow for recovery and optimal tissue health. If there is no sign of inflammation and the tissue appears healthy, immediate surgical correction can proceed.

Office cystoscopy and contrast studies, such as computed tomography (CT) urography, are commonly used for diagnosis. These methods help identify additional injuries and assist in surgical planning.

Attention to specific symptom details, such as leakage volume, vaginal fluid color, and smell, is necessary to distinguish urogenital fistula-related symptoms from other causes of urinary incontinence. Patients with a urogenital fistula often report more frequent changes of heavy pads. Complex fistulas involving ureters are also a possibility.

In imaging studies, cystoscopy is performed to evaluate residual bladder injury and to assess the number and characteristics of intravesical fistula orifices. Retrograde pyelography is utilized to examine ureteral integrity. Lower ureteric injuries associated with the large fistulas at the level of UV junction may be missed on CT Urography. They can be diagnosed at the time of Cystoscopy and DJ Stenting. At the time of DJ Stenting DJ stent may not pass through the Ureteric orifice or it gets coiled back in the bladder.

Pelvic MRI, being more sensitive than IVP or CT in diagnosing vesico-uterine fistula, provides higher soft-tissue contrast compared to CT cystogram. Specific institutional-based protocols, including combined cystoscopy and vaginoscopy, are available for evaluating suspicious or established vesicovaginal fistulas.

Another commonly performed test is the "double-dye" test, where the patient ingests oral phenazopyridine shortly before the office visit. Following this, a tampon or gauze is inserted into the vagina. After adequately filling the bladder, the tampon is removed and examined for orange staining. The presence of such staining indicates a genitourinary tract fistula, which could be a ureterovaginal or vesicovaginal fistula. Subsequently, the bladder is back-filled with dilute methylene. If only orange staining is observed without blue staining, a ureterovaginal fistula is likely. However, if both orange and blue staining are present, a vesicovaginal fistula is more probable.

Cystoscopy is especially beneficial for pinpointing the exact location of the fistula tract within the bladder. A small ureteric catheter or pediatric Foley catheter may be inserted through a suspected fistula tract to ascertain its entry point into the vagina. Vaginoscopy, conducted in the office using the cystoscope, assists in localizing the fistula opening on the vaginal side and is generally well-tolerated by most patients. Prior to surgical repair, contrast studies such as a multiphasic CT urogram are advised to detect any concurrent ureteral fistulas or abnormalities. Although more invasive techniques like endoanal ultrasound or subtraction magnetic resonance fistulography are usually unnecessary, they may be contemplated in specific cases.

23.3.3 Classification

- Simple vesicovaginal fistulas are singular, small in size (<0.5 cm), and are observed in non-radiated patients with no signs of malignancy involvement.
- Intermediate vesicovaginal fistulas ranges in size of 0.5–2.5 cm.
- Complex vesicovaginal fistulas are large in size (>2.5 cm) [1]

23.3.4 Differential Diagnosis

The possible causes of abnormal vaginal fluid leakage post-operatively or postpartum include infection, inflammation, malignancy, urgency or stress urinary incontinence, or other urogenital abnormalities [8] Sometimes ascitic/peritoneal fluid in cases of anaemic patients may leak through the vault.

We can send the leaking fluid for creatinine level for differential diagnosis with abdominal fluid or urine. If its value is equal or exceeds blood creatinine then its urine and if it is less, then it is peritoneal fluid.

23.4 Management

Managing patients with vesicovaginal fistula (VVF) requires immediate surgical intervention, often followed by additional procedures, while also taking into account nutritional and rehabilitative aspects of patient care. When choosing a delayed surgical approach, it's vital to address sanitary protection and skin care. Approximately 10% of cases experience spontaneous closure after 0.5–2 months of urethral catheterization and anticholinergic medication, especially when the fistula is small, detected early, or lacks epithelialization.

In cases of late diagnoses with epithelized fistulas, applying electrocoagulation to the mucosal layer, along with 2–4 weeks of catheterization, might promote closure [9]. However, patients with a thin vesicovaginal septum, large VVF or significant inflammation around the fistula tract may face risks and failures with fulguration. This process could potentially enlarge the fistula size and devitalize adjacent tissues. As an adjunctive measure fibrin sealant can be injected directly into the fistula tract following electrocoagulation. Positive outcomes have been attained using fibrin sealant combined with collagen as an additional "plug" [10]. Unfortunately, conservative methods are often ineffective, thus requiring surgical intervention.

Debates continue over whether the abdominal or vaginal route is more suitable for fistula repair. Typically, simple fistulas are addressed vaginally, whereas complex fistulas are often managed either vaginally using a myocutaneous flap or through an abdominal approach. Numerous gynaecological surgeons prefer the vaginal approach due to its capacity to reduce operative complications, hospital stay, blood loss, and post-procedural pain, all while achieving success rates comparable to the abdominal approach [11].

Nonetheless, the vaginal approach may be linked to issues such as vaginal shortening and the formation of a dead space prone to infection and inflammation [12]. Contraindications to the vaginal approach includes severely indurated vaginal epithelium, a small or poorly compliant bladder, repair necessitating ureteral reimplantation, involvement of other pelvic structures, vaginal stenosis, or difficulty in achieving adequate exposure [13, 14].

The transabdominal O'Connor's operation has gained widespread acceptance for repairing supratrigonal fistulas. This procedure entails suprapubic access for extraperitoneal dissection, a long sagittal cystotomy, excision of the fistulous tract, and a two-layer closure following tissue transposition between the bladder and vaginal walls. The abdominal approach is advocated for high-retracted fistulas in a narrow vagina, fistulas proximal to the ureters, cases with associated pelvic pathology, and multiple fistulas [15]. It has shown promising results with durable success rates ranging from 85% to 100% [16].

The transperitoneal approach permits extensive exploration and enables the utilization of peritoneal or omental grafts for larger fistulas. It becomes necessary in cases of associated intra-abdominal pathology, previous unsuccessful attempts, rigid vaginal walls, or when an abdominal interposed graft is required. Interposed tissues serve to create an additional layer in the repair, fill dead space, and introduce a new blood supply. They are commonly employed in repairing radiation fistulas or in reducing post-fistula repair stress incontinence in patients with urethral and bladder neck fistulas.

Repeated surgical failures may occur in some cases due to factors such as existing pelvic malignancy, severe radiation damage, or extensive soft tissue loss, especially in obstetric fistulas. Patients with coexistent medical morbidities may not be suitable candidates for repair, making urinary diversion, either through a conduit or continent reservoir, a viable option.

For individuals ineligible for surgical intervention, managing fistulas with percutaneous ureteral occlusion and permanent nephrostomy represents an alternative. Internal urinary diversion with ureterosigmoidostomy, although regarded as a last resort due to its metabolic and neoplastic risks, is applied in patients with unreconstructable lower urinary tracts.

Complex fistulas, especially those located high or large, close to ureteric orifices, or associated with hydronephrosis, hydroureter, urinary ascites, or an absent vaginal cuff, necessitate a transabdominal transvesical approach. Success predominantly relies on the prudent utilization of interposition flaps, with the omental flap being exceptionally versatile and suitable for both abdominal and combined abdominal–vaginal procedures. Complex vesicovaginal repairs demand a center of excellence with adequate surgical experience.

Robotic VVF repair, introduced in 2005, provides advantages such as three-dimensional visualization and wristed instrumentation have been pivotal in reducing angulation requirements and simpler intracorporeal knot tying. However, the best surgery for all VVF patients remains uncertain, given the condition's variability and the expertise of individual surgeons [17–20].

23.4.1 Surgical Management

When conservative measures prove ineffective for vesicovaginal fistula, surgery becomes the chosen course of action. Successful surgical fistula repairs vary, with success rates ranging between 70% and 100%, irrespective of whether transvaginal, transabdominal, or transperitoneal approaches are employed. In non-radiated patients, success rates are notably high, ranging from 91% to 97%, respectively [3]. The transvaginal approach is typically less invasive, enabling earlier repairs [2]. However, in radiated patients, repairs are less frequent and often more intricate, with success rates varying from 40% to 100%. Flaps, like those utilizing the labial fat pad or omentum, can serve as protective measures against recurrence in complex cases.

23.5 Steps of Surgery (Fig. 23.1)

Step 1 Insertion of Primary Port

Primary trocar of 5 mm placed at Jain point.

Advantages of Jain Point over Palmer point are

1. You can use this port as an operating port as it's lower than Palmer point
2. You can use this point even in moderate splenomegaly patients
3. We can use this entry point in all BMI patients

It is applicable in patients with previous surgical incisions in all quadrants of abdomen.

Step 2 Hysteroscopic visualisation as well as stenting of the fistula.

Stenting can be conducted through cystoscopy or vaginoscopy. In situations where the fistulous tract is not easily visible in small fistulas, filling the bladder with methylene blue can aid in visualization. Secure the bladder neck by gently pulling the Foley's catheter to prevent methylene blue leakage paraurethrally. Subsequently, perform vaginoscopy to identify the site of methylene blue leakage from the tract. For stenting, employ the flexible and hygroscopic Terumo™ guide wire.

Step 3 DJ Stenting

Opt for distinct-colored stents for the fistulous tract and DJ stent. Stenting is unnecessary for large-size fistulas. Decide on DJ stenting based on the distance from the ureteric orifice, with removal either post-procedure or after one month. DJ stenting guarantees optimal visualization of the ureteric orifice and prevents ureteric entrapment during cystostomy closure, typically using a 5 French DJ stent.

Step 4 Adhesiolysis

UVF cases with abdominal urine leakage lead to increased adhesion formation. The choice of energy source for adhesiolysis depends on adhesion type and viscera proximity (bowel, ureter). Opting for cold scissors is preferred for adhesiolysis near viscera. Occasionally, intentional opening of the rectovaginal space ensures tension-free closure of the vault.

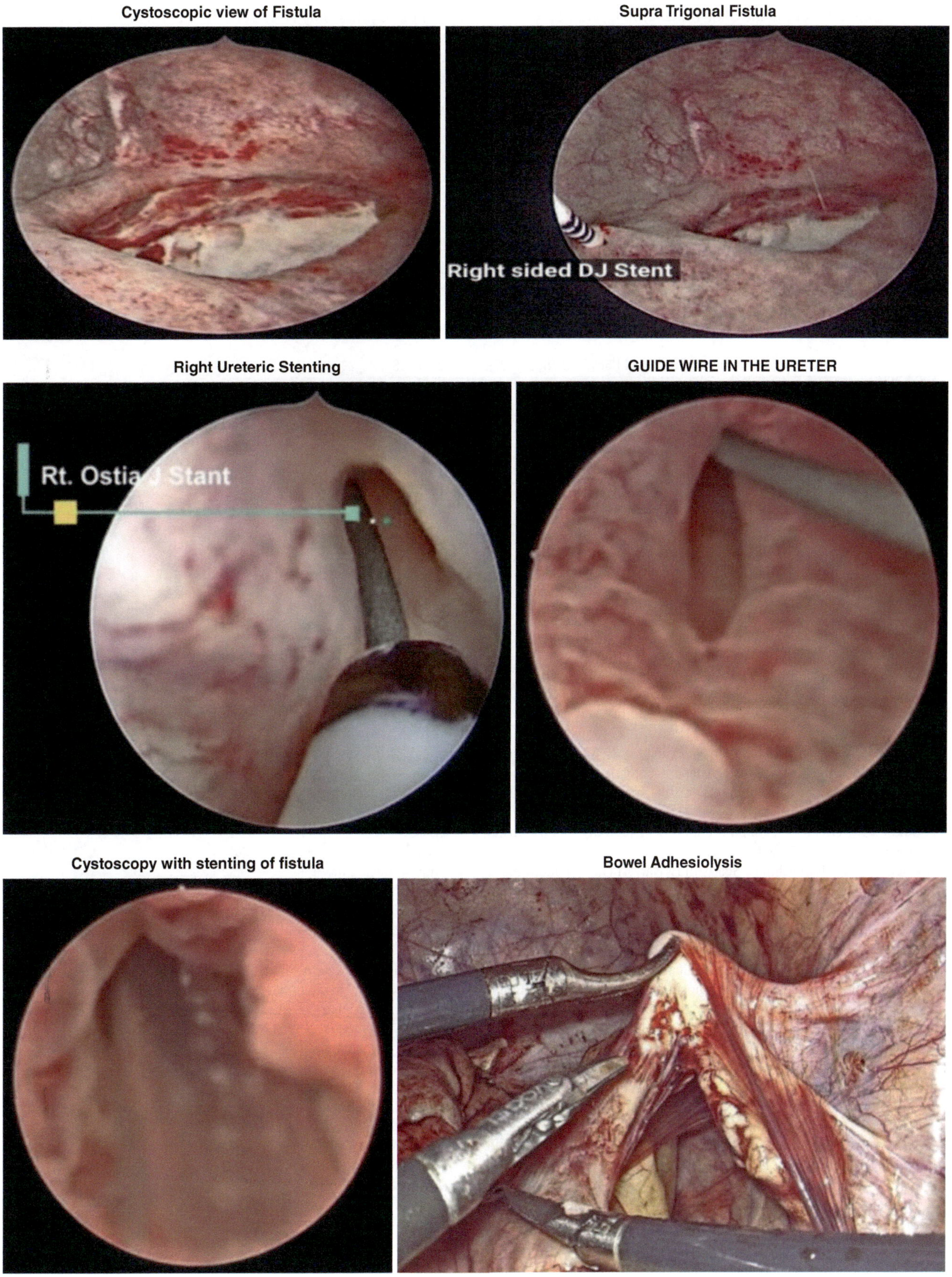

Fig. 23.1 Steps of VVF repair (Video.23.1 Large supra trigonal vesico vaginal fistula repair by transverse cystostomy) (▶ https://doi.org/10.1007/000-c9e)

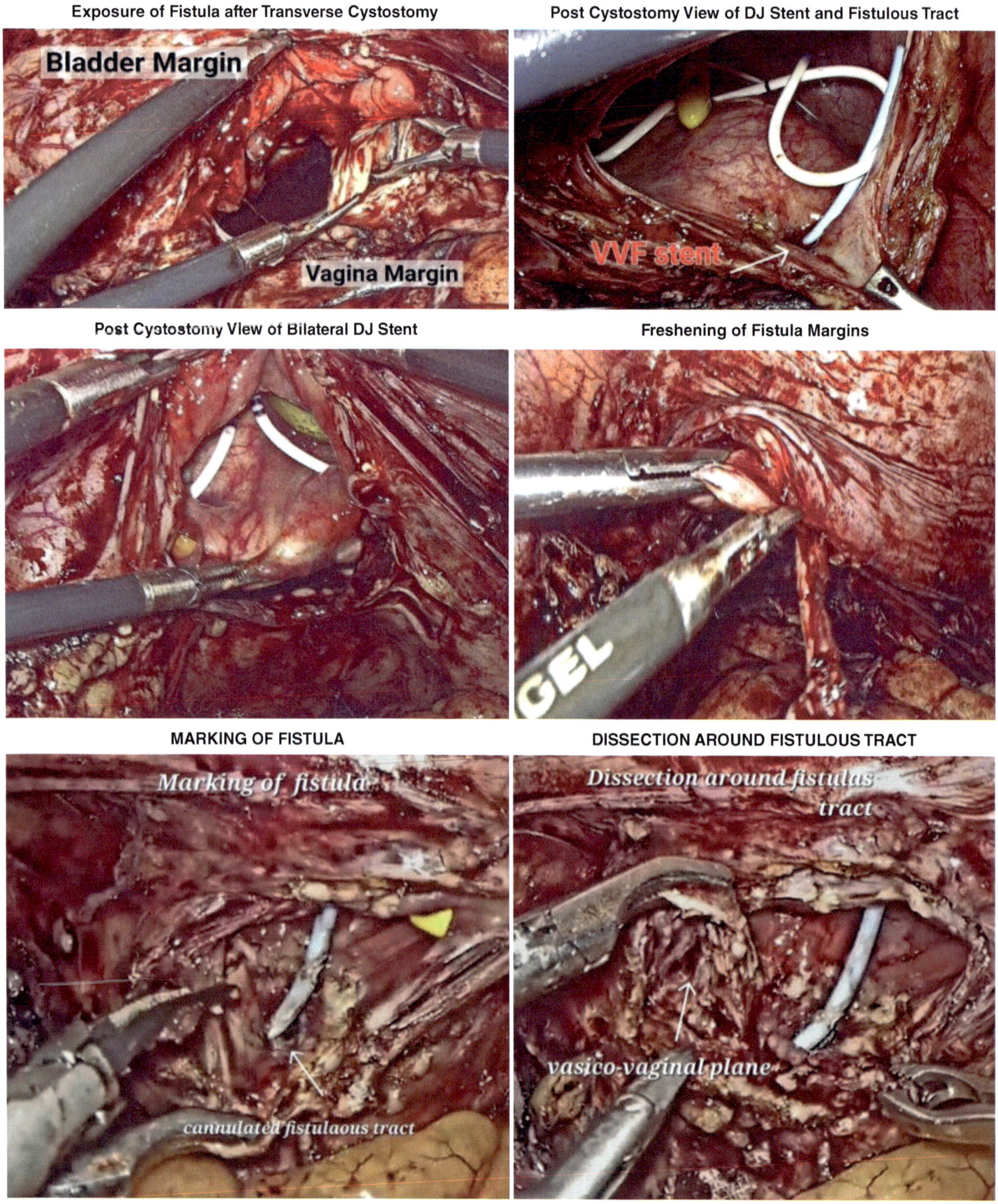

Fig. 23.1 (continued)

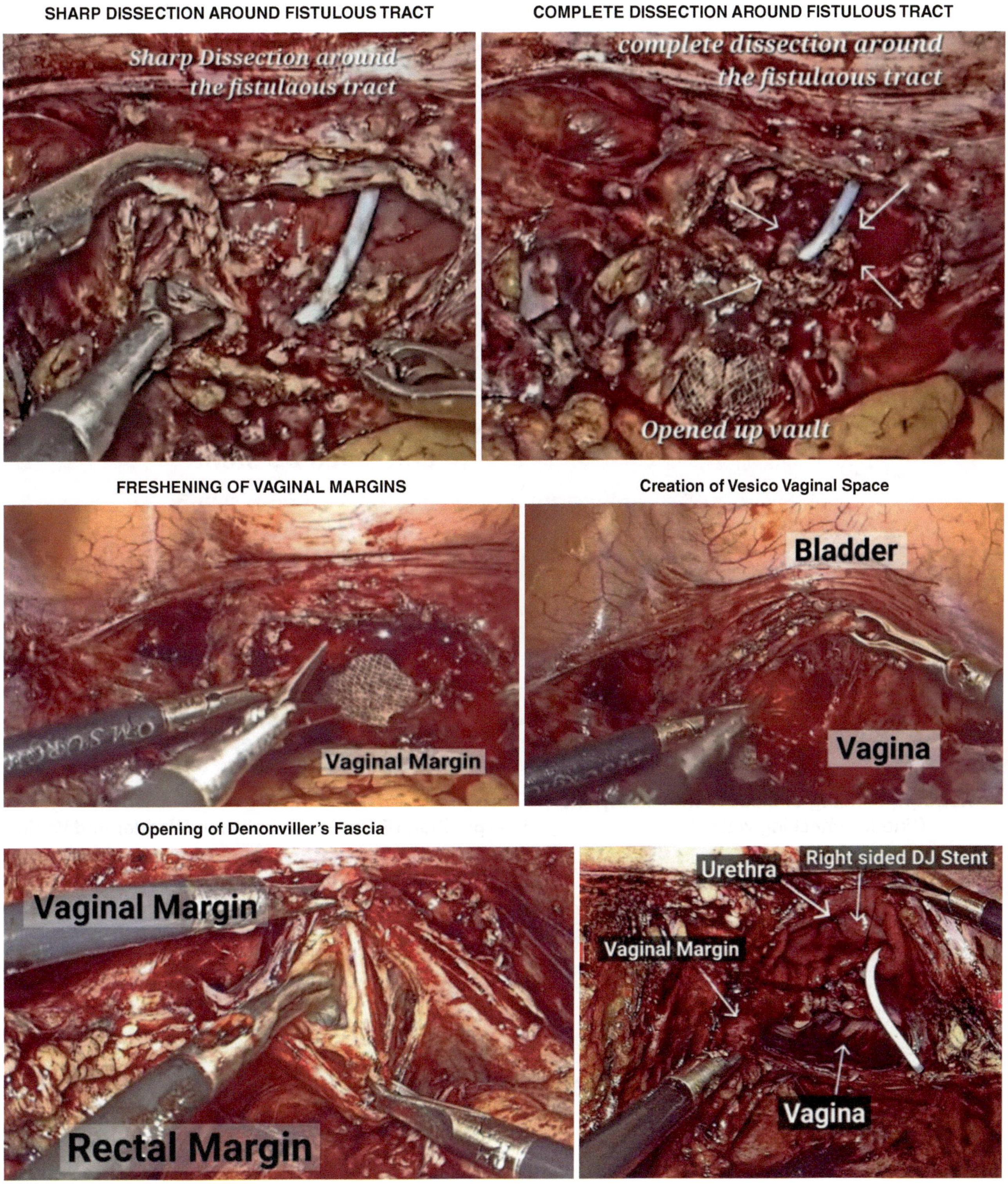

Fig. 23.1 (continued)

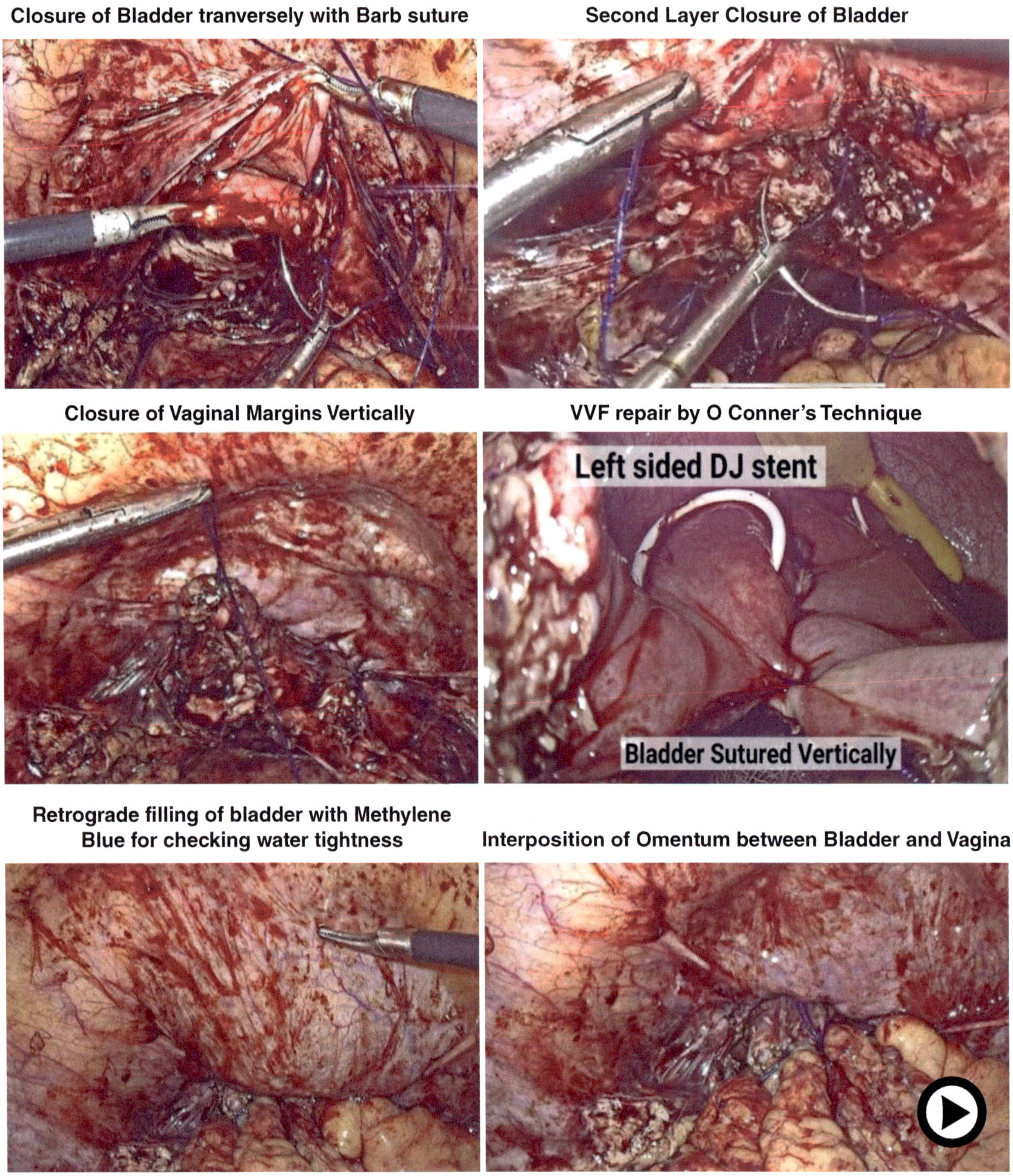

Fig. 23.1 (continued)

Step 5 Transverse Cystotomy Incision

Identify the bladder attachment over the vault for a transverse cystostomy near the fistulous tract or vault. Detect it by moving a swab stick inserted in the vagina. Opt for monopolar current or ultrasonic energy for transverse cystostomy due to its limited lateral spread.

Step 6 Marking of the fistula

Precision in tract excision is crucial. Apply a controlled amount of current to prevent bleeding upon entry into the vesicovaginal plane. Consider the use of vasopressin to minimize bleeding at this site.

Step 7 Dissection of the tract as well as bladder separation.

Merge the transverse cystostomy incision with the fistulous tract by providing traction on the vagina and making a bold nick on the bladder mucosa.

Use cold scissors to carefully dissect and locate the correct plane between the bladder and vagina. Ensure to dissect at least 1 cm around the marked fistula. Remove the stent initially inserted for fistulous tract identification from the vaginal portion at this stage.

Step 8 Excision of fistulous tract.

Following the identification of the appropriate plane between the bladder and vagina, proceed with the direct excision of the fistulous tract and any associated scarred tissue.

Step 9 Transverse Cystostomy closure with Barb suture.

Utilize Barb suture for its uniform tension distribution and self-locking mechanism. Opt for a two-layer closure of the transverse cystostomy. Employ the O'Conner stitch (Fig. 23.2), demonstrated in the diagram, for water-tight suturing. Begin with a bite away from the edge in the thick muscular portion, exiting close to the mucosa. Follow with a second bite close to the mucosa away from the edge with the full muscular portion. This continuous suturing ensures a water-tight closure. Remove the DJ stent at this step if certain of the distance from the cystostomy incision.

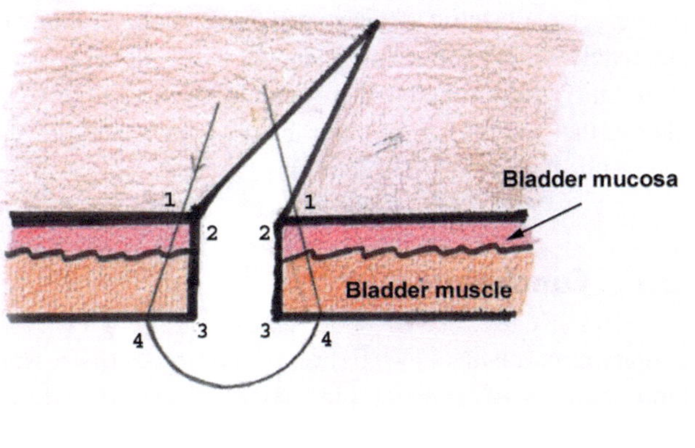

Fig. 23.2 Water tight suturing technique. Illustration by Dr Priyanka Sureddi

Step 10 Vaginal margin freshening with Vertical closure of vault.

Prevent suture line overlap by vertically closing the vaginal vault, complementing the transverse closure of the bladder.

Step 11 Interposition of omental graft.

The omentum enhances vascularity, aiding in the healing of the bladder and vagina, while also preventing leaks from the bladder to the vagina. If the omentum doesn't reach the fistulous site, trim it after a slight head-up position or consider using the appendix epiploica.

23.5.1 Rotational Flap Technique

The dome of the bladder, being well-vascularized, is rotated towards the site of the fistula. It is rotated on its own axis. Depending upon the amount of tissue loss in a fistula. Accordingly cystostomy is done so that we can bring in a large part of normal, healthy bladder to line the fistula. Now the dome of the bladder is pulled and perfect approximation is done to the apex. The bladder rests on the vaginal wall rather than the suture line. The suture lines moves anteriorly (Fig. 23.3).

23.5.2 Prognosis and Complications

The most common complication in vesicovaginal fistula surgery is the recurrence of fistula formation. Acute perioperative stages often see the emergence of urinary frequency and urgency. Long-term complications encompass urgency and stress urinary incontinence following vesicovaginal repair.

Stress incontinence, a well-acknowledged complication of vesicovaginal fistula (VVF), tends to manifest prominently in obstetric fistula patients, especially when the sphincter mechanism is affected, particularly due to tissue loss. This complication is observed in at least 10% of obstetric fistula cases and has also been documented in patients with surgical fistulas affecting the urethra or bladder neck [21]. Employing a labial musculo-fat graft in the initial repair may decrease the risk of this complication, and various other techniques have been explored to address it [22].

Notably, 30% of vesicovaginal repair cases experience failure and recurrence. In recurrent instances, consider delaying repair attempts by 2–3 months. The incorporation of flaps as a surgical technique should be considered to enhance the likelihood of a successful repair [23].

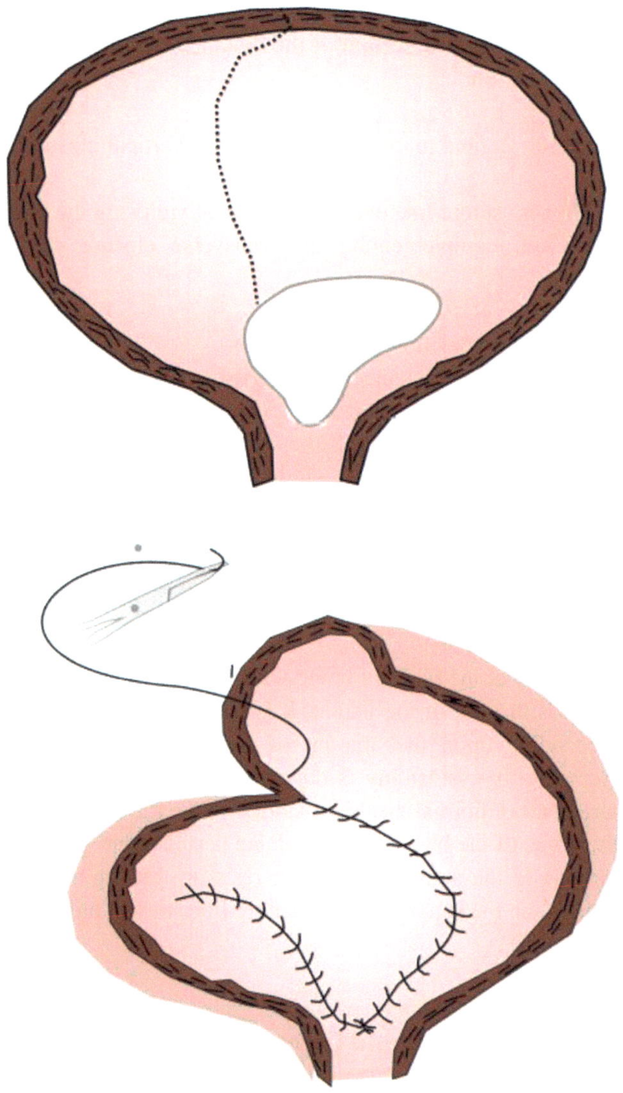

Fig. 23.3 Rotational flap technique(a) Fistulous tract(b) Cystostomy performed and dome of the bladder is pulled and approximated to the apex(c) Suturing of the flap

23.5.3 Postoperative Care

Ensuring continuous bladder drainage through a urethral Foley catheter is essential. In cases where the bladder neck is involved in the fistula, avoid inflating the balloon; instead, secure the catheter in place with sutures. Postoperative management holds paramount significance.

Maintaining a high fluid input and output until urine clears of blood is crucial, with continuous bladder drainage being indispensable. Blocked catheters pose a significant risk to repair failure. Catheterization should persist for 2–3 weeks after repair. Administer anticholinergic drugs for bladder spasms, as these contractions might compromise healing and cause discomfort to the patient. Regardless of the surgical approach to vesicovaginal fistulas (VVFs), the key to postoperative management lies in maintaining a dry, infection-free suture line. Consequently, a prolonged course of antibiotics is recommended after surgery, typically until all catheters are removed [23].

23.5.4 Recurrence

Success rates for fistula repair in non-radiated patients range from 70% to 100% in the literature, with comparable outcomes for vaginal or abdominal approaches—91% and 97%, respectively. Fistulas in radiated patients are repaired less frequently, with success rates ranging from 40% to 100%. Risk factors for recurrence typically include multiple fistulas (two or more), large size (>10 mm), fistula type (complex VVF involving the bladder cervix or urethra), urinary tract infection, and obstetrical etiology. The interposition of flaps is regarded as a protective factor against recurrence [24]. The omentum, in particular, offers excellent lymphatic drainage and helps maintain suppleness post-resolution of inflammation.

23.6 Healthcare Team to Enhance Outcomes and Prevention Measures

While a pelvic surgeon, whether a gynaecologist, urologist, or urogynaecologist, typically takes the lead in caring for a patient with a vesicovaginal fistula, achieving a successful repair hinges on the collaboration of a comprehensive interprofessional team of specialists.

Despite an optimistic prognosis when patients receive proper treatment, it is crucial to shift efforts towards preventing vesicovaginal formation.

This involves prioritizing women's reproductive health, guaranteeing access to emergency obstetric services, and promoting the training of proficient pelvic surgeons across the global medical community. Moreover, there should be an initiative to educate the general public about the prevalence and prevention of this devastating issue. This involves emphasizing women's reproductive health, ensuring access to emergency obstetric services, and fostering the training of adequately skilled pelvic surgeons within the global medical community. Additionally, there should be an initiative to educate the general public about the prevalence and prevention of this devastating problem [25].

23.7 Conclusion

Vesicovaginal fistulas (VVFs) represent highly distressing complications of gynecologic and obstetric procedures. Historically, clinical methods and dye testing have been the diagnostic cornerstones for this condition. The optimal opportunity for a successful repair lies in the initial attempt. Ongoing debates regarding the most suitable repair route lack clarity in existing publications. However, there is a consensus among respective authors regarding the favourable outlook on the role of interposition grafts in both abdominal and vaginal repairs. Adjuvant techniques become crucial for managing complex fistulas. Preventive measures must encompass universal education, enhanced women's status, and improved accessibility to medical services.

Learning Points

- Vesicovaginal Fistula (VVF) is an abnormal connection between the bladder and vagina, resulting in continuous urine leakage through the vagina.
- The etiology of VVF includes congenital and acquired factors, with gynaecological surgery being the most common cause in developed countries, while obstructed labor prevails in developing countries
- Risk factors for VVF in developing countries encompass poor socioeconomic status, malnourishment, low literacy rates, early marriage, childbearing, and inadequate obstetrical care.
- In developed countries, hysterectomy is the most common gynecological surgery leading to VVF, with rates varying depending on the surgical approach.
- Clinical presentation typically involves continuous urinary incontinence, usually following recent pelvic surgery. The severity and timing of symptoms can vary.
- Diagnostic approaches include history, clinical examination, tampon dye test, cystoscopy, and contrast studies such as CT urogram.
- VVF is classified as simple, intermediate, or complex based on size and involvement of surrounding structures.
- Surgical management is often necessary, with options including transvaginal, transabdominal, and transperitoneal approaches. Repair success rates range from 70% to 100%.
- Postoperative care emphasizes continuous bladder drainage, high fluid input and output, anticholinergic drugs, and prolonged antibiotic courses.
- Recurrence risk factors include multiple fistulas, large size, complexity, urinary tract infection, and obstetrical etiology.

Competing Interest The author declares no conflict of interest that are relevant to content of this chapter.

Ethical Approval Informed consent was obtained from individual participants and patients regarding publication and documentation without disclosing their identity.

References

1. Malik MA, Sohail M, Malik MT, Khalid N, Akram A. Changing trends in the etiology and management of vesicovaginal fistula. Int J Urol. 2018;25(1):25–9.
2. Hadley HR. Vesicovaginal fistula. Curr Urol Rep. 2002;3(5):401–7.
3. Stamatakos M, Sargedi C, Stasinou T, Kontzoglou K. Vesicovaginal fistula: diagnosis and management. Indian J Surg. 2014;76(2):131–6.
4. Penalver M, Angioli R. Urinary diversion. Chapter 11. In: Glenn HW, editor. Urogynecologic surgery. 2nd ed. New York: Lippincott-Raven; 2000. p. 193–206.
5. Eilber KS, Kavaler E, Rodríguez LV, Rosenblum N, Raz S. Ten-year experience with transvaginal vesicovaginal fistula repair using tissue interposition. J Urol. 2003;169(3):1033–6.
6. Härkki-Sirén P, Sjöberg J, Tiitinen A. Urinary tract injuries after hysterectomy. Obstet Gynecol. 1998;92(1):113–8.
7. Zoubek J, McGuire EJ, Noll F, DeLancey JOL. The late occurrence of urinary tract damage in patients successfully treated by radiotherapy for cervical cancer. J Urol. 1984;141:1347–9.
8. Srinivasan R, Cortes G, Richardson I, Guelfguat M. Salpingovesical fistula mimicking an enterovaginalfistula. Radiol Case Rep. 2020;15(9):1473–6.
9. Kursch ED, Stovsky M, Ignatoff JM, Nanniraga WF, O'Connor VJ. Use of fulguration in the treatment of vesicovaginal fistula. J Urol. 1993;149:292A.
10. Kumar U, Albala DM. Fibrin glue applications in urology. Curr Urol Rep. 2001;2(1):V79–82. https://doi.org/10.1007/s11934-001-0029-5.
11. Angioli R, Penalver M, Muzii L, Mendez L, Mirhashemi R, Bellati F, Crocè C, Panici PB. Guidelines of how to manage vesicovaginal fistula. Crit Rev Oncol Hematol. 2003;48(3):295–304. https://doi.org/10.1016/S1040-8428(03)00123-9.
12. Enzelseberger H, Gitsch E. Surgical management of vesicovaginal fistulas according to Chassar Moir's method. Surg Gynecol Obstet. 1991;173:183–6.
13. Carr LK, Webster GD. Abdominal repair of vesicovaginal fistula. Urology. 1996;48(1):10–1.
14. Kapoor R, Ansari MS, Singh P, Gupta P, Khurana N, Mandhani A, Dubey D, Srivastava A, Kumar A. Management of vesicovaginal fistula: an experience of 52 cases with a rationalized algorithm for choosing the transvaginal or transabdominal approach. Indian J Urol. 2007;23(4):372–6. https://doi.org/10.4103/0970-1591.36709.
15. Armenakas NA, Pareek G, Fracchia JA. Iatrogenic bladder perforations: long-term follow-up of 65 patients. J Am Coll Surg. 2004;198:78–82. https://doi.org/10.1016/j.jamcollsurg.2003.08.022.
16. Dalela D, Ranjan P, Sankhwar PL, Sankhwar SN, Naja V, Goel A. Supratrigonal VVF repair by modified O'Connor's technique: an experience of 26 cases. Eur Urol. 2006;49(3):551–6. https://doi.org/10.1016/j.eururo.2005.12.037.
17. Rizvi SJ, Gupta R, Patel S, Trivedi A, Trivedi P, Modi P. Modified laparoscopic abdominal vesico-vaginal fistula repair—"Mini-O'Conor" vesicotomy. J Laparoendosc Adv Surg Tech A. 2010;20(1):13–5. https://doi.org/10.1089/lap.2009.0176.
18. Zambon J, Batezini N, Pinto E, Skaff M, Girotti M, Almeida F. Do we need new surgical techniques to repair vesico-vaginal fistulas? Int Urogynecol J. 2010;21:337–42. https://doi.org/10.1007/s00192-009-1040-5.
19. Melamud O, Elehel L, Turbow B, Shanberg A. Laparoscopic vesicovaginal fistula repair with robotic reconstruction. Urol J. 2005;65:163–6. https://doi.org/10.1016/j.urology.2004.09.052.

20. Hemal A, Wadwa P. Robotic repair of vesico-vaginal fistula. In: Robotics in genitourinary surgery. London: Springer; 2011. p. 611–6.
21. Hilton P. The urodynamic findings in patients with urogenital fistulae. Br J Urol. 1998;81:539–42. https://doi.org/10.1046/j.1464-410x.1998.00596.x.
22. Hilton P, Ward A, Molloy M, Umana O. Periurethral injection of autologous fat for the treatment of post-fistula repair stress incontinence: a preliminary report. Int Urogynecol J Pelvic Floor Dysfunct. 1998;9:118–21. https://doi.org/10.1007/BF01982221.
23. Smith GL, Williams G. Vesicovaginal fistula. BJU Int. 1999;83:564–70. https://doi.org/10.1046/j.1464-410x.1999.00006.x.
24. Ockrim JL, Greenwell TJ, Foley CL, Wood DN, Shah PJR. A tertiary experience of vesico-vaginal and urethro-vaginal fistula repair: factors predicting success. BJU Int. 2009;103:1122–6. https://doi.org/10.1111/j.1464-410X.2008.08237.x.
25. Wall LL. Obstetric vesicovaginal fistula as an international public-health problem. Lancet. 2006;368(9542):1201–9.

Vaginal Cuff Dehiscence

24

Alison M. Zeccola and Suketu Mansuria

24.1 Introduction

Vaginal cuff dehiscence (VCD) is a rare but morbid complication of a total hysterectomy. It is defined as a separation of the anterior and posterior edges of the vaginal cuff incision with entry into the peritoneal cavity. Post-operative vaginal cuff dehiscence after hysterectomy is estimated to occur 0.14–4.1% and varies based on mode of hysterectomy [1–3]. It may be a complete or partial separation and may be accompanied by evisceration in its most severe form. Evisceration is estimated to occur with cuff dehiscence in 35–67% of cases (Fig. 24.1) [4]. For this reason, it is important to understand the clinical presentation, risk factors, techniques for prevention and clinical management of cuff dehiscence to reduce the morbidity associated with this postoperative complication.

Supplementary Information The online version contains supplementary material available at https://doi.org/10.1007/978-981-97-3226-5_24. The videos can be accessed individually by clicking the DOI link in the accompanying figure caption or by scanning this link with the SN More Media App.

A. M. Zeccola
Minimally Invasive Gynecologic Surgery, Magee-Womens Hospital, University of Pittsburgh Medical Center, Pittsburgh, PA, USA

S. Mansuria (✉)
Gynecologic Minimally Invasive Surgery, Magee-Womens Hospital, University of Pittsburgh Medical Center, Pittsburgh, PA, USA
e-mail: manssm@upmc.edu

N. Jain (ed.), *Complex Total Laparoscopic Hysterectomy (TLH) with Newer Approaches in Bladder Dissection*,
https://doi.org/10.1007/978-981-97-3226-5_24

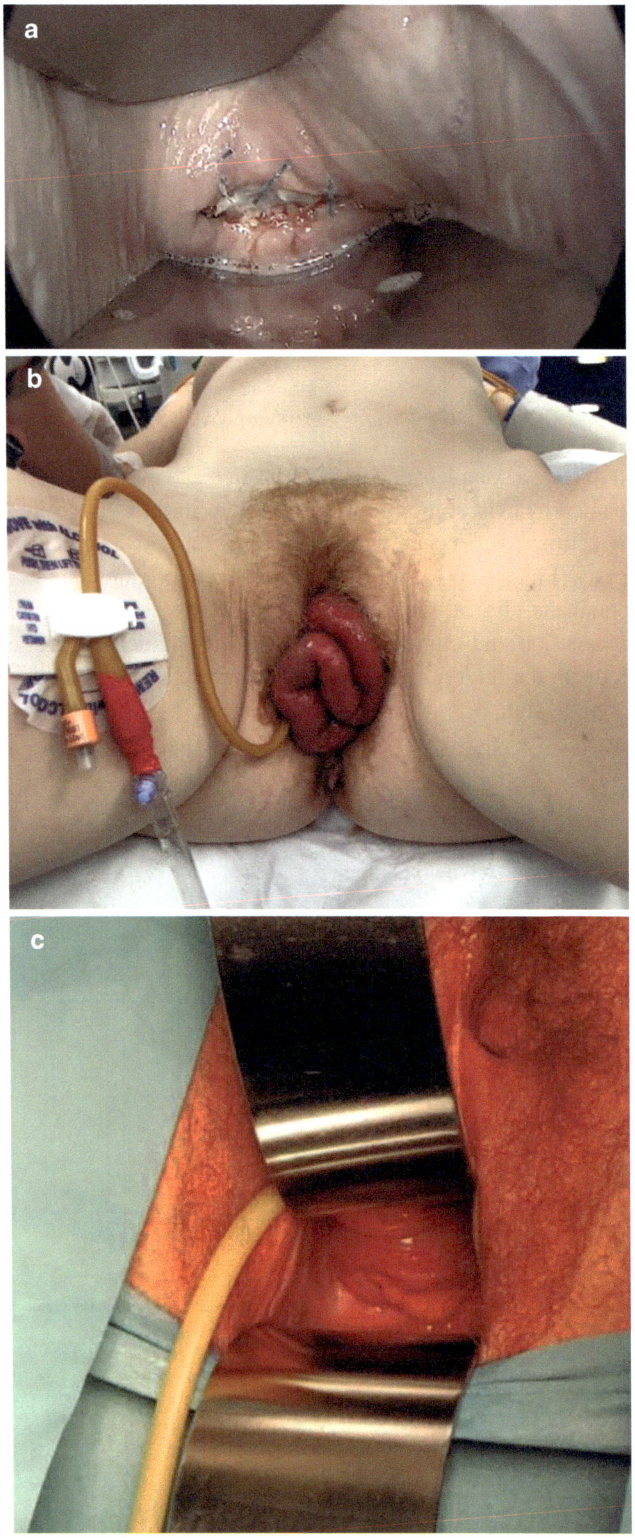

Fig. 24.1 **a** Cuff dehiscence without evisceration [16]. **b** Cuff dehiscence with evisceration. **c** Vaginal cuff dehiscence with subtle bowel evisceration [17]

24.2 Clinical Presentation

Patients typically present post-operatively with abdomino-pelvic pain, vaginal bleeding or discharge, or vaginal pressure or a mass [3, 5, 6]. Most commonly, vaginal cuff dehiscence occurs after first coitus post-operatively, so if this history is elicited then your index of suspicion for a cuff complication should increase [1, 3, 7]. Patients presenting with these symptoms need a thorough evaluation, including pelvic examination to assess the integrity of the vaginal cuff. Diagnosis is made clinically by visualizing or palpating a cuff separation. As previously discussed, evisceration may also be present. If clinical examination is suboptimal or inadequate, surgeons should have a low threshold to perform an examination under anesthesia to thoroughly evaluate the vaginal cuff and rule out a dehiscence.

24.3 Risk Factors

There are many risk factors for vaginal cuff dehiscence. It is important to consider both patient factors and surgical factors when assessing risk for dehiscence [7].

- **Patient factors—Wound Healing**

Factors that may negatively affect incisional wound healing theoretically put a patient at increased risk for cuff dehiscence. Patients with comorbidities that affect the healing property of the tissue such as diabetes, tobacco use, prior chemotherapy or radiation, pelvic organ prolapse, and post-menopausal vaginal atrophy are thought to put a patient at increased risk. The use of medications such as steroids or immunosuppressant increases a patient's risk, as well. Premenopausal age and obesity seem to be protective as there is a higher incidence of dehiscence in postmenopausal patients and those with lower BMIs [1, 7].

Additionally, post operative complications such as superficial or deep surgical site infections and hematomas predispose to further cuff complications, so infection prevention measures and achieving hemostasis intraoperatively are crucial [7].

- **Patient factors—Increased Intraabdominal pressure**

Medical comorbidities that predispose patients to increased abdominal pressure are at increased risk of cuff dehiscence. This includes conditions that produce chronic cough such as asthma, gastroesophageal reflux, and chronic obstructive pulmonary disease, among others. It also includes constipation, increased straining or Valsalva and heavy lifting post operatively. Additionally, precocious intercourse post operatively is highly associated with vaginal cuff dehiscence and most instances of cuff dehiscence occur upon resumption of intercourse post operatively [3, 7]. Optimum timing for pelvic rest is not known, but it has been suggested that abstaining from intercourse for 8–12 weeks post operatively may reduce risk of VCD [8].

- **Mode of hysterectomy**

Rates of vaginal cuff dehiscence vary based on mode of hysterectomy. TVH and TAH are thought to have the lowest risk of dehiscence, followed by laparoscopic (TLH) and robotic (RA-TLH) hysterectomies. One of the first studies to examine this was an observational study of 7286 patients who underwent hysterectomy performed at Magee Women's Hospital in Pittsburgh, PA, USA. The overall rate of vaginal cuff dehiscence was 0.14% (n = 10) and when separated by mode of hysterectomy and found highest rate after TLH (4.93%), followed by TVH (0.29%) and TAH (0.12%) [1]. The same group published a follow up study looking at 11,606 hysterectomies performed between 2000 to 2009 with a similar trend; however, the overall rates of dehiscence were much lower: TLH (1.35%) vs LAVH (0.28%), TAH (0.15%), TVH (0.08%) (Hur et al. in 2011). It was postulated that increased surgeon experience likely contributed to decreased rates of dehiscence as minimally invasive approaches were becoming much more prevalent [2].

Dr. Hur and colleagues published another follow up retrospective cohort study examining rates of vaginal cuff dehiscence in a population of over 4000 patients from 2010 to 2021 in New York City again with similar findings. Overall rate of VCD was 0.37% and <1% for all modes of hysterectomy. Rates of VCD after RA-TLH (0.66%) and TLH (0.32%) were still noted to be higher than that of TAH (0.27%) and TVH/LAVH (0%), but the overall rates of VCD are very low and significantly lower than previously reported. Of note, rates of minimally invasive hysterectomy (TLH, LAVH, RA-TLH) increased significantly over that time from 42% to 66%, as well [3]. Given the overall very low rates of VCD after minimally invasive hysterectomy, this is the recommended approach when feasible given the numerous benefits over open surgery.

24.4 Surgical Technique

24.4.1 Colpotomy

Other studies have tried to analyze specific procedural steps and surgical techniques to reduce the risk of VCD. This is a more difficult area to study given the heterogeneous methods of colpotomy and cuff closure between surgeons. It is thought that use of electrosurgical current for colpotomy versus cold cutting may be a contributing factor for increased risk of dehiscence after TLH due to the thermal effects on the tissue inhibiting healing [9]. When electrosurgical current is utilized for colpotomy, cutting over coagulation current is preferred, and it is recommended to limit tissue contact to minimize thermal effect on the surrounding vaginal tissue.

24.4.2 Suture

Suture material has also been examined as a variety of different suture types can be used for cuff closure: VICRYL™ (polyglactin 910), Maxon™ Monofilament Absorbable Sutures, PDS (polydioxanone), barbed suture, among others. A meta-analysis comparing cuff closure with barbed versus traditional suture concluded there was no difference in the risk of dehiscence between the two groups [10].

24.4.3 Cuff Closure

Previous studies recommended placement of full thickness suture bites, anterior and posterior, 0.5 to 1.5 cm beyond the coagulated edge to account for tissue necrosis due to thermal spread [7, 11].

A more recent study by Peters and Mansuria et al. in 2021 found decreased rates of VCD after a two-layer vaginal closure versus a one-layer closure. This retrospective study looked at 2973 patients undergoing minimally invasive hysterectomy by fellowship trained minimally invasive gynecologic surgeons at one institution in Pittsburgh, PA, USA. Hysterectomy and colpotomy technique were standardized in this study, including use of monopolar 60 watts cutting current for colpotomy, cuff angle suspension sutures, and use of 180 day delayed absorbable barbed suture; the only difference was one- versus two-layer vaginal cuff closure. They found decreased numbers of vaginal cuff complications in the two-layer closure group stemming from cuff complications (0.9 vs 2.6%, $P < 0.01$). There were 13 cases of cuff dehiscence in the one-layer closure group and there were no cases of vaginal cuff dehiscence in the two-layer closure group. All cases occurred after the patient's first postoperative resumption of insertional intercourse. The study concluded that the two-layer vaginal cuff closure leads to significant decreases in total post-operative complications and should be considered when feasible [12].

24.4.4 Two-Layer Vaginal Cuff Closure Technique

We will describe our two-layer vaginal cuff closure technique. After colpotomy is performed (Fig. 24.2), angle sutures are placed medial to the uterine artery pedicle (Fig. 24.3). We tie them down extracorporeally and then pass the suture to the assistant (Fig. 24.4a) to pull the suture through the lateral port, clamped externally with a straight clamp (Fig. 24.4b). The same procedure is then performed on the left side (Fig. 24.5) to suspend the cuff and place it on tension (Fig. 24.6). This angle stitch serves a few purposes. It achieves hemostasis by closing the dead space between the pedicle and cuff angle, and by placing the cuff on tension. Placing the cuff under tension often stops the small bleeding at the cuff edge, allowing us to minimize thermal energy application, and ensure the cuff is well vascularized for tissue healing and ultimately decreased rates of VCD. Hemostasis at the cuff is ultimately achieved with our suture at time of cuff closure. Additionally, the angle sutures serve to elevate the cuff away from the nearby bladder, bowel and ureters to minimize injury, and line up the anterior and posterior edges of the cuff for ease and efficiency of suturing.

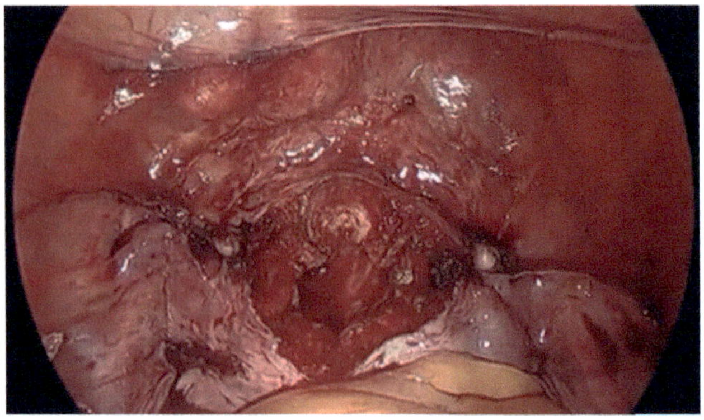

Fig. 24.2 Vaginal cuff after colpotomy, prior to cuff closure [13]

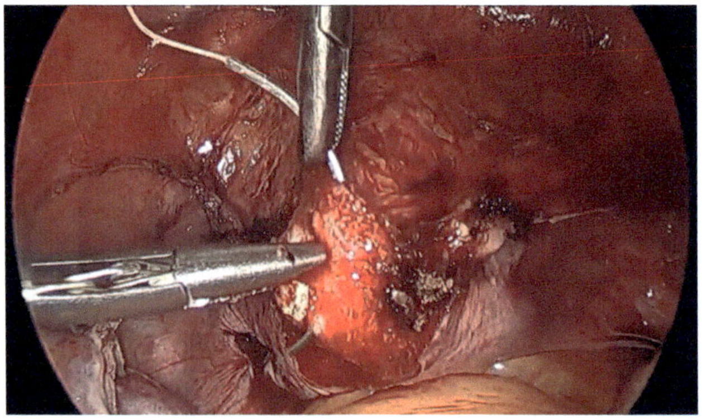

Fig. 24.3 Right vaginal cuff angle suture [13]

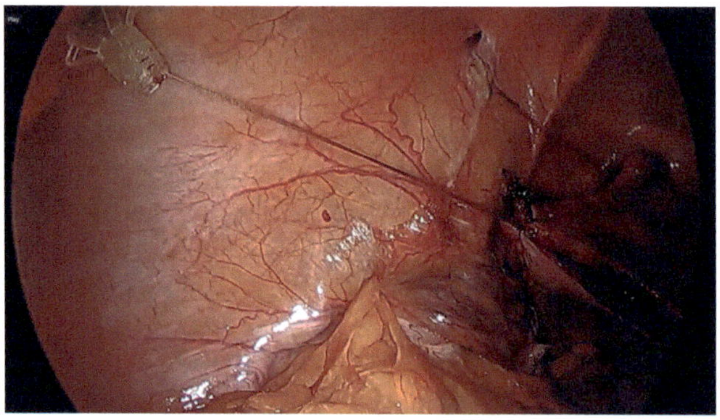

Fig. 24.5 Left angle suture pulled through left lower quadrant port [13]

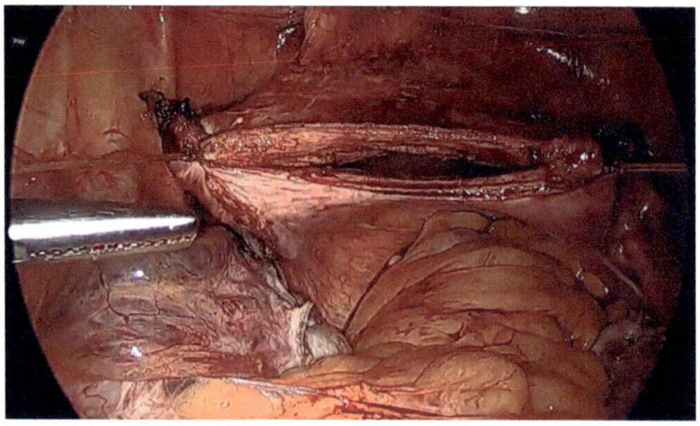

Fig. 24.6 Cuff placed on tension and suspended by two angle sutures [13]

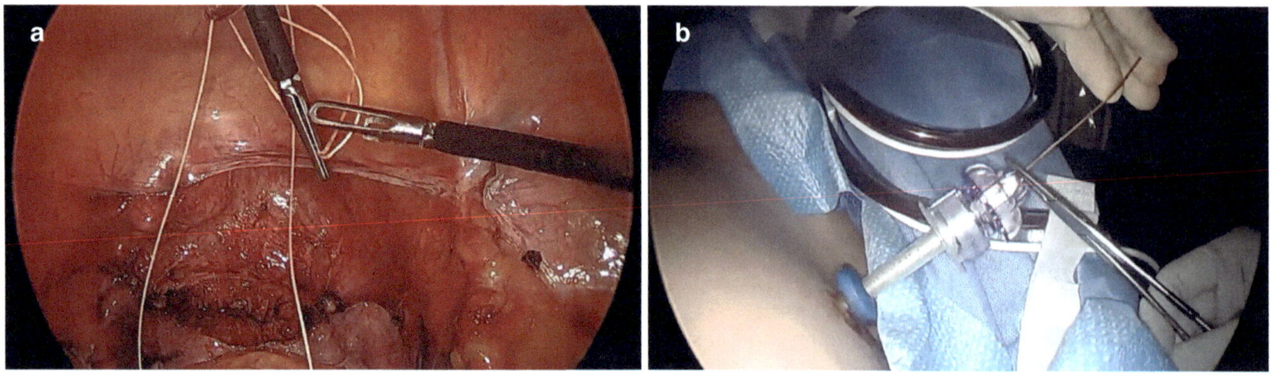

Fig. 24.4 **a** Passing angle suture to assistant on patient's right side. **b** Angle suture pulled out through lower quadrant port, assistant can place instrument in port despite suture presence [13]

We close our cuff with a 9-inch, 180 day delayed absorbable V-Loc suture. The first layer closes the vaginal mucosa (Fig. 24.7a). We suture in a running fashion, from right to left along the length of the cuff (Fig. 24.7b) and the same suture is then used for the second, imbricating layer. After the mucosal layer is closed, the left cuff angle is cut in order to reduce tension on the cuff, allowing us to better delineate the endopelvic fascia (Fig. 24.8). The second layer then imbricates the endopelvic fascia over the mucosal closure, which reduces tension in the first layer to facilitate cuff healing (Fig. 24.9). We lock our last stitch and place two additional tissue bites to secure the barbed suture and then cut it completely flush to the cuff upon completion (Fig. 24.10). The right-angle suture is cut, and we then confirm cuff hemostasis (Figs. 24.11 and 24.12) [12, 13].

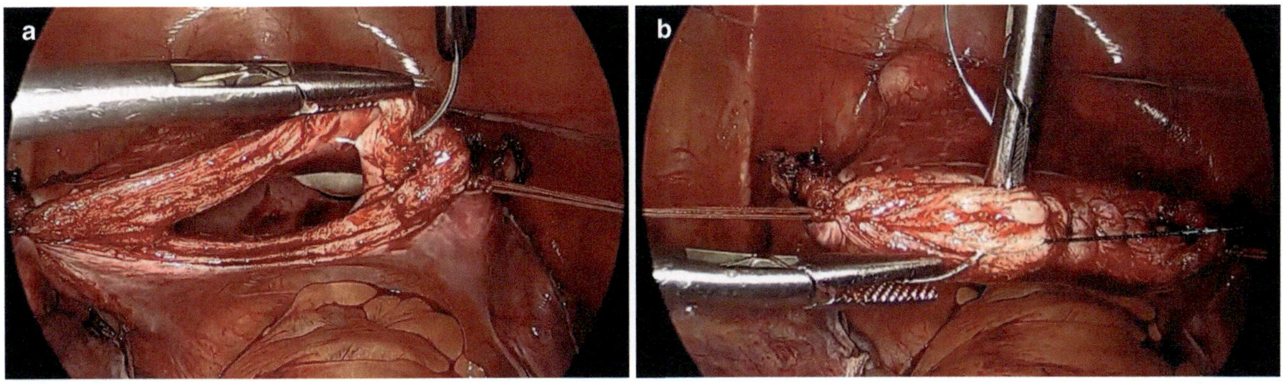

Fig. 24.7 **a** First layer of vaginal cuff closure—vaginal mucosa. **b** Continued first layer of closure [13]

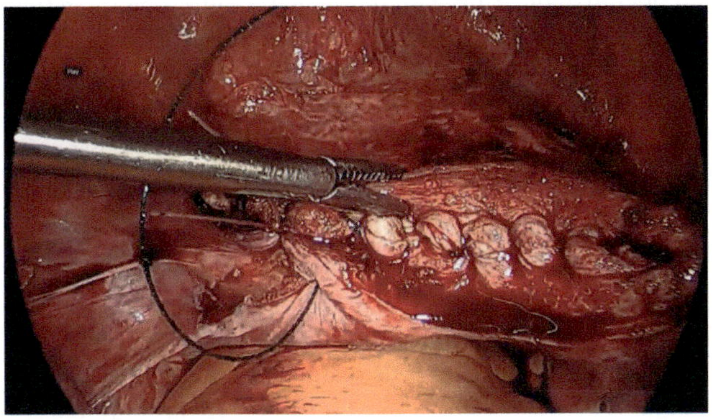

Fig. 24.8 After the mucosal closure is complete, the left angle suture is cut to release tension on the cuff for second imbricating layer [13]

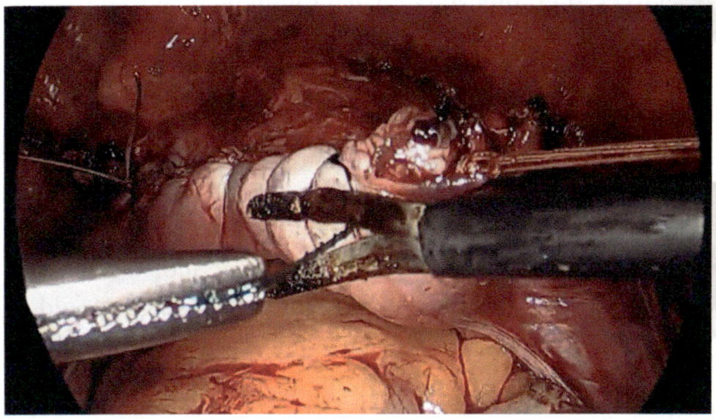

Fig. 24.10 After completion of the second layer, two additional tissue bites are taken and the suture is cut flush with the cuff [13]

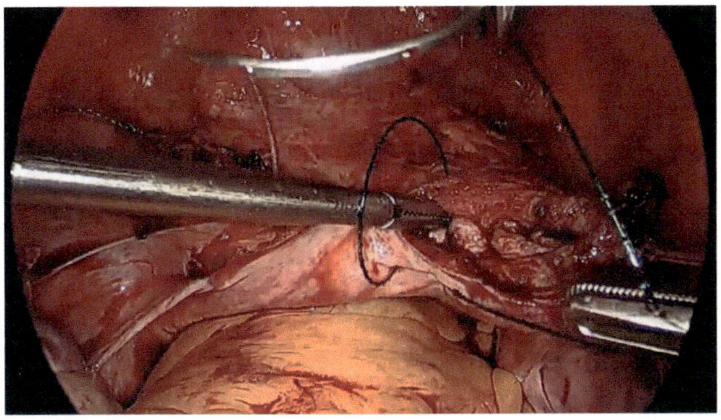

Fig. 24.9 Second layer of vaginal cuff closure—imbricating endopelvic fascia [13]

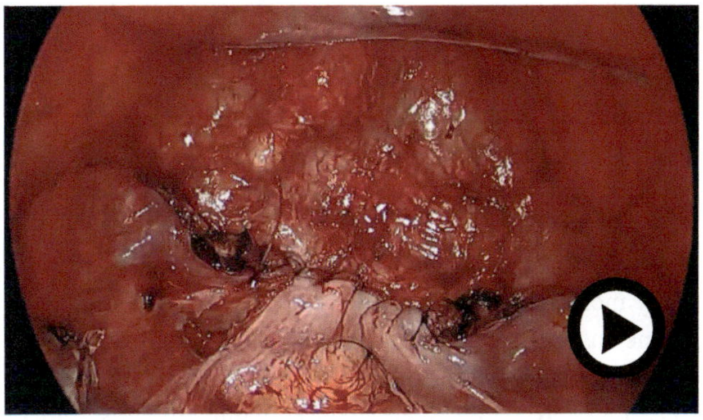

Fig. 24.11 Completed two layer vaginal cuff closure, after the right angle suture is cut [13] (Video.24.11Vaginal Cuff Dehiscence) (▶ https://doi.org/10.1007/000-c9f)

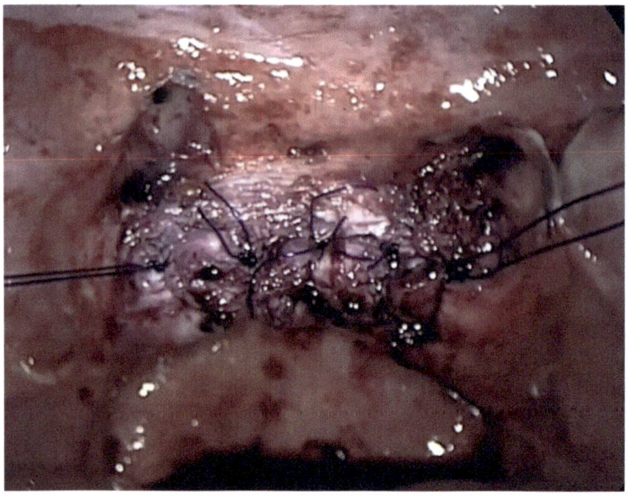

Fig. 24.12 Intraabdominal view of a vaginal cuff dehiscence after laparoscopic repair [18]

24.5 Management

If a patient is diagnosed with cuff dehiscence, we first recommend assessing clinical stability and presence or absence of evisceration. In a stable patient with no evidence of evisceration, after a pelvic speculum and bimanual examination is performed, the patient should remain supine or in Trendelenburg position and arrangements should be made for the patient to be transported to the operating room. The vagina can be packed with moist gauze to prevent evisceration. In a patient with evisceration, gentle attempts can be made to reduce the protruding viscera with moistened gauze upon diagnosis. If this is not possible, the viscera should be covered with moist, sterile gauze and the patient should be transported to the operating room immediately with consideration of general surgery consultation if concerned for bowel injury [7, 8]. Laboratory evaluation including a complete blood count and type and screen in preparation for the OR should be considered. If there is concern for an intraabdominal process prompting a VCD, such as a deep surgical site infection or hematoma, imaging via CT of the abdomen and pelvis can be performed as an adjunct; however, in the case of a surgical emergency, imaging should not delay operative management [8].

There is no consensus on an optimal route of repair for vaginal cuff dehiscence. All modalities have been reported: abdominal, vaginal, laparoscopic, robotic [2, 6]. A previously mentioned study looked at over 4000 hysterectomies at one institution with 15 cases of VCD. The majority of cases were repaired vaginally (53%) or laparoscopically (35%) [3]. If patients are hemodynamically unstable or with bowel necrosis, laparotomy is recommended; however, if the patient is stable then a minimally invasive approach may be reasonable depending on surgeon skill and comfort. Cystoscopy and proctoscopy can be performed in addition. More important than the route of repair are the surgical principles guiding the repair. It is important in these cases to restore normal anatomy, debride the cuff to healthy tissue, evaluate the bowel in the case of evisceration, proceed with copious irrigation and repeat closure of the vaginal vault [2, 8]. We recommend closure with a delayed absorbable suture.

Antibiotic prophylaxis and inpatient admission after surgical repair are recommended Typically, we use broad spectrum antibiotics to cover gram positives, gram negatives and anaerobes such as Piperacillin-Tazobactam, Ceftriaxone and metronidazole, or levofloxacin and metronidazole. Typically, we administer this inpatient for 24–48 hours with repeat clinical assessment for developing peritonitis and consideration of oral antibiotics upon discharge. Antibiotic prophylaxis may prevent peritonitis due to the breach of the vaginal cuff into the sterile abdominal cavity and may treat a subacute cuff infection that may have prompted the VCD.

24.6 Prevention

Preoperative measures can be taken to reduce risk of vaginal cuff dehiscence. This includes optimizing medical comorbidities such as glycemic control in diabetics and smoking cessation. Additionally, treatment of bacterial vaginosis when symptomatic and diagnosed preoperatively may reduce the risk of cuff complications [14]. Vaginal prep with chlorohexidine and preoperative antibiotics are recommended [7, 14]. First generation cephalosporins are typically first line as surgical prophylaxis [15].

Intraoperatively, judicious use of electrosurgery for hemostasis and meticulous surgical technique are paramount. As we reviewed, a two-layer vaginal cuff closure should be considered when feasible.

Currently there is no evidence-based recommendation regarding appropriate time to resume intercourse post operatively. Many suggest a period of pelvic rest for 8–12 weeks to reduce the risk of VCD [1, 8]. Additionally, aggressive prevention and treatment of constipation is recommended.

Learning Points

- Vaginal Cuff Dehiscence (VCD) is a rare but serious complication post-hysterectomy.
- Incidence varies (0.14–4.1%) with factors like mode of hysterectomy influencing rates.
- Clinical presentation includes abdominopelvic pain, bleeding, and vaginal pressure, often linked to post-op coitus.
- Risk factors encompass patient-related issues (diabetes, tobacco use) and surgical factors (infection, mode of hysterectomy).

- VCD rates differ based on the mode of hysterectomy, with laparoscopic approaches showing higher risks.
- Surgical techniques, like two-layer closure, impact VCD rates; consider suture material and colpotomy methods.
- Management varies (abdominal, vaginal, laparoscopic, or robotic) based on patient stability.
- Surgical principles for repair involve restoring normal anatomy, debriding the cuff, evaluating bowel, and thorough closure.
- Prevention strategies include optimizing patient health, meticulous surgical technique, and post-op management (infections, constipation).
- Overall, understanding clinical presentation, risk factors, and preventive measures is crucial for managing VCD effectively.

Competing Interest The author declares no conflict of interest that are relevant to content of this chapter.

Ethical Approval Informed consent was obtained from individual participants and patients regarding publication and documentation without disclosing their identity.

References

1. Hur HC, Guido RS, Mansuria SM, Hacker MR, Sanfilippo JS, Lee TT. Incidence and patient characteristics of vaginal cuff dehiscence after different modes of hysterectomies. J Minim Invasive Gynecol. 2007;14(3):311–7. https://doi.org/10.1016/j.jmig.2006.11.005.
2. Hur HC, Donnellan N, Mansuria S, Barber RE, Guido R, Lee T. Vaginal cuff dehiscence after different modes of hysterectomy. Obstet Gynecol. 2011;118(4):794–801. https://doi.org/10.1097/AOG.0b013e31822f1c92.
3. Polin M, Boone R, Lim F, et al. Hysterectomy trends and risk of vaginal cuff dehiscence: an update by mode of surgery. J Minim Invasive Gynecol. 2023;30(7):562–8. https://doi.org/10.1016/j.jmig.2023.03.005.
4. Ceccaroni M, Berretta R, Malzoni M, et al. Vaginal cuff dehiscence after hysterectomy: a multicenter retrospective study. Eur J Obstet Gynecol Reprod Biol. 2011;158(2):308–13. https://doi.org/10.1016/j.ejogrb.2011.05.013.
5. Ramirez PT, Klemer DP. Vaginal evisceration after hysterectomy: a literature review. Obstet Gynecol Surv. 2002;57(7):462–7. https://doi.org/10.1097/00006254-200207000-00023.
6. Cronin B, Sung VW, Matteson KA. Vaginal cuff dehiscence: risk factors and management. Am J Obstet Gynecol. 2012;206(4):284–8. https://doi.org/10.1016/j.ajog.2011.08.026.
7. Nezhat C, Kennedy Burns M, Wood M, Nezhat C, Nezhat A, Nezhat F. Vaginal cuff dehiscence and evisceration: a review. Obstet Gynecol. 2018;132(4):972–85. https://doi.org/10.1097/AOG.0000000000002852.
8. Hur HC, Lightfoot M, McMillin MG, Kho KA. Vaginal cuff dehiscence and evisceration: a review of the literature. Curr Opin Obstet Gynecol. 2016;28(4):297–303. https://doi.org/10.1097/GCO.0000000000000294.
9. Lawlor ML, Rao R, Manahan KJ, Geisler JP. Electrosurgical settings and vaginal cuff complications. JSLS. 2015;19(4):e2015.00088. https://doi.org/10.4293/JSLS.2015.00088.
10. Bogliolo S, Musacchi V, Dominoni M, et al. Barbed suture in minimally invasive hysterectomy: a systematic review and meta-analysis. Arch Gynecol Obstet. 2015;292(3):489–97. https://doi.org/10.1007/s00404-015-3653-x.
11. Kho RM, Akl MN, Cornella JL, Magtibay PM, Wechter ME, Magrina JF. Incidence and characteristics of patients with vaginal cuff dehiscence after robotic procedures. Obstet Gynecol. 2009;114(2 Pt 1):231–5. https://doi.org/10.1097/AOG.0b013e3181af36e3.
12. Peters A, Ali R, Miles S, et al. Two-layer compared with one-layer vaginal cuff closure at the time of total laparoscopic hysterectomy to reduce complications. Obstet Gynecol. 2021;138(1):59–65. https://doi.org/10.1097/AOG.0000000000004428.
13. Mansuria S. Two layer closure of the vaginal cuff with barbed suture. SurgeryU by AAGL; 2017, June 30. https://surgeryu.aagl.org/view?m=G0XWNqDYN. Accessed 10 Jan 2024.
14. Soper DE, Bump RC, Hurt WG. Bacterial vaginosis and trichomoniasis vaginitis are risk factors for cuff cellulitis after abdominal hysterectomy. Am J Obstet Gynecol. 1990;163(3):1016–23. https://doi.org/10.1016/0002-9378(90)91115-s.
15. ACOG Practice Bulletin No. 195: prevention of infection after gynecologic procedures. Obstet Gynecol. 2018;131(6):e172–89. https://doi.org/10.1097/AOG.0000000000002670.
16. Hur H-C. FMIGS webinar: intraop/postoperative complications part 2 (risk of vaginal cuff dehiscence, mitigating risk, and techniques for dehiscence repair). SurgeryU by AAGL; 2024, January 11. https://surgeryu.aagl.org/view?m=rPHQfVzls
17. Jaime Moens B, Buonomo A, De Sutter P. Vaginal cuff dehiscence: two case reports and a review of the literature. J Clin Med. 2023;12(13):4187. https://doi.org/10.3390/jcm12134187.
18. Hur H-C. AAGL FMIGS webinar: intraop/postoperative complications part 2 (risk of vaginal cuff dehiscence, mitigating risk, and techniques for dehiscence repair). SurgeryU; 2024. Retrieved January 24, 2024, from https://surgeryu.aagl.org/view?m=rPHQfVzls

GPSR Compliance

The European Union's (EU) General Product Safety Regulation (GPSR) is a set of rules that requires consumer products to be safe and our obligations to ensure this.

If you have any concerns about our products, you can contact us on ProductSafety@springernature.com

In case Publisher is established outside the EU, the EU authorized representative is:

Springer Nature Customer Service Center GmbH
Europaplatz 3
69115 Heidelberg, Germany

Batch number: 10731528

Printed by Printforce, the Netherlands